2003
YEAR BOOK OF
OBSTETRICS, GYNECOLOGY,
AND WOMEN'S HEALTH®

The 2003 Year Book Series

Year Book of Allergy, Asthma, and Clinical Immunology™: Drs Rosenwasser, Boguniewicz, Milgrom, Routes, and Spahn

Year Book of Anesthesiology and Pain Management™: Drs Chestnut, Abram, Black, Lang, Roizen, Trankina, and Wood

Year Book of Cardiology®: Drs Gersh, Graham, Kaplan, and Waldo

Year Book of Critical Care Medicine®: Drs Dellinger, Parrillo, Balk, Bekes, Roberts, and Ross

Year Book of Dentistry®: Drs Zakariasen, Boghosian, Dederich, Hatcher, Horswell, and McIntyre

Year Book of Dermatology and Dermatologic Surgery™: Drs Thiers and Lang

Year Book of Diagnostic Radiology®: Drs Osborn, Birdwell, Dalinka, Groskin, Maynard, Oestreich, Pentecost, and Ros

Year Book of Emergency Medicine®: Drs Burdick, Cone, Cydulka, Hamilton, Kassutto, and Niemann

Year Book of Endocrinology®: Drs Mazzaferri, Becker, Horton, Kannan, Kennedy, Kreisberg, Meikle, Molitch, Osei, Poehlman, and Rogol

Year Book of Family Practice®: Drs Bowman, Apgar, Dexter, Gilchrist, Neill, and Scherger

Year Book of Gastroenterology™: Drs Lichtenstein, Dempsey, Ginsberg, Katzka, Kochman, Morris, Nunes, Rosato, and Stein

Year Book of Hand Surgery®: Drs Berger and Ladd

Year Book of Medicine®: Drs Barkin, Frishman, Klahr, Loehrer, Mazzaferri, Phillips, and Pillinger

Year Book of Neonatal and Perinatal Medicine®: Drs Fanaroff, Maisels, and Stevenson

Year Book of Neurology and Neurosurgery®: Drs Bradley, Gibbs, and Verma

Year Book of Nuclear Medicine®: Drs Gottschalk, Blaufox, Coleman, Strauss, and Zubal

Year Book of Obstetrics, Gynecology, and Women's Health®: Drs Mishell, Kirschbaum, and Miller

Year Book of Oncology®: Drs Loehrer, Arceci, Glatstein, Gordon, Johnson, Morrow, and Thigpen

Year Book of Ophthalmology®: Drs Rapuano, Cohen, Eagle, Grossman, Myers, Nelson, Penne, Regillo, Sergott, Shields, and Tipperman

Year Book of Orthopedics®: Drs Morrey, Beauchamp, Peterson, Swiontkowski, Trigg, and Yaszemski

Year Book of Otolaryngology-Head and Neck Surgery®: Drs Paparella, Keefe, and Otto

2003

Year Book of
OBSTETRICS, GYNECOLOGY, AND WOMEN'S HEALTH

Editors

Daniel R. Mishell, Jr, MD

The Lyle G. McNeile Professor and Chairman, Department of Obstetrics and Gynecology, Keck School of Medicine, University of Southern California School of Medicine, Women's and Children's Hospital, Los Angeles County; University of Southern California Medical Center, Los Angeles, California

Thomas H. Kirschbaum, MD

Professor of Obstetrics and Gynecology, Maternal-Fetal Medicine Division, Department of Obstetrics and Gynecology, University of Alabama at Birmingham, Alabama

David Scott Miller, MD

Director and Dallas Foundation Chair in Gynecologic Oncology, Professor of Obstetrics and Gynecology, University of Texas Southwestern Medical Center at Dallas; Medical Director of Gynecologic Oncology, Parkland Health and Hospital System, Dallas, Texas

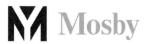 Mosby

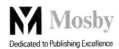
Dedicated to Publishing Excellence

Vice President, Continuity Publishing: Glen P. Campbell
Managing Editor: David Orzechowski
Senior Manager, Continuity Production: Idelle L.Winer
Issue Manager: Donna M. Skelton
Composition Specialist: Betty Dockins
Illustrations and Permissions Coordinator: Chidi C. Ukabam

2003 EDITION

Printed in the United States of America
Composition by Thomas Technology Solutions, Inc.
Printing/binding by Sheridan Books, Inc.

Editorial Office:
Elsevier
The Curtis Center
Suite 300
Independence Square West
Philadelphia, PA 19106-3399

International Standard Serial Number: 1090-798X
International Standard Book Number: 0-323-01588-3

Contributing Editors

Raquel D. Arias, MD

Associate Dean of Women, Associate Professor of Obstetrics and Gynecology, Keck School of Medicine, University of Southern California; Women's and Children's Hospital, Los Angeles County; University of Southern California Medical Center, Los Angeles, California

William H. Hindle, MD

Professor Emeritus, Department of Obstetrics and Gynecology, University of Southern California, Keck School of Medicine; Founder, Breast Diagnostic Center, Women's and Children's Hospital, Los Angeles County and University of Southern California Medical Center, Los Angeles, California

Morton A. Stenchever, MD

Professor and Chair Emeritus, University of Washington School of Medicine, Seattle, Washington

Table of Contents

Journals Represented

Mosby and its editors survey approximately 500 journals for its abstract and commentary publications. From these journals, the editors select the articles to be abstracted. Journals represented in this YEAR BOOK are listed below.

Acta Cytologica
Acta Obstetricia et Gynecologica Scandinavica
Acta Paediatrica
American Journal of Clinical Pathology
American Journal of Epidemiology
American Journal of Gastroenterology
American Journal of Medicine
American Journal of Neuroradiology
American Journal of Obstetrics and Gynecology
American Journal of Pathology
American Journal of Perinatology
American Journal of Physiology
American Journal of Roentgenology
Anesthesia and Analgesia
Annals of Internal Medicine
Archives of Ophthalmology
Archives of Surgery
Australian and New Zealand Journal of Obstetrics and Gynaecology
Breast Disease
Breast Journal
British Journal of Cancer
British Journal of General Practice
British Journal of Obstetrics and Gynaecology
British Journal of Radiology
British Journal of Surgery
British Journal of Urology International
British Medical Journal
Canadian Medical Association Journal
Cancer
Cancer Epidemiology, Biomarkers and Prevention
Circulation
Clinical Chemistry
Clinical Endocrinology (Oxford)
Clinical Infectious Diseases
Contraception
Current Women's Health Reports
Developmental Medicine and Child Neurology
Diabetes Care
Diseases of the Colon and Rectum
European Journal of Obstetrics, Gynecology and Reproductive Biology
Family Planning Perspectives
Fertility and Sterility
Gynecologic Oncology
Human Reproduction
International Journal of Cancer
International Journal of Gynaecology and Obstetrics
International Journal of Obesity

International Journal of Radiation, Oncology, Biology, and Physics
Journal of Clinical Endocrinology and Metabolism
Journal of Clinical Epidemiology
Journal of Clinical Oncology
Journal of Clinical Pathology
Journal of Infectious Diseases
Journal of Pediatrics
Journal of Reproductive Medicine
Journal of Sex and Marital Therapy
Journal of Stroke and Cerebrovascular Diseases
Journal of Surgical Research
Journal of Ultrasound in Medicine
Journal of Urology
Journal of the American College of Surgeons
Journal of the American Geriatrics Society
Journal of the American Medical Association
Journal of the National Cancer Institute
Kidney International
Lancet
Nature
Nature Medicine
New England Journal of Medicine
Obstetrics and Gynecology
Pediatric Neurology
Pediatric Research
Pediatrics
Pharmacotherapy
Placenta
Prenatal Diagnosis
Science
Transfusion
Ultrasound in Obstetrics and Gynecology
Urology
Women's Health Issues (WHI)

STANDARD ABBREVIATIONS

The following terms are abbreviated in this edition: acquired immunodeficiency syndrome (AIDS), cardiopulmonary resuscitation (CPR), central nervous system (CNS), cerebrospinal fluid (CSF), computed tomography (CT), deoxyribonucleic acid (DNA), electrocardiography (ECG), health maintenance organization (HMO), human immunodeficiency virus (HIV), intensive care unit (ICU), intramuscular (IM), intravenous (IV), magnetic resonance (MR) imaging (MRI), and ribonucleic acid (RNA) and ultrasound (US).

NOTE

materials. The editors' comments are their own opinions. Mention of specific products within this publication does not constitute endorsement.

To facilitate the use of the YEAR BOOK OF OBSTETRICS, GYNECOLOGY, AND WOMEN'S HEALTH as a reference tool, all illustrations and tables included in this publication are now identified as they appear in the original article. This change is meant to help the reader recognize that any illustration or table appearing in the YEAR BOOK OF OBSTETRICS, GYNECOLOGY, AND WOMEN'S HEALTH may be only one of many in the original article. For this reason, figure and table numbers will often appear to be out of sequence within the YEAR BOOK OF OBSTETRICS, GYNECOLOGY, AND WOMEN'S HEALTH.

Introduction

The YEAR BOOK OF OBSTETRICS, GYNECOLOGY, AND WOMEN'S HEALTH contains abstracts of the most clinically relevant scientific articles published during the preceding year in the area of women's health, followed by editorial comments discussing the relevance of each article for the reader. Topics covered include care of the pregnant, parturient and postpartum woman, and diagnosis and treatment of disorders of the female reproductive organs. Articles reviewed include those involving endocrinologic disorders and infertility as well as benign and malignant neoplasias. Other areas covered include breast disease, disorders of the urinary tract, contraception, and surveillance and treatment of the post-menopausal woman.

Throughout the year, the editors of the YEAR BOOK OF OBSTETRICS, GYNECOLOGY, AND WOMEN'S HEALTH periodically review articles published in medical journals focusing upon obstetrics, gynecology, and other areas of women's health, as well as relevant articles appearing in other medical journals. The editors select those articles that provide the most pertinent clinical information for clinicians, and write comments discussing the relevance of the findings for the reader. Once abstracts are written, they are sent for final review to the editor who selected the article for placement in the YEAR BOOK.

By reading the YEAR BOOK, clinicians with limited time will gain knowledge of the most important articles on women's health published in the previous year.

As in the past years, Dr Thomas Kirschbaum, a specialist in maternal and fetal medicine reviewed the articles concerning obstetrics for articles in this volume. Dr David Miller, an oncologist, reviewed and selected articles on gynecologic oncology and pelvic surgery, and I have reviewed and selected articles in the areas of reproductive endocrinology, infertility, menopause, contraception, and gynecologic infection. Drs William Hindle and Morton Stenchever are experts in the field of breast disease and gynecologic urology, respectively, and have selected the most relevant articles published in these areas.

During the past year, after receiving numerous scientific journals the authors selected 316 articles from 81journals for publication in this volume of the YEAR BOOK.

The editors believe that reading this volume will enhance each clinician's knowledge of advances in women's health. We welcome suggestions to improve our efforts in providing clinically relevant information to our readers.

Daniel R. Mishell, Jr, MD

OBSTETRICS

1 Maternal-Fetal Physiology

Evidence for Genetic Factors Explaining the Association Between Birth Weight and Low-Density Lipoprotein Cholesterol and Possible Intrauterine Factors Influencing the Association Between Birth Weight and High-Density Lipoprotein Cholesterol: Analysis in Twins
Ijzerman RG, Stehouwer CDA, van Weissenbruch MM, et al (Vrije Universiteit, Amsterdam)
J Clin Endocrinol Metab 86:5479-5484, 2001   1–1

Background.—Fetal growth parameters are inversely associated with cardiovascular morbidity and mortality in adulthood. It has recently been demonstrated that risk factors for cardiovascular disease—such as total cholesterol, low-density lipoprotein (LDL) cholesterol, and apolipoprotein B—are inversely related to birth size. This linkage has been considered to be a response to intrauterine malnutrition that induces permanent metabolic changes, resulting in an atherogenic lipid profile in adulthood. It is also possible that genetic factors influencing both birth weight and lipid profile could explain this relationship. A twin study was performed to examine the influence of both genetic and intrauterine factors on the relationship between birth weight and lipid profile in adulthood.

Study Design.—The study was part of a larger twin study of cardiovascular risk factors. This study included 53 dizygotic and 61 monozygotic same-sex adolescent twin pairs. Height and weight of each twin were measured. Total cholesterol, triglycerides, high-density lipoprotein (HDL) and LDL cholesterol, apolipoprotein A1 and B levels were assessed. Linear regression analysis was utilized to examine the influence of birth weight on serum lipids.

Findings.—Regression analysis revealed that low birth weight was associated with high levels of total cholesterol, LDL cholesterol, and apolipoprotein B and with low levels of HDL cholesterol, after adjustment for age, sex, and body mass index. Intrapair birth weight differences were significantly associated with differences in total cholesterol, LDL cholesterol, and apolipoprotein B in dizygotic twins after adjustment for differences in current body mass index. This indicated that the greater the birth weight difference, the greater the risk factors in the twin with the lower birth weight in dizygotic twins. In monozygotic twins, these associations went in the opposite direction. The association between intrapair birth weight and differences in HLD cholesterol were not significant in dizygotic twins and were of borderline significance in monozygotic twins.

Conclusion.—These findings suggest that genetic factors are responsible for the association between low birth weight and high levels of total cholesterol, LDL cholesterol, and apolipoprotein B. Intrauterine factors may play a role in the association between low birth weight and low levels of HDL cholesterol.

▶ This study, done in adolescent like-sex twins of known zygosity and their parents, offers a further refutation to the Barker hypothesis[1] (see also Abstract 10–2). Barker's hypopthesis is that low–birth-weight infants are, by virtue of fetal adjustment to impaired nutritional access or utilization, programmed to a state of increased probability of hypertension, arteriosclertoic heart disease, dyslipidemia, and myocardial infarction in later life. The few references above pertain to the cardiovascular risks; this one deals with the purported increased risk of dyslipidemia.

Barker's error of omission is to ignore the likelihood that parents with a genetic predisposition to dyslipidemia, arteriosclerotic heart disease, hypertension, and myocardial infarction are likely to transfer these characteristics to their offspring and also to produce growth-retarded newborns as results of their own pathology. In that way, parent-child genetic inheritance is a confounding variable between neonatal growth retardation and infant hypertensive cardiovascular disease and dyslipidemia in later life in a sense that it determines both growth retardation and its spurious direct relationship to later life disease. Here, comparisons are made between birth weight and dyslipidemia (increased cholesterol, LDL cholesterol, apolipoprotein concentrations, and decreased HDL cholesterol) in monozygotic and dizygotic twins. When adjusted for adult body mass index, in dizygotic twins, the larger the difference in birth weight the greater the evidence of dyslipidemia in the smaller–birth-weight twin compared with its co-twin, reflecting nongenetic influences.

For monozygotic twins, the greater the difference in lipid profiles between twins, the lower the risk factors in the low–birth-weight twin, reflecting their common genome. Differences in HDL cholesterol were not significant in dizygotic twins, suggesting that in utero events may play a role only in the determination of the association between low birth weight and HDL cholesterol. There have, to date, been no effective counterarguments to this reasonable alternative to the Barker hypothesis.

T. H. Kirschbaum, MD

Reference

1. 2002 YEAR BOOK OF OBSTETRICS, GYNECOLOGY, AND WOMEN'S HEALTH, pp 73-77; pp 254-256.

Prenatal Leptin Production: Evidence That Fetal Adipose Tissue Produces Leptin

Lepercq J, Challier J-C, Guerre-Millo M, et al (Hôpital Cochin-Saint Vincent-de-Paul, Paris; Université P & M Curie, Paris; INSERM U 465, Paris; et al)
J Clin Endocrinol Metab 86:2409-2413, 2001   1–2

Introduction.—In adults, circulating leptin is highly associated with adipose tissue mass. It is not known whether such a relationship exists prenatally since the actual source of fetal leptin has not been determined. The placental contribution to fetal and maternal circulating leptin concentrations was examined in 74 nonobese, nondiabetic women, as was whether fetal adipose tissue produces leptin.

Methods.—Placentas from uncomplicated pregnancies were obtained after cesarean sections and underwent placental perfusion evaluations. Maternal, placental, and umbilical blood and tissue sampling were performed for biochemical assays, RNA isolation, reverse transcriptase–polymerase chain

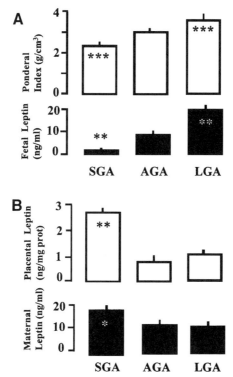

FIGURE 2.—Relationship between plasma leptin concentrations, ponderal index of infants, and placenta leptin content. Results are presented as mean ± SEM. Statistically significant differences: *Triple asterisk*, P < .0001; *double asterisk*, P < .001; *single asterisk*, P < .01 compared with AGA. *Abbreviations: SGA,* Small for gestational age; *AGA,* average for gestational age; *LGA,* large for gestational age. (Courtesy of Lepercq J, Challier J-C, Guerre-Millo M, et al: Prenatal leptin production: Evidence that fetal adipose tissue produces leptin. *J Clin Endocrinol Metab* 86(6):2409-2413, 2001. Copyright, The Endocrine Society.)

reaction, and quantitative reverse transcriptase–polymerase chain reaction analysis.

Results.—The rate of leptin production in the dually perfused placentas was 0.036 ng/min/g. Ninety-five percent of the leptin released was delivered into the maternal circulation, compared with 5% on the fetal side. Leptin messenger RNA and protein were identified in adipose tissue biopsy specimens of 20- to 38-week fetuses. The leptin concentration was twice as high in adult versus fetal adipose tissue (0.49 vs 0.22 ng/mg protein). The umbilical leptin levels closely reflected the ponderal index at birth over a wide range of birth weights (1.6-4.1 kg) (Fig 2). Both maternal and placental leptin concentrations were increased in pregnancies associated with fetal growth retardation.

Conclusion.—Umbilical leptin levels are independent of placental leptin production and can be considered a marker of fat mass in human fetuses. The placental leptin production makes a marked contribution to maternal circulating leptin levels during pregnancy.

▶ Maternal blood leptin concentration increases in pregnancy, primarily as the result of placental production, although maternal leptin concentration reflects maternal fat deposits and weight change better than it does newborn birth weight.[1,2] This study dissects human fetal from placental leptin production using 3 techniques. The first employs isolated placental cotyledon area perfusion with separate maternal and fetal perfusion circuits in measuring leptin production in perfusates collected over 2 hours. The results show that with a mean placental leptin production rate of 14 ng/min (0.84 μ/h), 95% of the protein product is distributed into the maternal circuit.

Second, when reverse transcriptase–polymerase chain reaction is used to measure leptin mRNA, it is found present in equal concentrations per unit protein in placenta and maternal and fetal adipose tissue, demonstrating the placenta to be an important site of the synthesis of the protein. Finally, when maternal and fetal leptin concentrations are compared in newborns with varying birth weights, fetal, but not maternal, leptin concentrations are directly related to newborn ponderal index, whereas the maternal levels are not. This is first evidence for leptin production by fetal fat, an important component of placental leptin transfer to the maternal circulation in pregnancy. The same procedures now need to be applied to preeclamptic gravidas in hopes of discerning the meaning of the decreased maternal leptin concentrations seen in such women.

T. H. Kirschbaum, MD

References

1. 1999 YEAR BOOK OF OBSTETRICS, GYNECOLOGY, AND WOMEN'S HEALTH, pages 13-15 and 2002 YEAR BOOK, pp 5-7.
2. 2001 YEAR BOOK OF OBSTETRICS, GYNECOLOGY, AND WOMEN'S HEALTH, pp 169.

Antepartum, Intrapartum, and Neonatal Significance of Exercise on Healthy Low-Risk Pregnant Working Women

Magann EF, Evans SF, Weitz B, et al (Univ of Mississippi, Jackson; Univ of Western Australia, Perth)

Obstet Gynecol 99:466-472, 2002   1–3

Background.—The effects of exercise on pregnancy and pregnancy outcomes are still unclear. An effort was made to determine the influence of exercise on maternal and perinatal outcomes in a low-risk, healthy obstetric population.

Methods and Findings.—Data were collected on 750 women, who were divided into 4 groups on the basis of levels of exercise during pregnancy. The groups did not differ in maternal demographic characteristics, antenatal illnesses, stress levels, social support, or smoking. Women who exercised heavily were older, had higher incomes, and were exercising more at conception. Women who were exercising heavily were more likely to need labor induction or induction or augmentation with oxytocin, and they had longer first-stage labors, which resulted in longer total labors. Although fewer umbilical cord abnormalities occurred with exercise, women who exercised had more colds and flu. Women who exercised heavily had smaller infants than did sedentary women.

Conclusions.—Exercising heavily during pregnancy is associated with lower birth weights, an increased number of inductions and augmentations of labors, and longer labor. Women who exercised more frequently had colds and flu.

▶ This controlled observational study provides some useful data concerning the impact of exercise on abnormal pregnancy. Seven hundred fifty active-duty women receiving care at the San Diego Naval Medical Center were segregated into 4 exercise groups based on questionnaire inquiry. The groups ranged from no pregnancy-associated exercise (group 1), those taking mandatory exercise for 30 minutes 3 times a week to 28 weeks' gestation coupled with aerobic exercise (group 2), to women continuing mandatory involuntary exercise to and after 28 weeks (group 4). A long list of pregnancy, labor, and delivery variables were evaluated for differences among the 4 groups. It is not entirely clear how univariate statistics were employed and, though the authors indicate that multivariate analyses were used to explore the many possible confounding relationships here, the results of those analyses are not provided. In this relatively homogeneous population that may be a less serious omission than usual. No significant impact of exercise on either maternal weight gain or infant birth weight was exhibited.

The length of the first stage of labor was less in nonexercising group 1 women than in those who were exercising. Antepartum oxytocin use for induction or augmentation was more common in exercisers than in abstainers. The lack of data concerning epidural analgesia and labor anesthesia among the 4 groups precludes full evaluation of those findings. What is most interesting is the failure to find evidence of any adverse impact of exercise over this range of intensity on pregnancy hypertension, preterm labor and delivery, fetal growth retardation, and neonatal morbidity and mortality. That's a useful basis for support for recommendations for intrapartum exercise in normal pregnant women who are so inclined.

T. H. Kirschbaum, MD

Absorption of Amniotic Fluid by Amniochorion in Sheep

Faber JJ, Anderson DF (Oregon Health Sciences Univ, Portland)
Am J Physiol 282:H850-H854, 2002   1–4

Background.—Sheep are said to have insignificant quantities of amniotic fluid exchanged with the maternal plasma, and under experimental conditions, the control of amniotic fluid volume is not regulated by either lung fluid production or urination. It appears that amniochorionic absorption increases when swallowing is not possible and when amniotic fluid inflow is supplemented by the infusion of Ringer solution. How amniochorionic absorption is effected remains unclear, with possible mechanisms being responses to a hypo-osmotic condition of the fetal plasma or to the difference in colloid osmotic pressures. These possibilities were explored by measuring amniochorionic absorption in the presence of induced changes in the osmolar and oncotic gradients between amniotic fluid and fetal plasma.

Methods.—The ability to swallow amniotic fluid and lung fluid inflow were eliminated operatively in 10 sheep fetuses. Ligation of the allantoic end of the urachus was performed, then fetal urine was drained to the outside. Amniotic fluid was drained to the outside for quantification and sampling, then 21 experiments were performed, and the fluid was again drained, measured, and sampled. During the experiments, which lasted a mean of 66 hours, amniotic fluid osmolalities and oncotic pressures were managed by the experimenters.

Results.—Based on the measurements obtained on various parameters, the experiments did not adversely affect the health of the fetuses. The control value for mean fluid absorption was 21.9 mL/h. When sodium solutions of varying concentrations were infused, the osmolality of the amniotic fluid depended most on electrolyte concentrations. A strong effect on the rate of fluid absorption or production by the amniochorion was exerted by the crystalloid osmolalities of the amniotic fluid. However, at zero osmolality difference, the mean absorption rate was 23.8, indicating that another mechanism must also be at work. When bovine albumin solutions were infused into the amnion, the oncotic gradient that usually favors fetal plasma was reversed, so that mean protein concentration was +14.1, higher in the amniotic fluid than plasma. This was compared to a value of −29.0 when no protein was infused into the amnion. Infused bovine albumin was absorbed at a rate of 1.8 g/h, for a flow volume of 33.8 mL/h.

Conclusion.—Fluid absorption by the amniochorion was strongly influenced by the osmolality difference between amniotic fluid and fetal plasma, thus indicating that crystalloid osmotic pressures drive amniotic fluid absorption. However, an additional method must also be at work because absorption continues even with a zero osmolality difference, and plasma albumin was significantly absorbed by a nondiffusional method.

▶ There has been considerable confusion introduced into the study of amniotic fluid dynamics by the introduction and misuse of the term "intramembranous pathway" to describe a poorly defined route for water and solute transfer between the fetus and amniotic fluid compartment.[1] Regrettably, these authors perpetuate the confusion in part. They study a chronic fetal sheep preparation based on a 2-compartment model of fetus and amniotic fluid. By ligating and connecting the trachea to the esophagus, they ablate swallowing which depletes and lung fluid expulsion that normally augments amniotic fluid volume.

They then catheterize the bladder, remove and measure amniotic fluid volume and osmolality, and hold amniotic fluid volume constant with infusions of amniotic fluid, urine, or a synethetic mixture into the amniotic fluid compartment. At the completion of an experiment with a mean duration of 6 hours, amniotic fluid volume was remeasured and the difference, initial minus final amniotic fluid volume, plus additions attributed to an intramembranous pathway.

What in reality happened to that fluid flux, averaging 25 mL per hour here, was that it was transferred from fetus to mother across the placenta intact during the studies. To this point, the authors misquote one of their references.[2] Dr Brace describes placental transfer of water through the placenta occurring in sheep fetuses and provides data estimating its flow at 400 to 500 mL/d, depending on fetal weight, roughly the same rate of efflux as the 600 mL/d rate identified here. Brace neglects water flux through fetal skin and umbilical cord because it remains unmeasured.

The contribution of transplacental water transport in the human and primate placenta has been measured and is known to be very large.[3] The purported role of a mysterious amniochorionic transfer site, the intramembranous path, is a reflection of failure to consider fetal-maternal transplacental water transfer in conceptual models that omit it.

T. H. Kirschbaum, MD

References

1. Mann SE, Nijland, MJM, Ross MG: Mathematical modeling of human amniotic fluid dynamics. *Am J Obstet Gynecol* 175:937, 1996.
2. Brace RA: Physiology of amniotic fluid volume regulation, in WM Gilbert (ed): *Clinical Obstetrics and Gynecology*, vol 210. Philadelphia, Lippincott-Raven, 1997.
3. Fredman EA, Gray MG, Hutchinson DL, et al: The role of the monkey fetus in exchange of water and sodium of the amniotic fluid. *J Clin Invest* 38:961, 1959.

Immunoelectron Microscopic Localization of Endothelial Nitric Oxide Synthase in Human Placental Terminal Villous Trophoblasts: Normal and Pre-eclamptic Pregnancy

Matsubara S, Takizawa T, Takayama T, et al (Jichi Med School, Tochigi, Japan)
Placenta 22:782-786, 2001   1–5

Introduction.—Several trials have reported the presence of nitric oxide synthase (NOS) in the human placental villi. Placental NOS is primarily of the endothelial type (eNOS), and syncytiotrophoblasts are the primary sources of placental eNOS. The subcellular localization within the syncytiotrophoblasts has not been determined. The subcellular localization of syncytial eNOS was examined in the human placental trophoblasts. The distribution pattern was compared with that from the preeclamptic placental trophoblasts by using immunogold electron microscopy. There was a focus

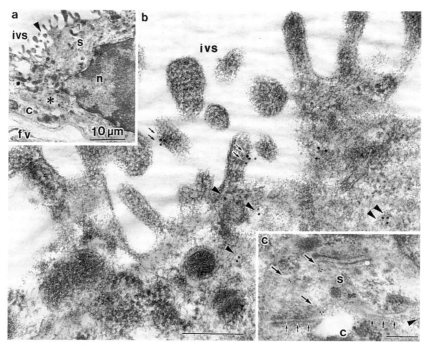

FIGURE 1.—Subcellular immunohistochemical localization of eNOS in the normal term human placental terminal villi without preeclampsia. Bar = 0.2 μm except for **a**. **a**, Electron micrograph at a low magnification. The areas marked by an *arrowhead* or by an *asterisk* are shown at a higher magnification in **b** and **c**, respectively. *Abbreviations: n*, Nucleus of the syncytiotrophoblast; *ivs*, intervillous space; *s*, syncytiotrophoblast; *c*, cytotrophoblast; *fv*, fetal vessel. **b**, Gold particles for eNOS were observable in microvilli (*arrows*) and in the cytoplasm of the syncytiotrophoblasts (*arrowheads*). **c**, Particles were distributed in the syncytial cytoplasm (*arrows*). A few particles (*arrowhead*) were also observable in the cytoplasm of cytotrophoblasts. *Small arrows* indicated the intercellular space between syncytium (*s*) and the cytotrophoblast (*c*). (Courtesy of Matsubara S, Takizawa T, Takayama T, et al: Immunoelectron microscopic localization of endothelial nitric oxide synthase in human placental terminal villous trophoblasts: Normal and pre-eclamptic pregnancy. *Placenta* 22:782-786, 2001.)

on the terminal villi, which are considered to be functioning villi in several placental functions.

Methods.—Five placentas from term or preterm pregnant women at 34 to 38 weeks' gestation and 5 from women with severe preeclampsia at 34 to 39 weeks' gestation were examined. Severe preeclampsia was characterized by a blood pressure of 160/110 mm Hg or higher on at least 2 seperate occasions, and a urinary protein level of 300 mg/dL or higher. All 5 infants in the preeclampsia group were light for their gestation age, and all 5 in the group without preeclampsia had weights appropriate for their gestational age. The latter acted as controls for the preeclampsia group. All placentas were examined via immunohistochemistry and semiquantitative analysis.

Results.—Immunolabeling for eNOS was visible notably in the syncytial microvilli and synctial cytoplasm (Fig 1). Semiquantitative analysis demonstrated that the concentration and distribution pattern of gold particles for eNOS did not significantly vary between normal and preeclamptic placental trophoblasts.

Conclusion.—Syncytiotrophoblastic microvilli and cytoplasm were the subcellular localization sites of syncytium-derived eNOS in terminal villi. There were no significant differences in this eNOS subcellular distribution pattern between normal and preeclamptic syncytiotrophoblasts in terms of immunohistochemically discernable eNOS.

▶ NOS catalyzes the conversion of arginine to citrulline and leads to liberation of nitric oxide (NO). NO is an important modulator of parts of the inflammatory reaction and platelet aggregation and induces vasodilatation, as well as serving as a signaling intermediate for a wide range of biochemical reactions. It is known to be present in the placenta in its endothelial isoform (eNOS) and is also abundant in vascular endothelium. Interest in its role in preeclampsia stems from observations that it exists in higher blood concentrations in preeclamptics than in normotensive women.[1-3] In this study, its subcellular localization in the human placenta was sought as well as its relative concentration in normal and preeclamptic pregnancy.

Sections of placenta from 5 preeclamptics were compared with sections from 5 normal control gravidas. Sections of placental tissue were exposed to rabbit antihuman antibody for eNOS and labeled with colloidal gold particles, which then render eNOS discernable on transmission electron microscopy. The concentration of eNOS is expressed in terms of number of gold particles per unit surface area, apical versus basal segments of villi, and its relative distribution in syncytium versus cytotrophoblast with or without hypertensive disease. In syncytial cells, normal controls averaged 9.5 gold particles per square meter versus 9.1 in preeclamptics, indicating no increase in eNos in preeclamptic villi. Roughly 30% of eNOS in villi is located in the apical syncytial microvilli; cytotrophoblast averages 1.3 gold granules per square meter.

It is important to recall the work of Redman et al,[4] who demonstrated that plasma but not serum from preeclamptics inhibited endothelial cell growth in vitro and was capable of resulting in endothelial injury. The same investigators found syncytial apical microvillous segments present in plasma but caught in the fibrin mesh works of the coagulum, and found that they exist in larger concentrations in preeclamptics than in normals.[5] It's possible then that part of the increased NO production found in the preeclamptic blood comes from an increase in trophoblastic microvilli shed into the circulation, leaving the concentration of unshed enzyme in maternal placenta tissue unchanged by the disease. Preeclamptic gravidas also likely increase NO production on the basis of increased vascular endothelial shear stress as blood velocity in constricted arterioles stimulates its production.[6] The immediate role of NO in preeclampsia remains obscure but may represent a compensation for the increased peripheral vascular resistance of preeclampsia produced by an as yet obscure additional mechanism.

T. H. Kirschbaum, MD

References

1. 1997 YEAR BOOK OF OBSTETRICS, GYNECOLOGY, AND WOMEN'S HEALTH, pp 24-25.
2. 1998 YEAR BOOK OF OBSTETRICS, GYNECOLOGY, AND WOMEN'S HEALTH, pp 23-25.
3. 2001 YEAR BOOK OF OBSTETRICS, GYNECOLOGY, AND WOMEN'S HEALTH, pp 6-8.
4. 1997 YEAR BOOK OF OBSTETRICS, GYNECOLOGY, AND WOMEN'S HEALTH, pp 37-39.
5. 1999 YEAR BOOK OF OBSTETRICS, GYNECOLOGY, AND WOMEN'S HEALTH, pp 31-33.
6. 2002 YEAR BOOK OF OBSTETRICS, GYNECOLOGY, AND WOMEN'S HEALTH, pp 128-131.

Preeclampsia and Maladaptation to Pregnancy: A Role for Atrial Natriuretic Peptide?

Spaanderman M, Ekhart T, van Eyck J, et al (Academic Hosp Maastricht, The Netherlands; Sophia Hosp Zwolle, Maastricht, The Netherlands)
Kidney Int 60:1397-1406, 2001   1–6

Background.—Most women with a history of preeclampsia have an underlying vascular disorder. Whether the adaptation to pregnancy would differ depending on the underlying condition present in these women was examined.

Study Design.—Women who had experienced severe preeclampsia and were planning another pregnancy were eligible to be included in the study group. The initial study group consisted of 63 nondiabetic women with a history of preeclampsia and 15 normal controls. Final analysis included 37 women with a history of preeclampsia and 10 controls who became pregnant with singleton pregnancies within the year. All study participants were white and none smoked during the pregnancy.

All participants were tested for thrombophilia and hemodynamic function. This was used to divide the 37 women with a history of preeclampsia into 10 with hypertension (HYPERT), 13 who were normotensive and thrombophilic (THROMB), and 14 who were normotensive and non-thrombophilic (NONTHROMB). Mean arterial pressure, heart rate, cardiac output, central cardiovascular dimensions, plasma volume, glomerular filtration rate, effective renal plasma flow, 17-β estradiol, progesterone, the renin-angiotensin-aldosterone axis hormones, catecholamines and α-atrial natriuretic peptide were assessed at least 5 months postpartum at about day 5 of the menstrual cycle and again at 5 and 7 weeks amenorrhea in the next pregnancy.

Findings.—The early pregnancy increase in cardiac output, renal variables, renin-angiotensin-aldosterone activity, and plasma volume did not differ significantly among the 4 groups. The HYPERT and NONTHROMB groups differed from control subjects by having a lower plasma volume between pregnancies and by increasing the level of circulating α-atrial natriuretic peptide during early pregnancy. At 7 weeks, women in the HYPERT and NONTHROMB groups had the lowest plasma volume. Plasma volume was inversely correlated with the level of circulating α-atrial natriuretic peptide.

Conclusion.—Women with hypertension and normotensive nonthrombophilic women with a history of severe preeclampsia differed from healthy control subjects and thrombophilic women with a history of preeclampsia by having an increase in circulating α-atrial natriuretic peptide in early pregnancy, together with a lower plasma volume.

▶ The relationship of hypovolemia to preeclampsia in recurrent pregnancy hypertension has been attributed to altered production and release rates of atrial naturetic peptides (ANPs), but whether there is a cause and effect relationship between the two and, if so, what its significance is, remains uncertain. This group reports some interesting but somewhat controversial data and an arguable hypotheseis. Their premises are that, following a preeclamptic pregnancy, those with underlying chronic cardiovascular renal disease will, in the 7 weeks after the amenorrheic onset of a next pregnancy, behave differently than those who showed evidence of thrombophilia or a third group of women with neither evidence of cardiovascular disease, nor coagulopathy.

Baseline measurements in singlet pregnancies were done in the early follicular phase of a cycle at last 5 months after delivery of the initial preeclamptic pregnancy. Thirty-seven women with singlet pregnancies who conceived within 1 year after the initial hypertensive pregnancy and were not taking antihypertensives, were admitted for longitudinal studies at 5 and 7 weeks gestational age for comparisons and prepregnancy assays. Several assays of cardiovascular renal and endocrine variables were performed. Of the 37, 10 showed evidence of cardiovascular disease, 13 had 1 test of a series positive for thrombophilia, and 14 had neither cardiovascular nor thrombophilic positive assays. One comparison is between the 10 normal secundagravidas and those with evidence of cardiovascular disease after a preeclamptic first pregnancy.

Of the latter, those with chronic hypertension showed elevated maternal arterial pressures, renal vascular resistance, angiotensin-2 concentrations, and reduced plasma volume as well as elevated ANP compared with controls, as expected. Normals showed the usual increase in cardiac output, glomerular filtration rate, renal plasma flow, plasma volume, and reduced maternal arterial pressure and peripheral vascular resistance during the first trimester. These findings agree with measurements in later pregnancy, the third trimester, and 6 days post partum. In that case, ANP was elevated in the third trimester and for as long as 6 days post partum compared with normals,[1] apparently in response to the hypervolemia of the early postpartum state and the need to produce diuresis to decrease the elevated venous return postpartum.

Roughly 20% of patients with preeclampsia may be expected to show chronic hypertensive findings after a first episode of severe preeclampsia.[2] In a later study,[3] ANF was shown to exist in decreased concentrations as early as 8 weeks through 36 weeks of pregnancy, compared with normotensive women, the opposite of what was found here.

A more puzzling comparison is between controls and the 14 women with neither cardiovascular or neurothrombophilic findings, called NONTHROMB this study. In this latter group, plasma volume was decreased and ANF significantly increased in earlier pregnancy. At least 1 assay among antiphospholipid antibodies, proteins S and C, lupus anticoagulants, and homocystine concentrations was positive in this group. The Leiden V mutation was regrettably not sought. Two groups of investigators have failed to find evidence supporting a tendency for repeat pregnancy-induced hypertension among women with thrombophilia defined only in this way.[4] The NONTHROMB subset showed lesser body mass indexes, low sodium excretion on 100 mmol/d sodium intake, low plasma volume, and mean body weight at the 18th percentile. The cause of the increased ANP and reduced plasma volume in this subset is simply obscure.

What is clear is that preeclamptic women showed decreased plasma volume and increased ANP as early as 5 to 7 weeks into a following pregnancy, with a 20% risk of pregnancy-induced hypertension. Which is cause and which effect is uncertain, nor is it certain what happens to plasma volume regulation past the seventh week of pregnancy until delivery. That is a critical concern in view of the evidence of changes in cardiac output and peripheral vascular resist in preeclampsia after 34 to 36 weeks' gestation, as shown earlier.[5] If women with pregnancy hypertension are relatively hypovolemic near term, one would expect a low ANP acting to impede diuresis and closure values in duration. What occurs to ANP during mid-pregnancy is clearly important in evaluating the volume changes of preeclampsia.

T. H. Kirschbaum, MD

References

1. 1998 YEAR BOOK OF OBSTETRICS, GYNECOLOGY, AND WOMEN'S HEALTH, pp 13-16.
2. 2002 YEAR BOOK OF OBSTETRICS, GYNECOLOGY, AND WOMEN'S Health, pp 133-134.
3. 2001 YEAR BOOK OF OBSTETRICS, GYNECOLOGY, AND WOMEN'S HEALTH, pp 108-110.
4. 2002 YEAR BOOK OF OBSTETRICS, GYNECOLOGY, AND WOMEN'S HEALTH, pp 133-134; pp 227-229.
5. 2001 YEAR BOOK OF OBSTETRICS, GYNECOLOGY, AND WOMEN'S HEALTH, pp 105-108.

Effect of Ro 61-1790, a Selective Endothelin-A Receptor Antagonist, on Systemic and Uterine Hemodynamics and Fetal Oxygenation in Sheep

McElvy S, Greenberg S, Baker RS, et al (Univ of Cincinnati, Ohio)
Am J Obstet Gynecol 186:55-60, 2002   1–7

Background.—Endothelin-1 has been shown to be increased in preeclampsia. Previous laboratory studies have shown that infusion of endothelin-1 increases mean arterial pressure, hemoconcentration, and proteinuria and reduces uterine blood flow. If endothelin-1 plays a role in preeclampsia, selective endothelin-A receptor blockers may be a promising treatment. The effects of a selective endothelin-A receptor inhibitor, Ro 61-1790, on mean arterial pressure, heart rate, and uteroplacental blood flow in pregnant and nonpregnant sheep were investigated.

Methods.—Seven pregnant and 7 nonpregnant sheep were studied. Indwelling femoral artery and vein catheters and bilateral uterine artery flow probes were placed to assess mean arterial pressure, heart rate, and uteropla-

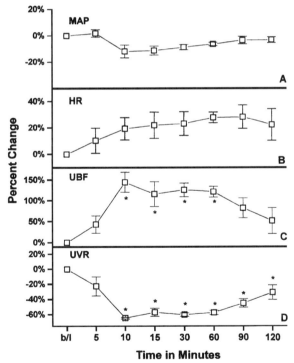

FIGURE 2.—Effect of endothelin-A (ET$_A$) receptor antagonist Ro 61-1790 (3 mg/kg IV) on systemic and uterine hemodynamics over time in nonpregnant sheep. Data are presented as percent change from baseline (*b/l*). **A**, Mean arterial pressure (*MAP*). **B**, Heart rate (*HR*). **C**, Uterine blood flow (*UBF*). **D**, Uterine vascular resistance (*UVR*). *Asterisk, P < .05* versus baseline. (Courtesy of McElvy S, Greenberg S, Baker RS, et al: Effect of Ro 61-1790, a selective endothelin-A receptor antagonist, on systemic and uterine hemodynamics and fetal oxygenation in sheep. *Am J Obstet Gynecol* 186:55-60, 2002.)

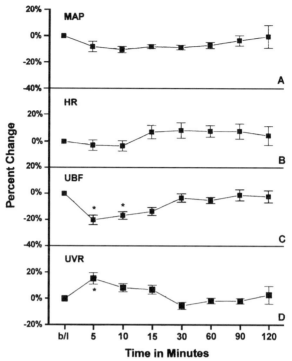

FIGURE 3.—Effect of endothelin-A (ET$_A$) receptor antagonist Ro 61-1790 (3 mg/kg IV) on systemic and uterine hemodynamics over time in pregnant sheep. Data are presented as percent change from baseline (*b/l*). A, Mean arterial pressure (*MAP*). B, Heart rate (*HR*). C, Uterine blood flow (*UBF*). D, Uterine vascular resistance (*UVR*). *Asterisk, P* < .05 versus baseline. (Courtesy of McElvy S, Greenberg S, Baker RS, et al: Effect of Ro 61-1790, a selective endothelin-A receptor antagonist, on systemic and uterine hemodynamics and fetal oxygenation in sheep. *Am J Obstet Gynecol* 186:55-60, 2002.)

cental blood flow. Sheep were given IV Ro 61-1790, 1 or 3 mg/kg. Hemodynamic responses were monitored for 120 minutes.

Findings.—The administration of 1 mg/kg of Ro 61-1790 did not affect the parameters studied. However, the infusion of 3 mg/kg of Ro 61-1790 increased total uterine blood flow in nonpregnant sheep from a mean of 22 mL/min to 51 mL/min. No significant changes in mean arterial pressure occurred (Fig 2). In pregnant sheep, 3 mg/kg of Ro 61-1790 reduced mean uteroplacental blood flow by 20% and transiently increased uterine vascular resistance. Fetal mean arterial pressure, heart rate, and oxygenation were unaffected (Fig 3).

Conclusions.—Endogenous endothelin-1 may play an important role in regulating uterine vascular tone in sheep. Inhibiting endogenous endothelin-1 may result in decreased uteroplacental perfusion in pregnant sheep.

▶ Endothelin (ET-1) is a very potent vasoconstrictor produced largely by endothelial cells. After an initial claim that its increased presence in pregnancy hypertension might explain the increased peripheral vascular resistance in that disorder,[1] subsequent work has shown no evidence of a significant functional role for ET-1 in the altered hemodynamics either of normal or hypertensive human pregnancy.[2,3] Rather, it appears to play a role in vascular adjustments of peripheral vascular resistance in chronic hypertensive states in nonpregnant women. Here, the results of IV administration of a selective blocker of endothelin-A (ET-A), the ET-1 receptor, are studied in pregnant and nonpregnant sheep using Doppler flow probes for measuring right and left uterine artery blood flow, and using indwelling external artery and vein catheters in mother and fetus to measure changes in pulse and heart rate. The results confirm the inferences described above. The receptor blocker results in decreased uterine vascular resistance in nonpregnant ewes but showed a modest insignificant 10% reduction in maternal arterial pressure and a slight but statistically significant decrease in uterine artery blood flow, at most by 20%. Bear in mind that the syndesmochorial sheep placenta differs from the human hemochorial placenta in that the uterine vasculature is closed in the sheep with intact arteriolar vasoregulating elements, compared with the dilated patulous human arterioles that empty into the intervillous space, a nonendothelial lined compartment lacking vascular autoregulation. This work does suggest, however, that the ET-A blocker might be useful as a maternal antihypertensive agent, leaving the fetal circulation largely unaltered. Clearly, the work would benefit from some observations in human beings.

T. H. Kirschbaum, MD

References

1. 1992 Year Book of Obstetrics, Gynecology, and Women's Health, pp 42-43.
2. 1998 Year Book of Obstetrics, Gynecology, and Women's Health, pp 21-22.
3. 2001 Year Book of Obstetrics, Gynecology, and Women's Health, pp 108-110.

Connexin 43 Expression in Normal Versus Dysfunctional Labor
Pierce BT, Calhoun BC, Adolphson KR, et al (Madigan Army Med Ctr, Fort Lewis, Wash; Univ of Hawaii, Honolulu)
Am J Obstet Gynecol 186:504-511, 2002   1–8

Background.—Gap junctions are believed to be one of several essential components necessary for effective labor and delivery. Gap junctions mediate cell-to-cell communication, maintain normal cell function, and have an important role in embryonic development and possibly control of growth. Connexins are a family of gap junction proteins named for their molecular weights. The major gap junction protein present in myometrium is connexin 43 (Cx43), with a molecular weight of 43 kd. Gap junction plaques are undetectable or present in very low numbers for most of pregnancy, which is consistent with the presence of poorly coordinated, low-amplitude contractions (Braxton Hicks) during pregnancy. At the onset of labor, there is a dramatic increase in the number and size of the plaques, an increase in the electrical conductivity of the myometrium, and the development of spontaneous, well-coordinated labor contractions. Cx43 mRNA levels increase in the myometrium toward term, in correlation with the appearance of gap junction plaques, and are highest during delivery. Whether Cx43 is differentially expressed in normal versus dysfunctional labor was investigated.

Methods.—Myometrial biopsy specimens were obtained from 28 patients who were undergoing cesarean section. The patients were grouped into the following categories: no labor, dysfunctional labor, and normal labor. Cx43 mRNA and protein expression were evaluated with Northern and Western analyses, respectively. Localization of Cx43 protein was determined by immunohistochemistry.

Results.—Labor was associated with an increase in Cx43 mRNA expression but not with an increase in protein expression. There was no difference in mRNA or protein expression between patients with normal labor and those with dysfunctional labor. There was no significant difference among the groups in the extent of Cx43 immunohistochemical staining.

Conclusions.—There were no indications of aberrant Cx43 mRNA or protein expression or a reduction in immunodetectable Cx43 gap junctions in association with dysfunctional labor.

▶ Gap junctions are intracytoplasmic bridges that form between adjoining smooth muscle cells in the mammalian uterus that serve to facilitate ion transfers, and therefore electropotential transmission among the cells. They form as a result of gene activation progressively through labor and are assembled in 2 cylindrical segments (connexons), 1 from each adjoining cell. Each connexin is formed in turn by 6 protein molecules (connexins), the most common Cx43, named for its molecular weight. They are needed because the rate of electrical potential decay along the smooth muscle fiber is large and requires short-circuiting to allow cell-to-cell communication of action potentials. The progressive production of gap junctions during pregnancy, under endocrine control, is thought to be responsible for the progressive coordination of uterine muscle contractile activity involving larger and larger myometrial segments with time in the transition from isolated events to Braxton-Hicks–like contractions to full-scale labor. It has long been thought that dysfunctional labor might well be related to deficient or suboptimally effective gap junction formation. This study uses analysis of myometrial segments obtained at the time of cesarean section in women not in labor, in normal labor, and in dysfunctional labor to exclude deficient numbers of connexin molecules, connexons, and gap junctions as a cause of subnormal labor. Connexin mRNA was measured by Northern blot, connexin protein by Western blot, and gap junctions were identified by immunohistochemistry by using anti-Cx43 antibody. Although mRNA was more prevalent in labor than without, no differences between normal and dysfunctional labor were seen. Clearly, this fails to support a role for deficient gap junction numbers as a cause of dysfunctional labor, but the possibility that gap junctions may be less effective in ion transfer in such cases despite their normal numbers persists.

T. H. Kirschbaum, MD

Adhesion Molecules Expression in the Placental Bed of Pregnancies With Pre-eclampsia

Tziotis J, Malamitsi-Puchner A, Vlachos G, et al (Univ of Athens, Greece)
Br J Obstet Gynaecol 109:197-201, 2002   1–9

Introduction.—Platelet endothelial cell adhesion molecule-1 (PECAM-1) is a 130-kd member of the immunoglobulin superfamily. It is expressed on the surface of circulating platelets, monocytes, neutrophils, and certain T-cell subsets. It is an important constituent of the endothelial cell intercellular junction and is implicated in several functions as a result of its cellular expression pattern. The expression of intracellular adhesion molecule-1 (ICAM-1), vascular cell adhesion molecule-1 (VCAM-1), PECAM-1, and E-selectin in placental bed biopsies (endothelium of spiral arteries as well as trophoblastic cells) from both normal and preeclamptic pregnancies was evaluated prospectively.

Methods.—Placental bed biopsy specimens were obtained immediately after delivery from 16 preeclamptic and 20 uncomplicated normotensive pregnant females. Tissue samples from preeclamptic and control females were embedded in paraffin and underwent immunocytochemical staining for ICAM-1, VCAM-1, PECAM-1, and E-selectin. The percentage of positive cells were compared with the total number of cells lining the vessel wall in each section.

Results.—The PECAM-1, VCAM-1, and ICAM-1 adhesion molecules had similar expression in the placental bed of both normotensive and preeclamptic groups (Table 2). E-selectin was not identified in the placental bed of either group. PECAM-1 was expressed throughout the vascular tree of the placental bed and not in the interstitial trophoblastic tissue. This was also true regarding staining of VCAM-1 and ICAM-1. Negative staining was observed for VCAM-1 and E-selectin on the trophoblastic tissue.

Conclusion.—Adhesion molecules ICAM-1, VCAM-1, and PECAM-1 but not E-selectin were expressed in the placental bed of normal and pre-

TABLE 2.—Expression of Adhesion Molecules in the Placental Bed
Vasculature. Percentage of Positive Blood Vessels in the
Preeclamptic and Control Group

	Groups		*P*
	Pre-eclamptic (*n* = 16)	Control (*n* = 20)	
PECAM	60 (22)	73 (27)	NS
ICAM-1	62 (23)	72 (22)	NS
VCAM-1	31 (13)	27 (11)	NS
E-selectin	0	0	NS

Values are mean (SD).
Abbreviations: PECAM, Platelet endothelial cell adhesion molecule-1; *ICAM-1,* intercellular adhesion molecule-1; *VCAM-1,* vascular cell adhesion molecule-1.
(Courtesy of Tziotis J, Malamitsi-Puchner A, Vlachos G, et al: Adhesion molecules expression in the placental bed of pregnancies with pre-eclampsia. *Br J Obstet Gynaecol* 109:197-201, 2002. With permission from Elsevier Science.)

eclamptic pregnancies. It appears that these adhesion molecules are not likely to be implicated in the etiology of preeclampsia.

▶ This important set of findings deals with the arcane world of intercellular junction formations between cells and extracellular matrix or among components of the matrix itself. The subject derives its significance from the striking changes that take place during implantation, placentation, and placental development. Trophoblastic epithelium is able to bind to spiral arteriolar endothelium, penetrate down those intervillous space inflow channels, and alter their morphology.[1] It also transiently acquires the ability to invade maternal spiral arterioles and to incorporate that vasculature into the developing intervillous space.[2] At the depth of placental attachment, trophoblastic epithelial cells enter into anchoring functions with matrix to hold cotyledons in place, and others penetrate into more depth in the form of wandering trophoblast cells. Defects in the depth of implantation have been implicated as a covariant of preeclampsia, preterm labor, and fetal growth retardation.[3] A current hypothesis regarding the origin of preeclampsia posits interference with vascular endothelial cell functions and, in particular, the role of intact endothelium in arteriolar vasoregulation.

Protein molecules that form anchoring functions do so by connecting actin fibers between intercellular attachment proteins with transmembrane linkage proteins. Adherence between cells is carried on by cadherins. Integrins bind cellular adhesion plaques to surface receptors or matrix molecules, or join 2 or more elements of matrix components together. Endothelium expresses adhesion molecules to bind intracellular elements of leukocytes and especially T cells (ICAM) to other epitopes on blood-formed elements (VCAM) and platelets (PEACM) active in regulation of inflammation and immune reactivity. Here their presence and concentration is used to detect active endothelial functions in the presence of preeclampsia. E-selectin is a cell surface carbohydrate-binding protein that performs transient low-intensity binding to endothelium in, for example, leukocyte margination, and penetration into the extracellular connective tissue matrix. Adhesion molecules by virtue of their position and expression determine the position, motility, structure, and function of the cellular composition of tissues and organs.

In this study, placental bed biopsy specimens were obtained at the time of cesarean section in 16 patients with preeclampsia and compared with samples from 20 normal control gravidas. The relative abundance of PECAM, ICAM-1, VCAM-1, and E-selectin were measured by immunocytochemistry. Although E-selectin was not found in placental bed biopsy specimens, all the other adhesion molecules were abundant in the maternal vasculature in equal amounts in normal and hypertensive patients. This is a convincing piece of evidence supporting normal function and the lack of maternal endothelial pathology at the site of maternal vascularization of the placenta in preeclampsia, as measured by alterations in the expression of adhesion molecules.

T. H. Kirschbaum, MD

References

1. 1994 YEAR BOOK OF OBSTETRICS, GYNECOLOGY, AND WOMEN'S HEALTH, pp 59-60.
2. 1998 YEAR BOOK OF OBSTETRICS, GYNECOLOGY, AND WOMEN'S HEALTH, pp 18-21.
3. 1988 YEAR BOOK OF OBSTETRICS, GYNECOLOGY, AND WOMEN'S HEALTH, pp 50-51.

IGF-I, Osteocalcin, and Bone Change in Pregnant Normotensive and Pre-Eclamptic Women

Sowers M, Scholl T, Grewal J, et al (Univ of Michigan, Ann Arbor; Univ of Medicine and Dentistry of New Jersey, Piscataway)
J Clin Endocrinol Metab 86:5898-5903, 2001   1–10

Background.—From 5% to 10% of pregnant women are affected by preeclampsia, a disorder of uncertain cause. The symptoms of preeclampsia commonly present around or after 20 weeks' gestation. The hypothesis that insulin-like growth factor I (IGF-I), osteocalcin, and bone loss would differ in pregnant women with preeclampsia compared with normotensive pregnant women was studied.

Methods.—The study group was composed of 962 pregnant healthy women between the ages of 12 and 35 years. The women were assessed for osteocalcin and IGF-I concentrations at entry to care (baseline), at 28 weeks, and at delivery. Bone US was measured at baseline and at 6 weeks postpartum, and bone mineral density was measured at delivery by dual radiograph densitometry.

Results.—A total of 64 women (6.7%) had preeclampsia develop. In these women, IGF-I concentrations in the third trimester were 74% greater compared with the first trimester, but there was little change in the concentration of osteocalcin. In comparison, the IGF-I concentrations in normotensive women increase by an average of 43%, whereas there was a 63% decline in osteocalcin concentrations. There was a significant correlation between IGF-I and osteocalcin concentrations in women with preeclampsia in both the first and third trimester time points, but this correlation was only seen in the third trimester among normotensive women. There was no statistically significant difference in bone change between the 2 groups.

Conclusions.—It would appear that women with preeclampsia have an exaggerated IGF-I responsiveness compared with normotensive women. The strong correlation between IGF-I and osteocalcin observed in women with preeclampsia suggests that IGF-I retains its ability to act as a local regulator of bone remodeling.

▶ IGF-I clearly plays a role in the regulation of fetal growth, and possible changes in preeclamptic women have been reported, but with conflicting observations.[1] This longitudinal study of 869 gravidas provides some authoritative answers concerning calcium metabolism in preeclampsia. Maternal IGF-I serum concentrations in pregnancy were slightly lower than in nonpregnant women in early pregnancy but progressively increased slightly to term in comparison to nonpregnant normals. In the 64 women with preeclampsia, three fourths of them nulliparas, mean IGF-I concentration increased significantly in the second and third trimesters and exceeded values in normotensive gravidas at that time. Maternal serum osteocalcin concentration increased in parallel with IGF-I, indicating increased sensitivity to IGF and in excess of values for normotensive gravidas. Such increases, usually taken to mean new bone production, were not confirmed by serial bone density dual radiographic densitometry. Rather, densitometry suggested maternal bone density in preeclampsia decreased compared with normal pregnancy, though not significantly.

The findings suggest increased demand for maternal skeletal calcium release through an uncertain mechanism and for an unknown purpose. The existence of IGF binding proteins, each with distinct effects and anatomic locations, complicates the picture at present.

T. H. Kirschbaum, MD

Reference

1. Giudice LC, Martina NA, Crystal RA, et al: Insulin-like growth factor binding protein-1 at the maternal-fetal interface and insulin-like binding growth factor I in the circulation of women with severe preeclampsia. *Am J Obstet Gynecol* 176:751, 1997.

Stimulation of Human Extravillous Trophoblast Migration by IGF-II Is Mediated by IGF Type 2 Receptor Involving Inhibitory G Protein(s) and Phosphorylation of MAPK

McKinnon T, Chakraborty C, Gleeson LM, et al (Univ of Western Ontario, London, Canada)
J Clin Endocrinol Metab 86:3665-3674, 2001   1–11

Background.—Previous research has shown that migration and invasiveness of first-trimester human extravillous trophoblast cells are stimulated by IGF-II, independently of IGF type 1 receptor. In addition, migration stimulation is the main reason for increased IGF-II–induced extravillous trophoblast cell invasiveness. An effort was made to determine the functional role of IGF type II receptor in IGF-II stimulation of extravillous trophoblast cell migration and the underlying signal transduction pathways, including the participation of inhibitory G protein(s) and MAPK.

Methods and Findings.—A Transwell migration assay was used to quantitate the migratory ability of a well-characterized in vitro propagated human first-trimester extravillous trophoblast cell line expressing the phenotype of extravillous trophoblast cells in situ under different experimental conditions. Extravillous trophoblast cells were found to express an abundance of IGF type 2 receptor, as detected by immunostaining and Western blots. Recombinant human IGF-II promoted their migration in a dose-dependent and time-dependent fashion. Polyclonal and monoclonal IGF type 2 receptor-blocking antibodies blocked the migration-stimulating effects of IGF-II. Two synthetic IGF-II analogues—1 that can bind to IGF type 2 receptor and IGF-binding proteins but not IGF type 1 receptors and 1 that can bind to IGFR-II but not IGFR-I or IGF-binding proteins—stimulated extravillous trophoblast cell migration to levels greater than those induced by wild-type IGF-II. Thus, IGF type 2 receptor mediated IGF-II action, independently of IGF type I receptor and IGF-binding proteins. When extravillous trophoblast cell membrane preparations were treated with IGF-II, adenylyl cyclase activity declined in a concentration-dependent fashion, demonstrating the participation of inhibitory G proteins in IGF-II action. Treatment with IGF-II rapidly stimulated phosphorylation of extravillous trophoblast cells with the MAPK kinase inhibitor PD98059. In addition, extravillous trophoblast cell migration was blocked in the presence or absence of IGF-II.

Conclusions.—IGF-II stimulates extravillous trophoblast cell migration by signaling through IGF type 2 receptor. This involves inhibitory G proteins and activation of the MAPK pathway.

▶ In the process of placentation, dedicated cytrotrophoblast stem cells produce syncytial trophoblast cells, which invade the decidua in controlled fashion, setting up columns of cells that anchor villi to the decidual extracellular matrix via cell surface integrins and invade endometrial glands and arterioles.[1] In arterioles they have the capacity to remodel maternal arterioles, converting them into dilated thin-walled structures of low vascular resistance, which facilitate the high-flow-rate circulation in the intervillous space.[2] Where a trophoblast cell exists in decidua or other tissues remote from villous cores, it is called an extravillous trophoblast. Extravillous trophoblasts may be seen in myometrial layers and maternal vessels in remote organs, characteristically evoking no inflammatory response because of their immune privilege and producing no degenerative changes in normal maternal tissue. The role of extravascular trophoblasts is apparently defective in preeclampsia and some forms of fetal growth retardation.[3] Loss of the ability to coexist with normal host tissues results in invasive mole and trophoblastic malignancies. Clearly, the mechanisms that regulate extravascular trophoblast growth are very important.

This is an in vitro experience in the cell biology of extravillous trophoblasts obtained and maintained in cell culture. Reactions to reagents are measured by visually noting cell margin migration rates over millipore membranes and identifying protein cell products by immunohistochemistry, using measurements of adenylyl cyclase and cAMP activity. The authors show that IGF-II is produced by extravillous trophoblast, stimulates its growth and metabolic activity, and is blocked by an antibody directed at its receptor, IGFR II. IGF-II is produced by trophoblasts and stimulates cell growth, in part by upregulating transport of nutrients and intermediates by endosomal migration. Others[4-6] have shown that decidual production of a high-infinity binding protein, IGFBP-1, also enhances the growth and migration of extravillous trophoblasts. Other locally active growth factors among them TGF (produced by decidua) provide negative control of extravascular trophoblast migration, proliferation, and invasiveness.

This glimpse of trophoblast cell regulation opens new areas to research in the pathophysiology of some forms of pregnancy in hypertension and growth retardation.

T. H. Kirschbaum, MD

References

1. 1998 YEAR BOOK OF OBSTETRICS, GYNECOLOGY, AND WOMEN'S HEALTH, pp 18-21.
2. Brosnes I, Robertson WB, Dixon HG: The physiological response of vessels of the placental bed to normal pregnancy. *J Pathol Bacteriol* 93:569, 1967.
3. 1994 YEAR BOOK OF OBSTETRICS, GYNECOLOGY, AND WOMEN'S HEALTH, pp 59-60.
4. Irving JA, Lala PK: Functional role of cell surface integrins on human trophoblast cell migration: Regulation by TGF-β, IGF-II and IGFBP-1. *Exp Cell Res* 217:419-427, 1995.
5. Han VKM, Bassett N, Walton J, et al: The expression of IGF and IGFBP genes in the human placenta and membranes: Evidence for IIGF-IGFBP interactions at the feto-maternal interface. *J Clin Endocrinol Metab* 81:2680-2693, 1996.
6. Hamilton GS, Lysiak JJ, Han VKM, et al: Autocrine-paracrine regulation of human trophoblast invasiveness by IGF-II and IGFBP-I. *Exp Cell Res* 244:147-156, 1998.

Reduced Binding of Progesterone Receptor to Its Nuclear Response Element After Human Labor Onset

Henderson D, Wilson T (Dundee Univ, Scotland)
Am J Obstet Gynecol 185:579-585, 2001   1–12

Background.—In most mammals, labor is initiated by withdrawal of progesterone, but there is little evidence for progesterone reduction as the cause of labor in humans. Progesterone acts by binding to a specific cellular receptor. This study tested the hypothesis that there is decreased progesterone receptor binding to its specific DNA progesterone-responsive element in human laboring tissues.

Study Design.—Placental membranes were obtained from 52 women who were term, preterm, in labor, and not in labor. Homogenates of the maternal component of the membranes (decidua) were compared for progesterone receptor/response element binding by electrophoretic mobility shift, supershift, and immunoaffinity assays.

Findings.—Progesterone receptor/response element binding was decreased ninefold in maternal decidua tissue obtained after the onset of labor, compared with before the onset of labor (Fig 4). Binding was significantly higher in both preterm and term tissues from mothers who were not in labor, compared with in-labor tissues.

Conclusion.—The significant decrease in progesterone receptor/DNA progesterone responsive element binding in laboring tissues suggests a major role for progesterone in the induction of labor in humans. Further work is required to understand the mechanism of decreased binding at labor onset.

▶ Among nonhuman mammals, reduction in progesterone blood concentrations is a precursor to the onset of labor. Though some have claimed to show

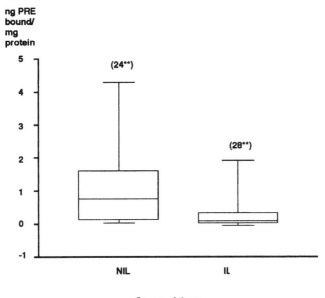

Source of tissue

FIGURE 4.—Comparison of labeled progesterone-responsive element (*PRE*) binding to receptor from tissue taken before (*NIL*) and after (*IL*) the onset of labor. The *horizontal lines in the boxes* are medians; the *vertical sides of the boxes* represent the 25th and 75th percentiles. The *error bars* show the entire range of data. The number of replicates is shown in *brackets*. *Double asterisk* indicates significance of *P* < .01 by the Mann-Whitney U test. (Courtesy of Henderson D, Wilson T: Reduced binding of progesterone receptor to its nuclear response element after human labor onset. *Am J Obstet Gynecol* 185:579-585, 2001.)

reductions in serum progesterone concentration over the weeks preceding the onset of human labor, the finding is controversial and certainly far different from the sharp decrease that takes place over a few days in sheep, for instance. It has been difficult to prove any consistent decrease in cytoplasmic progesterone receptor in human reproductive tissues, yet inhibition of progesterone synthesis with RV486 is a potent stimulant to labor. Release from the inhibitory effect of progesterone on oxytocin receptor expression and gap junction protein formation seem likely precursors to labor despite miniscule, if any, decrease in progesterone concentration in maternal blood. Certainly, exogenous progesterone fails to inhibit labor in the human. This study, spawned by the increased knowledge of intracellular regulation of gene expression by hormones, offers a possible explanation.

Progesterone in blood readily crosses cell membranes and complexes with cytoplasmic receptors. But the ligand-receptor complex then undergoes structural modification, often dimerization, and reacts with specific DNA sequences in the genome called hormone response elements. Those elements then direct gene expression in a highly specific way, to reduce oxytocin receptor activity for example. Here the DNA response element activity is measured in maternal decidua obtained at cesarean section before or after the onset of premature or term labor. Measurements were made on gel electrophoresis of biotin-labeled, double-stranded oligonucleotides derived from progesterone response elements of a murine tumor virus and its specificity demonstrated in comparison to rabbit polyclonal progesterone receptor antibody.

The results, shown in Figure 4, show a clear reduction in the progesterone response element after the onset of labor. This could well be the manner in which the human phylogeny of progesterone inhibition in labor is carried out, rather than through reduction of serum progesterone concentration seen in other mammals.

T. H. Kirschbaum, MD

Chemokine Ligand and Receptor Expression in the Pregnant Uterus: Reciprocal Patterns in Complementary Cell Subsets Suggest Functional Roles

Red-Horse K, Drake PM, Gunn MD, et al (Univ of California, San Francisco; Duke Univ, Durham, NC)
Am J Pathol 159:2199-2213, 2001   1–13

Background.—The maternal immune system in a successful pregnancy defies all known laws of transplantation by tolerating the presence of a conceptus expressing paternal antigens. There is a great deal of research being performed as to the mechanisms behind this immunologic paradox. Currently, there is evidence to indicate that multiple levels of regulation are involved in supporting maintenance of the fetal hemiallograft. Maternal leukocytes coexist with fetal cytotrophoblasts that occupy the decidua and uterine blood vessels. The immune cells are known as decidual granulated leukocytes and are composed predominately of the CD56[bright] subset of natural killer cells. These decidual leukocytes are accompanied by T cells and macrophages. The mechanisms underlying the recruitment of these cells to the uterus were studied.

Methods.—Placental and decidual tissue from elective termination of pregnancy or from normal-term delivery was collected within 1 hour, washed in phosphate-buffered saline with antibiotics, and placed on ice. The tissue to be used for in situ hybridization was immediately placed in 10% buffered formalin. The tissue was then subjected to overnight fixation and prepared for sectioning. Investigators evaluated the expression patterns of 14 chemokines in the decidualized uterine wall by in situ hybridization. RNase protection was used to investigate the expression of chemokine receptors on decidual leukocytes.

Results.—There was an impressive concordance between the expression of chemokines in the uterus and their receptors on decidual leukocytes. This concordance facilitated the identification of numerous receptor-ligand pairs that may recruit leukocytes to the uterus during pregnancy. The potential for other nonimmune functions for these molecules was indicated by the chemokine expression patterns.

Conclusions.—These findings indicated that there may be an important role for chemokine networks in the maternal-fetal interface.

▶ This group has been interested in exploring the details of the relations between trophoblastic epithelium and decidua at the site of early implantation of the human conceptus, in part because abnormalities in that relation appear to be an integral part of the origin of preeclampsia. They have described the progressive expression of adhesion molecules and their receptor sites for laminin, fibronectin, and collagens as trophoblastic columns penetrating the decidua in early implantation.[1] At greater depth, integrins of αV and VE-cadherin families are expressed that enable trophoblastic cells to establish intimate relations with and inside maternal vascular tissues.[2,3] They are now exploring the broader role of the decidua leukocytes that infiltrate the decidua and, at 6 to 10 weeks' gestation, comprise roughly 75% to 80% of its cellular content.[4] To some extent these immune cells appear to be associated with the immune protection of the fetal allograft and to introduce cell-cell adhesion molecules that serve to form and progressively adjust the implantation site tissues for growth and altered function of the conceptus. One mechanism involves expression of semisoluble molecules (chemokines) that attract and incorporate migrating cells through pathway guidance. In the development of the immune system, the initially enormous range of each cell's repertoire is limited by exposure to antigen that fixes its specificity and begins development of a clone of cells, designated by CD number, which is uniquely capable of responding to the sensitizing antigen, now an epitope. The general function of each clone is reasonable well known. Any of these decidual immune cells express CD69 and CD71 as well as Fas, an activation marker for apoptosis, but the cytolytic properties of such clones are relatively low and they appear to impede immune rejection. But other properties are revealed by in vitro immune hybridization using known plasmid clones to synthesize probes to 14 chemokines and archival cDNAs to enable Northern blot hybridization used to identify chemokine receptor mRNA. The latter step proves gene expression of the receptor gene; its CD number identifies some of the properties of the corresponding chemokines.

The authors found abundant, diffuse distribution of chemokine mRNA in decidua, cytotrophoblast, floating and anchoring trophoblastic villi, wandering trophoblast cells in the placental bed, and uterine blood vessels. The majority of chemokine receptor expression is similar to those for activated T and natural killer cells of native or innate immunity. The presence of decidual leukocytes with properties other than immune suppression specifically recruited in large numbers continually through pregnancy indicates that nonimmune functions involving altered properties of decidua stroma with trophoblastic cells are being carried out in a specific, highly controlled manner. Looking for changes in chemokine receptor expression patterns in pregnancy complicated by preterm labor, chorioamnionitis, and deciduitis then becomes an important future research aim. This work marks the opening of a new door to understanding the normal and pathologic cellular biology of the maternal-fetal interface and has enormous potential.

T. H. Kirschbaum, MD

References

1. 1994 YEAR BOOK OF OBSTETRICS, GYNECOLOGY, AND WOMEN'S HEALTH, pp 59-60.
2. 1998 YEAR BOOK OF OBSTETRICS, GYNECOLOGY, AND WOMEN'S HEALTH, pp 18-21.
3. 1998 YEAR BOOK OF OBSTETRICS, GYNECOLOGY, AND WOMEN'S HEALTH, pp 50-51.
4. 1994 YEAR BOOK OF OBSTETRICS, GYNECOLOGY, AND WOMEN'S HEALTH, pp 3-4.

2 Maternal Complications of Pregnancy

Failure of Metronidazole to Prevent Preterm Delivery Among Pregnant Women With Asymptomatic *Trichomonas Vaginalis* Infection
Klebanoff MA, and the National Institute of Child Health and Human Development Network of Maternal-Fetal Medicine Units (Natl Inst of Child Health and Human Development, Bethesda, Md; et al)
N Engl J Med 345:487-493, 2001   2–1

Background.—Preterm delivery has been associated with infection with *Trichomonas vaginalis* during pregnancy. Whether treating asymptomatic trichomoniasis in pregnant women decreases the occurrence of preterm delivery was investigated.

Methods.—Six hundred seventeen women with asymptomatic trichomoniasis who were 16 to 23 weeks pregnant were assigned to two 2-g doses of

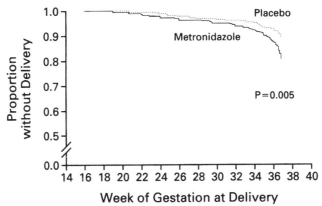

FIGURE 2.—Length of gestation at delivery according to treatment group. (Reprinted by permission of *The New England Journal of Medicine* courtesy of Klebanoff MA, and the National Institute of Child Health and Human Development Network of Maternal-Fetal Medicine Units: Failure of metronidazole to prevent preterm delivery among pregnant women with asymptomatic *Trichomonas vaginalis* infection. *N Engl J Med* 345:487-493, 2001. Copyright 2001, Massachusetts Medical Society. All rights reserved.)

metronidazole or placebo 48 hours apart. At 24 to 29 weeks' gestation, the women were treated again with the same 2-dose regimen.

Findings.—Trichomoniasis resolved in 92.6% of the women in the treatment group and in 35.4% in the placebo group. Delivery before 37 weeks occurred in 19% of the metronidazole-treated women and in 10.7% of the placebo-treated women (Fig 2). This difference was explained mainly by an increase in preterm delivery resulting from spontaneous preterm labor, which occurred in 10.2% and 3.5% of the women, respectively.

Conclusion.—Treating asymptomatic trichomoniasis in pregnant women does not prevent preterm birth. Thus, routine screening and treatment for this condition in asymptomatic pregnant women is not justified.

▶ The relationship between infection and preterm birth is clearly apparent in some pregnancies complicated by acute chorioamnionitis, maternal bacteremia, and septicemia, but such cases compose a minor subset of the overall problem of preterm births: obstetrics' unsolved problem. Prematurity rates vary widely among groups with different ages, past reproductive histories, racial backgrounds, socioeconomic status, and habits, but overall rates vary from 4% to 28% and have not proven amenable to prophylactic antibiotic therapy which might prevent the infectious stimulus. This is a companion study to an Australian study which found no value in metronidazole treatment of gravidas with bacterial vaginosis,[1] and another which showed no value in preventing preterm birth.[2]

A series of 617 gravidas with cultural evidence of *Trichomonas vaginalis* without symptoms were randomly assigned to receive metronidazole, 2 g twice at 48 hours intervals. Their sexual partners received a single 2-g dose and used condoms for the duration of the treatment regimen. Follow-up examination at 24 to 30 weeks of pregnancy showed 71.8% to be free of the organism on culture, the same percentage incidence as present in controls. The incidence of preterm delivery was not decreased but increased statistically significantly in women receiving the drug, compared with controls. The reason for the increased preterm birth rate with therapy is conjectural, but may represent a therapeutic paradox as lysed tricomonads release viruses or other degradation products of the organism, which then impact on continuing pregnancy. The recommendation from this authoritative source is that routine testing for *T vaginalis* in asymptomatic pregnant women is not warranted.

T. H. Kirschbaum, MD

References

1. 1999 YEAR BOOK OF OBSTETRICS, GYNECOLOGY, AND WOMEN'S HEALTH, pp 38-40.
2. 1995 YEAR BOOK OF OBSTETRICS, GYNECOLOGY, AND WOMEN'S HEALTH, pp 62-64.

Revisiting the Short Cervix Detected by Transvaginal Ultrasound in the Second Trimester: Why Cerclage Therapy May Not Help

Rust OA, Atlas RO, Reed J, et al (Lehigh Valley Hosp and Health Network, Allentown, Pa)
Am J Obstet Gynecol 185:1098-1105, 2001   2–2

Background.—Sonographic criteria for diagnosing cervical incompetence include dilatation of the internal os, prolapse of the membranes into the endocervical canal, shortening of the distal cervical segment, and exacerbation of findings associated with transfundal pressure. The risk factors correlated with increased neonatal morbidity in patients treated for sonographic evidence of internal os dilatation and distal cervical shortening in the second trimester were investigated.

Methods.—One hundred thirteen patients between 16 and 24 weeks' gestation were assigned randomly to McDonald cerclage or no cerclage. All had internal os dilatation and either membrane prolapse into the endocervical canal of at least 25% of the total cervical length but not beyond the external os, or a shortened distal cervix of less than 2.5 cm. Before randomization, all patients underwent amniocentesis, multiple urogenital cultures, and indomethacin and clindamycin therapy for 48 to 72 hours.

Findings.—Fifty-five patients received cerclage, and 58, no cerclage. Four rescue cerclage procedures were needed in each group. In a regression analysis, factors consistently associated with early gestational age at delivery and increased morbidity were readmission for preterm labor, chorioamnionitis, and abruption. Cerclage had no effect on perinatal outcomes (Table 2).

Conclusions.—The findings of second trimester internal os dilatation, membrane prolapse, and distal cervical shortening on sonography probably represent a common pathway of several pathophysiologic processes. Cer-

TABLE 2.—Group Comparison*

	Cerclage Group (n = 55 Women; 63 Infants)	No Cerclage Group (n = 58 Women; 67 Infants)	P Value
Previous preterm birth (%)	54.4	36.2	.1
Previous second trimester loss (%)	12.1	27.3	.07
Multiple gestation (%)	12.3	12.1	.8
Dilation of internal os (cm)†	1.6 ± 0.7	1.8 ± 0.9	.2
Depth of prolapse (cm)†	1.7 ± 1.1	1.7 ± 1.0	.9
Distal cervical length (cm)†	2.1 ± 1.0	2.0 ± 0.9	.6
Total cervical length (cm)†	3.7 ± 1.1	3.6 ± 1.0	.4
Gestational age at diagnosis (wk)	21.1 ± 2.1	22.7 ± 2.1	.2
Gestational age at delivery (wk)	33.8 ± 6.0	33.8 ± 5.5	.9
Delivery less than 34 wks (%)	34.9	36.2	.8
Readmission for preterm labor (%)	51.9	53.4	.2
Placental abruption (%)	10.9	13.8	.8
Chorioamnionitis (%)	20.0	10.3	.2
Perinatal death (%)	12.7	11.9	.9

*Interval data expressed as mean ± SD; categoric data expressed as a percentage.
†Correspond with measurements depicted in Fig 1 in original journal article.
(Courtesy of Rust OA, Atlas RO, Reed J, et al: Revisiting the short cervix detected by transvaginal ultrasound in the second trimester: Why cerclage therapy may not help. *Am J Obstet Gynecol* 185:1098-1105, 2001.)

clage did not affect any perinatal outcome variables. Increased neonatal morbidity appeared to be related to subclinical infection, preterm labor, and abruption.

▶ This is the larger of 2 recent prospective randomized studies designed to evaluate the role of cerclage, using contemporary criteria for treatment. It is an extension of earlier work with fewer patients done as a feasibility study (Abstract 7–3). Women from 16 to 24 weeks' gestation with sonographic evidence of cervical change were admitted to the study. Criteria for admission included dilation of the internal cervical os, prolapse of membranes into at least the proximal one fourth of the cervical canal but not through the external os, and cervical length less than 2.5 cm. Further, fundal pressure was required to exacerbate all 3 findings viewed on ultrasound. Candidates were admitted for 48 to 72 hours of evaluation, given clindamycin and indomethacin, and treated for any positive urogenital cultures; they then underwent amniocentesis to rule out latent chorioamnionitis. Randomization was then done, and 55 women received cerclage after McDonald, and 58 were managed without cerclage. Antibiotics and indomethacin were then withdrawn within 24 hours of randomization, bedrest was liberalized, and patients eventually were discharged to modified bedrest at home. Eight women at less than 24 weeks' gestation in the control group who showed membrane prolapse in the vagina were treated with cerclage, and the results were reported by intent to treat. There was no significant difference in gestational age at delivery or neonatal morbidity between the 2 groups. Multivariate analysis found an identical pattern of associated independent variables in the 2 groups, and when all 113 cases were combined and cerclage was assessed as an independent variable, it proved to have no significant impact on major outcome variables.

A similar study is reported in the same journal issue with the opposite conclusion.[1] It suffers primarily in presenting data from only 35 cases evaluated only by univariable methods, and is therefore less authoritative than the report by Rust et al.

T. H. Kirschbaum, MD

Reference

1. Althuisius FM, Dekker GA, Hummel P, et al: Final results of the cervical incompetence prevention randomized cervical trial. *Am J Obstet Gynecol* 185:1106, 2001.

Mid-Trimester Endovaginal Sonography in Women at High Risk for Spontaneous Preterm Birth

Owen J, for the National Institute of Child Health and Human Development, Maternal-Fetal Medicine Units Network (Univ of Alabama, Birmingham; et al)
JAMA 286:1340-1348, 2001   2–3

Background.—Shortened cervical length is consistently associated with spontaneous preterm birth. However, at what point during gestation this risk factor becomes apparent is unknown. Whether sonographic cervical findings between 16 weeks' and 18 weeks 6 days' gestation can predict spontaneous preterm birth was determined. Also determined was whether serial evaluations up to 23 weeks 6 days' gestation improve prediction in women at high risk.

Methods.—Between 1997 and 1999, 9 university-affiliated US medical centers enrolled a total of 183 women with singleton gestations in the study. All women had previously given birth spontaneously before 32 weeks' gestation. A total of 590 endovaginal sonographic examinations were performed at 2-week intervals. Cervical length was measured, and funneling and dynamic cervical shortening were recorded.

Findings.—Twenty-six percent of the women gave birth spontaneously before 35 weeks' gestation. A cervical length of less than 25 mm at initial sonography correlated with a relative risk of 3.3 for spontaneous preterm birth. After adjusting for cervical length, neither funneling nor dynamic shortening significantly, independently, predicted spontaneous preterm birth. However, the relative risk of a cervical length of less than 25 mm increased to 4.5 when the shortest ever observed cervical length on serial evaluations, after any dynamic shortening, was used. A receiver operating characteristic curve analysis indicated that, compared with a single cervical measure at 16 weeks' to 18 weeks 6 days' gestation, serial measures at up to 23 weeks 6 days significantly improved the prediction of spontaneous preterm birth.

Conclusion.—Augmented by serial assessments, cervical length determined on endovaginal sonography between 16 weeks' and 18 weeks 6 days' gestation can be used to predict spontaneous preterm birth before 35 weeks' gestation in high-risk women. Further research is needed.

▶ Clearly, there is an inverse relationship between the US length of the cervical canal prior to the last trimester and the risk of preterm birth,[1-3] but whether the relationship is strong enough to warrant surgical intervention is unsettled. This product of 9 maternal fetal medicine units, part of the National Institute of Child Health and Human Development Maternal-Fetal Medicine Network, provides a careful, scholarly attempt to revisit this problem following an earlier effort.[4]

The authors largely eliminate earlier problems stemming from cervical canal measurements after 20 weeks' gestational age in low risk populations without comparisons with controls. Study entry in this case occurred between 16 and 18 6/7 weeks during the interval from March 1997 to November 1999 and was limited to women with singlet pregnancies and a prior spontaneous birth at less than 32 weeks' gestational age. Comparisons were made with women spontaneously delivering infants weighing less than 1.5 kg without evidence of chronic medical or obstetrical complications or prior cerclage, not followed by cervical US.

Sonograms were done by well-trained sonographers of objectively proven adequacy. Cervical length measurements in triplicate were made through the anterior vaginal fornix and supplemented by observations with fundal pressure and longitudinal repeat observations done until 23 6/7 weeks. The primary outcome was the incidence of preterm birth at less than 35 weeks' gestational age and sample size was guided by power analysis. One hundred eighty three such women completed the study, 26% of them delivering prior to 35 weeks' gestational age.

Some women (16%) had a lower uterine segment so poorly developed in the early second trimester that the canal could not be measured accurately . This proved often to be a transient phenomenon and was not associated with an increased risk of preterm birth. The inverse relationship between cervical length and the risk of preterm birth was again confirmed, and neither the result of uterine pressure or longitudinal studies added to the predictability of that finding. Receiver operating curves showed improved predictability using the shortest cervical length noted throughout the course of the examinations but failed to show clear evidence of a single "abnormal" cervical length, demonstrating instead a continuous monotonic inverse relationship between cervical length and preterm delivery. As demonstrated earlier, funneling is not a significant additional risk indicator.

The authors correctly ascribe their findings to preterm labor being a function of multiple variables largely independent of cervical length. Their recommendation is that cervical length measurements be used only for investigative purposes and lack the accuracy needed to be employed for decisions in patient care.

T. H. Kirschbaum, MD

References

1. 1998 YEAR BOOK OF OBSTETRICS, GYNECOLOGY, AND WOMEN'S HEALTH, pp 54-86.
2. 2000 YEAR BOOK OF OBSTETRICS, GYNECOLOGY, AND WOMEN'S HEALTH, pp 39-43.
3. 2001 YEAR BOOK OF OBSTETRICS, GYNECOLOGY, AND WOMEN'S HEALTH, pp 157-158.
4. 1997 YEAR BOOK OF OBSTETRICS, GYNECOLOGY, AND WOMEN'S HEALTH, pp 27-28.

Recurrence of Preterm Birth in Singleton and Twin Pregnancies
Bloom SL, Yost NP, McIntire DD, et al (Univ of Texas, Dallas)
Obstet Gynecol 98:379-385, 2001   2–4

Background.—The history of preterm birth is a significant risk factor for recurrence in future pregnancy, with an odds ratio (OR) of 5.8, which is high compared to other markers (OR 5.2 for detection of fetal fibronectin in cervical secretions, OR 4.1 for ultrasonic shortening of the cervix, and OR 1.3 for colonization of the genital tract with bacterial vaginosis). Data are presented on more than 15,000 women from their first delivery through all subsequent consecutive pregnancies. Recurrent preterm birth risk was determined from whether the initial preterm pregnancy was a singleton or twin birth, whether labor was spontaneous or induced, when the recurrence occurred, and the overall contribution of these women to preterm birth data in the study cohort.

Methods.—A total of 15,945 women were studied. Their first pregnancy was classified according to delivery time (between 24 and 34 weeks' gesta-

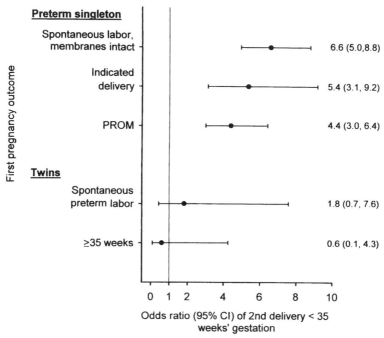

FIGURE 2.—Odds ratios and 95% CIs for recurrent delivery less than 35 weeks according to first pregnancy outcome and using women whose first delivery was at least 35 weeks as the referent group. (Reprinted with permission from The American College of Obstetricians and Gynecologists, courtesy of Bloom SL, Yost NP, McIntire DD, et al: Recurrence of preterm birth in singleton and twin pregnancies. *Obstet Gynecol* 98:379-385, 2001.)

tion or 35 weeks or beyond) and type of labor (spontaneous or induced). Analysis was done to determine their risk of preterm delivery in subsequent pregnancies.

Results.—Six categories were formulated based on the result of the first pregnancy. A statistically significantly increased risk for recurrence (OR 5.6) was found for women whose previous singleton births were at less than 35 weeks' gestation (Fig 2). No increased risk was found for women with twin preterm deliveries (OR 1.9). Those women who had a history of a spontaneous preterm birth, a preterm delivery, or preterm ruptured membranes had similar ORs for recurrence of a singleton birth before 35 weeks' gestation. Women whose first birth was a singleton and occurred at less than 35 weeks' gestation had a significantly increased risk for recurrence independent of the timing of their first preterm delivery (Fig 3). No significant effect on subsequent birth timing accompanied a previous twin delivery. Recurrent preterm birth occurred within 1 week of the gestational age of the first delivery in 49% of women, with 70% delivering within 2 weeks of their previous delivery. A 7.9 OR for recurrent spontaneous preterm birth was found for women with intact membranes; this was 5.5 for women with ruptured membranes. Overall, history of preterm birth in a subsequent pregnancy for women who

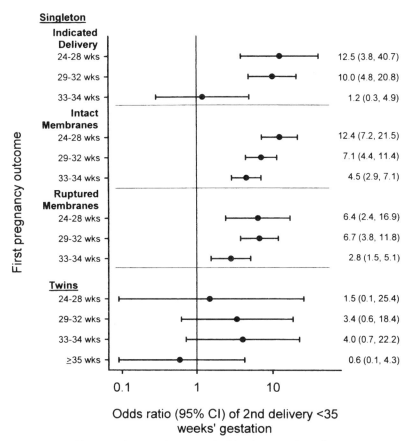

FIGURE 3.—Odds ratios and 95% CIs for recurrent birth less than 35 weeks in relation to categorization and gestational age of the first delivery. The referent group is women whose first delivery occurred beyond 35 weeks. (Reprinted with permission from The American College of Obstetricians and Gynecologists, courtesy of Bloom SL, Yost NP, McIntire DD, et al: Recurrence of preterm birth in singleton and twin pregnancies. *Obstet Gynecol* 98:379-385, 2001.)

had preterm singleton births previously was predictive in only 10% of the preterm births occurring in the study population.

Conclusions.—Assessment of future risk for preterm delivery must include the consideration of type of pregnancy (singleton or twin, with a higher risk accompanying prior singleton births). Risk also increases with number of previous preterm births. Gestational age of the previous delivery is a good predictor of gestational age at delivery in subsequent pregnancies. Only 10% of the premature births could be predicted based on previous historical risk factors.

▶ One of the several problems that complicate the study of preterm birth is that it occurs uncommonly enough that it is wasteful to apply possible prophylaxis to all pregnant women. It is also difficult to identify a population subset at sufficiently high risk to allow controlled studies of moderate size to be conducted without dilution of results by women predestined to deliver in fact at term.[1,2] This review of data collected over 10 years at the University of Texas Southwestern Medical Center containing the results of the first 2 or more pregnancies in 15,935 women helps explain the errors introduced by accepting the history of a preterm delivery as a good predictive risk characteristic for repeat preterm delivery. The overall chance of preterm delivery for a singlet pregnancy was 4% and for a twin pregnancy 33%. Preterm delivery was defined as delivery after 24 weeks gestational age but prior to the completion of the 34th week (less than 35 and 0/7th weeks) because of the infrequency of newborn morbidity when birth occurs after the onset of the 35th week of gestation.

Given an initial singlet preterm delivery, the mother is at increased risk of a second preterm delivery regardless of whether the first occurred spontaneously, was associated with premature rupture of membranes, or was a medically indicated birth. Further, the increased risk was independent of a gestational age at which the first preterm delivery occurred, or whether or not premature preterm rupture of membranes preceded it. Although such events are positive risk factors they are unlikely and a history of preterm delivery has a predictive value of a positive finding of 10%, and hence a false-positive rate of 90%. Preterm delivery of a twin pregnancy carries no increased risk of a second preterm delivery thereafter. Given a woman with 1, 2, or 3 prior preterm deliveries, the chances of a repeat preterm delivery thereafter were 16%, 41%, and 67%, respectively, although the last figure is based on only 3 cases. Clearly we overestimated the predictive value of the history of preterm delivery in choosing groups of women at high risk of a repeat event.

T. H. Kirschbaum, MD

References

1. 2002 YEAR BOOK OF OBSTETRICS, GYNECOLOGY, AND WOMEN'S HEALTH, pp 167-170.
2. 2001 YEAR BOOK OF OBSTETRICS, GYNECOLOGY, AND WOMEN'S HEALTH, pp 43-47.

The Preterm Prediction Study: Toward a Multiple-Marker Test for Spontaneous Preterm Birth
Goldenberg RL, for the Maternal-Fetal Medicine Units Network (Maternal-Fetal Medicine Units Network)
Am J Obstet Gynecol 185:643-651, 2001   2–5

Objective.—The Preterm Prediction Study evaluated 28 potential biologic markers for spontaneous preterm birth in asymptomatic women at 23 to 24 weeks gestational age. This analysis compares those markers individually and in combination for an association with spontaneous preterm birth at <32 and <35 weeks gestational age.

Study Design.—With the use of a nested case-control design from an original cohort study of 2929 women, results of tests from 50 women with a spontaneous preterm birth at <32 weeks and 127 women with a spontaneous preterm birth at <35 weeks were compared with results from matched-term control subjects.

Results.—In the univariate analysis, the most potent markers that are associated with spontaneous preterm birth at <32 weeks by odds ratio were a positive cervical-vaginal fetal fibronectin test (odds ratio, 32.7) and <10th percentile cervical length (odds ratio, 5.8), and in serum, >90th percentiles of α-fetoprotein (odds ratio, 8.3) and alkaline phosphatase (odds ratio, 6.8), and >75th percentile of granulocyte colony-stimulating factor (odds ratio, 5.5). Results for spontaneous preterm birth at <35 weeks were generally similar but not as strong. Univariate and multivariate logistic regression analyses demonstrated little interaction among the tests in their association with spontaneous preterm birth (Table 3). Combinations of the 5 markers were evaluated for their association with <32 weeks spontaneous preterm birth (Table 5). Ninety-three percent of case patients had at least 1 positive test result versus 34% of control subjects (odds ratio, 24.0; 95% CI, 6.4-93.4). Among the case patients, 59% had ≥2 positive test results versus 2.4% of control subjects (odds ratio, 56.5; 95% CI, 7.1-451.7) (Table 6). If a cutoff of 3 positive test results was used, 20% of case patients and none of the control subjects had positive test results (P < .002). With the use of only the 3 serum tests (alkaline phosphatase, α-fetoprotein, and granulocyte colony-stimulating factor), any positive test identified 81% of cases versus 22% of control subjects (odds ratio, 14.7; 95% CI, 5.0-42.7). For spontaneous preterm birth at <35 weeks gestation, any 2 positive tests identified 43% of cases and 6% of control subjects (odds ratio, 11.2; 95% CI, 4.8-26.2).

Conclusion.—Overlap among the strongest biologic markers for spontaneous preterm birth is small. This suggests that the use of tests such as maternal serum α-fetoprotein, alkaline phosphatase, and granulocyte colony-stimulating factor as a group or adding their results to fetal fibronectin test and cervical length test results may enhance our ability to predict spontaneous preterm birth and that the development of a multiple-marker test for spontaneous preterm birth is feasible.

TABLE 3.—The Adjusted Odds Ratio for a Spontaneous Preterm Birth at <32 or <35 Weeks That Was Associated With a Specific Risk Factor, Based on Regression Analysis

| | Preterm Birth | | | |
| | < 32 wks | | < 35 wks | |
Factor	Odds Ratio (%)	95% CI	Odds Ratio (%)	95% CI
α-fetoprotein (>90th %ile)	33.7	5.0-229.7	3.9	1.7-8.7
Alkaline phosphatase (>90th %ile)	—	—	4.0	1.1-14.9
Granulocyte colony-stimulating factor (>75th %ile)	12.7	2.8-56.5	3.1	1.4-6.9
Defensins (>90th %ile)	13.1	1.6-104.5	—	—
Fetal fibronectin (≥50 ng/mL)	12.2	1.1-135.2	6.6	1.7-25.5
Cervical length (≤25 mm)	3.7	0.7-19.4	3.9	1.7-9.2
History of previous spontaneous preterm birth	2.1	0.5-9.4	4.0	1.9-8.4
Vaginal bleeding	—	—	2.2	1.1-4.4

(Courtesy of Goldenberg RL, for the Maternal-Fetal Medicine Units Network: The Preterm Prediction Study: Toward a multiple-marker test for spontaneous preterm birth. *Am J Obstet Gynecol* 185:643-651, 2001.)

TABLE 5.—The Correlations Among the Strongest Predictors of Spontaneous Preterm Birth

	Alkaline Phosphatase	α-Fetoprotein	Granulocyte Colony-Stimulating Factor	Defensins	Fetal Fibronectin	Cervical Length
Serum alkaline phosphatase	—	0.10	0.14*	0.09	0.10	−0.01
Serum α-fetoprotein	0.10	—	−0.03	0.05	−0.04	−0.03
Serum granulocyte colony-stimulating factor	0.14*	−0.03	—	0.10	0.15*	−0.09
Serum defensin	0.09	0.05	0.10	—	0.05	0.17*
Fetal fibronectin	0.10	−0.04	0.15*	0.05	—	−0.23*
Cervical length	−0.01	−0.03	−0.09	0.17*	−0.23*	—

*P < .05.
(Courtesy of Goldenberg RL, for the Maternal-Fetal Medicine Units Network: The Preterm Prediction Study: Toward a multiple-marker test for spontaneous preterm birth. *Am J Obstet Gynecol* 185:643-651, 2001.)

TABLE 6.—Test Values for the Prediction of Spontaneous Preterm Birth at <32 Weeks, Comparing Single Versus Multiple Markers

Test	Sensitivity	Specificity	Odds Ratio (%)	95% CI
Fetal fibronectin (≥50 ng/mL)	40.0	98.0	32.7	4.2-256.1
Cervix (≤25 mm)	44.9	87.8	5.8	2.1-16.2
α-fetoprotein (>90th %ile)	36.2	93.6	8.3	2.2-30.9
Granulocyte colony-stimulating factor (>75th %ile)	48.9	85.1	5.5	2.0-14.7
Defensins (> 90th %ile)	20.9	95.4	5.4	1.1-26.8
1/5 Tests positive	92.7	65.9	24.4	6.4-93.4
2/5 Tests positive	58.5	97.6	56.5	7.1-451.7
3/5 Tests positive	19.5	100	∞*	—
1/3 (serum) Tests positive	80.5	78.1	14.7	5.0-42.7
2/3 (serum) Tests positive	26.8	100	∞*	—

*Odds ratio cannot be calculated with specificity of 100%.
(Courtesy of Goldenberg RL, for the Maternal-Fetal Medicine Units Network: The Preterm Prediction Study: Toward a multiple-marker test for spontaneous preterm birth. *Am J Obstet Gynecol* 185:643-651, 2001.)

▶ Causal factors in the production of human preterm labor appear to be multiple, discrete, and diverse but to operate with relatively low prevalence. Therapy aimed at prevention of preterm labor has not been proven effective because it often affects only a relatively few potential victims, most of whom do not enter preterm labor or did not respond to the particular therapy chosen for trial. The Preterm Prediction Study is aimed at defining criteria useful in selecting a subset of gravidas often enough likely to respond to therapy. Several such attempts have been reviewed here previously (see 1997 YEAR BOOK OF OBSTETRICS, GYNECOLOGY, AND WOMEN'S HEALTH, pp 27-28; 1999 YEAR BOOK, pp 35-37; 2001 YEAR BOOK, pp 23-31, 43-47; and 2002 YEAR BOOK, pp 167-171). In general, they show low sensitivity in the range of 20% to 50%, large false-positive rates, and high specificity based predominantly on the low prevalence of preterm labor.

This article reviews many of the earlier studies and data and explores the prospects for use of multiple indicators (see 2002 YEAR BOOK, pp 43-45 and 167-171). The general approach is a familiar one. Twenty-eight risk factors and test results were analyzed on the basis of risk ratios of positive findings compared with the results in women with preterm labor at 32 and 35 weeks' gestational age versus normal controls. Multivariant regression was used to reduce the impact of confounding variables, and 8 variables were identified as important ones (Table 3). Simple correlation demonstrated the 6 strongest predictors to be discrete without tendency to vary together in any of several paired relationships (Table 5). Using 107 of 2929 original cohort who experienced spontaneous preterm labor at less than 32 or less than 35 weeks and using data for all the tests in Table 5, the investigators calculated sensitivity and specificity values, and these are shown for delivery at less than 32 weeks in Table 6. Note that if 1 of the 5 is positive, 92.7% of the women who deliver preterm are identified; however, as more positive tests are added as predictive criteria, the incidence of women with preterm labor decreases as sensitivity decreases, reflecting the lack of intercorrelations among variables. What is crucial here is the failure to calculate, or to provide the data needed to calculate, the predictive value of positive findings. That statistic indicates the chances of preterm labor, given a positive test result and reflects the false-positive rate embedded in it. Given a prospective value of a positive finding of 10%, to identify 109 women with preterm labor among 2929 gravidas, for example, one would have to deal with 1090 apparent positives, most of which were false-positives, a hopeless prospect for clinical application. Without knowledge of false-positive rates, preditability cannot be evaluated. These statistics were done by competent people; I am sure they know that.

T. H. Kirschbaum, MD

Third-Trimester Unexplained Intrauterine Fetal Death Is Associated With Inherited Thrombophilia
Many A, Elad R, Yaron Y, et al (Tel Aviv Univ, Israel)
Obstet Gynecol 99:684-687, 2002   2–6

Background.—Placental changes associated with hypercoagulability are found in many women with unexplained intrauterine fetal death (IUFD). The risk of thrombophilia in such women was investigated.

Methods.—During a 26-month period, all women with IUFD at 27 weeks' gestation or more were evaluated. After exclusions, 40 women with unexplained IUFD were matched by age and ethnicity to 80 healthy women who had had at least 1 normal pregnancy. At least 2 months after delivery, all participants were tested for mutations of factor V Leiden; prothrombin gene; methylenetetrahydrofolate reductase; and deficiencies of protein-S, protein-C, and antithrombin III. The women were also tested for and determined to be negative for anticardiolipin antibodies.

Findings.—Women in the study group had a significantly lower gestational age at delivery and lower birth weight. The prevalence of inherited thrombophilia in the study and control groups were 42.5% and 15%, respectively. Prothrombin mutations and protein-S deficiency rates were significantly greater in the study group.

Conclusion.—Third-trimester IUFD correlated significantly with thrombophilia. Thus, thrombophilia workups should be included in IUFD investigations. These findings may have therapeutic and prognostic implications for future pregnancies.

▶ The unexpected appearance of inexplicable IUFD in utero in the last trimester of an otherwise normal pregnancy is a tragedy familiar to all obstetricians and occurs in roughly 0.2% to 0.5% of pregnancies. In the absence of hypertensive disease, diabetes mellitus, infectious disease, congenital anomalies, cord accidents, or findings on fetal placental necropsy, both doctor and patient share distress over the unexplained loss. A few studies point to the possible surplus of evidence of genetically determined thrombophilia in such cases, that is, the presence of Factor V Leiden mutation, deficiencies in proteins C and S, anti-thrombin III, and mutational interference with methylene tetrahydrofolate reductase or prothrombin production.

Previous studies have been marked by small patient numbers and failure of exclusion of known maternal pathology. These authors are careful in managing case exclusions and, though only 40 cases and 80 controls are reported, the data seem to suffice to support their conclusions. The incidence of unexplained fetal death was 0.36%, and some forms of thrombophilia occurred in 42.5% of the aggregate of women with fetal death compared to 15% in controls. Only the prothrombin mutation, protein-S deficiency, and the aggregate of all thrombophilias showed individual statistical significance of prevalence. The authors reasonably suggest that a search for such mutational defects should be made instances of unexplained fetal death on the basis of the associative relationships they have found.

T. H. Kirschbaum, MD

Leptin Stimulates Fatty-Acid Oxidation by Activating AMP-Activated Protein Kinase
Minokoshi Y, Kim Y-B, Peroni OD, et al (Harvard Med School, Boston; Imperial College School of Medicine, London)
Nature 415:339-342, 2002   2–7

Background.—The impairment of fuel metabolism is an early pathogenic factor in obesity and type 2 diabetes mellitus. Increased lipid stores in non-adipose tissues such as muscle have been linked to functional impairments, called lipotoxicity, which lead to insulin resistance and impaired secretion of insulin. In vivo treatment with leptin has been shown to significantly improve insulin sensitivity, possibly a result in part of the depletion of triglyceride stores in skeletal muscle. Leptin stimulates the oxidation of fatty acids and the uptake of glucose and prevents the accumulation of lipid in nonadipose tissues. However, the signaling pathways that mediate the metabolic effects of leptin have not been elucidated. The 5'-AMP-activated protein kinase (AMPK) is a potent stimulator of fatty-acid oxidation in muscle through the inhibition of activity of acetyl coenzyme A carboxylase (ACC). AMPK is conserved from yeast to human beings and can serve as a indicator of the status of cellular energy. This study attempted to identify signaling pathways for leptin in a mouse model.

Methods.—Leptin injections were administered to male FVB and db/db mice that were unilaterally surgically denervated in 1 hind limb. A group of control mice were not given leptin injections. Enzyme activities, fatty-acid utilization in muscles in vivo, and in vitro studies of isolated soleus muscle were performed.

Results.—Leptin acts directly on muscle to stimulate early activation of AMPK, whereas later activation of AMPK depends on leptin functioning through the hypothalamic-sympathetic nervous system axis. While activating AMPK, leptin also suppresses the activity of ACC and thus stimulates the oxidation of fatty acid in muscle. The phosphorylation of ACC stimulated by leptin is inhibited by blocking the AMPK activation.

Conclusions.—This study identifies a previously unknown signaling pathway for leptin by showing that leptin selectively stimulates phosphory-lation and activation of the α2 catalytic subunit of AMPK in skeletal muscle. AMPK is identified as the principal mediator of the effects of leptin on the metabolism of fatty acid in muscle.

▶ Leptin, a product of adipocytes, stimulates glucose uptake and fatty-acid oxidation and helps regulate the relations among fat storage, food intake, and energy expenditure. Obesity, through stimulating leptin release, is often asso-ciated with insulin resistance, excessive fat storage in adipose tissue, liver, and muscle, and predisposes to the development of type 2 diabetes. The mechanisms by which obesity changes the signaling function of leptin in reg-ulating energy metabolism are the subject of this letter. This work was carried out in transgenic mice with a knockout of acetyl coenzyme A carboxylase (ACC) in surgically and pharmacologically denervated soleus muscles in the hind limb. The authors "lipotoxicity hypothesis" is that insulin resistance stems from excessive lipid deposition, not in adipocytes, but in insulin-sensitive cells of the liver and skeletal muscle. A likely intermediate in this ef-fect is the phosphorylation of protein kinase C by leptin, which in turn phos-phorylates ACC and diacyl-glycerol. Normally these intermediates, acting through malonyl coenzyme A, serve to direct cytoplasmic fatty acid into mito-chondria where they are metabolized to yield adenosine triphosphate. When melonyl coenzyme A is inhibited, fatty acid cell metabolism is reduced and fat-ty acids are instead diverted into skeletal muscle and liver. In those storage sites, that storage results in insulin resistance. The normal role of hyperlep-tinemia to prevent lipotoxicity in nonadipose cells is therefore lost. This work brings focus on the prevention of inactivation of AMPK as a therapeutic goal in the prevention and treatment of obesity-linked type 2 diabetes mellitus block-ing this new obesity-linked pathway, which impedes mitochondrial oxidation of fatty acids.

T. H. Kirschbaum, MD

Maternal and Neonatal Outcome of 100 Consecutive Triplet Pregnancies
Devine PC, Malone FD, Athanassiou A, et al (Columbia Univ, New York; Tufts Univ, Boston)
Am J Perinatol 18:225-235, 2001   2–8

Background.—In the past several decades, the incidence of multiple ges-tations has increased dramatically, mainly because of the use of ovulation-inducing drugs and assisted reproductive technologies. Maternal and neo-natal outcomes in 1 series of triplet gestations were reported.

Methods.—One hundred triplet gestations managed and delivered be-tween 1992 and 1999 by 1 perinatal group were included in the analysis. All were managed on an outpatient basis, with no prophylactic interventions.

Findings.—At least 1 complication occurred in 96% of the pregnancies. Preterm labor was the most common complication. The median gestational

TABLE 6.—Comparison of Previously Published Series of Triplet Gestations

Author	Study Period	No. of Patients	GA at Delivery*	PNM†
Itzkowic[8]	1946-1976	59	33.5	232
Daw[9]	1958-1977	14	34.7	310
Holcberg et al[10]	1960-1979	31	31.8	312
Loucopoulos et al[11]	1965-1981	27	35.8	83
Lipitz et al[12]	1975-1988	78	33.2	93
Gonen et al[13]	1978-1988	24	32.4	52
Newman et al[14]	1985-1988	198	33.2	66
Seoud et al[15]	1982-1990	15	31.8	0
Boulot et al[16]	1985-1990	33	34.1	42
Santema et al[17]	1981-1991	40	32.0	200
Peaceman et al[18]	1988-1991	15	34.7	0
Albrecht et al[19]	1989-1994	57	33.0	41
Kaufman et al[4]	1992-1996	55	32.1‡	121
Skrablin et al[20]	1986-1997	52	32.8	167
Current study	1992-1999	100	33.0‡	103

Note: All reference numbers refer to references in original journal article.
*Mean gestational age at delivery (week).
†Crude perinatal mortality rate.
‡Median gestational age at delivery.
(Reprinted with permission from *American Journal of Perinatology*, courtesy of Devine PC, Malone FD, Athanassiou A, et al: Maternal and neonatal outcome of 100 consecutive triplet pregnancies. *Am J Perinatol* 18:225-235, 2001. Thieme Medical Publishers, Inc.)

age at delivery was 33 weeks. Fourteen percent of pregnancies were delivered before 28 weeks' gestation. The corrected perinatal mortality rate was 97 in 1000. Babies delivered after 27 weeks' gestation had minimal long-term morbidity. Pregnancy outcomes did not vary by birth order or conception mode.

Conclusion.—Triplet pregnancy carries a high rate of antenatal complications. The use of prophylactic interventions will lead to more favorable neonatal outcomes in such gestations (Table 6).

▶ This large, uncontrolled cohort study of 100 triplet pregnancies is important, given the increasing incidence of multiple pregnancies and for what it says about their antenatal care. Management occurred in a single institution with a stable medical staff and a uniform approach to care. Serial sonographs were performed monthly and biophysical profiles and umbilical artery Doppler studies were used when growth retardation was detected. Tocolysis, cerclage, bedrest, and hospitalization were not employed as routines. Women with threatened preterm labor were admitted for magnesium sulfate tocolysis, adrenal steroids, and group B streptococcus antibiotic prophylaxis.

Abdominal delivery was carried out electively at 37 weeks. As expected, the major maternal complications were preterm labor (78%), preeclampsia (26%), anemia (24%), and premature preterm rupture of membranes (24%). Magnesium tocolysis was offered to 73% of women in preterm labor, and there were 2 cases of pulmonary edema following administration of corticosteroids and magnesium sulfate. Abdominal delivery was carried out in 89%; perhaps this was the reason that no impact of birth order was seen in neonatal outcomes.

Four women exhibited acute fatty liver of pregnancy at about 32 weeks' gestational age. A 4% incidence rate for this disorder is high, perhaps because of enhanced awareness in the 1990s, but without controls, only supposition is possible. Four cases of fetal demise occurred at from 24 to 32 weeks' gestational age, and 21 live-born fetuses at 20 to 24 weeks' gestational age expired after delivery. Corrected perinatal mortality was 97 per 1000 live births, a low rate attributable largely to improvements in neonatal care, in comparison with perinatal mortality rates cited in a series of 14 earlier case report summarized in Table 6.

All infants delivered past 26 weeks' gestational age survived. It is important that despite alert, intensive efforts to detect preterm labor and aggressive use of tocolytics, no improvement in the ability to prolong mean gestation in comparison with earlier studies was noted (see Table 6). The authors point out our failure to impact preterm delivery incidence in this group of women and observe that efforts at tocolysis offered more potential harm than benefit.

The results are as good as those offering prophylactic tocolysis, extended bedrest, home uterine activity monitoring, repeated corticosteroid therapy, and routine hospitalization. The authors' experience makes these seem to be efforts of dubious merit.

T. H. Kirschbaum, MD

Extreme Grandmultiparity: Is It An Obstetric Risk Factor?
Kumari AS, Badrinath P (Al-Mafraq Hosp, Abu Dhabi, United Arab Emirates; UAE Univ, Abu Dhabi, United Arab Emirates)
Eur J Obstet Gynecol Reprod Biol 101:22-25, 2002   2–9

Background.—Traditionally, grandmultiparity (GMP) has been considered an independent obstetric risk factor linked to an increased number of adverse perinatal outcomes. With the extensive and rapid advances in biotechnology, pharmacology, and obstetric practices, and improved socioeconomic conditions, better access to high-quality perinatal care has been achieved, yet GMP has maintained its reputation as a risk-increasing factor. By basing a study in Abu Dhabi—a Persian Gulf oil-rich emirate with a per capita income among the highest in the world, where modern medical care is comparable to that provided in Western nations and free to all residents—the high incidence of GMP permitted examination of its actual risks in the light of high-quality care.

Methods.—Mothers having had 10 or more previous viable pregnancies (1015 women) were considered extreme grandmultiparas (EGMPs); those having 5 to 9 (1662 women) were considered GMPs; and those having 2 to 4 (2044 women) were considered nongrandmultiparas. Antepartum, intrapartum, and postpartum complications were evaluated, especially as they related to previously reported adverse effects of GMP.

Results.—The maximum parity documented was 19 children. Gestational diabetes and macrosomia developed in EGMPs at a greater rate than in the other groups, whereas preterm delivery and induced labor occurred less frequently. None of the women suffered a ruptured uterus. The incidences of antepartum hemorrhage, cesarean section, and adverse neonatal outcome were essentially the same among the various groups.

Conclusion.—With the excellent medical care available in Abu Dhabi, EGMP appears to have no adverse effect on perinatal outcome.

▶ It is important to understand the United Arab Emirates in interpreting this review of the outcomes of 4721 multiparous pregnancies. Endowed with abundant natural resources, the Emirates benefit by one of the world's highest per capita incomes and lavish governmental provisions for social support and medical facilities and services, generally supplanted by an extensive system of contractural agreements from neighboring and other nations. An Islamic country, reproduction there is held as an important element of femininity, encouraged by governmental incentives. Early marriages are common, abortion is prohibited, and contraception is rarely practiced.

It was therefore not surprising that in 7 years time, records of 1015 women para 10 or greater than 1662 with parity 5 to 9 could be collected and compared to 2044 women with parity that ranged from 2 to 4 inclusively. Since age and parity are such strong covariates, it is not surprising to find increases in pregnancy-induced hypertension, except for those women with parity 10 or greater, diabetes mellitus, gestational diabetes mellitus, and chronic hypertension associated with progressively advanced parity.

What is interesting is that preterm delivery and labor induction became decreasingly prevalent with advanced parity and that growth retardation, malpresentation, fetal distress, cesarean section, and operative birth remain unchanged as a function of extraordinary parity. Granted it is not easy to generalize from this unique population. The data do suggest that much of the host of problems associated with advanced parity noted in the past in other settings may well have been a reflection of socioeconomic and environmental factors rather than biological limits on the capacity to reproduce repeatedly with safety.

T. H. Kirschbaum, MD

3 Fetal Complications of Pregnancy

Rapid and Radical Amniodrainage in the Treatment of Severe Twin-Twin Transfusion Syndrome
Jauniaux E, Holmes A, Hyett J, et al (Royal Free and Univ College, London; Hosp for Sick Children, London)
Prenat Diagn 21:471-476, 2001   3–1

Background.—Twin-twin transfusion is a severe complication of multiple pregnancies which occurs in 10% to 20% of monochorionic twins. It is caused primarily by the presence of 1 or more unbalanced arteriovenous anastomoses between the placental branches of the umbilical circulations. In twin-twin transfusion, a shift of blood volume may occur from one twin to the other, depending on the type and number of anastomoses and the balance of placental sharing between the twins. In typical cases, the "donor" becomes hypovolemic and oliguric, while the "recipient" becomes hypervolemic and polyuric. Some cases may resolve spontaneously, but usually the oliguria in the donor leads to oligohydramnios, and the twin becomes compressed in its own amniotic sac, which slows its growth velocity. Meanwhile, polyhydramnios and increased myocardial overload develop in the recipient, which leads eventually to cardiac failure and fetal hydrops. From 70% to 90% of fetuses die either during pregnancy or immediately after delivery in the absence of medical intervention. The role of a rapid and radical method of amniodrainage using a vacuum bottle system in treating severe twin-twin tranfusion was evaluated.

Methods.—The outcomes for 15 patients with severe twin-twin transfusion who were treated with amniodrainage via a vacuum bottle system (study group) were compared with outcomes of 15 patients who were treated with a standard procedure with a syringe system. The patients were matched for gestational age at the time of the initial procedure. For the women in the study group, the amniodrainage ended when no amniotic fluid could be aspirated. For women in the standard group, fluid was removed until the deepest amniotic fluid pool was less than 8 cm.

Results.—At the initial procedure, women in the study group had a significantly higher mean volume of amniotic fluid drained (3252 mL vs 2153 mL) compared with women in the standard procedure group, and the length of

47

TABLE 2.—Comparison of the Technical Characteristics of the Radical Versus the Standard Amniodrainage Procedure*

Variable	Radical Amniodrainage	Standard Amniodrainage	p
Procedures (n)	1.5 (1.1, 1.9)	5.4 (4.2, 6.6)	< 0.001
Time (min)	21 (17, 26)	41 (33, 49)	< 0.001
Volume/time (ml/min)	143 (108, 178)	55 (42, 68)	< 0.001
Post-procedure AFI (cm)	2.9 (2.3, 3.5)	7.7 (6.3, 9.2)	< 0.001

*Data are presented as mean and 95% CI.
Abbreviation: AFT, Amniotic fluid index.
(Courtesy of Jauniaux E, Holmes A, Hyett J, et al: Rapid and radical amniodrainage in the treatment of severe twin-twin transfusion syndrome. *Prenat Diagn* 21:471-476, 2001. Copyright John Wiley & Sons. Reproduced by permission.)

the procedure was significantly shorter for women in the study group (21 minutes vs 41 minutes). The mean postprocedure index was significantly smaller (2.9 vs 7.7) after radical amniodrainage than after standard amniodrainage, and the women in the study group had a significantly lower mean number of procedures (1.5 vs 5.6) (Table 2). There was a significant increase in the mean placental thickness in the study group, from 9 mm before the procedure to 49 mm after the procedure. The overall perinatal survival rate was 80% for the study group, with a survival rate of 93% for at least 1 survivor.

Conclusion.—Early, rapid, and radical amniodrainage is an effective and low-cost means for treating severe twin-twin transfusion syndrome.

▶ The principal approaches to managing severe twin-twin transfusion syndrome in monochorionic twins includes fetocide, laser coagulation of umbilical vessels on the chorionic plate,[1,2] and repeated amniocenteses.[3,4] The infants survival rate for the latter approach clusters around 60%, clearly surpassing the maximum of 50% survival with fetocide. This is an approach to exploring rapid, large volume amniocentesis as a means of improving results.

Fifteen women with severe twin-twin transfusion syndrome were treated with a total of 22 procedures with a mean volume of 3.25 L of amniotic fluid removed. All had acute onset of maternal symptoms, evidence of "stuck" twins, amniotic fluid index greater than 40, growth retardation, and dilated fetal hearts with tricuspid insufficiency. Historical controls matched for gestational age and entry for care over the 2 years prior to this new approach were constructed. The rapid treatment used vacuum bottles to remove amniotic fluid from the recipient to a level at which the deepest amniotic fluid pocket was less than 8 cm.

The mean time of entry for both groups into this study was 23 weeks' gestation, and rapid evacuation required 22 aspirations compared with 81 procedures using the standard more deliberate approach to amnioreduction. Fetal survival was 80% compared with 63% of the controls.

Use of historical controls always leaves time and the experience of the operators uncontrolled and is likely to bias toward improved later results. What is most impressive here is the reduction in the number of aspirations apparently required for results which, if anything, are slightly superior. The authors suggestion is worth considering.

T. H. Kirschbaum, MD

References

1. 1996 YEAR BOOK OF OBSTETRICS, GYNECOLOGY, AND WOMEN'S HEALTH, pp 180-181.
2. 1999 YEAR BOOK OF OBSTETRICS, GYNECOLOGY, AND WOMEN'S HEALTH, pp 160-163.
3. 1995 YEAR BOOK OF OBSTETRICS, GYNECOLOGY, AND WOMEN'S HEALTH, pp 130-131.
4. 1996 YEAR BOOK OF OBSTETRICS, GYNECOLOGY, AND WOMEN'S HEALTH, pp 116-119.

Maternal Antecedents for Cerebral Palsy in Extremely Preterm Babies: A Case-Control Study

Gray PH, Jones P, O'Callaghan MJ (Mater Mothers' Hosp, South Brisbane, Australia; Mater Children's Hosp, South Brisbane, Australia)
Dev Med Child Neurol 43:580-585, 2001   3–2

Background.—As increasing numbers of preterm infants survive, those antenatal risk factors that contribute to cerebral palsy (CP) become increasingly important. A matched case-control designed study was performed to identify significant antenatal risk factors for CP.

Study Design.—The study group was derived from all infants born at 24 to 27 weeks' gestation from 1989 through 1996 at Mater Mother's Hospital. Infants with a proven syndrome or chromosomal abnormality were excluded, as were those from triplet or larger multiple births. At the age of 2

TABLE 2.—Maternal Factors Among Infants With Cerebral Palsy and Control Infants: Unmatched and Matched Analysis

	Infants With CP, % (n = 30)	Control Infants, % (n = 120)	Odds Ratio (95% CI) Matched Analysis
Maternal age < 20 or > 35 y	4 (13.3)	22 (18.3)	0.6 (0.2-1.8)
Primigravidity	7 (23.3)	36 (30.0)	0.7 (0.3-1.8)
Parity ≥ 3	6 (20.0)	14 (11.7)	1.9 (0.7-5.4)
Preterm labour	9 (30.0)	42 (35.0)	0.8 (0.3-1.8)
PPROM	12 (40.0)	47 (39.2)	1 (0.5-2.4)
Antepartum haemorrhage	6 (20.0)	36 (30.0)	0.6 (0.3-1.5)
Vaginal bleeding	11 (37.9)	49 (40.8)	0.8 (0.4-2)
Chronic hypertension	1 (3.3)	2 (1.7)	2 (0.2-23.2)
Preeclampsia	2 (6.7)	14 (11.7)	0.5 (0.1-2.5)
Clinical chorioamnionitis	9 (30.0)	26 (21.8)	1.7 (0.8-3.9)
Maternal fever	5 (16.6)	13 (10.8)	1.6 (0.5-5)
Maternal infection	0. (0.0)	5 (4.2)	
IUGR	5 (16.7)	3 (2.5)	6.6 (1.8-25.2)
Time to delivery > 24 h	21 (70.0)	71 (59.1)	1.6 (0.7-3.9)
Antenatal treatment			
Corticosteroids	21 (70.0)	102 (85.0)	0.4 (0.1-0.98)
Antibiotics	7 (23.3)	28 (23.3)	1 (0.4-2.5)
Tocolytics	7 (23.3)	43 (35.8)	0.6 (0.2-1.4)

(Courtesy of Gray PH, Jones P, O'Callaghan MJ: Maternal antecedents for cerebral palsy in extremely preterm babies: A case-control study. *Dev Med Child Neurol* 43:580-585, 2001.)

years (corrected for prematurity), 293 infants were available for follow-up. These children underwent a detailed neurologic evaluation. Thirty were identified as having CP and all but 1 had spasticity. There were no cases of both twins in a pregnancy receiving a diagnosis of CP. For each child with CP, the next 4 mothers who delivered an infant at the same hospital served as controls. Data on risk factors (Table 2) were obtained from obstetric notes by a practitioner blinded to neurologic status. A matched analysis was performed for maternal predictors of CP.

Findings.—Antenatal growth restriction was associated with increased risk of CP. Maternal administration of corticosteroids was associated with a reduced risk of CP. No relationship was observed between chorioamnionitis or funisitis and CP. Maternal preeclapsia was not associated with a significant reduction in CP (Table 2).

Conclusion.—Antenatal administration of corticosteroids was significantly associated with a reduction in CP in preterm infants. Therefore, it is recommended that corticosteroids be considered when preterm birth is anticipated.

▶ Among the antecedents of CP, it is common to list preterm birth, chorioamnionitis, antepartum bleeding, and birth trauma.[1-4] In many respects however, evaluation of data such as these leads to uncertainties based on differences between term, preterm, and immature births; cerebral palsy and more diffuse neurologic impairment; the role of premature rupture of membranes; and uncertainty about the relative role of magnesium sulfate in contrast to the purportedly diminished risk of CP in preeclamptic pregnancies. Some authors have recently shown differences in risk factors for CP versus spastic diplegia and between births at less than 28 weeks' gestation versus infants born at from 28 to 31 weeks.

This is a case-control study of infants born between 24 and 27 weeks gestational age referred to a Brisbane Tertiary Care unit between 1989 and 1996. Of 444 such births, 310 infants survived, and 293 were followed up to at least 2 years of age to allow the evaluation of possible CP and/or spastic diplegia.

The specific goals were to evaluate risk factors in this gestational age range; the role of chorioamnionitis, membrane rupture, and preeclampsia on those factors; and possible differences between CP and spastic diplegia as outcome measurements. The authors' approach was to use univariate analysis, calculating risk ratios for the presence of dependent variables between 30 pregnancies with the diagnosis of infant CP, 18 with spastic diplegia, and 120 normals serving as controls matched for age. Univariate analysis is an appropriate first step in exploring causal associations, but the approach here generates large confidence intervals because of the small individual case numbers.

As Table 2 displays, the diagnosis of growth retardation antepartum is a strong and significant risk factor for CP in this gestational age range. Neither maternal age, parity, membrane rupture, preterm labor, or antepartum bleeding showed associative links. The risk ratio for preeclampsia is only 0.5 and for chorioamnionitis and maternal infection in pregnancy, 1.7 and 1.6, respectively, but none of these show a statistically significant association between the variable and brain injury. Use of antenatal corticoids employed in 70% to

85% of these preterm births was associated with significantly reduced likelihood of CP (RR 0.4), clearly the most notable finding in this study. No difference in results was seen when spastic diplegia was replaced as an outcome variable for CP.

T. H. Kirschbaum, MD

References

1. 1996 YEAR BOOK OF OBSTETRICS, GYNECOLOGY, AND WOMEN'S HEALTH, pp 124-126.
2. 1997 YEAR BOOK OF OBSTETRICS, GYNECOLOGY, AND WOMEN'S HEALTH, pp 115-117.
3. 1999 YEAR BOOK OF OBSTETRICS, GYNECOLOGY, AND WOMEN'S HEALTH, pp 123-128.
4. 2001 YEAR BOOK OF OBSTETRICS, GYNECOLOGY, AND WOMEN'S HEALTH, pp 62-63.

Congenital Abnormalities Among Children With Cerebral Palsy: More Evidence for Prenatal Antecedents

Croen LA, Grether JK, Curry CJ, et al (California Birth Defects Monitoring Program, Oakland, Calif; Valley Children's Hosp, Madera, Calif; Univ of California, San Francisco; et al)
J Pediatr 138:804-810, 2001   3–3

Objectives.—To investigate the association between cerebral palsy (CP) and congenital abnormalities among children with very low, low, and normal birth weight.

Study design.—A population-based, case-control study among the cohort of 155,636 live births delivered between 1983 and 1985 in 4 California counties. Children with moderate or severe congenital CP (n = 192) diagnosed by age 3 were identified from 2 California State service agencies, and 551 control children were randomly sampled from birth certificate files. Information on congenital abnormalities diagnosed by the age of 1 year was obtained from the California Birth Defects Monitoring Program registry. Odds ratios (OR) and 95% CIs were calculated to estimate risk for CP associated with congenital abnormalities (Table 2).

Results.—Among singletons, congenital abnormalities were present in 33 (19.2%) children with CP and 21 (4.3%) control children (OR = 5.2, 95% CI 2.8-9.7). For each birth weight group, the percent of children with congenital abnormalities among children with CP exceeded that among control children. Structural abnormalities of the central nervous system were more common among children with CP (OR = 16.2, 95% CI 5.8-49.3) than control children. In contrast, the percent of children with non–central nervous system abnormalities only was similar between case patients and control subjects.

Conclusion.—These findings provide further evidence that factors operating in the prenatal period contribute significantly to the etiology of CP.

▶ The tendency for infants and children with CP to have an increased likelihood of other congenital anomalies has long been recognized, but the magnitude of the associations is uncertain. Further, the large variety both of anoma-

TABLE 2.—Odds Ratios (OR) and 95% CIs for Congenital Abnormalities Among Singleton Children With CP Compared With Control Subjects Within Strata of Selected Child and Maternal Characteristics

	Children With CP		Control Children			
	Congenital Abnormality	No Congenital Abnormality	Congenital Abnormality	No Congenital Abnormality	OR	95% CI
Sex						
Male	22	71	9	232	8.0	3.3-19.7
Female	11	68	12	230	3.1	1.2-7.9
Birth weight						
<1500 g	6	36	8	75	1.6	0.4-5.5
1500-2499 g	8	25	2	16	2.6	0.4-13.3
≥2500 g	19	78	11	371	8.2	3.5-19.3
Maternal age						
<20 y	6	16	3	44		
20-34 y	25	104	16	372	5.6	2.7-11.4
≥35 y	2	19	2	46		
Maternal race/ethnicity						
White, non-Hispanic	17	73	11	224	4.7	2.0-11.4
White, Hispanic	8	31	5	94	4.8	1.3-18.7
Black	4	20	5	51		
Asian	3	9	0	43		
Other	1	5	0	47		
Parity						
Primiparous	14	69	5	203	8.2	2.6-27.3
Multiparous	19	70	16	259	4.4	2.0-9.5

(Courtesy of Croen LA, Grether JK, Curry CJ, et al: Congenital abnormalities among children with cerebral palsy: More evidence for prenatal antecedents. *J Pediatr* 138:804-8110, 2001.)

lous development options and of CNS abnormalities and differences in defining and categorizing congenital anomalies and data from infants with CP has led to inconsistent reported results. These authors attempt to deal with the complex problems of categorization in a very rich data matrix of CP and birth defects from 4 counties in the San Francisco Bay area occurring from 1983 to 1985. Analysis of these data has been reported here previously (see 1995 YEAR BOOK OF OBSTETRICS, GYNECOLOGY, AND WOMEN'S HEALTH, pp 135-138; 1996 YEAR BOOK, pp 126-128; 1997 YEAR BOOK, pp 115-117, 162-164; and 1999 YEAR BOOK, pp 125-126).

Only patients in whom moderate to severe CP was diagnosed by age 3 were selected, to avoid diluting associations by marginal case selections. CP related to trauma as well as infection or events occurring after 1 month of age were excluded as well. One hundred ninety-two children with CP were segregated among very low and normal birth weight subsets. Instances of anomalous development were further subdivided into CNS anomaly alone, non–CNS anomaly alone, and a combination of the 2. A 2:1 control group of 151 newborns matched for birth weight ranges, gender, maternal age, ethnicity, and parity, was constructed. ORs were struck between CP and control groups for demographic data and CNS and other abnormalities.

The results reflect the complexity of the data analysis. Children with CP were 3 times more likely to be in the 1.5 to 2.5K birth weight range, but the greatest risk ratio existed among infants with birth weight greater than 2.5 kg, indicating that birth weight is not a strong covariant of CP risk in these data. The infants with CP had an increased likelihood of being boys born to women in the age range from 20 to 34 years of age who were white and primiparous. Among singletons in whom CP was diagnosed by the age of 1 year, 19.2% had a diagnosable congenital anomaly versus 4.3% of the controls, across the full range of maternal demographic variables. By the age of 1 year, 14.5% of the children with CP exhibited structural abnormalities, versus 1% of the controls. There was no difference in the incidence of non–CNS anomalies between cases and controls, and among 20 twins with CP only 1 anomaly was reported by the age of 1 year. This analysis makes clear the association between congenital CNS anomaly and the diagnosis of CP and strongly supports the prominent part that anomalous development before delivery plays in the ultimate diagnosis of CP.

T. H. Kirschbaum, MD

Antenatal Magnesium Exposure and Neonatal Demise

Farkouh LJ, Thorp JA, Jones PG, et al (Obstetrix Med Group of Colorado, Denver; Obstetrix Med Group of Kansas and Missouri, Kansas City; Analytic Consultants of Lee's Summit, Mo; et al)
Am J Obstet Gynecol 185:869-872, 2001   3–4

Background.—Recent research suggests that tocolytic magnesium use may increase perinatal mortality. However, this research included small study populations, which make the findings difficult to interpret. The possible association between antenatal magnesium exposure and neonatal death was investigated.

Methods.—Data on 12,876 live births gathered prospectively at 100 tertiary centers between May 1997 and January 2000 were analyzed retrospectively. The data included nonanomalous newborns admitted to the neonatal ICU between 23 and 34 weeks' gestation. In a univariate analysis of 24 candidate variables, predictors of neonatal death were determined. In addition, a multivariate predictive model for mortality was developed by using variables with significant interactions with the death rate.

Findings.—When the neonates were stratified according to gestational age, magnesium correlated with a significant decrease in neonatal death, with an odds ratio of 0.67. This association persisted after adjustment for gestational age and indication for treatment. In the final model, after controlling for additional antenatal factors, the effect was similar.

Conclusions.—Antenatal magnesium exposure did not increase neonatal death, after adjustment for other variables and regardless of treatment indication. This study is of greater magnitude than recent research suggesting that such exposure may increase neonatal death.

▶ A signal retrospective multicenter study designed to demonstrate relationships between obstetric and neonatal events and cerebral palsy studying 189 such cases resulting from more than 46,000 births between 1955 and 1966 failed to demonstrate an important role of risk factors during labor and delivery on the ultimate diagnosis of cerebral palsy.[1,2] Because antepartum fetal heart rate monitoring was not a regular part of obstetric care for those patients, a later study of 192 cases of cerebral palsy resulting from 155,636 births between 1983 and 1985 using data from the California Birth Defects Monitoring program essentially repeated the earlier study. This time, the impact of fetal monitoring and some other independent variables, among them magnesium for tocolysis or convulsion prophylaxis, led to the same results.[3] Incidentally, an inverse correlation between magnesium ion dosage during pregnancy and labor, and eventual cerebral palsy was demonstrated.[4] A still later study based on 170 infants with cerebral palsy delivered from 1988 to 1994 in the San Francisco Bay area and metropolitan Atlanta failed to confirm a protective trend associated with magnesium use (Abstract 5–7). Subsequently, a study designed to explore the putative effects of magnesium ion in preterm fetuses was halted when a cluster of fetal and perinatal deaths occurred in women tocolyzed with magnesium sulfate (Abstract 4–29).[5] In a subsequent study of infants weighing less than 1.5 kg at birth, no surplus mortality was seen among infants whose mothers received magnesium compared with those who did not,[6] but infant follow-up was terminated at 120 days of life, too early to reliably exclude the development of cerebral palsy, which might appear as late as 2 to 3 years of age. It is important that these investigators separated women receiving magnesium as a tocolytic from preeclamptic women receiving convulsion prophylaxis in view of the significant reduction of risk of cerebral palsy apparently associated with hypertensive disease of pregnancy. As a result, they studied only patients receiving tocolytic magnesium sulfate.

The current study brings to bear the records of 12,876 nonanomalous new-borns delivered at 23 to 34 weeks of gestational age between 1997 and 2000, who were admitted to neonatal ICUs in Colorado, Missouri, and Kansas. The dependent variable here is neonatal death, not cerebral palsy. Crude neonatal mortality rates were 3.9% in magnesium-treated pregnancies versus 3.2% in controls. When data were adjusted for variable gestational ages, a statistically significantly decreased risk of neonatal mortality appeared in the magnesium recipients (RR 0.67). However, when a multivariate regression model was used to consider the impact of 7 other variables, no significant impact of magnesium therapy was discernable. The authors offer a firm conclusion that neonatal mortality is not increased by magnesium therapy, and a somewhat less robust conclusion that it is also of no benefit. This latter conclusion appears to be fair from what data now exists.

T. H. Kirschbaum, MD

References

1. 1987 YEAR BOOK OF OBSTETRICS, GYNECOLOGY, AND WOMEN'S HEALTH, pp 243-245.
2. 1988 YEAR BOOK OF OBSTETRICS, GYNECOLOGY, AND WOMEN'S HEALTH, pp 116-118.
3. 1995 YEAR BOOK OF OBSTETRICS, GYNECOLOGY, AND WOMEN'S HEALTH, pp 135-138, 202-204.
4. 1996 YEAR BOOK OF OBSTETRICS, GYNECOLOGY, AND WOMEN'S HEALTH, pp 126-128.
5. 1999 YEAR BOOK OF OBSTETRICS, GYNECOLOGY, AND WOMEN'S HEALTH, pp 56-57.
6. 2000 YEAR BOOK OF OBSTETRICS, GYNECOLOGY, AND WOMEN'S HEALTH, pp 230-231.

Fetal Leptin Influences Birth Weight in Twins With Discordant Growth
Sooranna SR, Ward S, Bajoria R (Univ of Manchester, England; Imperial College, London; Chelsea Hosp, London; Chelsea and Westminster Hosp, London)
Pediatr Res 49:667-672, 2001   3–5

Background.—Many researchers have found markedly lower plasma leptin levels in newborns with intrauterine growth retardation than in those with normal growth. Plasma leptin levels in twin pregnancies in relation to chorionicity and discordant fetal growth were studied.

Methods.—Fifty-three twin pregnancies were analyzed. In 27, growth was concordant, and in 26, growth discordance of 20% or greater was found.

Findings.—In discordant monochorionic pregnancies, the growth-restricted twins had lower fetal plasma leptin concentrations than did the co-twins with normal growth. Concordant monochorionic twin pairs did not have this difference. Fetal plasma leptin levels in appropriate-for-gestational-age twins were greater than in the growth-restricted twins of discordant dichorionic pregnancies. These differences were not found in the concordant dichorionic twin pairs. In all 4 groups, maternal plasma leptin concentrations were comparable and greater than fetal levels. Fetal plasma leptin levels were comparable in the growth-restricted twins of discordant monochorionic and dichorionic pregnancies (Figs 1 and 2). Cord plasma leptin levels were positively correlated with the birth weight of twin pairs.

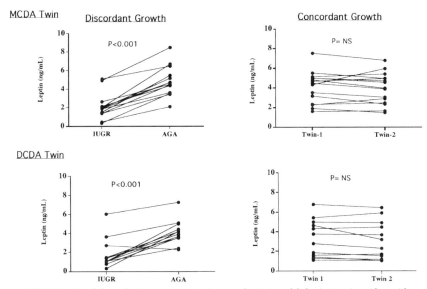

FIGURE 1.—Fetal plasma leptin concentrations in monochorionic and dichorionic twins with or without growth disturbance. *Abbreviations: IUGR,* Intrauterine growth retardation; *AGA,* appropriate growth for gestational age. (Courtesy of Sooranna SR, Ward S, Bajoria R: Fetal leptin influences birth weight in twins with discordant growth. *Pediatr Res* 49(5):667-672, 2001.)

Percentage differences in birth weight and fetal delta plasma leptin levels of the discordant monochorionic and dichorionic twin pairs were significantly, positively associated.

Conclusion.—Regardless of chorionicity, plasma leptin levels in twins with intrauterine growth retardation are 2-fold lower than in their normally growing co-twins. Placental factors appear to explain these differences.

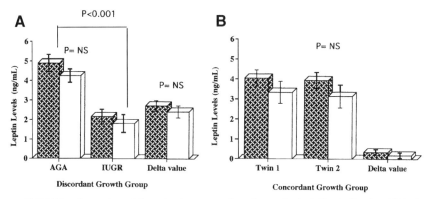

FIGURE 2.—Comparison of plasma leptin concentrations of monochorionic (*hatched bars*) and dichorionic (*open bars*) twin pairs with (**A**) and without (**B**) discordant growth. *Abbreviations: IUGR,* Intrauterine growth retardation; *AGA,* appropriate growth for gestational age. (Courtesy of Sooranna SR, Ward S, Bajoria R: Fetal leptin influences birth weight in twins with discordant growth. *Pediatr Res* 49(5):667-672, 2001.)

▶ The relationship between fetal plasma leptin and birth weight is potentially confounded by gestational age, birth order, gender, parental genetic factors, and diurnal, and seasonal variations. In comparing leptin concentrations between concordant and discordant weight twins from monochorionic and dichorionic twin placentas with collection of blood samples from mother and newborn simultaneously at birth around 32 to 35 weeks' gestational age, the authors were able to exclude the influence of most confounding variables. Having excluded the potential effects of maternal pregnancy—hypertension, diabetes mellitus, overt twin-twin transfusion syndromes, and fetal structural and genetic abnormalities—they strove to examine fetal weight regulation in remaining normal pregnancies.

Choice of a weight discrepancy of at least 20% as indicative of weight discordance and, by inference, growth retardation in 1 twin introduces some surplus variability since about 10% to 20% of normal twins exhibit differences of this size. Further, surplus fetal and newborn morbidity is not seen regularly until weight discrepancies greater than 30% are present, and below that level abnormal outcome measurements are rare.

Granting these reservations, the results are fairly clear. Maternal leptin is unrelated to fetal leptin concentration. Growth retarded twins, whether monochorionic or dichorionic, have significantly reduced leptin concentrations compared with twins of appropriate growth for gestational age. Newborn leptin is independent of gender. Since intrapair fetal leptin differences in discordant monochorionic and dichorionic dyzgotic twins are similar, it is unlikely, or at least uncommon, that growth retardation in monochorionic twins is a function of differential distribution of nutrients and blood supply of the placental vascular shunts. Newborn leptin concentration is, as expected, directly proportional to birth weight. The authors leave us with the conclusion that maternal environmental and familial genetic factors are not important in growth retardation in twins mediated by changes in leptin concentration, but that placental factors are among the most likely determinants.

T. H. Kirschbaum, MD

Decreased Amniotic Fluid Index in Low-Risk Pregnancy
Kreiser D, El-Sayed YY, Sorem KA, et al (Stanford Univ, Calif)
J Reprod Med 46:743-746, 2001   3–6

Introduction.—A finding of diminished amniotic fluid volume at antepartum US may indicate impaired placental function. The perinatal outcomes of pregnancies complicated by isolated decreased amniotic fluid index (AFI) after 30 weeks' gestation were examined retrospectively.

Methods.—Included in the analysis were 150 singleton, nonanomalous pregnancies with decreased AFI (≤5 cm or >5 cm but <2.5th percentile) and intact membranes. Previous perinatal loss, previous cesarean section, suspected fetal growth restriction, and decreased fetal movement were among the indications for fetal surveillance. Seven pregnancy outcomes were assessed: fetal heart rate abnormalities before labor, induction of labor be-

TABLE 3.—Neonatal Outcomes

Outcome	Study Group (Total) (n = 150) (%)	AFI ≤ 5 (n = 57) (%)	AFI > 5 But < 2.5th Percentile (n = 93) (%)
Gestational age (wk) at delivery	38.9 ± 1.8	39.2 ± 2.2	38.8 ± 1.6
Birth weight (g)	3174 ± 536	3111 ± 585	3213 ± 503
Apgar score <7	1 (0.66)	0	1 (1.1)
Perinatal mortality	0	0	0
Admissions to neonatal intensive care unit	0	0	0

Data presented as mean ± SD, number, and %.
No statistically significant differences between groups.
(Courtesy of Kreiser D, El-Sayed YY, Sorem KA, et al: Decreased amniotic fluid index in low-risk pregnancy. J Reprod Med 46:743-746, 2001.)

cause of an abnormal nonstress test (NST), emergency cesarean section because of fetal heart rate abnormalities, the presence of meconium, Apgar score <7 at 5 minutes, admission to neonatal ICU, and perinatal mortality.

Results.—Fifty-seven pregnancies had an AFI ≤5 cm, and 93 had an AFI >5 but <2.5th percentile. On average, the women remained undelivered for more than 2 weeks from diagnosis. The 2 groups did not differ significantly in mean maternal age, parity, gestational age at the start of testing, or number of antenatal NSTs performed. Antepartum fetal heart rate changes, intrapartum outcomes, and neonatal outcomes (Table 3) were also similar in the 2 groups, except that variable decelerations on NST were significantly more common among patients in the AFI ≤5 cm group.

Discussion.—The association between low AFI and poor pregnancy outcome is uncertain, and opinions vary regarding the actual threshold for defining a low AFI. But in otherwise-uncomplicated pregnancies, intensive antepartum monitoring is an alternative to immediate delivery in cases of low or borderline AFI.

▶ It is not clear that more data regarding the innocuous nature of uncomplicated oligohydramnios diagnosed by US are needed, but since the condition appears persistently to be a frequent indication for labor induction and the increased risk of cesarean section that ensues, it may be worth citing another.[1,2] This is a report of 150 such patients collected over 2 years at Stanford University. All represent singlet pregnancies past 30 weeks of gestational age with low amniotic fluid indices and intact membranes. Two criteria for the diagnosis of oligohydramnios by US are used. In 57 cases, Phalens definition of AFI (≤5 cm is used). In 93 cases, a more-liberal definition based on the study of amniotic fluid index in pregnancies followed for acardiac monochorionic twins is used.[3] Generally, those deemed to have oligohydramnios by virtue of an amniotic fluid index at or below the 2.5th percentile for gestational age by the Moore criteria have AFIs in the range of 6 to 9 cm. Exclusions from this study, an important item to remember, are premature preterm rupture of membranes, diabetes, preeclampsia, growth retardation, or maternal medical disease. There is no control group here, and management varied among cases, but this becomes of less concern when one notes that there was no perinatal morbidity as reflected in low birth weight notes, reduced Apgar scores, perinatal mortality, or neonatal ICU admission. Granted the exclusionary criteria, oligohydramnios defined by contemporary US criteria in otherwise-normal pregnancies, lacking other risk factors for perinatal mortality, appears to be of no obstetrical consequence whatsoever.

T. H. Kirschbaum, MD

References

1. 2001 YEAR BOOK OF OBSTETRICS, GYNECOLOGY, AND WOMEN'S HEALTH, pp 35-38.
2. 2002 YEAR BOOK, pp 252-254.
3. Moore TR, Gale S, Benirschke K: Perinatal outcome of 49 pregnancies complicated by acardiac twinning. *Am J Obstet Gynecol* 163:907, 1990.

Effect of Twin-to-Twin Delivery Interval on Umbilical Cord Blood Gas in the Second Twins
Leung T-Y, Tam W-H, Leung T-N, et al (Chinese Univ, Hong Kong)
Br J Obstet Gynaecol 109:63-67, 2002   3–7

Introduction.—Vaginal delivery of the second twin continues to be challenging because of uterine inertia, abnormal lie, or high presenting part of the second twin. It has been widely accepted that the intertwin delivery interval should occur within 15 to 30 minutes. Scientific evidence concerning the safe time limit for twin-to-twin delivery interval is lacking. The effect of twin-to-twin delivery interval on the umbilical cord blood gas status of the second twin was retrospectively examined.

Methods.—The association between the twin-to-twin delivery interval, and both the umbilical arterial and venous blood gas parameters of the second twin, including pH, partial pressure of CO_2, and base excess, was examined in twin deliveries at or beyond 34 weeks' gestation during a period of 5 years, with the first twin delivered vaginally. Twins with any antepartum complications were excluded.

Results.—The mean gestational age at delivery was 37.1 weeks for 118 cases reviewed; the median twin-to-twin delivery interval was 16.5 minutes. The mode of delivery of the second twin varied for different twin-to-twin intervals (Fig 2). There were significant negative correlations between twin-to-twin delivery interval and both the umbilical cord arterial and venous pH and base excess of the second twin ($P < .05$). There were also significant positive associations between both arterial and venous partial pressure of CO_2 and the delivery interval ($P < .05$). Similar changes were detected even when analyses were restricted to those who had normal vaginal deliveries. The umbilical arterial pH of twin 2 was below 7.00 in 0% of cases delivered within 15 minutes of the birth of twin 1, 5.9% if within 16 to 30 minutes, and 27% if more than 30 minutes. Among cases with an intertwin delivery

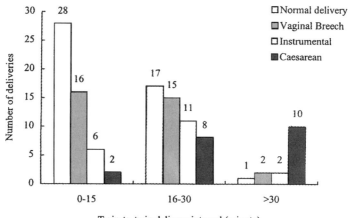

FIGURE 2.—Mode of delivery of second twin at different twin-to-twin delivery intervals. (Courtesy of Leung T-Y, Tam W-H, Leung T-N, et al: Effect of twin-to-twin delivery interval on umbilical cord blood gas in the second twins. *Br J Obstet Gynaecol* 109:63-67, 2002. With permission from Elsevier Science.)

interval of more than 30 minutes, 73% had cardiotocographic evidence of fetal distress that necessitated operative delivery.

Conclusion.—Umbilical cord arterial and venous values of pH, partial pressure of CO_2, and base excess of the second twin worsen with increasing twin-to-twin delivery interval. The risks of fetal distress and acidosis in the second twin are high in the presence of a twin-to-twin delivery in excess of 30 minutes.

▶ There is no question that second twins are disadvantaged compared to first twins in terms of a number of functions, but it is by no means clear why that is so. Changing the mode of delivery doesn't affect the disadvantage of being second born. The pattern is independent of vaginal versus abdominal birth[1] or whether twin 2 is born by version and extraction or section.[2] The second twin has an increased risk for respiratory distress syndrome independent of malpresentation or depression at birth.[3] Since the incidence of intracranial hemorrhage is not increased in the second born, independent of birth order, birth weight, mode of delivery or presentation,[4] some have suggested that both RDS and intracranial hemorrhage are determined primarily by neonatal, not prenatal and intrapartum events. Even in the birth weight range of 1500 to 2500 g, the sharp increase in abdominal birth occurring during 1973-1983 resulted in no benefit as judged by second trimester status at birth or neonatal mortality,[5] and no differences in outcome were noted from services devoted to the vaginal birth of twins,[6] where the cesarean section rate was only 28%. Clearly, the incidence of congenital anomaly is nearly 3 times greater in twin pregnancies than in singlets and has a tendency for greater incidences in second twins.[7,8] Twinning increases the incidence of cerebral palsy 12-fold, and though the incidence rate is larger in second than in first twins, the difference is not statistically significantly so and appears to be a function primarily of the differential occurrence of low birth weight in second twins. The data on singlet pregnancies and cerebral palsy are important because of the work of Nelson and Ellenberger[9] in term pregnancy, who showed that breech presentation was a significant risk factor but that breech delivery was not.[10] This led to an active hypothesis that some genetic or environmental factor is operating in patients with cerebral palsy that covertly interferes with central nervous system function and development, and reduces fetal motor activity in utero, an important factor in determining cephalic presentation at term and second twin position in utero. Changes in intrauterine geometry in twin pregnancy also increases the chances for malpresentation. Some behavioral studies, subjective with little control for observer bias, suggest motor activity in newborn second twins is less than that in first twins.

In this study, the time between deliveries of infants 1 and 2 is inversely correlated with cord blood P_{O_2} and base excess, and directly with cord blood P_{CO_2}. As Figure 2 shows, most second twins are sectioned after more than 30 minutes has elapsed after the first. That latter population includes both normal second twins and those with clinical findings suggesting fetal compromise, howsoever imprecise that diagnosis may be. Cesarean section also introduces potential problems in cardiovascular and respiratory control, which may have influenced the findings in second twins significantly. Clearly, there are several alternative explanations to what was observed here, and the problem seems oversimplified by the authors' interpretation that the interval greater than 30 minutes between delivery 1 and 2 solely determines the observations in cord blood.

T. H. Kirschbaum, MD

References

1. 1987 YEAR BOOK OF OBSTETRICS, GYNECOLOGY, AND WOMEN'S HEALTH, pp 201-202.
2. 1988 YEAR BOOK OF OBSTETRICS, GYNECOLOGY, AND WOMEN'S HEALTH, pp 170-171.
3. 1989 YEAR BOOK OF OBSTETRICS, GYNECOLOGY, AND WOMEN'S HEALTH, pp 99-100.
4. 1989 YEAR BOOK OF OBSTETRICS, GYNECOLOGY, AND WOMEN'S HEALTH, pp 107-108.
5. 1992 YEAR BOOK OF OBSTETRICS, GYNECOLOGY, AND WOMEN'S HEALTH, pp 103-104.
6. 1994 YEAR BOOK OF OBSTETRICS, GYNECOLOGY, AND WOMEN'S HEALTH, pp 138-139.
7. 2002 YEAR BOOK OF OBSTETRICS, GYNECOLOGY, AND WOMEN'S HEALTH, pp 57-60.
8. Grethen JK, Nelson KB, Cummings SK: Twinning in cerebral palsy: Experience in 4 northern California counties in 1983 to 1985. *Pediatrics* 92:854, 1993
9. 1988 YEAR BOOK OF OBSTETRICS AND GYNECOLOGY, pp 116-118.
10. 2001 YEAR BOOK OF OBSTETRICS AND GYNECOLOGY, pp 67-68.

4 Medical Complications of Pregnancy

The HLA A2/6802 Supertype Is Associated With Reduced Risk of Perinatal Human Immunodeficiency Virus Type 1 Transmission

MacDonald KS, Embree JE, Nagelkerke NJD, et al (Univ of Toronto; Mount Sinai Hosp, Toronto; Univ of Manitoba, Winnipeg, Canada; et al)
J Infect Dis 183:503-506, 2001
4–1

Background.—Certain HLAs may partly account for differences in HIV-1 susceptibility, presenting conserved immunogenic epitopes for T-cell recognition. The HLA supertype A2/6802 has been associated with reduced susceptibility to HIV-1 among prostitutes. In some cases, the alleles in this supertype present the same HIV-1 peptide epitopes for T-cell recognition. Whether this HLA supertype is associated with protection from HIV-1 in an independent population with another transmission mode was determined.

Methods and Findings.—The population studied was a prospective cohort of 171 children and 135 mothers in Kenya. All the women were infected with HIV-1. Nineteen children were classified as infected perinatally, and 152 as not infected at birth. Of the latter group, 12 were infected subsequently from prolonged breast-feeding. Reduced perinatal HIV-1 infection risk correlated strongly with the presence of a functional cluster of related HLA alleles—the A2/6802 supertype. This effect was found to be independent of the protection afforded by maternal-child HLA discordance.

Conclusion.—These data support the notion that HLA supertypes are associated with differential susceptibility to HIV-1 transmission. In this cohort, the A2/6802 supertype in infants was associated with an estimated 7-fold protective effect from perinatal HIV-1 transmission.

▶ Studies of uninfected individuals with likely regular exposure to HIV-1 are very important in the search for prophylactic, protective, and possibly therapeutic modifications of this disease. For example, a homozygous gene deletion mutation in the chemokine receptor CCR5 clearly inhibits maternal-to-fetal infection in HIV positive gravidas.[1] In this case, the study of sex workers in sub-Saharan Africa who are HIV-1 negative, despite repeated presumed exposures to the virus, has demonstrated that many have genotypes containing a series of 6 exceptional alleles in the class I HLA portion of the major histocompatibility complex located on chromosome 6.

Known as the HLA A2/6802 subtype or supertype, this portion of the major histocompatibility complex gene allows the expression of epitopes that avoid the immunosuppression of HIV infection and allow the generation of a population of cytotoxic T cells that facilitate clearance of the virus-infected immune cells potentially or actually transferred to the fetus during pregnancy and labor. What results is a 7-fold protective effect against maternal-to-fetal infection in HIV positive gravidas. No protection against infant infection through breast feeding is afforded, presumably because of issues of dosage and route of infection from this holocrine secretion. This is the sort of observation uniquely valuable in HIV vaccine development.

T. H. Kirschbaum, MD

Reference

1. 1999 YEAR BOOK OF OBSTETRICS, GYNECOLOGY, AND WOMEN'S HEALTH, pp 77-78.

Antiretroviral Resistance Mutations Among Pregnant Human Immuno-deficiency Virus Type 1–Infected Women and Their Newborns in the United States: Vertical Transmission and Clades
Palumbo P, for the Perinatal AIDS Collaborative Transmission Study (Univ of Medicine and Dentistry of New Jersey, Newark; et al)
J Infect Dis 184:1120-1126, 2001   4–2

Background.—Pregnant HIV-1–infected women have been offered zidovudine (AZT) to decrease perinatal transmission since 1994 in the United States. It is not known how the emergence of drug resistance will affect the prevention of perinatal transmission. To examine the prevalence of antiretroviral drug resistance mutations in HIV-1–infected pregnant women and its effect on perinatal transmission, genotypic resistance testing was performed.

Study Design.—The study group consisted of 220 HIV-infected pregnant women from 4 American cities who participated in the 1991 to 1997 Perinatal AIDS Collaborative Transmission Study and received AZT during their pregnancy. These women and 24 of their HIV-infected newborns were genotyped, using a chip assay that targeted both the viral reverse transcriptase and protease genes.

Findings.—AZT-associated mutations were detected in 17% of these pregnant HIV-infected women by genotyping. Mutations to nonnucleoside reverse-transcriptase inhibitors and protease inhibitors were not common. There was no significant association between the presence of antiretroviral drug resistance mutations and perinatal transmission. AZT resistance mutations were detected in 8% of the neonates, but these mutations were different from those detected in the maternal samples.

Conclusion.—Genotyping of HIV-infected women who had received AZT therapy during their pregnancies revealed that about 17% had mutations specific for AZT resistance. Despite the emergence of antiretroviral drug mutations, no effect on perinatal transmission was detected. Surveillance remains important to detect the emergence of resistance mutations and to track their effect on perinatal transmission.

▶ As antiretroviral agents are used in increasing numbers and amounts in treating HIV-infected women, the problem of drug resistance has loomed in treatment and in the risk of maternal-to-fetal transmission. A group of 220 HIV-positive women who received AZT during pregnancy and 217 of their infants were studied from that viewpoint. Requirements for entry included maternal plasma HIV RNA counts of at least 1000/mL, a history of antiretroviral use during pregnancy, and determinable fetal status. In both maternal and infant cases, quantitative HIV RNA counts were performed; polymerase chain reaction was done on cDNA both for reverse transcriptase and protease genes; and both gene segments were sequenced, looking for possible inactivating mutations. Only 3 women received protease inhibitors in addition to AZT.

In general, though the incidence of mutational events was considerable, there was little evidence that they were functionally important. In infected women, the incidence of mutated genes was 17.3% and on univariate analysis, the presence of mutations correlated inversely with the decrease in CD4 counts and directly with the duration of AZT use. Mutations were noted in 15.2% of the infants, unrelated to CD4 counts or duration of maternal drug use. There were no relationships between mutated reverse transcriptase or protease gene segments and the risk of maternal-to-fetal transmission. Among clinical parameters, only the duration of ruptured membranes before delivery appeared to be associated with an increased risk of maternal-to-fetal transmission. Many more data will emerge with time as investigators continue to work on these important issues.

T. H. Kirschbaum, MD

Efficacy of Three Short-Course Regimens of Zidovudine and Lamivudine in Preventing Early and Late Transmission of HIV-1 From Mother to Child in Tanzania, South Africa, and Uganda (Petra Study): A Randomised, Double-Blind, Placebo-Controlled Trial
Lange JMA, for the Petra Study Team (Mulago Hosp, Kampala, Uganda; et al)
Lancet 359:1178-1186, 2002   4–3

Introduction.—The use of antiretrovirals are responsible for large decreases in the transmission of HIV-1 from mother to child in more developed countries. Short-course regimens, appropriate for resource-poor countries, also significantly diminish peripartum HIV-1 transmission. The efficacy of short-course regimens with zidovudine and lamivudine were examined in a predominately breast-feeding population in a randomized, double-blind, placebo-controlled trial in South Africa, Uganda, and Tanzania.

TABLE 4.—Early Efficacy of HIV-1 Infection and HIV-1 Infection or Death

	n (%)	Early Efficacy at Week 6 (Relative Risk [95% CI])	p
HIV-1 infection only			
Regimen A	16 (5·7%)	0·37 (0·21-0·65)	0·001
Regimen B	24 (8·9%)	0·58 (0·36-0·94)	0·025
Regimen C	40 (14·2%)	0·93 (0·62-1·40)	0·74
Placebo	40 (15·3%)	1·00	··
HIV-1 infection or death			
Regimen A	20 (7·0%)	0·39 (0·24-0·64)	0·001
Regimen B	32 (11·6%)	0·64 (0·42-0·97)	0·003
Regimen C	51 (17·5%)	0·97 (0·68-1·38)	0·85
Placebo	49 (18·1%)	1·00	··

(Courtesy of Lange JMA, for the Petra Study Team: Efficacy of three short-course regimens of zidovudine and lamivudine in preventing early and late transmission of HIV-1 from mother to child in Tanzania, South Africa, and Uganda [Petra Study]: A randomised, double-blind, placebo-controlled trial. *Lancet* 359:1178-1186, 2002. Reprinted with permission from Elsevier Science.)

Methods.—Between June 1996 and January 2000, HIV-1-infected mothers were randomly assigned to receive treatment with 1 of 4 regimens: (1) zidovudine plus lamivudine beginning at 36 weeks' gestation followed by oral intrapartum dosing and by 7 days' postpartum dosing of mothers and infants (regimen A); (2) same as regimen A, without the prepartum component (regimen B); (3) intrapartum zidovudine and lamivudine only (regimen C); or (4) placebo. From February 18, 1998 onward, females were only randomly assigned to 1 of the active treatment groups. The main outcome measures were HIV-1 infection and child mortality at week 6 and month 18 after birth. Analysis was by intention to treat of females who underwent randomization before February 18, 1998.

Results.—A total of 1797 HIV-1-infected females were identified. The HIV-1 transmission rates at week 6 were 5.7% for group A, 8.9% for group B, 14.2% for group C, and 15.3% for the placebo group. The respective relative risks for HIV-1 transmission in the treatment groups versus the placebo group were 0.37 (95% CI, 0.21-0.65), 0.58 (0.36-0.94), and 0.93 (0.62-1.40), respectively. For the combined end point of HIV-1 infection and infant mortality at week 6, the rates were 7.0%, 11.6%, 17.5%, and 18.1%, respectively; relative risks were 0.39 (0.24-0.64), 0.64 (0.42-0.97), and 0.97 (0.68-1.38) (Table 4 and Fig 2). A total of 1081 (74%) females initiated breast-feeding. Transmission of HIV-1 was rarely observed among children who were not breast-fed and was primarily observed in breast-fed infants (Fig 3). An interval-censored survival analysis demonstrated that HIV infection rates at 18 months were 15% (95% CI, 9-23), 18% (12-26), 20% (13-30), and 22% (16-30), respectively.

Conclusion.—At week 6 after birth, regimens A and B were effective in decreasing the transmission of HIV-1. Benefits are considerably lower after 18 months of follow-up. The introduction of short-course regimens for prevention of mother-to-child transmission of HIV-1 in less developed countries

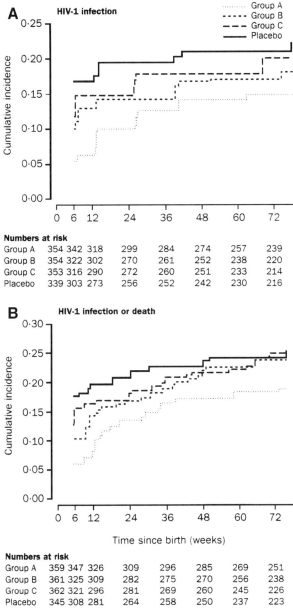

Numbers at risk

Group A	354	342	318	299	284	274	257	239
Group B	354	322	302	270	261	252	238	220
Group C	353	316	290	272	260	251	233	214
Placebo	339	303	273	256	252	242	230	216

Time since birth (weeks)

Numbers at risk

Group A	359	347	326	309	296	285	269	251
Group B	361	325	309	282	275	270	256	238
Group C	362	321	296	281	269	260	245	226
Placebo	345	308	281	264	258	250	237	223

FIGURE 2.—Kaplan-Meier curves for time to HIV-1 infection (**A**) and HIV-1 infection or death (**B**) among infants randomized to regimens A, B, C, and placebo. (Courtesy of Lange JMA, for the Petra Study Team: Efficacy of three short-course regimens of zidovudine and lamivudine in preventing early and late transmission of HIV-1 from mother to child in Tanzania, South Africa, and Uganda [Petra Study]: A randomised, double-blind, placebo-controlled trial. *Lancet* 359:1178-1186, 2002. Reprinted with permission from Elsevier Science.)

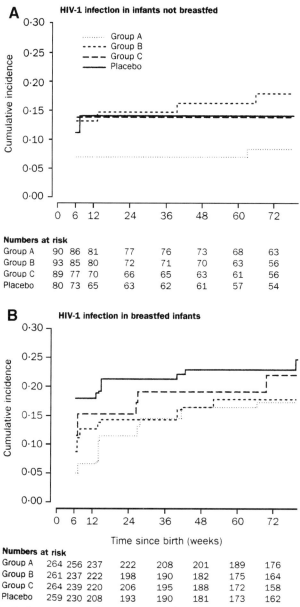

A   HIV-1 infection in infants not breastfed

Cumulative incidence

.... Group A
----- Group B
--- Group C
——— Placebo

Time axis: 0 6 12 24 36 48 60 72

Numbers at risk

Group A	90	86	81	77	76	73	68	63
Group B	93	85	80	72	71	70	63	56
Group C	89	77	70	66	65	63	61	56
Placebo	80	73	65	63	62	61	57	54

B   HIV-1 infection in breastfed infants

Cumulative incidence

Time since birth (weeks)

Time axis: 0 6 12 24 36 48 60 72

Numbers at risk

Group A	264	256	237	222	208	201	189	176
Group B	261	237	222	198	190	182	175	164
Group C	264	239	220	206	195	188	172	158
Placebo	259	230	208	193	190	181	173	162

FIGURE 3.—Kaplan-Meier curves for time to HIV-1 infection in each of the four treatment groups for infants who have never been breastfed (**A**) and those who were breastfed (**B**). (Courtesy of Lange JMA, for the Petra Study Team: Efficacy of three short-course regimens of zidovudine and lamivudine in preventing early and late transmission of HIV-1 from mother to child in Tanzania, South Africa, and Uganda [Petra Study]: A randomised, double-blind, placebo-controlled trial. *Lancet* 359:1178-1186, 2002. Reprinted with permission from Elsevier Science.)

needs to be accompanied by interventions to minimize the risk of subsequent transmission by breast-feeding.

▶ Zidovudine (AZT) has been shown to reduce the incidence of newborn and infant HIV infection by nearly 70% when given to HIV-1-positive gravidas in the last half of pregnancy, during labor and delivery, and continuously to both mother and infant to 6 weeks postpartum.[1] The AZT drug regimen makes demands on funding and available health care systems and workers that usually cannot be met in the African continent where a majority of early infant HIV-1 infections, an estimated 500,000 cases per year, occur. For this reason, the administration of nevirapine to women in labor and to newborn infants within 72 hours after birth for the first 4 days of life has stimulated exploration of short-term therapy with reverse transcriptase inhibitors in various treatment regimens.[2] At the end of 2 months, treated mothers, 98% of whom lactated, showed a rate of infant infection of 15% compared with 40% in the placebo-treated group. This rate corresponds well with that attributable to transmission through breast milk in infancy.[3-5]

In this South African prospective, randomized, blinded trial of 3 dosage regimen, placebo-controlled for the first 20 months of the study, AZT was combined with lamivudine, a non-nucleoside reverse transcriptase inhibitor which works by incorporating a nucleoside analogue that stops DNA replication at its incorporation site. A pilot study showed its adjunctive effect coupled with AZT. Dosage varied from regimen A (36 weeks of gestational age, through labor, and maternal and infant administration for the first 7 days postpartum) to regimen C (drug administration during labor and no therapy postpartum). Infants were followed up for 18 months by quantitative polymerase chain reaction (PCR) for infant blood HIV-1 DNA, and by nucleotide sequence–based amplification for HIV-1 RNA prevalence. After 15 to 18 months of age, ELISA was used to test for newborn infection. The results showed progressively increasing infant infection and death rates with time through that period in nursing infants to the point that the advantage to drug therapy decreased to become equal to the rates after placebo administration by 18 months of life. Infants who received regimen C showed little difference from untreated controls. Through follow-up among infants not breast-fed by HIV-1–positive mothers, HIV-1 transmission past 6 weeks was rare. The authors claim that either scheduled or emergency cesarean section significantly lowered infant transmission rates as measured at 6 weeks postpartum. This is an impressive reminder that the benefits of short-term therapy of HIV-1 infection in the gravidas who nurse must be evaluated for at least 24 weeks after delivery. Past that time, HIV-1 DNA recoverable from breast milk begins progressively to decline, and nursing becomes somewhat safer.[3,4]

T. H. Kirschbaum, MD

References

1. 1996 Year Book of Obstetrics, Gynecology, and Women's Health, pp 84-85.
2. 2001 Year Book of Obstetrics, Gynecology, and Women's Health, pp 87-89.
3. 1994 Year Book of Obstetrics, Gynecology, and Women's Health, pp 38-39.

4. 1997 YEAR BOOK OF OBSTETRICS, GYNECOLOGY, AND WOMEN'S HEALTH, pp 89-91.
5. 2000 YEAR BOOK OF OBSTETRICS, GYNECOLOGY, AND WOMEN'S HEALTH, pp 122-123.

Impact of Human Immunodeficiency Virus Type 1 (HIV-1) Subtype on Women Receiving Single-Dose Nevirapine Prophylaxis to Prevent HIV-1 Vertical Transmission (HIV Network for Prevention Trials 012 Study)

Eshleman SH, Becker-Pergola G, Deseyve M, et al (Johns Hopkins Med Institutions, Baltimore, Md; Fred Hutchinson Cancer Research Ctr, Seattle; Univ of Washington, Seattle)
J Infect Dis 184:914-917, 2001   4–4

Background.—Little is known regarding the relationship between HIV-1 subtype (clade) and HIV-1 transmission or pathogenesis. Most HIV-1 infections in Uganda are attributable to subtypes A and D, which have similar prevalence rates. The HIV Network for Prevention Trials (HIVNET) 012 study in Uganda recently demonstrated that single-dose nevirapine (Nvp) prophylaxis is effective in preventing mother-to-child transmission of HIV-1. In that study, pregnant Ugandan women received a single dose of Nvp at the onset of labor, and infants received a single dose of Nvp within 72 hours of birth. That regimen significantly reduced the rate of HIV-1 mother-to-child transmission. In addition, the efficacy, simplicity, and low cost of the HIVNET 012 Nvp regimen make it an attractive regimen for use in areas in which resources are limited. The relationships among HIV-1 subtype, mother-to-child transmission, and the development of Nvp resistance were examined in women who received Nvp prophylaxis during the HIVNET 012 study.

Methods.—In the HIVNET 012 study, plasma samples were collected from women at 7 days and at 6 to 8 weeks after delivery. These same samples were used for HIV-1 subtyping.

Results.—Samples were available from 102 women. Infants from 32 of these women were HIV-1 infected by age 6 to 8 weeks, and infants from 70 women were uninfected. HIV-1 subtypes included 50 subtype A (49%), 35 subtype D (34%), 4 subtype C (4%), 12 recombinant subtype (12%), and 1 subtype unclassified. There appeared to be no difference in the rate of mother-to-child transmission among women with subtype A versus D. Nvp resistance mutations were detected more frequently at 6 to 8 weeks postpartum in women with subtype D than in women with subtype A.

Conclusions.—The distribution of HIV-1 subtypes in this cohort is similar to the distribution found in Uganda in recent epidemiologic studies. Further studies are needed to more clearly define the relationship between HIV-1 subtype and Nvp resistance among women receiving Nvp prophylaxis.

▶ The demonstration that a single oral dose of Nvp given to HIV-1–positive women at the onset of labor coupled with a newborn dose of 2 mg/kg within 72 hours of life resulted in a decrease in the maternal-to-fetal infection transfer rate of HIV from 40% to 15% was an important step.[1] This together with the reduction in cost from $48,000 per patient in Europe and North America to $4 in Uganda was important in increasing the prospects for pediatric control of the infection.[1] Much of the residual pediatric infection is attributable to breast-feeding, which for cultural reasons and the absence of adequate facilities for formula feeding, is nearly universal among Ugandan women. The agent Nvp has the advantage of rapid absorption and fetal transfer where it is immediately available without further biological processing to destroy both intracellular and extracellular virus. This is an ancillary part of the HIV prevention trial (HIV-NET O12) designed to explore among HIV-1 subtypes possible specific differences in maternal-to-fetal transfer rates and in mutational development of Nvp resistance. Typing is based on the detection of changes in normal nucleoside composition and alignment in amino acids corresponding to the HIV protease and reverse transcriptase–responsive elements of the HIV-1 virus. The results, though preliminary, show some promise in the ability to match drug therapy to the development of drug resistance among viral types.

Blood samples obtained from parturients 6 to 8 weeks postpartum, from 102 women whose HIV-I subtypes were determined and whose infants were exposed through pregnancy and compared subtypes of 32 infected with 70 who were uninfected, demonstrated subtype A in 49%, subtype D in 34%, subtype C in 4%, and recombinant forms in 12%. The latter represent recombinations among types A and D, likely resulting from a high incidence of coinfection with both types, which is commonplace in sub-Saharan Africa. The overall maternal-to-fetal transfer rates in this population receiving Nvp was 15.3%. No difference in maternal-to-fetal transcription rates were seen among HIV-1 types, but the incidence of viral mutations with the effect of decreasing Nvp responsiveness was 18% in parturients 6 to 8 weeks postpartum, and 2.93 times more common among type D compared with type A infected women. There is suggestive evidence that the interval from HIV-1 infection to the development of AIDS is briefer with subtype D HIV-1 infection, but a more definitive answer will follow long-term follow-up of these women. This study certainly shows the striking mutability of HIV-1, which is a substantive challenge to its chemotherapeutics.

T. H. Kirschbaum, MD

References

1. 2001 Year Book of Obstetrics, Gynecology, and Women's Health, pp 87-89.

Perinatal Transmission of Human Immunodeficiency Virus Type 1 by Pregnant Women with RNA Virus Loads <1000 Copies/mL
Ioannidis JPA, Abrams EJ, Ammann A, et al (Univ of Ioannina, Greece; Tufts Univ, Boston; Harvard School of Public Health, Boston; et al)
J Infect Dis 183:539-545, 2001   4–5

Background.—The maternal viral load of HIV-1 is a strong predictor of perinatal HIV transmission. Current antiretroviral therapy aims to maintain viral load at less than 1000 copies/mL, but whether this prevents HIV transmission to the neonate is not known. A collaborative registry of 7 large European and American prospective trials was established to investigate this issue.

Study Design.—There were 5 cohort studies and 2 randomized trials included in the collaborative registry. The study group consisted of 1202 mother-infant pairs from these 7 studies, in which the mother had viral loads of less than 1000 copies/mL. Of these, there were 44 mother-infant pairs with perinatal transmission who formed the basis of the study. Transmission rates were estimated for mothers who received antiretroviral therapy and for those who did not. Unadjusted risk ratios for transmission were calculated. Multivariate logistic regression analyses were performed to consider other potential prognostic factors. The efficacy of maternal antiretroviral therapy in preventing perinatal transmission in this low-risk patient group was analyzed.

Findings.—For those HIV+ mothers with low virus loads who received antiretroviral therapy during pregnancy, the perinatal transmission rate was 1.0%. For those HIV+ mothers with low virus loads who did not receive antiretroviral therapy during pregnancy, there was a 10% perinatal transmission rate. Multivariate analysis indicated that lower transmission rates were associated with antiretroviral therapy, cesarean section, higher birth weight and higher maternal CD4 cell count. In 12 of the 44 cases, serial RNA measurements were available. In 10 of the 12 cases, viral load was greater than 500 copies/mL.

Conclusion.—Antiretroviral therapy is effective in preventing perinatal transmission of HIV from mothers with low viral loads (less than 1000 copies/mL) to their infants. This therapy should be continued during pregnancy, even for mothers with low viral loads.

▶ This is a test of the presumption that it is appropriate that highly effective antiretroviral therapy (HART) for HIV infection—including proteinase inhibitors—aims at reducing maternal viral loads to 1000 HIV-1 RNA copies/mL[3] of blood as a test of adequate therapy. Though anecdotal accounts of maternal-to-fetal infection below this copy number are clear, they are so rare as to prevent meaningful rate estimates. That was the purpose of this collaborative data collection from 7 European and American treatment centers. Stringent criteria for newborn infection helped avoid laboratory errors and confusion between passive versus active fetal antibody. All 1201 women were required to have HIV-1 RNA concentrations less than 1000/mL in studies performed in Europe or the United States.

Of the 70% of women untreated with HART, newborn transmission occurred in 9.8% at birth, and in the 30% of women treated with HART, the transmission rate was 0.96%. As usual, the identifiable risk factors for newborn infection were maternal CD4 count equal to or less than 500/mL, prematurity by gestational age or low birth weight, and ruptured membranes at least 4 hours prior to birth. As the authors point out, the primary limitation of the study was that maternal blood measurements at delivery were sometimes lacking but more than 80% were sampled either in the last month of pregnancy or within 3 days of newborn life. This is a reassuring demonstration of the appropriateness of the therapeutic goals defined above, and objective evidence of the virtue of proteinase inhibitors in the prevention of fetal HIV infection.

T. H. Kirschbaum, MD

Randomized Trial of Presumptive Sexually Transmitted Disease Therapy During Pregnancy in Rakai, Uganda
Gray RH, Wabwire-Mangen F, Kigozi G, et al (Johns Hopkins Univ, Baltimore, Md; Makerere Univ, Kampala, Uganda; Uganda Virus Research Inst, Entebbe; et al)
Am J Obstet Gynecol 185:1209-1217, 2001   4–6

Background.—Controlling sexually transmitted diseases (STDs) is especially important in developing nations, where the rates of such infection are high. The effects of presumptive STD treatment on pregnancy outcome and HIV transmission were assessed in a community, randomized trial conducted in the rural Rakai district of southwestern Uganda.

Methods and Findings.—In this district, 2070 pregnant women were assigned to presumptive STD treatment one time during pregnancy at varying gestational ages, and 1963 control subjects received iron and folate and referral for syphilis. The rate ratio for *Trichomonas vaginalis* was 0.28; for bacterial vaginosis, 0.78; for *Neisseria gonorrhoeae/Chlamydia trachomatis*, 0.43; and for infant ophthalmia, 0.37. The rates of neonatal death were also reduced, with a rate ratio of 0.83. The rate ratios for low birth weight and preterm delivery were 0.68 and 0.77, respectively (Table 6). However, maternal HIV acquisition and perinatal HIV transmission were unaffected (Tables 5A and 5B).

Conclusions.—Reducing maternal STD improved pregnancy outcomes in this rural district in Uganda. Unfortunately, it did not decrease maternal HIV acquisition or perinatal HIV transmission.

▶ There is strong epidemiologic evidence that acute and chronic STD serve as cofactors to HIV-1 infection and presumably that STD treatment might be expected to reduce the rate of new HIV infection. In this prospective, controlled, randomized study in Uganda, it was not possible to demonstrate a resultant decrease in HIV infections. Women aged 15 to 59 years were enrolled and randomly assigned to receive azithromycin, cefixine, and metronidazole; those with serologic evidence of syphilis were treated with benzathine penicillin regardless of random assignment. Gravidas were enrolled at various durations of pregnancy and, therefore, the time of possible protection conferred by STD treatment was an uncontrolled variable. Treatment and follow-up data were obtained during 3 surveys each 1 month apart. The prevalence of HIV-1 infection was greater in the intervention than the control arm (15.5% vs 12.0%,) but not significantly so (Table 5). The impact of antibiotic treatment was evident from significant reductions in vaginal infections and infant ophthalmia as well as lesser early infant mortality and low birth weight. No significant decrease in

TABLE 6.—Low Birth Weight and Preterm Birth

	Intervention Arm		Control Arm		
	Infections/ Tested (n)	Prevalence (%)	Infections/ Tested (n)	Prevalence (%)	Cluster Adjusted RR (95% CI)*
Chest circumference <30 cm	131/1438	9.1	136/1236	11.0	0.68 (0.53-0.86)
Head circumference <31 cm and/or chest circumference <30 cm	178/1478	12.0	172/1266	13.6	0.76 (0.59-0.99)
Preterm delivery ≤36 weeks, based on Ballard score	141/1438	9.8	145/1228	11.8	0.77 (0.56-1.05)
Preterm (<36 wk) and chest circumference <30 cm	41/1425	2.9	44/1223	3.6	0.59 (0.30-1.21)

*Variables included in the model: month of pregnancy at enrollment, infant sex, maternal age, parity, education, marital status, number of sex partners during pregnancy, and HIV status.
(Courtesy of Gray RH, Wabwire-Mangen F, Kigozi G, et al: Randomized trial of presumptive sexually transmitted disease therapy during pregnancy in Rakai, Uganda. *Am J Obstet Gynecol* 185:1209-1217, 2001.)

TABLE 5A.—Maternal and Infant HIV Infection

	Intervention Arm		Control Arm		
Maternal HIV Incidence	Incidence (n)/ Person y	Rate/100 Person y	Incidence/ Person y	Rate/100 Person y	Cluster Adjusted RR (95% CI)
All maternal seroconversions	28/833	3.4	15/657	2.3	1.44 (0.64-3.25)*
During pregnancy	17/425	4.0	9/368	2.5	1.16 (0.31-4.32)*
After delivery	11/408	2.7	6/289	2.1	1.12 (0.75-1.71)*

*Adjusted for age and number of sexual partners by Poisson regression, with the use of cluster-paired analyses (with cluster pairing based on baseline HIV prevalence).
(Courtesy of Gray RH, Wabwire-Mangen F, Kigozi G, et al: Randomized trial of presumptive sexually transmitted disease therapy during pregnancy in Rakai, Uganda. *Am J Obstet Gynecol* 185:1209-1217, 2001.)

TABLE 5B.—Maternal and Infant HIV Infection

	Intervention Arm		Control Arm		
	Infections/ Tested (n)	Proportion (%)	Infections/ tested (n)	Proportion (%)	Cluster Adjusted RR (95% CI)
Maternal HIV prevalence	254/1640	15.5	176/1374	12.8	1.14 (0.73-1.77)†
Maternal-to-child HIV transmission					
All	38/207	18.4	30/144	20.8	1.05 (0.40-2.79)‡
0-6 d	13/75	17.2	7/41	17.1	0.74 (0.08-6.53)‡
7 d-6 wk	25/132	18.9	23/103	22.3	0.92 (0.29-2.91)‡

†Adjusted for age and number of sex partners in the past year by logistic regression, with the use of cluster-paired analyses.
‡Adjusted for paired clusters.
Abbreviation: RR, Rate ratio.
(Courtesy of Gray RH, Wabwire-Mangen F, Kigozi G, et al: Randomized trial of presumptive sexually transmitted disease therapy during pregnancy in Rakai, Uganda. *Am J Obstet Gynecol* 185:1209-1217, 2001.)

preterm birth occurred, nor were there significant decreases in maternal HIV-1 serologic conversions during or after pregnancy. Maternal-to-fetal transmission rates (18.5% and 20.8% in infant intervention and control groups, respectively) were not significantly different. The incidence of chorioamnionitis was not effected by treatment, and both groups had a roughly 50% incidence of HIV-1 testing and counseling.

The purpose of this study was to evaluate the merits of widespread STD treatment on HIV-1 acquisition during pregnancy. The results were clearly negative. Other more focused research is needed to evaluate other possible benefits of this widespread approach to STDs.

T. H. Kirschbaum, MD

Pregnancy Outcome in Type 1 Diabetic Women With Microalbuminuria
Ekbom P, Feldt-Rasmussen U, Damm P, et al (Natl Univ Hosp (Rigshospitalet), Copenhagen; Steno Diabetes Ctr, Gentofte, Denmark)
Diabetes Care 24:1739-1744, 2001   4–7

Background.—Pregnant women with type 1 diabetic nephropathy are at increased risk for preeclampsia and preterm delivery associated with increased perinatal morbidity. Microalbuminuria is an early sign of diabetic microvascular disease that precedes diabetic nephropathy in patients with type 1 diabetes. The influence of microalbuminuria on maternal complications and fetal outcome in patients with type 1 diabetes was examined in this prospective cohort study.

Study Design.—The study group consisted of 240 white women with type 1 diabetes who entered obstetric care before 17 weeks of gestation from January 1996 to November 1999. These women were categorized by their urinary albumin excretion levels. There were 203 women with normal urinary albumin excretion (<30 mg/24 h), 26 women with microalbuminuria (30-300 mg/24 h), and 11 women with diabetic nephropathy (>300 mg/24 h). These women were also classified according to the system of White. Multivariate logistic regression analysis was employed to identify those variables independently associated with preterm delivery and preeclampsia.

Findings.—Preterm deliveries occurred in 91% of women with diabetic nephropathy, 62% of those with microalbuminuria, and 35% of those with normal urinary albumin excretion. Preeclampsia developed in 64% of the women with diabetic nephropathy, 42% of those with microalbuminuria, and 6% of those with normal urinary albumin excretion (Table 2). Urinary albumin excretion level was independently associated with preterm delivery and preeclampsia.

Conclusion.—In pregnant women with type 1 diabetes, microalbuminuria is associated with an increased risk of preterm delivery associated with preeclampsia. Classification according to urinary albumin excretion and metabolic control in the first trimester is superior to the White system of

TABLE 2.—Pregnancy Course and Outcome in 240 Women With Type 1 Diabetes and Normal Urinary Albumin Excretion, Microalbuminuria, and Nephropathy

	Normal Urinary Albumin Excretion	Microalbuminuria	Nephropathy	$P*$
n	203	26	11	—
HbA_{1c}, weeks 10-34 (%)*	6.5 ± 0.7	6.7 ± 0.6	7.3 ± 0.6	<0.01
Preeclampsia	12 (6)	11 (42)	7 (64)	<0.001
Pregnancy-induced hypertension without proteinuria	11 (5)	1 (4)	—	NS
Proteinuria >3 g/24 h	1 (0.5)	6 (23)	6 (55)	<0.001
Preterm delivery before week 37	71 (35)	16 (62)	10 (91)	<0.001
Preterm delivery before week 34	12 (6)	6 (23)	5 (45)	<0.001
Perinatal mortality	3 (1.5)	1 (4)	0	NS
Singleton small-for-gestational-age infants (<10%)†	4 (2)	1 (4)	5 (45)	<0.001
Birth weight, singletons (g)†	3,553 ± 672	3,124 ± 767	2,235 ± 1038	<0.001
Major congenital malformations	5 (2.5)	1 (4)	1 (9)	NS
Tachypnea continuous positive pressure <1 h, singletons‡	42 (21)	4 (15)	6 (55)	NS
Jaundice requiring treatment, singletons‡	30 (15)	2 (8)	8 (73)	<0.01

Note: Data are number (percentage) or means ± standard deviation.
*Mean of HbA_{1c} values in weeks 10, 14, 20, 28, and 34.
†n = 197, 23, and 11, respectively.
‡n = 195, 23, and 11, respectively. The statistics applied are χ^2 trend test when comparing categorical data and linear trend test (regression) for 1-way analysis of variance when comparing continuous data.
Abbreviation: NS, Not significant.
(Courtesy of Ekbom P, Feldt-Rasmussen U, Damm P, et al: Pregnancy outcome in type 1 diabetic women with microalbuminuria. *Diabetes Care* 24:1739-1744. Copyright 2001 American Diabetes Association. Reprinted with permission from The American Diabetes Association.)

classification for the prediction of preterm delivery in women with type 1 diabetes.

▶ Microalbuminuria—that is, urinary albumin excretion in the range of 30 to 300 mg for 24 hours—is a frequent intermediate stage in the development of diabetic nephropathy in type I diabetics. Though albuminuria at this excretion rate is usually considered normal, when it is part of a pattern of progressive increase prior to and during pregnancy, it carries with it the same increase in risk of development of pregnancy hypertension, preterm delivery, and growth retardation as seen in White's class F women with full-blown nephropathy, albeit not as frequently. It is a point obstetricians often miss because it was not a part of the original White classification.

Here, a group of 240 type I diabetics were reviewed in light of measurements of blood pressure, hemoglobin A_{1c}, and albuminuria over the 2 years prior to presentation in pregnancy. In this way, 26 women, or about 10% of type I diabetics, were found to have microalbuminuria preceding pregnancy, and 11, or 5%, of those had established diabetic nephropathy. Thirty five percent were already receiving antihypertensive agents, though most of them were normotensive.

Table 2 shows their 42% incidence of pregnancy hypertension, their 62% incidence of preterm delivery, and decrease in mean birth weight based on trend analysis using chi-square. It is well to look for microalbuminuria in pregnancy type I diabetics since it offers a strong hint of the likelihood of pregnancy complications and the need for even more careful antenatal monitoring than usual in those usually normotensive women.

T. H. Kirschbaum, MD

Sonographic Estimation of Fetal Weight in Macrosomic Fetuses: Diabetic Versus Non-Diabetic Pregnancies
Wong SF, Chan FY, Cincotta RB, et al (Mater Mothers' Hosp, South Brisbane, Queensland, Australia)
Aust N Z J Obstet Gynaecol 41:429-432, 2001   4–8

Background.—Fetal weight is frequently estimated with US scanning. In women with diabetes and macrosomic fetuses, the estimated fetal weight (EFW) often influences mode of delivery. Macrosomic babies of diabetic women had anthropometric features that differ from macrosomic babies of women without diabetes. This study was conducted to compare the accuracy of sonographic estimation of fetal weight of macrosomic babies in diabetic versus nondiabetic pregnancies.

Methods.—This retrospective study included all babies weighing 4000 g or more at birth who had US scans performed within 1 week of delivery. Pregnancies with diabetes were compared with pregnancies without diabetes mellitus. Comparisons were made between the 2 groups for mean simple error, which was defined as the actual birth weight minus the estimated fetal weight; mean standardized absolute error (which was defined as the absolute value of simple error [grams]/actual birth weight [kilograms]); and the percentage of estimated birth weight falling within 15% of the actual birth weight. From a total of 9516 deliveries during the study period, a total of 56 nondiabetic pregnancies and 19 diabetic pregnancies were compared.

Results.—Among the diabetic pregnancies, the average sonographic estimation of fetal weight was 8% less than the actual birth weight; by comparison, the average sonographic estimation of fetal weight in the nondiabetic group was 0.2% less than the actual birth weight. The estimated fetal weight was within 15% of the birth weight in 74% of the diabetic pregnancies and in 93% of the nondiabetic pregnancies. Underestimation of the birth weight by more than 15% occurred in 26.3% of the diabetic group compared with 5.4% of the nondiabetic group.

Conclusions.—These findings demonstrate significantly worse predictive accuracy for estimation of fetal weight with standard formulas in macrosomic fetuses when the pregnant woman has diabetes compared with pregnant women who do not have diabetes. A more conservative measure should be considered when sonographic fetal weight estimation is used to influence the mode of delivery for women with diabetes.

▶ This retrospective cohort study provides a clear reminder of the problems of ultrasonic estimated fetal weight determinations specific to infants of diabetic mothers. It contains comparative data from infants born with birth weights more than 4 kg who had ultrasonic weight determinations done 1 week or less before delivery. Nineteen were infants of diabetic mothers and 85 were born to nondiabetics. Estimated fetal weight is frequently calculated by Hadlock's method or a derivative. The problem in estimating macrosomic diabetic fetuses ultrasonically arises because their femur lengths and head transverse or circumferential measurements tend to be the same, or smaller than, those of normal fetuses. Because increased abdominal circumference, the most distinctive finding in these infants, tends to be underrepresented in the estimated fetal weight calculation compared with the other variables, these infants tend to have estimated fetal weights underestimated by US. In this experience the diabetic newborn mean biparietal and head circumference values (93 and 339 mm, respectively) were significantly smaller than those of newborns of nondiabetic mothers (96 and 349 mm, respectively). Comparing projected with actual newborn weight measurements, the mean difference for infants with diabetic mothers was an underestimate of 378 g compared with 16 g for nondiabetic pregnancies. Ultrasonic estimations of fetal weight were 8% less than the actual birth weight compared with 0.2% in nondiabetics. This is only a particular case in the general proposition that ultrasonic birth weight is faulty in the upper range of birth weight at and above 4 kg. It is part of the general unsolved problem of diabetic fetal weight at term and part of the rationale for early delivery for these infants, all other things being equal.

T. H. Kirschbaum, MD

Maternal and Fetal Inherited Thrombophilias Are Not Related to the Development of Severe Preeclampsia

Livingston JC, Barton JR, Park V, et al (Univ of Tennessee, Memphis)
Am J Obstet Gynecol 185:153-157, 2001   4–9

Objective.—Thrombotic vascular disease may predispose patients to the development of preeclampsia. The purpose of this study was to determine whether maternal or fetal genotype frequencies of the inherited thrombophilic gene mutations (factor V Leiden, methylenetetrahydrofolate, and prothrombin) are altered in severe preeclampsia.

Study Design.—We performed a prospective cross-sectional study to compare the maternal and fetal genotype frequencies of factor V Leiden, methylenetetrahydrofolate, and prothrombin. One hundred ten patients with severe preeclampsia were matched for gestational age to 97 normotensive pregnancies. Umbilical cord blood was obtained from 92 control patients and 75 patients with preeclampsia. Deoxyribonucleic acid was extracted from leukocytes and polymerase chain reaction was performed. Polymerase chain reaction products were digested with the appropriate restriction enzyme and fractionated by gel electrophoresis. Genotype frequencies were calculated. Statistical significance was determined by the χ^2 test.

Results.—There were no significant differences between patients with severe preeclampsia and control patients regarding frequency of maternal factor V Leiden G/506/A mutation (4.4% vs 4.3%; $P = .96$), methylenetetrahydrofolate CC/667/TT mutation (9.6% vs 6.3%; $P = .54$), or prothrombin G/20210/A mutation (0% vs 1.1%; $P = .92$). In addition, no statistical difference could be found between fetal thrombophilias and the development of preeclampsia. Findings were similar in both white (n = 47) and African American (n = 63) preeclamptic subsets. Moreover, there was no association between any of the maternal or fetal genetic polymorphisms and the incidence of hemolysis, elevated liver enzymes, and low platelet count syndrome (n = 21); eclampsia (n = 12); or intrauterine growth restriction (n = 9).

Conclusion.—Inherited thrombophilias are not associated with severe preeclampsia.

▶ When the Leiden mutation of clotting factor V was first identified, it was promptly held suspect for a role in the pathogenesis of preeclampsia.[1] This mutation renders factor V resistant to activation by protein C and induces a state of maternal hypercoagulability. Because the microscopic pathology of preeclampsia consists dominantly of small vessel thrombosis, ischemia, and hemorrhage, this supposition was reasonable. As other thrombogenic mutations have been identified over the past 5 years, they have been added to the list of suspects.

This cohort study compares 110 women with severe preeclampsia with 97 normotensive gravidas as well as umbilical blood from 75 preeclamptic pregnancies and 92 normal pregnancies with respect to the presences of the Leiden V mutation, the methylenetetrahydrofolate reductase and prothrombin

III mutations, all determined by maternal and fetal genomic polymerase chain reaction and diagnostic restriction enzyme application. There were no significant differences in the frequencies of these specific gene mutations in either preeclamptic women or their fetuses in comparison with controls. As the authors point out, these findings lack the assurance that might come from the prospective longitudinal study of a larger number of suspects, but it should suffice to dissuade those who do costly screening or prophylactic therapy for preeclamptic prevention on women who carry one of these mutations.

T. H. Kirschbaum, MD

Reference

1. 1998 YEAR BOOK OF OBSTETRICS, GYNECOLOGY, AND WOMEN'S HEALTH, pp 211-212.

Pregnancy Outcomes After Peripheral Blood or Bone Marrow Transplantation: A Retrospective Survey

Apperley JF, for the Late Effects Working Party of the European Group for Blood and Marrow Transplantation (Hammersmith Hosp, London)
Lancet 358:271-276, 2001   4–10

Introduction.—Some patients who undergo transplantation of hemopoietic stem cells (peripheral blood or bone marrow) become permanently infertile, whereas others retain or recover fertility. The outcome of conception in females and partners of males previously treated by autologous or allogenic stem cell transplantation (SCT) was examined in a retrospective, multicenter investigation.

Methods.—Questionnaires were sent to 229 centers of the European Group for Blood and Marrow Transplantation. Data were gathered concerning the original disease, transplant procedure, and outcome of conception for both male and female patients.

Results.—One hundred ninety-nine centers responded with information regarding 19,412 allogeneic and 17,950 autologous transplant patients. There were 232 (0.6%) patients who conceived after SCT. The crude annual birth rate for 4-month survivors of SCT was lower, compared with the national average for England and Wales, at 1.7/1000 patients. There were 312 conceptions reported in 113 patients (74 allograft) and partners of 119 patients (93 allograft). Most pregnancies were uncomplicated and produced 271 live births. Twenty-eight (42%) of 67 allograft recipients underwent cesarean section, compared with 16% in the normal population (difference, 26%; 95% CI, 15-38); 12 (20%) of 59 had preterm delivery compared with a normal rate of 6% (difference, 14%; CI, 4-24), and 12 (23%) of 52 had low birth weight singleton offspring, compared with a normal rate of 6% (difference,17%; CI, 6-29) (Table 5).

Conclusion.—Pregnancy after SCT is likely to result in live birth. Pregnancies in patients who undergo allograft and have received high total body

TABLE 5.—Characteristics of Offspring

	Female		Male
	Autograft	Allograft	Both Groups
Total singleton livebirths (*)	32 (26)	73 (52)	132 (112)
LBW (1·8-2·5 kg)	3	9	5
VLBW (<1·8 kg)	0	3	1
Birthweight (median [range], kg)	3·14 (2-4·57)	3·13 (0·87-3·47)	3·34 (1·2-4·6)
All livebirths (*)	38 (34)	84 (73)	149 (136)
F:M	16/18	42/31	71/65
Congenital anomalies	0	3†	4‡
Perinatal problems	0	2§	3‖

*Number for which data were available are given in parentheses.
†One case each of cerebral palsy and patent ductus arteriosus, dislocation of the hip, and umbilical hernia.
‡ Everted feet (3 siblings), congenital hemangioma.
§Two deaths from pulmonary failure at 6.5 weeks and 3 months of age.
‖One case each of acute respiratory distress syndrome, death from vitamin K deficiency at age 2 months, and sudden infant death syndrome.
Abbreviations: LBW, Low birth weight; *VLBW,* very low birth weight; *F:M,* female-to-male child ratio.
(Courtesy of Apperley JF, for the Late Effects Working Party of the European Group for Blood and Marrow Transplantation: Pregnancy outcomes after peripheral blood or bone marrow transplantation: A retrospective survey. *Lancet* 358:271-276, 2001. Reprinted with permission from Elsevier Science.)

irradiation should be considered at high risk for both maternal and fetal complications.

▶ The use of SCT from blood or bone marrow sources has grown over the past 2 decades and prospects for its continued growth are very good. This retrospective review of data from 229 European centers operating prior to July 1995 provides a comprehensive comparison to pregnancy outcomes from national statistical data from England, Wales, France, and Nordic countries, and some other European nations. The data matrices are complex and involve allografts and autografts in 232 women and 312 pregnancies for differing indications, pretransplant treatment (chemotherapy with or without total body radiation), and both natural and artificial reproductive techniques. Included among the latter were in vitro fertilization, using frozen partner's sperm, cryopreserved embryo transplants, and menopausal gonadotropin therapy. Since women pregnant by male patients had normal pregnancies, some simplification of results is possible.

Among the 312 pregnancies of patients or partners of patients, the birth rate, based on newborn survival to 4 months, was 1.7/1000 live births compared to a norm of 12.5 per 1000 live births. This difference reflected the impact of underlying disease (malignancy, aplastic anemia, thalasemia major) and pre-implantation therapy. Of 21 of 74 women who received total body x-radiation prior to allografts or malignant disease, 12 conceived normally with 9 using artificial reproductive therapy. The incidence of multiple pregnancy was 6%, reflecting the use of artificial reproductive therapy. Pregnancy-induced hypertension occurred in 15%, and the cesarean section rate of 38% reflected the concern for high risk pregnancies. Both the incidences of preterm births and low birth weight were increased compared to the norms, but there was no increase in the incidence of spontaneous abortion and congenital anomalies among the stem cell recipients. In general, reproduction in female SCT is uncommon, clinically complicated but clearly possible. This study provides estimates of risks for enough permutations of independent variables that it deserves direct reading by those counseling a couple interested in post stem cell transplant therapy.

T. H. Kirschbaum, MD

Is There an Increased Maternal-Infant Prevalence of Factor V Leiden in Association With Severe Pre-eclampsia?

Currie L, Peek M, McNiven M, et al (Canberra Hosp, Garran, Australia; Univ of Sydney, Australia)
Br J Obstet Gynaecol 109:191-196, 2002   4–11

Introduction.—There is suspicion that the factor V Leiden mutation contributes to the development of obstetric complications by promoting the formation of microthrombi in the placenta and thus compromising fetomaternal circulation. It is possible that if placental infarction occurs before onset of disease or develops as a consequence, then factor V Leiden in the fetus could be a factor in the development of preeclampsia via placental compromise. The prevalence of factor V Leiden mutation in children and maternal-infant pairs in pregnancies affected by severe pre-eclampsia was compared with its prevalence in unmatched normal controls in a prospective cohort investigation.

Methods.—Samples of DNA were extracted from cheek swabs obtained from 48 maternal-infant pairs in whom the index pregnancy was affected by severe preeclampsia, and from 46 unmatched maternal-infant pairs in whom the index pregnancy was defined as normal. The main outcome measure was the prevalence of factor V Leiden mutation in mothers, infants, and maternal-infant pairs in association with severe preeclampsia compared with the prevalence in unmatched controls.

Results.—Two (4.2%) of 48 infants born in severe preeclamptic pregnancies were heterozygous for factor V Leiden mutation, compared with 6 (13.0%) of 46 children in the control group (P = .15). Four (8.3%) of the 48 women affected by severe preeclampsia were heterozygous for factor V Leiden mutation, compared with 6 (13.0%) of the 46 women in the control group (P = .52). The mutation was present in 2 maternal-infant pairs in

TABLE 3.—The Prevalence of the Factor V Leiden Mutation

	Severe Pre-eclamptic (n = 48)	Controls (n = 46)	P	OR (95% CI)
Infants	2(4.2)	6(13.0)	0.15	0.29 (0.06-1.52)
Women	4(8.3)	6(13.0)	0.52	0.61 (0.16-2.31)
Maternal–infant pairs	2(4.2)	5(10.9)	0.26	0.36 (0.07-1.94)

Values are n (%).
Abbreviation: OR, Odds ratio.
(Courtesy of Currie L, Peek M, McNiven M, et al: Is there an increased maternal-infant prevalence of factor V Leiden in association with severe pre-eclampsia? *Br J Obstet Gynaecol* 109:191-196, 2002. With permission from Elsevier Science.)

pregnancies affected by severe preeclampsia, and in 5 (10.9%) of the control pregnancies ($P = .26$) (Table 3).

Conclusion.—There was no evidence for increased prevalence of the factor V Leiden mutation in either mothers or children in the severe preeclamptic group. These findings do not support a factor V Leiden fetal or maternal contribution to the development of severe preeclampsia.

▶ With the demonstration that a point mutation in the gene for clotting Factor V that renders it resistant to activation by protein C, causes intravascular clotting, there was hope that this common mutation might bear a causal relationship to preeclampsia.[1,2] Its occurrence in 15% to 20% of Caucasians justified interest in that possibility. Related hypotheses included the production of placental infarction, and ischemic and obliterative endothelial injury. Although a few studies supported the presence of such a relationship and added concern that a fetus bearing the inherited gene defect might also play a role by partial obliteration of the umbilical circulation, the bulk of evidence weighs against the Leiden mutation and other genetic thrombophilias existing inordinately among women with severe preeclampsia.[3] Although this too is a negative study, its design and execution are very strong and worthy of review. In a series of 48 pregnancies marked with severe preeclampsia, DNA was obtained by buccal swab from mother and newborn, and 46 control pairs of unmatched mothers and infants with normal pregnancies were selected for comparisons. Gene amplification was done by polymerase chain reaction, and the mutated gene identified from restriction fragment polymorphisms manifest on column chromotography. The prevalence of the Leiden mutation was less among women and infants from pregnancies with severe preeclampsia than in controls, although not statistically significantly so. The same findings persist when possible faults in the control structures were tested. Regrettably, this study fails to support such a relationship and adds to the quantity of negative evidence. Regrettably, the Leiden mutation hypothesis appears to have been a false lead to the etiology of preeclampsia.

T. H. Kirschbaum, MD

References

1. 1998 Year Book of Obstetrics, Gynecology, and Women's Health, pp 210-211.
2. 1999 Year Book of Obstetrics, Gynecology, and Women's Health, pp 71-74.
3. 2002 Year Book of Obstetrics, Gynecology, and Women's Health, pp 227-229.

Preeclampsia in Multiple Gestation: The Role of Assisted Reproductive Technologies
Lynch A, McDuffie R Jr, Murphy J, et al (Kaiser Permanente, Denver; Natl Jewish Med and Research Ctr, Denver; Univ of Colorado, Denver)
Obstet Gynecol 99:445-451, 2002   4–12

Background.—Complications related to preeclampsia or eclampsia contribute to nearly 20% of pregnancy-related deaths, and the risk for develop-

TABLE 3.—Multivarable Logistic Regression Analysis Showing the Crude and Adjusted Odds Ratios of Assisted Reproductive Technology and Other Risk Factors for Preeclampsia

Risk Factor		Crude	Odds Ratio Adjusted	95% CI
Model A*				
Assisted reproductive technology	Yes	3.8	2.8	1.1, 7
	No†	1.0	1.0	
Clomiphene citrate	Yes	1.2	1.3	0.6, 3.1
	No†	1.0	1.0	
HMG	Yes	1.5	2.0	0.6, 6.7
	No†	1.0	1.0	
History of clomiphene citrate	Yes	1.9	0.9	0.4, 1.9
	No†	1.0	1.0	
History of HMG	Yes	1.3	0.6	0.2, 1.6
	No†	1.0	1.0	
Maternal age‡		1.1	1.0	0.9, 1.1
Parity	Nulliparity	2.3	2.0	1.2, 3.2
	Multiparity†	1.0	1.0	
Maternal race	Black	0.4	0.6	0.2, 2
	Other†	1.0	1.0	
Fetal number	Triplets/quadruplets	2.6	1.5	0.6, 4
	Twins†	1.0	1.0	
Preexisting hypertension	Yes	1.5	1.7	0.6, 5
	No†	1.0	1.0	
Model B§				
Assisted reproductive technology	Yes	3.8	2.1	1.1, 4.1
	No†	1.0	1.0	
Maternal age‡		1.1	1.1	1.0, 1.1
Parity	Nulliparity	2.3	2.1	1.3, 3.4
	Multiparity†	1.0	1.0	

*Model A is the fully adjusted multivariable logistic regression model containing the primary and secondary exposures and other risk factors.
†Referent group.
‡Maternal age examined as a continuous variable.
§Model B is the multivariable logistic regression model after backward selection of statistically unimportant variables (ovulation induction treatment with clomiphene citrate or human menopausal gonadotropin, previous ovulation induction with clomiphene citrate or human menopausal gonadotropin, maternal race, fetal number, and preexisting maternal hypertension) from model A.
Abbreviation: HMG, Human menopausal gonadotropin.
(Reprinted with permission from The American College of Obstetricians and Gynecologists courtesy of Lynch A, McDuffie R Jr, Murphy J, et al: Preeclampsia in multiple gestation: The role of assisted reproductive technologies. Obstet Gynecol 99:445-451, 2002.)

ment of hypertensive disorders during pregnancy is twice as high with multiple births as with singletons. The incidence of multiple births has increased with the assisted conception methods now more widely available. Whether assisted reproductive technology and the use of ovulation-inducing agents are related to the development of preeclampsia was assessed in 528 multiple births. Both established and new risk factors were analyzed for their possible contribution to this relationship.

Methods.—Data were obtained from a Colorado HMO and assessed retrospectively. Univariate and logistic regression analysis techniques were used to see whether women who conceived a multiple gestation through assisted conception ran a higher risk of preeclampsia than those whose multiple gestations were spontaneous.

Results.—Of the 528 multiple gestations, 95% were twins, 4.7% triplets, and 1 a set of quadruplets. Three hundred thirty were spontaneous and 198 were assisted; of the assisted gestations, 75% of the mothers were over age 35 years and more of these women were white, married, and nulliparous than among the spontaneous group. Preeclampsia developed in 94 women, with 74% mild cases and 26% severe. Delivery was induced because of preeclampsia in 85% of the cases.

The relative risk of development of preeclampsia among women who were assisted in conception was higher than among women whose multiple gestations were spontaneous, specifically, 4.8 and 2.7, respectively. When the other risk factors were assessed, assisted reproductive technologies and nulliparity were significantly associated with risk of preeclampsia. Older women also showed an increased incidence of preeclampsia. Thus, the only variables linked to preeclampsia were assisted reproductive technologies, maternal age, and nulliparity (Table 3), with mothers whose conception was assisted having a 2.1-fold higher likelihood of development of preeclampsia.

Conclusion.—Preeclampsia developed twice as often among women whose multiple gestation resulted from assisted reproductive technologies as among women whose gestations were spontaneous. Maternal age and nulliparity were also noted to be significant factors; women seeking assisted conception tend to be older than those who have spontaneous multiple gestations.

▶ The incidence of preeclampsia is increased in multiple gestations compared to singlets, and several investigators have reason to suggest there is an increased risk among pregnancies conceived by assisted reproductive technology (ART) involving manipulative procedures done on ova or embryos. This study deals with whether or not ART further increases the 2-fold risk of preeclampsia inherent in twin pregnancies, normally conceived. The authors explore a database reflecting 7 years obstetrical experience at Colorado's Kaiser Permanente facilities consisting of 28,905 births, 528 multiple births, 86 of them (16.2%) preeclamptic. The diagnosis was based on standard definitions but did not exclude multiparas who composed 30% of the study population. Preexisting hypertension was estimated by recording blood pressure of more than 140/90 prior to pregnancy or to the 20th gestational week in 21 women.

Comparisons were made among 69 women treated with ART, 91 with induction of ovulation using clomiphene or human menopausal gonadotropin (not ART), and 330 conceiving unassisted. Univariate comparisons showed significantly increased risk ratios for preeclampsia for women using ART but not ovulation stimulation. Using multivariate logistic regression, only ART (2.8-fold increase) and multiparity (2.0-fold increase) showed a significant independent relationship with the occurrence of preeclampsia. Neither maternal age, race, nor fetal number or any other potential confounders showed such a relationship.

This observation is consistent with the hypothesis that preeclampsia represents a failure of immune privilege of the fetal allograft by the maternal immune system. Exploration of the use of surgically obtained sperm in ART is consonant with the proposition that maternal contact with potential paternal epitopes contained in semen helps desensitize the mother to fetal antigens normally conveyed by the paternal halpotype of the father (see Abstract 4–14) and prevents preeclampsia. Failure of exposure to semen via donor insemination or embryo transfer ablates this hypothetical desensitization step and may increase the risk of preeclampsia. Leon Chesley would be proud of the affirmation of his recognition that preeclampsia is primarily a disease of the primigravid.[1]

T. H. Kirschbaum, MD

Reference

1. Chesley L: Recognition of the long term sequelae of eclampsia. *Am J Obstet Gynecol* 182:249, 2000.

Long Term Mortality of Mothers and Fathers After Pre-Eclampsia: Population Based Cohort Study
Irgens HU, Reisæter L, Irgens LM, et al (Univ of Bergen, Norway)
BMJ 323:1213-1217, 2001   4–13

Background.—The causes of preeclampsia are not well known. It has been established that there is a paradoxic preventive effect when the mother smokes, but the underlying mechanism has not been elucidated. It is likely that maternal and fetal genes, including paternal genes expressed in the fetus, also play a part. There is a high risk of preeclampsia recurrence in subsequent pregnancies and a strong association of risks between sisters as well as an increased occurrence in daughters of mothers who had preeclampsia, all of which provide further evidence of maternal genes for susceptibility. Paternal genes also seemed to be involved in preeclampsia. Recently it has been proposed that there are common risk factors for preeclampsia and atherosclerosis. The set of genes that expresses thrombophilia is a candidate for susceptibility to preeclampsia. Whether mothers and fathers have a higher long-term risk of death, particularly from cardiovascular disease and cancer, after the mother has had preeclampsia was assessed.

Methods.—This population-based study included mothers and fathers of all 626,272 births that were the mothers' first deliveries recorded in the Norwegian medical birth registry from 1967 to 1992. The parents were grouped on the basis of whether the mother had preeclampsia during the pregnancy. The subjects were also stratified as to whether the birth was term or preterm because preeclampsia might be more severe in preterm pregnancies. The main outcome measures were the total mortality rates and the mortality rate from cardiovascular causes, cancer, and stroke.

Results.—The long-term risk of death was 1.2-fold higher among women with preeclampsia than among women who did not have preeclampsia (Fig 1). Among women with preeclampsia and a preterm delivery, the risk was 2.71-fold higher than in women who did not have preeclampsia and whose pregnancies were term pregnancies. Of significance, the risk of death from cardiovascular causes among women with preeclampsia and a preterm de-

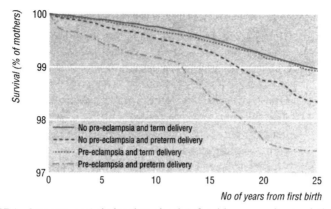

FIGURE 1.—Long term survival of mothers after their first delivery, according to whether they had preeclampsia and gestational age of baby at birth (term = ≥37 weeks). (Courtesy of Irgens HU, Reisæter L, Irgens LM, et al: Long term mortality of mothers and fathers after pre-eclampsia: Population based cohort study. *BMJ* 323:1213-1217, 2001, with permission from the BMJ Publishing Group.)

livery was 8.12-fold higher. However, these women also had a slightly but not significantly decreased risk of cancer. Among fathers, the long-term risk of death was no higher for fathers of preeclamptic pregnancies than for the fathers of pregnancies in which preeclampsia did not occur.

Conclusions.—There may be a link between the genetic factors that increase the risk of cardiovascular disease and preeclampsia. However, fathers did not have an increased risk of death from cardiovascular causes or cancer, and these findings did not indicate a possible genetic contribution from fathers to the risk of preeclampsia.

▶ Dr Leon Chesley, one of our pioneer investigators in primary hypertension in pregnancy, was able to show a marked difference in maternal mortality rate on follow-up of eclamptic women based on parity and age at the time of seizures.[1] Primigravid women have normal life expectancies on average, and an incidence of pregnancy-induced hypertension with later pregnancies reflecting the ultimate appearance of cardiovascular renal disease in later life seen as they age.[2] This cohort study of women with preeclampsia with the first pregnancy confirms those findings and adds some new information. The presence or absence of preeclampsia in first pregnancies delivered at term among more than 600,000 births recorded by the Norwegian Medical Birth Registry made no measurable difference in maternal mortality rate over the ensuing 25 years. On the other hand, preterm delivery in women without preeclampsia, 4.1% of all deliveries, was associated with an increased maternal mortality rate in later years. Presumably these were pregnancies with more serious, likely multisystem, disorders and contained among them women with underlying cardiovascular renal disease, recognized by Chesley in the form of late-life eclampsia. In this group, both preterm birth and primigravid preeclampsia were additive in increasing maternal mortality rate in the 0.4% of Norwegian parturients followed here. Primigravid preeclampsia is generally benign once the hazards of hypertensive pregnancy are negotiated and has a small chance of recurrence, its size depending largely on the risks of hypertension in the general population. Those women bear latent or subclinical cardiovascular renal disease. Those manifestations are destined to be manifest with greater age and parity in potentially life-threatening form, as this report indicates.

T. H. Kirschbaum, MD

References

1. Chesley LC: Recognition of the long-term sequelae of eclampsia. *Am J Obstet Gynecol* 182:249-250, 2000.
2. Chesley LC, Annitto JE, Cosgrove RA: The remote prognosis of preeclamptic women. *Am J Obstet Gynecol* 124:446, 1976.

Surgically Obtained Sperm, and Risk of Gestational Hypertension and Pre-eclampsia

Wang JX, Knottnerus A-M, Schuit G, et al (Adelaide Univ, Woodville, Australia)
Lancet 359:673-674, 2002   4–14

Background.—Preeclampsia is a common disorder among pregnant women, but the cause is unknown. It is probably multifactorial, but epidemiologic data have suggested that a partner-specific immune maladaptation may be involved, which might be initiated by regular exposure of the female genital tract to semen. In addition, a prospective study has indicated that the length of a sexual relationship is inversely proportional to the incidence of preeclampsia. Several other studies have also identified an increased rate of preeclampsia in pregnancies after gamete donation. Intracytoplasmic sperm injection (ICSI) is a technique that involves the injection of sperm into the cytoplasm of an oocyte. ICSI is used to help couples conceive in the absence of healthy sperm. Sometimes the sperm must be obtained surgically from the testis or epididymis. In couples who conceive by this method, there is little to no exposure of the female genital tract to sperm cells during intercourse, while there is exposure to seminal fluid. Thus, this group is an ideal model to test whether sperm cells provide a protective partner-specific immune tolerance that is independent of the protection provided by seminal fluid. Whether exposure to sperm cells before conception can protect against preeclampsia and hypertension was determined.

Methods.—From a cohort of all women treated with in vitro fertilization (IVF) or ICSI from 1986 to 1998 at a reproductive medicine unit of an Australian university, women whose pregnancies lasted longer than 20 weeks or resulted in the birth of an infant weighing 400 g or more were identified for study.

Results.—There were 1621 births during the study period, and 384 women (24%) had multiple births. Of this group, 195 women (12%) had gestational hypertension and 67 (4%) had preeclampsia. The risk of gestational hypertension was doubled in women treated with ICSI who used surgically obtained sperm, compared with women who underwent IVF with ejaculated sperm and those who underwent ICSI with ejaculated sperm. Women who underwent ICSI with surgically obtained sperm also had a 3-fold higher risk of preeclampsia when compared with the other 2 groups. These findings were not affected by multivariate logistic regression analysis to adjust for possible confounding effects of age and body mass index.

Conclusions.—Gestational hypertension and preeclampsia are more common in women who undergo implantation of an oocyte fertilized by surgically obtained sperm instead of their partner's ejaculated sperm. There may be a protective effect of semen exposure on the later development of gestational hypertension and preeclampsia that is associated with either exposure to sperm cells or a factor in the ejaculate that is closely linked with sperm.

▶ It's a persistent hypothesis that preeclampsia and gestational hypertension represent the results of failure of host immune tolerance of the fetal allograft. There is epidemiologic support from demonstrations that pregnancies conceived by gamete donation show an inordinately high incidence of pregnancy-induced hypertension and that the incidence of the hypertensive syndrome is inversely related to the duration of the sexual relationship that led to conception. Both data sets suggest that maternal exposure to semen acts to ameliorate the risks of pregnancy-induced hypertension, perhaps by resulting in immune tolerance based on repeated exposure to paternal antigens in seminal plasma, spermatozoa, or both. This study derived from 162 women treated with IVF or ICSI suggests that sperm may serve as the source for immune desensitization. Crucial to the observation are 82 women undergoing ICSI with sperm obtained by aspiration from the testis and epididymis in cases of total obstruction of the vas deferens. Such women have, for some time, been exposed to vaginal seminal fluid but not spermatozoa. By using the South Australian data registry to identify hypertensive pregnancies, those women had an 11% incidence of pregnancy-induced hypertension. For women undergoing IVF or ICSI with ejaculated sperm, having been exposed both to seminal plasma and spermatozoa, the incidence of pregnancy and hypertension was 4%. It is not possible to assay the impact of primiparity here. The data do, however, provide further support for this interesting hypothesis.

T. H. Kirschbaum, MD

Perinatal Outcome in Women With Recurrent Preeclampsia Compared With Women Who Develop Preeclampsia as Nulliparas
Sibai BM, for the National Institute of Child Health and Human Development Network of Maternal-Fetal Medicine Units (Univ of Cincinnati, Ohio)
Am J Obstet Gynecol 186:422-426, 2002   4–15

Background.—The overall rate of preeclampsia recurrence has been reported to be as high as 40%, 3 to 6 times the rate of preeclampsia in nulliparous women. The rates and perinatal outcomes in women with preeclampsia in a previous pregnancy were compared with those in nulliparas who develop preeclampsia.

Methods.—Data were obtained from 2 multicenter trials of aspirin for preventing preeclampsia. A total of 598 women who had had preeclampsia previously were compared with 2934 nulliparas.

Findings.—The rates of preeclampsia were 17.9% in the women with a history of preeclampsia and 5.3% in nulliparas. Severe preeclampsia occurred in 7.5% and 2.4%, respectively. Women with recurrent preeclampsia had more preterm deliveries before 37 and 35 weeks of gestation than did nulliparous women in whom preeclampsia developed. Among those with severe preeclampsia, women with recurrent disease had higher rates of preterm delivery than did nulliparous women both before 37 weeks' gestation (67% vs 33%) and before 35 weeks' gestation (36% vs 19%), and also had higher rates of abruptio placentae (6.7% vs 1.5%) and fetal death (6.7% vs 1.4%) than did nulliparous women.

Conclusions.—Compared with nulliparous women, women with preeclampsia in a previous pregnancy had significantly higher rates of preeclampsia. In addition, adverse perinatal outcomes associated with preterm delivery as a result of preeclampsia were significantly more common in women with a history of preeclampsia.

▶ This is a review of data derived from 2 prior prospective randomized trials that failed to demonstrate the value of low-dose aspirin in the prevention of preeclampsia.[1,2] Here, the data are used to explore the significance of recurrent pregnancy hypertension after the diagnosis of primigravid preeclampsia. Regrettably, the authors failed to realize that the issue has been explored previously and more productively by Chesley[3,4] and Tillman.[5] Preeclampsia is overwhelmingly, in Chesley's words, "a reversible syndrome appearing during a first pregnancy in previously normotensive women." In the absence of diabetes mellitus or multiple pregnancy, hypertension in subsequent pregnancies is related to the age-related increase in chronic hypertension, the tendency for pregnancy to serve as an evocative test of subclinical renovascular disease in later life, and the dramatic changes in blood pressure following the 40% likelihood of reduction to normotensive levels in women with hypertension antedating pregnancy. In such women, as Tillman showed so clearly, a woman hypertensive after pregnancy was almost surely hypertensive before pregnancy. The incidence of hypertensive pregnancies after initial preeclampsia is a reflection of the genetic predisposition to essential hypertension, age, increased body mass, and smoking, all of which are usually, as in this case, more likely in multiparas compared with the primigravid. Note that 71.4% of multiparas were African Americans compared with 49.3% of primigravidas, ensuring a higher incidence of chronic hypertension among the former. Nothing is demonstrated here that has not been reported 45 years ago. The failure to reference Chesley's work on this subject is a startling omission on the part of the authors and of the editorial review to which the paper was subjected.

T. H. Kirschbaum, MD

References

1. 1995 Year Book of Obstetrics, Gynecology, and Women's Health, pp 64-66.

2. 1999 YEAR BOOK OF OBSTETRICS, GYNECOLOGY, AND WOMEN'S HEALTH, pp 81-83.
3. Lindheimer MD, Roberts JM, Cunningham FG, et al: in Lindheimer MD, Roberts JM, Cunningham FG (eds): *Chesley's Hypertensive Disorders in Pregnancy.* Stamford, Conn, Appleton and Lange, 1999, pp 26-36.
4. Chesley LC: Recognition of the long term sequelae of eclampsia. *Am J Obstet Gynecol* 182:249, 2000.
5. Tillman AJB: The effect of normal and toxemic pregnancy on blood pressure. *Am J Obstet Gynecol* 70:589, 1955.

Adverse Perinatal Outcomes Are Significantly Higher in Severe Gestational Hypertension Than in Mild Preeclampsia

Sibai BM, for the National Institute of Child Health and Human Development Network of Maternal-Fetal Medicine Units, Bethesda, Maryland (Univ of Cincinnati, Ohio)
Am J Obstet Gynecol 186:66-71, 2002   4–16

Background.—About 7% of all pregnancies are complicated by hypertensive disorders, which are second only to thromboembolism as a cause of maternal death. Current literature emphasizes the increased risk of adverse outcomes in pregnancies complicated by proteinuria and hypertension. The frequency of adverse fetal outcomes was compared in women in whom hypertensive disorders developed with or without proteinuria.

Methods.—A secondary analysis was performed for data from 598 women who had preeclampsia in a previous pregnancy and were enrolled in an ongoing multicenter trial of aspirin for the prevention of preeclampsia. None of the women had a history of chronic hypertension or renal disease, and all were normotensive at enrollment. This study assessed preterm delivery at less than 37 weeks and less than 35 weeks of gestation, rate of small-for-gestational-age infants, and abruptio placenta. Data were analyzed by using the χ^2 test. Women who continued to be normotensive or who had mild gestational hypertension were evaluated as a single group because their outcomes were similar.

Results.—Women with severe gestational hypertension (without proteinuria) had higher rates of both preterm delivery at less than 37 weeks' gestation and small-for-gestational-age infants than women with mild preeclampsia. In women with severe gestational hypertension, both gestational age and birth weight were significantly lower at delivery than in women with mild preeclampsia (Table 3). Women in whom severe gestational hypertension developed had higher rates of preterm delivery at less than 37 weeks of gestation (54.2% vs 17.8%) and also at less than 35 weeks of gestation (25% vs 8.4%), as well as a higher incidence of delivery of small-for-gestational-age infants (20.8% vs 6.5%) compared with normotensive women or those in whom mild gestational hypertension developed. No statistically significant differences in perinatal outcomes emerged between women in the normotensive/mild gestational hypertension group and those in the mild preeclampsia group.

TABLE 3.—Relative Risk of Adverse Outcomes (Severe Gestational Hypertension Versus Severe Preeclampsia)

Outcome	Relative Risk	95% CI
Delivery at <37 wk	0.81	0.53-1.24
Delivery at <35 wk	0.70	0.32-1.56
SGA infant	1.83	0.56-5.71
Abruptio placenta	0.63	0.07-5.69
LGA infant	1.87	0.28-12.49
NICU admission	0.55	0.23-1.31
Respiratory distress syndrome	0.75	0.21-2.63

The severe gestational hypertension group is the reference group.
Abbreviations: LGA, Large for gestational age; *NICU,* neonatal ICU; *SGA,* small for gestational age.
(Courtesy of Sibai BM, for the National Institute of Child Health and Human Development Network of Maternal-Fetal Medicine Units: Adverse perinatal outcomes are significantly higher in severe gestational hypertension than in mild preeclampsia. *Am J Obstet Gynecol* 186:66-71, 2002.)

Conclusions.—Among women with gestational hypertension or pre-eclampsia, only women with severe hypertension have increased rates of preterm delivery and delivery of small-for-gestational-age infants. However, in these women, the presence of proteinuria does not affect perinatal outcome.

▶ This is yet another secondary analysis of data obtained at the time of the negative evaluation of the possible role of aspirin in the prevention of pre-eclampsia[1] conducted by the NICHD Maternal Fetal Medicine Network. Five hundred ninety eight women with pregnancies following an initial diagnosis of preeclampsia were compared with respect to 32% who showed pregnancy hypertension with a subsequent pregnancy. If associated with proteinuria of at least 0.3 g per day, a subsequent hypertensive episode was called preeclampsia; if albuminuria was less than 0.3 g per day, the diagnosis was gestational hypertension. Both classes of patients were subclassified with respect to severity (blood pressure greater than 160/110, use of antihypertensive agents, albuminuria greater than 5 g per day, etc). A variety of perinatal outcomes were compared among the 4 groups, preeclamptic, gestationally hypertensive, mild and severe, and the normotensive parous women as controls.

It is well to remember what is known about the women chosen for entry into the study, all with the diagnosis of preeclampsia with albuminuria in a prior pregnancy. Preeclampsia is largely but not wholly exclusively confined to primigravidas. Many of the 197 women would be expected to show cardiovascular renal hypertension in later life, variously reflecting their racial and genetic predispositions.[2] Of 131 women with either preeclampsia or severe gestational hypertension, 72% were black. Albuminuria occurs at various times during pregnancy, may diminish in amount with progressive gestation or appear for the first time after delivery, even in eclampsia.[3] When women with hypertensive pregnancies lack albuminuria, the chances of the eventual diagnosis of hypertension are doubled compared with those who have albuminuria.[4]

The women at interest here were heterogeneous, many having chronic hypertension and others destined to qualify for that diagnosis at a later age. Given severe hypertension, the results of this study showed that the presence or absence of albuminuria makes no difference in outcome; nor is there a difference in perinatal outcome between those with mild hypertension with or without alubuminuria and those two thirds of women with subsequent normotensive pregnancies after an initial preeclamptic episode. Only 1 fetal death was noted among 45 women with severe proteinuric preeclampsia, and 4 were noted among the 460 normotensive controls. The results show a tendency to growth retardation and preterm delivery related to severe hypertension regardless of albuminuria, likely related to iatrogenic preterm deliveries. The authors conclude that women with severe hypertension deserve careful surveillance, whether they had albuminuria or not. Certainly they are correct.

T. H. Kirschbaum, MD

References

1. 1999 Year Book of Obstetrics, Gynecology, and Women's Health, pp 81-83.
2. Chesley CL: Recognition of the long term sequelae of eclampsia. *Am J Obstet Gynecol* 182:249, 2000.
3. Chesley CL: *Hypertensive disorders of pregnancy.* New York, Appleton-Century-Crofts, 1978, pp 157-162.
4. Berman CS: Observations in the toxemia clinic, Boston Lying-in Hospital in 1929-30. *N Engl J Med* 203: 361, 1930.

Treatment of Hypertension in Pregnancy: Effect of Atenolol on Maternal Disease, Preterm Delivery, and Fetal Growth
Easterling TR, Carr DB, Brateng D, et al (Univ of Washington, Seattle)
Obstet Gynecol 98:427-433, 2001   4–17

Background.—The control of blood pressure during pregnancy, while it reduces the risk of severe maternal hypertension, the incidence of preeclampsia, and the incidence of respiratory distress syndrome in neonates, may also negatively influence fetal growth. This study focused on a population of women identified as being at risk for the development of preeclampsia for whom antihypertensive therapy was initiated in early pregnancy. The program was intended to prevent severe maternal hypertension and the need for preterm delivery due to maternal hypertension while maintaining an environment appropriate for fetal growth.

Methods.—Atenolol was given as deemed appropriate based on measurements of cardiac output (measured by Doppler technique) (Fig 1). The references used in analyzing fetal growth were previous pregnancy outcome, treatment inconsistent with standards existing at the study period's conclusion, and year when treatment was given. The analysis techniques included paired and unpaired *t*-test, variance analysis for multiple comparisons, and linear regression.

Results.—Therapy with atenolol was initiated before 18 weeks' gestation in the 235 women studied, most of whom were treated for chronic hypertension (Fig 3). Additional therapy included furosemide (used in 10% of cases) and hydralazine (used in 20%). Treatment inconsistencies were found in 6.5% of cases. At baseline, 55% of these women had more than 100 mg of

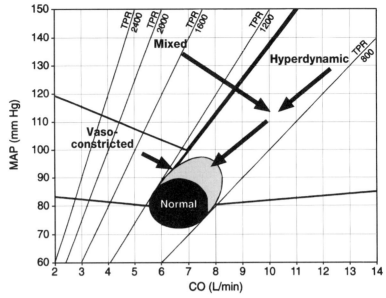

FIGURE 1.—Mean arterial pressure is plotted against cardiac output. Isometric lines of vascular resistance permit visualization of each hemodynamic variable. Vasodilators such as hydralazine produce vectors of change perpendicular to lines of resistance. Drugs such as atenolol and furosemide produce vectors of change roughly parallel to lines of resistance but with some increase in resistance. (Reprinted with permission from The American College of Obstetrics and Gynecology, courtesy of Easterling TR, Carr DB, Brateng D, et al: Treatment of hypertension in pregnancy: Effect of atenolol on maternal disease, preterm delivery, and fetal growth. *Obstet Gynecol* 98:427-433, 2001.)

proteinuria, and severe preeclampsia developed in 1 patient. Delivery before 32 weeks occurred in 2.1% of cases and before 34 weeks in 4.7%. A strong association was found between lower percentile birth weight and previous pregnancy with intrauterine growth restriction, treatment inconsistency, and earlier pregnancy. Fetal growth was less than would have been expected in a normal population. At the beginning of the study, percentile birth weight was at 20%; by the end of the study, it had increased to 40%.

Conclusions.—The therapy given to control blood pressure in this group of women prevented severe maternal hypertension and prevented preterm delivery in most cases, but fetal growth rate continued to be less than expected among a normal pregnant population. Factors associated with reduced growth included previous pregnancy with intrauterine growth restriction and treatment inconsistencies.

▶ The major determinants of central cardiovascular function—blood pressure, cardiac output (that is pulse rate times stroke volume), and vascular resistance—are all nicely depicted in the Poiseuille-Hagan diagram that these University of Washington investigators use. A 4th variable, blood volume, is omitted, and one needs to remember that increasing blood volume tends to lower vascular resistance but increases cardiac output with variable effects on blood pressure in pregnancy hypertension. What is offered here is an account

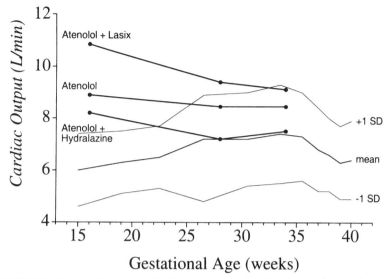

FIGURE 3.—Mean cardiac output is plotted against gestational age for 3 groups of patients determined by antihypertensive therapy at delivery. Normal cardiac output (mean ± SD) over gestation is included for reference. (Reprinted with permission from The American College of Obstetrics and Gynecology, courtesy of Easterling TR, Carr DB, Brateng D, et al: Treatment of hypertension in pregnancy: Effect of atenolol on maternal disease, preterm delivery, and fetal growth. *Obstet Gynecol* 98:427-433, 2001.)

of a systematic, physiologic approach to the management of hypertensive gravidas, two thirds of them chronic hypertensives, which evolved with the authors' experience with 235 such women. Their approach is to begin β adrenergic blockers before 18 weeks of pregnancy, slowing the heart rate and reducing cardiac output in what they believe is the dominant problem in early pregnancy, a hyperdynamic heart. For years they have differed with Henk Wahlenburg, a Rotterdam investigator, whose approach is based largely on right heart catheterization proximate to labor when he finds reduced cardiac output. Recently, Irish investigators have demonstrated both to be correct [1] in their longitudinal studies of hypertensive women that tend to show increased cardiac output early in pregnancy, decreasing to lower values close to the onset of labor. The University of Washington group uses early pregnancy ultrasonic evaluation of aortic blood flow velocity as a measure of cardiac output, a method proven accurate in comparison to more classic techniques.[2,3] From this, using blood pressure, they calculate vascular resistance, and in 70% of their patients, control blood pressures solely with a β blocker. The hazard of course is uterine hypoperfusion and fetal compromise. They learned to guard against this by maintaining cardiac output at least at the mean value for gestational age and keeping peripheral vascular resistance less than 1150 dyne · sec · cm^{-5}. With measurements later in pregnancy, Wahlenburg finds normal peripheral vascular (PVR) to be 1500 dyne · sec · cm^{-5}. In the event those limits were exceeded, a diuretic was used to lower plasma volume in 10% of patients or a vasodilator was used in 20%, both of which have the impact of reducing peripheral vascular resistance. Wahlenburg, more concerned with hypovolemia closer to term, first expands plasma volume and then uses vasodilators to reduce PVR and blood pressure.

This experience, although uncontrolled and unrandomized, compares well with historic controls. The occurrence of superimposed pregnancy-related hypertension is not identified but 1 patient with what is described as severe preeclampsia is noted. Preterm delivery less than 34 weeks occurred in 4.7% and the incidence of growth retardation, perhaps a consequence of marginal uterine hypoperfusion, was 19.8%. Those who practice obstetrics should read this approach to management and compare it with Wahlenburg's.[4] This is a rational approach to managing this important complication of pregnancy.

T. H. Kirschbaum, MD

References

1. 2001 Year Book of Obstetrics, Gynecology, and Women's Health, pp 105-108.
2. 1988 Year Book of Obstetrics, Gynecology, and Women's Health, pp 54-57.
3. 1992 Year Book of Obstetrics, Gynecology, and Women's Health, pp 133-134.
4. Wahlenburg HCS: Hemodynamics in hypertensive pregnancy, in Rubin PC (ed): *The Handbook of Hypertension*, vol 10. *Hypertension in Pregnancy*. New York, Elsevier, 1988, pp 66-101.

Increased AT_1 Receptor Heterodimers in Preeclampsia Mediate Enhanced Angiotensin II Responsiveness

AbdAlla S, Lother H, el Massiery A, et al (Ain Champs Univ, Cairo; Heinrich-Pette-Institut, Hamburg, Germany; Institut für Pharmakologie und Toxikologie, Würzburg, Germany)
Nat Med 7:1003-1009, 2001   4–18

Background.—Preeclampsia and eclampsia are the leading causes of maternal mortality in developed countries, with an incidence of 3% to 10%. Hypersensitivity to the vasoconstrictor angiotensin II has been considered the most effective predictor of preeclampsia, although the mechanism of the increased pressor response to angiotensin II in preeclamptic women has not been elucidated. Angiotensin-II–mediated signaling is known to increase with AT_1-B_2-receptor heterodimerization. Whether altered AT_1-receptor dimerization mediated an increased angiotensin II response in preeclampsia was investigated..

Methods.—The study included 34 pregnant women, 19 of whom had preeclampsia as defined by hypertension after week 20 of pregnancy and the appearance of proteinuria. AT_1- and B2-receptor protein levels on platelets from these women were determined by immunoblot analysis with antibodies specific for the AT_1 or the B_2 receptors.

Results.—In the preeclamptic hypertensive women, a significant increase in heterodimerization occurred between the AT_1-receptor for angiotensin II and the B_2 receptor for bradykinin. Heterodimerization of AT_1-B_2 receptors in preeclampsia correlated with a fourfold to fivefold increase in B_2-receptor protein levels. The expression of the AT_1-B_2 heterodimer increased the responsiveness to angiotensin II and conferred resistance in AT_1-receptors to inactivation by reactive oxygen species in both normotensive and preeclamptic pregnant women.

Conclusion.—The findings suggest that AT_1-B_2 heterodimers play a contributing role in the development of angiotensin II hypersensitivity in pregnant women with preeclampsia. Preeclampsia is identified as the first disorder associated with alteration of G-protein–coupled receptor heterodimerization.

▶ Guanosine triphosphate–binding proteins, or G proteins, constitute a family of proteins that serve as part of the extracellular assemblage of transmembrane receptors, to provide specificity to the regulation of cell membrane transactions. Widely distributed, they act when coupled with a specific activating molecule by generating cyclic guanylate cyclase, adenylyl cyclase, and phospholipases, or directly regulate ion channels. Although usually monomeric, this group has identified a 2-part G protein aggregate coupling an angiotensin receptor (AT_1) to a bradykinin receptor (B_2), the properties of which suffice to provide an explanation for the increased peripheral vascular resistance in preeclampsia. Instead of balancing the vasoconstrictor properties of angiotensin II with the vasodilating properties of bradykinin, the dimer strongly increases the vasoconstrictive effect of angiotensin II.

Using platelets and omental vessels, comparing primigravid preeclamptic women with normotensive controls, the authors were able to identify the AT_1/B_2 dimer in preeclamptic tissues using receptor-specific immunoaffinity chromatography and failed to identify the complex in tissues from normal gravidas. The dimer was associated with a 4-fold to 5-fold increase in B_2 receptor G protein content and enhanced calcium channel flux on coupling with angiotensin II in both cell types. Further, the AT_1/B_2 dimer was resistant to oxidative stress, sometimes noted in preeclampsia (see Abstract 1–2) mediated by H_2O_2 but resulted in activation of AT_1 G protein monomers and had no effect on tissues from normal women or cell cultures without dimer formation.

This is important in view of the protection it provides the AT_1/B_2 dimer from the regular appearance of circulating markers of oxidative stress. The formation of the dimer is known to be stimulated by uteroplacental ischemia, sympathetic hyperactivity, proteolytic enzymes resulting in bradykinin production, or other pro-inflammatory cytokines.

The authors provide strong evidence that this alteration of guanosine triphosphate–binding proteins occurs and can explain both the angiotensin II sensitivity and the increased peripheral vascular resistance that occurs in preeclampsia. The comparisons between 19 primigravidas with preeclampsia and a return to normal blood pressure postpartum with 15 normals are convincing. The implicit assumption that changes in mesenteric vessels represent changes in the general arterial circulation needs confirmation. The uncertain impact of gestational age needs to be clarified as well. This is a new, provocative, potentially very valuable approach to the pathophysiology of preeclampsia which deserves wide attention.

T. H. Kirschbaum, MD

Fas and Fas Ligand Expression in Maternal Blood and in Umbilical Cord Blood in Preeclampsia

Kuntz TB, Christensen RD, Stegner J, et al (Univ of Florida, Gainesville)
Pediatr Res 50:743-749, 2001   4–19

Background.—The Fas–Fas ligand (FasL) pathway of apoptosis is abnormally activated in diseases associated with impaired intolerance or chronic inflammation. Pregnancy-related hypertension typically causes significant morbidity in both women and newborn infants. Pregnancy-related hypertension is associated with generalized inflammation, and there may be a causal link between pregnancy-related hypertension and impaired maternal-fetal intolerance. Enhanced trophoblast expression of FasL has been observed in 1 form of pregnancy-related hypertension. The hypothesis that pregnancy-related hypertension may be associated with abnormal activation of the Fas–Fas ligand (FasL) pathway was studied.

Methods.—Enzyme-linked immunoassay and flow cytometric analyses were used to prospectively study soluble and leukocyte-associated Fas receptor and FasL in the maternal and umbilical cord blood (CB) sera in 20 gestations complicated by preeclampsia and in 18 normal control gestations.

Results.—Higher soluble FasL levels were noted in paired maternal and CB sera of hypertensive gestations compared with control gestations; however, the 2 groups had similar soluble Fas levels (Fig 1). Surface expression of FasL was lower on maternal and CB neutrophils from hypertensive gestations, but surface Fas expression was lower on maternal neutrophils and leukocytes but not on CB neutrophils and leukocytes (Fig 2).

Conclusions.—Gestations complicated by preeclampsia demonstrated altered expression of Fas and FasL in sera and on leukocytes. It is speculated

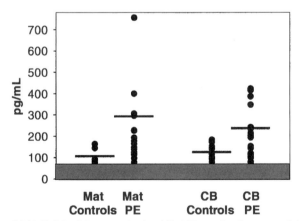

FIGURE 1.—Soluble FasL levels in maternal and umbilical CB sera. Results represent individual soluble FasL concentrations (pg/mL) in paired samples of maternal (*Mat*) and CB sera from control gestations and gestations complicated by preeclampsia (*PE*). *Horizontal lines* represent mean values for each group; *P* < .02, controls vs PE (Mann Whitney). *Shaded area* represents limit of sensitivity for assay, and proportion of values falling within this area varied for each group. (Courtesy of Kuntz TB, Christensen RD, Stegner J, et al: Fas and Fas ligand expression in maternal blood and in umbilical cord blood in preeclampsia. *Pediatr Res* 50(6):743-749, 2001.)

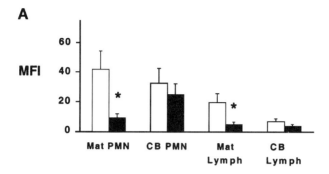

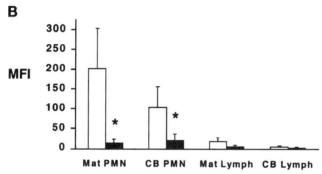

FIGURE 2.—Surface Fas and FasL expression on maternal (*Mat*) and CB leukocytes. Results represent mean fluorescence intensity *(MFI)* of surface Fas receptor (**A**) and surface FasL (**B**) on Mat and CB neutrophils (*PMN*) and lymphocytes (*Lymph*) from control (*open bars*) and hypertensive gestations (*solid bars*). *P < .02, **P < .05, preeclampsia vs controls (analysis of variance). (Courtesy of Kuntz TB, Christensen RD, Stegner J, et al: Fas and Fas ligand expression in maternal blood and in umbilical cord blood in preeclampsia. *Pediatr Res* 50(6):743-749, 2001.)

that in preeclampsia the activation of the Fas-FasL pathway mediates associated pathologic processes in affected women and their neonates.

▶ Fas receptor is an integral membrane protein located on the surface of numerous cell types, among them hematopoietic cells. FasL is a transmembrane structure limited to leukocytes and tissues expressing immune privilege. Fas-FasL interactions are related to graft tolerance and reduction of macrophages active in antigen presentation as well as the initiation of apoptosis. Transgenic mice lacking FasL show increased transfers from mother to fetus of activated leukocytes and fetal growth retardation, an expression of apoptosis or genetically regulated cell death or inflammation in shared tissues. Hoping to confirm the presence of apoptosis[1,2] and primary or secondary inflammatory changes,[3] the authors measured Fas and FasL in maternal and CB obtained at delivery, comparing results in 20 women with preeclampsia with 18 controls. Both soluble serum forms and surface expression on maternal and CB leukocytes were measured immunologically. Because only about half of the women labeled preeclamptic were primigravid, it is perhaps better to describe them as showing pregnancy-induced hypertension. Serum soluble Fas-L was significantly elevated in maternal and CB serum from hypertensive pregnancies compared with controls. Surface Fas and FasL were decreased in hypertensive pregnancies in maternal and CB hematopoietic cells.

Although the findings support prior observations of apoptosis and inflammatory activation in preeclampsia, there are a lot of currently active and unresolved hypotheses in this area. Membrane-bound FasL may be lost from trophoblast cells to both maternal and fetal blood. Activated inflammatory cells may release surface FasL to both maternal and fetal serum or, indirectly, through their production of inflammatory cytokines, which would have the same effect. These data demonstrate and confirm that something is happening in hypertensive pregnancies that affects the Fas-FasL system. It is not yet clear precisely what that something is.

T. H. Kirschbaum, MD

References

1. 1999 YEAR BOOK OF OBSTETRICS, GYNECOLOGY, AND WOMEN'S HEALTH, pp 19-21.
2. 2001 YEAR BOOK OF OBSTETRICS, GYNECOLOGY, AND WOMEN'S HEALTH, 119-123.
3. 2002 YEAR BOOK OF OBSTETRICS, GYNECOLOGY, AND WOMEN'S HEALTH, pp 200-202.

Endothelial Function in Myometrial Resistance Arteries of Normal Pregnant Women Perfused With Syncytiotrophoblast Microvillous Membranes

Van Wijk MJ, Boer K, Nisell H, et al (Univ of Amsterdam; Huddinge Univ, Stockholm; Univ of Oxford, England)
Br J Obstet Gynaecol 108:967-972, 2001   4–20

Introduction.—Although the cause of preeclampsia remains unclear, defective placentation appears to be the central feature in early pregnancy. Factors in the maternal circulation, as yet unidentified, may cause the generalized maternal endothelial dysfunction seen in late-phase preeclampsia, when clinical symptoms appear. Syncytiotrophoblast microvillous membranes (STBM) have been proposed as a factor linking defective placentation to endothelial dysfunction in the disease. Biopsies of myometrial resistance arteries from healthy term women were analyzed to determine the effects of STBM on endothelial function.

Methods.—Biopsies were obtained from 18 women at the time of elective cesarean section. The site of the biopsies was the upper edge of the transverse incision in the lower uterine segment. Twenty-nine myometrial resistance arteries were isolated, mounted in a pressure arteriograph, and perfused intraluminally for 3 hours with STBM (20 to 2000 ng/mL) or with erythrocyte membranes or physiologic salt solution as controls, all substituted with 0.5% bovine serum albumin. Bradykinin concentration-response curves performed before and after perfusion were fitted to the Hill equation, and maximal dilation and the pEC_{50} values were calculated from these fits.

Results.—The experimental groups did not differ in the passive diameter of the arteries. The bradykinin concentration-response curves for STBM 20,

200, and 2000 ng/mL and control substances erythrocyte membranes 200 and 2000 ng/mL all exhibited bradykinin-mediated dilation before and after perfusion. Neither STBM nor erythrocyte membrane perfusion affected maximal dilation or the pEC_{50} values of the bradykinin concentration-response curves at any concentration. Electron microscopy examination revealed no obvious damage to the endothelium after perfusion with STBM or erythrocyte membranes.

Conclusion.—In these experiments, perfusion with STBM in concentrations up to 100 times those reported in preeclampsia did not significantly affect bradykinin-mediated dilation in isolated myometrial arteries. The endothelial dysfunction observed in preeclampsia does not appear to be caused by a direct effect of STBM on the endothelial cells.

▶ In the vigorously ongoing search for a placental factor responsible for endothelial cell dysfunction and resultant changes in the cardiovascular and other organ systems in preeclampsia, investigators from Oxford University's Nuffield Institute have been important contributors. They have demonstrated that preparations of syncytiotrophoblastic microvillous membranes (STBM) found in plasma but not in serum are capable of inducing endothelial cell injury in vitro.[1] Further, transmission electron microscopy shows endothelial cell injury after perfusion of STBM of subcutaneous arterioles preparations as well as loss of capacity of acetylcholine to produce vasodilatation, presumably by inhibiting endothelial nitric oxide production.[2] Subsequent work demonstrated increased shedding of STBM into the maternal circulation in preeclampsia, compared with normals,[3] and measured average concentration in preeclampsia of about 30 g of protein per mL plasma in this form. This work, done by investigators at Stockholm's Karolinska Institute together with Oxford collaboration is aimed at refining the perfusion experiments, using concentrations of STBM known to exist in vivo in preeclamptics.

Vessels from myometrial biopsies at cesarean sections were used because of the experimental evidence of decreased blood flow in vivo in preeclamptic humans and ease of access. Bradykinin-mediated vessel dilatation after maximum constriction by norepinephrine after 3 hours of perfusion of STBM versus erythrocyte membranes as controls were then studied. Technical expertise was extraordinary. Arteriole segments 2.5 to 3.0 mm in length were perfused in a pressure arteriograph at 60 mm Hg and were studied before and after 3 hours of perfusion with membrane preparations, using STBM concentrations of 20, 200, and 2000 ng of protein per mL perfusate. No significant impact of STBM perfusion, nor of erythrocyte membrane perfusion could be noted.

The authors' data indicate the absence of a direct role of STBM fragments alone in producing endothelial cell injury in vitro. One could argue that longer perfusion times would be desirable, but 3 hours is well within the range of time that yielded the opposite results in subcutaneous vessels. Bovine serum albumin 0.5% was used to prevent fragment clumping in vitro, but this is less than the albumin concentration noted in vivo. Though this finding may well change the directions of future research in this area, these remain very interesting observations in the functional pathology of preeclampsia.

T. H. Kirschbaum, MD

References

1. 1997 YEAR BOOK OF OBSTETRICS, GYNECOLOGY, AND WOMEN'S HEALTH, pp 57.
2. 1998 YEAR BOOK OF OBSTETRICS, GYNECOLOGY, AND WOMEN'S HEALTH, pp 47.
3. 1999 YEAR BOOK OF OBSTETRICS, GYNECOLOGY, AND WOMEN'S HEALTH, pp 31.

Endothelial Junctional Protein Redistribution and Increased Monolayer Permeability in Human Umbilical Vein Endothelial Cells Isolated During Preeclampsia
Wang Y, Gu Y, Granger DN, et al (Louisiana State Univ, Shreveport; Magee-Womens Research Inst, Pittsburgh, Pa)
Am J Obstet Gynecol 186:214-220, 2002   4–21

Background.—Increased endothelial monolayer permeability in preeclampsia may indicate altered monolayer barrier properties resulting from disorganization of endothelial cell junction proteins. Monolayer permeability and junctional protein distribution and expression were examined in endothelial cells isolated from women with preeclampsia and with normal pregnancies.

Methods.—Endothelial cells were obtained from umbilical veins in 9 women with normal pregnancies and from 9 with preeclampsia immediately after delivery. In the first passage of endothelial cells, permeability was assessed by measuring horseradish peroxidase passage through confluent cell monolayers grown on transwell filters. Distribution and protein expression of vascular endothelial cadherin and occludin were assessed by means of immunofluorescent staining of the proteins and Western blot analysis. In addition, vascular endothelial cadherin distribution was evaluated in the second and third passage endothelial cells. Reverse transcriptase polymerase chain reaction was used to study messenger ribonucleic acid expression of vascular endothelial cadherin and occludin.

Findings.—Endothelial cells isolated from preeclamptic women had a significantly higher relative monolayer permeability than those from women with normal pregnancies (Fig 1). Vascular endothelial cadherin expression in normal endothelial cells had a continuous staining of the junctional protein surrounding cell borders. However, vascular endothelial cadherin in endothelial cells from women with preeclampsia showed disorganized staining, and vascular endothelial cadherin fibrils were retracted, with gaps observed at the cell borders. Occludin expression had a pattern comparable to that of vascular endothelial cadherin in normal and preeclamptic pregnancies. In the Western blot analysis of expression of vascular endothelial cadherin and occludin, expression of junctional proteins was also reduced. By the time cells reached the third passage in vitro, the endothelial cell junctional protein distribution and expression of vascular endothelial cadherin

**Normal
Endothelial Cells**

**Preeclampsia
Endothelial Cells**

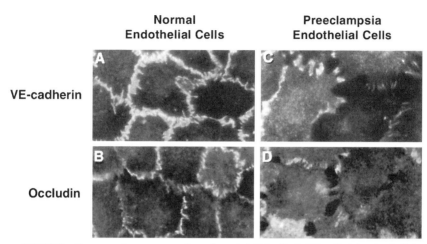

VE-cadherin

Occludin

FIGURE 1.—Representative appearance of vascular endothelial cadherin (VE-cadherin) and occludin in the first-passage endothelial monolayer. Panels **A** and **C** were stained for VE-cadherin; panels **B** and **D** were stained for occludin. Panels **A** and **B** were endothelial cells isolated from women with normal pregnancies; panels **C** and **D** were endothelial cell samples isolated from women with preeclampsia. In normal endothelial cells, VE-cadherin expression showed a continuous staining around cell borders. In comparison, VE-cadherin staining in endothelial cells isolated from women with preeclampsia showed that junctional fibers were contracted, density was decreased, and intercellular gaps were present at cell contact regions. The expression of occludin revealed a pattern similar to that described for VE-cadherin in endothelial cells from both normal and preeclamptic pregnancies. These results indicate that endothelial cell monolayer morphology and junctional protein distribution are significantly altered in preeclampsia. (Courtesy of Wang Y, Gu Y, Granger DN, et al: Endothelial junctional protein redistribution and increased monolayer permeability in human umbilical vein endothelial cells isolated during preeclampsia. *Am J Obstet Gynecol* 186:214-220, 2002.)

and occludin seen in the first passage of endothelial cells from preeclamptic pregnancies was normalized. mRNA expression for the vascular endothelial cadherin and occludin did not differ significantly between normal and preeclamptic endothelial cells.

Conclusions.—Increased endothelial cell monolayer permeability in preeclamptic pregnancies appears to indicate disorganized and reduced expression of endothelial cell junctional proteins. The mediation of the latter occurs at the posttranscriptional level.

▶ The thrust of this study is to confirm the presence of endothelial dysfunction in preeclampsia by studying the biochemistry of proteins responsible for endothelial cell-cell junction formations. Integrins are proteins responsible for recognition of like cells, formation of cell-cell adhesion relationships and intimate cytoskeletal constructs which mark more or less permanent cell junctions. The latter are discernible in electronmicroscopy in mature tissue; integrins are developmental constructs most easily recognizable by immunohistochemistry using specific antibody. These investigators look to vascular endothelial cell cadherin, a calcium-dependent adhesion molecule, and occludin, a protein responsible for water-tight junctions as, for example, in the anchoring of placental villi or the formation of the membranous sheets of cells, which are active in selective permeability. Using cell cultures of human umbilical vein endothelial cells obtained from umbilical cord vessels, and comparing placentas with and without preeclampsia, they find fragmentation and discontinuity of both proteins in specimens from preeclamptics. Using a 2-chamber perfusion system with an intervening monolayer cell culture and employing horseradish peroxidase as a marker for perfusion, they find enhanced perfusion in endothelial cells derived from preeclamptic pregnancies.

The problem is that the experimental substrate consists of fetal cells and that fetuses fail to show the vascular pathophysiology of preeclampsia, that is, proteinuria, increased extracellular fluid volume, plasma contraction, increased peripheral vascular resistance, and hypertension. Though the authors conjecture that what damages maternal endothelium in preeclampsia must pass the placenta and damage fetal endothelium as well, there is no substantive support for that hypothesis. No one has demonstrated, using fetal blood, the counterpart to the evidence that maternal preeclamptic serum induces changes in endothelial cell cultures.[1,2] It is becoming very clear that these studies must be repeated using maternal endothelium from preeclamptics, difficult though it may be to obtain, before such work can be accepted as reflecting the maternal pathology of the disease.

T. H. Kirschbaum, MD

References

1. 1997 YEAR BOOK OF OBSTETRICS, GYNECOLOGY, AND WOMEN'S HEALTH, pp 37-39.
2. 2000 YEAR BOOK OF OBSTETRICS, GYNECOLOGY, AND WOMEN'S HEALTH, pp 117-119.

No Evidence for Lipid Peroxidation in Severe Preeclampsia

Regan CL, Levine RJ, Baird DD, et al (Univ of Pennsylvania, Philadelphia; Natl Inst of Child Health and Human Development, Bethesda, Md; Natl Inst of Environmental Health Services, Research Triangle Park, NC; et al)
Am J Obstet Gynecol 185:572-578, 2001   4–22

Objective.—This study was undertaken to address the role of oxidative stress in preeclampsia.

Study Design.—We measured urinary 8,12-*iso*-iPF$_{2\alpha}$-VI, a chemically stable, free-radical catalyzed product, in a case control study of severe preeclampsia nested within the trial of Calcium for Preeclampsia Prevention. Cases included 29 women who developed severe preeclampsia and from whom urine had been obtained 10 to 20 weeks before the diagnosis of preeclampsia, 3 to 9 weeks before, and 1 day before through delivery (Fig 1). Controls did not develop hypertension or proteinuria and were matched to cases by center, gestational age at each of 3 corresponding urine collections, and date of enrollment.

Results.—Urinary 8,12-*iso*-iPF$_{2\alpha}$-VI did not differ significantly between cases and controls before or at diagnosis of preeclampsia, nor did it vary with gestational age.

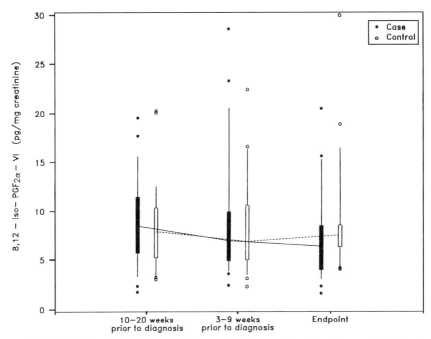

FIGURE 1.—Urinary 8,12-*iso*-iPF$_{2\alpha}$-VI pg/mg creatinine in case patients (*closed boxes and circles*) and control subjects (*open boxes and circles*) is depicted within each time interval with respect to the diagnosis of preeclampsia, as follows: 10 to 20 weeks before, 3 to 9 weeks before, and from 1 day before until delivery. *Boxes* represent 25th to 75th percentiles; *whiskers* represent 10th to 25th and 75th to 90th percentiles; and *circles* represent outlying values. Medians are connected with *solid lines* (case patients) or *dotted lines* (control subjects). End point specimens were those collected at diagnosis of preeclampsia, from 1 day before diagnosis through delivery. (Courtesy of Regan CL, Levine RJ, Baird DD, et al: No evidence for lipid peroxidation in severe preeclampsia. *Am J Obstet Gynecol* 185:572-578, 2001.)

Conclusions.—These results call into question the importance of oxidative stress in the disease and the biochemical rationale for clinical trials of antioxidants to prevent and treat preeclampsia.

▶ This is another example of the use of archival samples stored in connection with the Calcium for Preeclampsia Prevention trial reported earlier.[1] In this case, development of the ability to measure directly the products of lipid peroxidation by free radicals of prostaglandin isomers formed from arachidonic acid becomes an important new step. The urinary metabolite 8,12 iso-iPF$_{2\alpha}$-VI, an F$_2$ isoprostane, can be measured in urine with use of chromatography and mass spectroscopy. The advantage over measurement of malandialdehyde is that the latter reflects thromboxane production, which is often increased in preeclampsia, in addition to lipid peroxidation. Other immune assays for iPF$_{2\alpha}$III reflect general cyclooxygenase activity, including platelet enzyme activity, in addition to lipid peroxidation.

Among 4589 gravidas followed through pregnancy prospectively, 29 developed severe preeclamspia and had frozen urine samples obtained at the time of delivery and during the interval from 3 to 9 weeks and 10 to 20 weeks prior to the delivery date. Urine samples from healthy control subjects were matched for center of origin, gestational age, and time from randomization to delivery to compensate for degeneration in storage. Analysis of the F_2 isoprostane failed to show evidence of increased lipid peroxidation associated with the development of severe preeclampsia. The peroxidation hypothesis has been so widely embraced by investigators that interest is likely to continue for awhile. Nonetheless, this is a strong argument against a valid role for lipid peroxidation in the production of preeclampsia.

T. H. Kirschbaum, MD

Reference

1. 1998 YEAR BOOK OF OBSTETRICS, GYNECOLOGY, AND WOMEN'S HEALTH, pp 45-47.

Expression of Inflammatory Cytokines in Placentas From Women With Preeclampsia

Benyo DF, Smarason A, Redman CWG, et al (Univ of Pittsburgh, Pa; Magee-Womens Research Inst, Pittsburgh, Pa; Univ of Oxford, England)
J Clin Endocrinol Metab 86:2505-2512, 2001   4–23

Introduction.—The failure of the uterine vasculature to undergo sufficient physiologic remodeling in women with preeclampsia leads to speculation that a consequence of decreased placental perfusion is the generation of cytotoxic factors that circulate and injure the maternal endothelium. A comparison was made of tumor necrosis factor α (TNFα), interleukin (IL)-1α, IL-1β, and IL-6 levels in the placenta of patients with preeclampsia and those with normal term pregnancies.

Methods.—Multiple sites per placenta were sampled since the placenta is a large heterogeneous organ. Semiquantitative reverse transcriptase–polymerase chain reaction and enzyme-linked immunosorbent assay analyses of placental homogenates were performed. Peripheral and uterine venous blood samples were evaluated for TNFα.

Results.—There were no significant differences among normal term, preeclamptic, or preterm placentas of women without preeclampsia (Table

TABLE 2.—Cytokine Protein Levels in Placental Homogenates

Cytokine	Normal Term Pregnant	Preeclamptic
TNFα	0.79 ± 0.12	0.80 ± 0.16
IL-1β	6.00 ± 2.21	4.98 ± 0.73
IL-1α	2.36 ± 0.30	3.49 ± 1.73
IL-6	7.52 ± 0.97	8.98 ± 1.96

Note: Values are in picograms per milogram protein.
Values are the mean ± SEM, average of 8 sites assayed in duplicate per placenta for normal term (5 patients) and preeclampsia (4 patients). There are no significant differences between groups.
(Courtesy of Benyo DF, Smarason A, Redman CWG, et al: Expression of inflammatory cytokines in placentas from women with preeclampsia. *J Clin Endocrinol Metab* 86(6):2505-2512, 2001. Copyright, The Endocrine Society.)

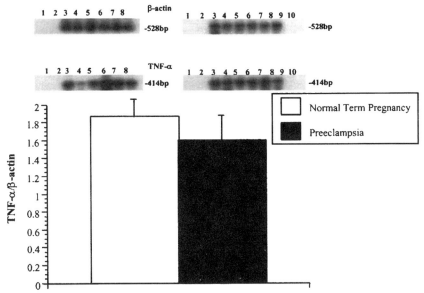

FIGURE 4.—Tumor necrosis factor α (*TNFα*) gene expression in normal term and preeclamptic placentas (6 each). Total RNA was pooled from 4 biopsy sites per placenta and reverse transcribed. β-Actin and TNFα polymerase chain reaction products were visualized by Southern blotting. **Left insets:** Lanes 1 and 2, no RNA; lanes 3, 5, and 7, 3 different normal term placentas; lanes 4, 6, and 8, 3 different preeclamptic placentas. **Right insets:** Lanes 1 and 2, no RNA; lanes 3, 5, and 7, 3 additional different normal term placentas; lanes 4, 6, and 8, 3 additional different preeclamptic placentas. Lanes 9 and 10 are without reverse transcriptase. The data are summarized in the graph (mean ± SEM). (Courtesy of Benyo DF, Smarason A, Redman CWG, et al: Expression of inflammatory cytokines in placentas from women with pre-eclampsia. *J Clin Endocrinol Metab* 86(6):2505-2512, 2001. Copyright, The Endocrine Society.)

2). A 3-fold variation was observed overall in cytokine protein levels across the 8 sites sampled for each placenta. No significant differences were observed in TNFα mRNA between the normal term and preeclamptic placentas (Fig 4). The TNFα mRNA levels were lower in placentas of preterm women without a diagnosis of preeclampsia versus the normal term placentas. In vitro, hypoxia stimulated the production of TNFα, IL-1α, and IL-1β, but not of IL-6, by placental villous explants from both groups of patients. This was not exaggerated in preeclampsia (Fig 6). Although peripheral and uterine venous levels of TNFα were increased among preeclamptic women compared with those in the normal term group, the ratio of uterine to peripheral venous TNFα levels was not significantly different from 1.0 for either patient group.

Conclusion.—Sources other than the placenta contribute to the higher concentrations of TNFα and IL-6 observed in the circulation of women with preeclampsia.

▶ It has long been a viable hypothesis that preeclampsia begins with defective placentation and vascularization, resulting in ischemic hypoxia and the production of inflammatory cytokines that subsequently result in increased maternal peripheral vascular resistance.[1-3] Indeed, 2 of these authors have

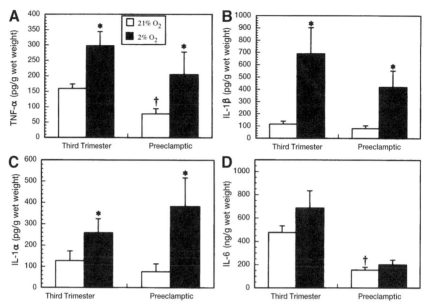

FIGURE 6.—Cytokine production by villous explants prepared from normal term and preeclamptic placentas. Villous explants were maintained for 24 hours under standard tissue culture conditions (21% oxygen; *white squares*; 5 patients) or hypoxia (2% oxygen; *black squares*; 5 patients). The cytokines evaluated were tumor necrosis factor (*TNFα*) (A), IL-1β (B), IL-1α (C), and IL-6 (D). Cytokine concentrations in the conditioned medium were corrected for wet weight of the villous tissue and are expressed as the mean ± SEM. *Asterisk* indicates statistical difference between 21% and 2% oxygen; *dagger* indicates significant difference between incubations of normal term and preeclamptic villous explants (*P* < .05). (Courtesy of Benyo DF, Smarason A, Redman CWG, et al: Expression of inflammatory cytokines in placentas from women with preeclampsia. *J Clin Endocrinol Metab* 86(6):2505-2512, 2001. Copyright, The Endocrine Society.)

supported that concept, reporting, among other investigators, increased maternal blood concentrations of TNFα, IL-1β, and IL-6 in preeclamptic women. Here, measuring protein cytokine concentration and mRNA in placental homogenates, they find no significant difference in the concentration of any cytokine in 8 preeclamptic specimens compared with 6 controls.

Preeclampsia is correctly defined at the University of Pittsburgh as including only primigravid women with evidence of increased blood creatinine concentration. Criteria are less rigorous at the University of Oxford, but those samples were used only for determining maternal blood concentrations. Cytokines were quantitatively measured by enzyme-linked immunosorbent assay and mRNA by reverse transcriptase–polymerase chain reaction, with Southern blotting for confirmation. Table 2 shows placental homogenate cytokine concentrations and Figure 4 shows TNF-mRNA gene expression in placental biopsy specimens. Since gestational age was an uncontrolled variable, the authors show that normal preterm deliveries were associated with less than term pregnancy controls with respect to both cytokine protein and messenger. They confirmed in these placentas their earlier finding that placental explants have the capacity to increase cytokine production in 2% oxygen (see Fig 6).

This study refutes the claim, based on human tissue, that increased cytokine concentration in preeclampsia is the cause of maternal pathophysiology.

It suggests strongly that increased cytokine expression in the presence of hypoxia arises because of changes in vascular epithelium, circulating immune cells, or parenchymal organ injury—an effect not a cause of preeclampsia.

T. H. Kirschbaum, MD

References

1. 1996 YEAR BOOK OF OBSTETRICS, GYNECOLOGY, AND WOMEN'S HEALTH, pp 48-49.
2. 2000 YEAR BOOK OF OBSTETRICS, GYNECOLOGY, AND WOMEN'S HEALTH, pp 105-107.
3. 2001 YEAR BOOK OF OBSTETRICS, GYNECOLOGY, AND WOMEN'S HEALTH, pp 124-126.

The Relationship Between Hemodynamics and Inflammatory Activation in Women at Risk for Preeclampsia
Carr DB, McDonald GB, Brateng D, et al (Univ of Washington, Seattle; Columbia Univ, New York; Merck & Co Inc, Rahway, NJ)
Obstet Gynecol 98:1109-1116, 2001   4–24

Background.—Preeclampsia is an important cause of maternal and neonatal morbidity and mortality. The preclinical phase of preeclampsia is characterized by a hyperdynamic circulation and elevated markers of endothelial and inflammatory activation. The relationship of these 3 markers of preeclampsia during pregnancy and the effect of hemodynamic therapy were investigated in a longitudinal study.

Study Design.—The study group consisted of 46 pregnant women with clinical risk factors for preeclampsia (high-risk group) and 25 pregnant women at low-risk for preeclampsia (control group). Those women in the high-risk group who had a second trimester cardiac output greater than 7.4 L/min were treated with the β-blocker, atenolol. At enrollment, data on age, parity, weight, gestational age, and blood pressure were obtained. Blood was drawn to assess tumor necrosis factor (TNF)-α, TNF-α receptors, vascular cell adhesion molecule-1, and fibronectin. Blood pressure was evaluated.

TABLE 1.—Maternal and Pregnancy Characteristics at Enrollment Described as Means ± Standard Deviations or Number of Subjects and Percentage (in Parentheses)

	High Risk (n = 46)	Control (n = 25)	CI	P
Age (y)	28.3 ± 5.4	30.3 ± 5.5	−4.68, 0.74	.2*
Weight (kg)	100.7 ± 23.5	67.2 ± 13.8	24.3, 42.8	<.001*
Primigravida, n (%)	23 (50)	18 (72)	0.14, 1.11	.07†
Gestational age (wk)	17.3 ± 4.3	16.1 ± 4.2	−1.01, 3.23	.3*
MAP (mmHg)	91.8 ± 10.6	79.6 ± 7.3	7.9, 16.5	<.001*

Abbreviations: MAP, Mean arterial pressure; *CI*, confidence interval for *t* test (mean difference between groups) or χ^2 test (risk ratio).
*t test
†χ^2 test
(Reprinted with permission from The American College of Obstetricians and Gynecologists courtesy of Carr DB, McDonald GB, Brateng D, et al: The relationship between hemodynamics and inflammatory activation in women at risk for preeclampsia. *Obstet Gynecol* 98: 1109-1116, 2001.)

TABLE 2.—Hemodynamic Measurements and Biochemical Markers of Endothelial and Inflammatory Activation at Enrollment

	High Risk ($n = 46$)	Control ($n = 25$)	Slope* (CI)	P
CO (L/min)	9.7 ± 1.7	7.3 ± 1.7	−2.39 (−3.22, −1.56)	<.001
TPR (dyne · sec · cm^{-5})	777.7 ± 165.6	914.5 ± 237.4	153.81 (51.96, 255.67)	.004
TNF-α (pg/mL)	LLD (LLD, 2089.6)	LLD (LLD, 5846.6)	−0.23 (−0.98, 0.53)	.6
TNFR1 (pg/mL)	509.3 (205.3, 861.0)	413.2 (117.2, 1469.5)	−0.028 (−0.11, 0.06)	.5
TNFR2 (ng/mL)	6.14 (1.77, 112.2)	5.24 (LLD, 2559.4)	0.053 (−0.26, 0.36)	.7
VCAM-1 (ng/mL)	491.7 ± 133.7	441.4 ± 75.9	−0.059 (−0.11, −0.01)	.02
cFN (mg/L)	485.0 (217.4, 1928.0)	391.2 (226.0, 892.0)	−0.06 (−0.14, 0.02)	.1

Abbreviations: CO, Cardiac output; *TPR,* total peripheral resistance; *TNF-α,* tumor necrosis factor-α; *TNFR1,* tumor necrosis factor-α receptor 1; *TNFR2,* tumor necrosis factor-α receptor 2; *VCAM-1,* vascular cell adhesion molecule-1; *cFN,* cellular fibronectin; *LLD,* lower limit of detection.

*The slope indicates the average difference in the baseline parameter between the control and high-risk groups.

(Reprinted with permission from The American College of Obstetricians and Gynecologists courtesy of Carr DB, McDonald GB, Brateng D, et al: The relationship between hemodynamics and inflammatory activation in women at risk for preeclampsia *Obstet Gynecol* 98: 1109-1116, 2001.)

Multivariable linear regression analysis was utilized to examine the association between each group and both hemodynamic measurements and biochemical markers.

Findings.—Maternal age, gestational age, and parity did not differ significantly between the 2 groups. As expected, the high-risk women weighed significantly more than the control women (Table 1). Both cardiac output and vascular cell adhesion molecule-1 were significantly increased in the high-risk group at baseline, compared with the control group (Table 2). Of the 46 women in the high-risk group, 42 were given atenolol during pregnancy for high cardiac output. TNF-α receptor 1 increased more slowly in these treated women than in the control group.

Conclusion.—This longitudinal study examined the relationship between maternal hemodynamics and biochemical markers of endothelial and inflammatory activation in women at high and low risk for preeclampsia. Women at high-risk for preeclampsia had a hyperdynamic circulation and elevated levels of vascular cell adhesion molecule-1, compared with low-risk women. Women with a hyperdynamic circulation who were treated with a β-blocker had a slower increase in TNF-α receptor 1 compared with untreated women. This suggests a relationship between hemodynamic status during pregnancy and markers of endothelial and inflammatory activation.

▶ These authors attempt, generally unsuccessfully, to add weight to 3 hypotheses concerning the pathogenesis of preeclampsia. They continue to espouse increased cardiac output, that is, greater than 7.4 L/min, using Doppler analysis of maternal aortic cardiac output as the primary determinant of hypertension. As before,[1] they decline to follow the lead of most clinicians and physiologists who recognize the role of body mass and/or surface area in determining cardiac output.

Most investigators handle this by calculating the cardiac index, obtained by dividing cardiac output by body surface area, yielding units of liters per minute per square meter to correct for the role of body mass. The customary calculation of body mass surface area uses the formula of DuBois and DuBois[2] based on weight and height measurements. Although the authors do not provide height data for their high risk and control groups, it is possible to calculate cardiac indexes assuming all women are 5 ft 6 inches tall. That leaves mean cardiac indexes of 4.31 and 4.11 L/min/m² for high-risk versus low-risk groups, that is, between high cardiac output and low cardiac output groups in the authors' terminology. The difference is not statistically significant. The same calculations at 4 other reasonable mean body heights yield the same results.

In seeking women at high risk of preeclampsia, these authors appear simply to have selected for a large body mass among a high-risk group of 46 women with a mean body weight of 221 lb and compared them with a control group averaging 148 lb during pregnancy. The authors continue to ignore longitudinal studies showing hyperdynamic cardiac function to be a feature of mid-pregnancy hypertensives, reverting to normal or low cardiac output past the 34th week of gestational age. Additional concerns are with relationship of peptides produced by endothelial changes and concomitants of the inflammatory reaction. Neither of these has a proven relationship to preeclampsia, and it is uncertain whether they are an effect of or contribute to the hypertensive process. Ultimately, this is a cohort study with patients segregated by cardiac output uncorrected for body mass selected on the basis of prior preeclampsia, obesity, or suspected hypertension, excluding patients on either antihypertensives and without evidence of autoimmune disease or infection.

The "high risk" group received a β-blocker (atenolol), and comparisons were made with the slimmer untreated group. Atenolol appeared not unexpectedly to provide some blood pressure control in the group with the high likelihood of chronic cardiovascular disease. No significant differences between the groups were noted in the concentration of TNF-α or its receptor or in the concentration of endothelial adhesion molecules or cellular fibronectin. The authors hold that fibronectin represents an inflammatory component to the presence of preeclampsia. "High-risk" pregnancies produced infants of normal body weight but slightly less than the control group, and there were no differences in the incidence of growth retardation or preeclampsia between the 2 groups. Without additional controls, not much can be said about the effects of the β-blocker nor in support of any of the hypotheses that the authors purport to test.

T. H. Kirschbaum, MD

References

1. 1992 Year Book of Obstetrics and Gynecology, pp 40-42.
2. DuBois D, DuBois EF: A formula to estimate the approximate surface area if height and weight be known. *Arch Intern Med* 17:863-871, 1916.

Association of a Woman's Own Birth Weight With Subsequent Risk for Gestational Diabetes

Innes KE, Byers TE, Marshall JA, et al (Univ of Colorado, Denver; Univ of Virginia, Charlottesville)
JAMA 287:2534-2541, 2002
4–25

Background.—Birth weight has been inversely related to the risk of development of type 2 diabetes mellitus and related endocrine disorders. Gestational diabetes (GDM), an important complication occurring during pregnancy, is strongly predictive of development of type 2 diabetes mellitis later in life. GDM can reveal information supportive or nonsupportive of the fetal origins hypothesis in young adult populations, yet markers of a woman's personal fetal development related to her later risk for GDM remain largely unexplored. The markers of fetal growth and subsequent risk of GDM were evaluated in a population of young women in New York.

Methods.—In testing the hypothesis that a woman's own fetal growth inversely reflects her risk of GDM, vital record data and linked hospital discharge information were analyzed. The women evaluated had completed their first pregnancies. Four hundred forty women had a record of GDM and 22,955 having no evidence of GDM served as control subjects.

Results.—A strong positive link was shown between the risk for GDM in a woman's first pregnancy and her age. An inverse relationship was noted between her educational level and risk for GDM. A U-shaped relationship to risk for GDM was noted with birth weight alone and birth weight adjusted for gestational age. Therefore, both high birth weight and low birth weight carried a higher risk for GDM. After adjustment for gestational age, a birth weight under 2000 g carried an odds ratio of 2.16 and a birth weight of over 4000 g carried an odds ratio of 1.53. With adjustments for confounding factors, the odds ratio for low birth weight increased but that for high birth weight declined. Thus, there was a strong inverse dose-response relationship between birth weight and risk for GDM.

Conclusion.—Women with low birth weights and high birth weights were at increased risk for development of GDM later in life. This occurred when assessed alone and when adjusted for gestational age. While the relationship between large birth size and GDM risk could be explained by the mother's prepregnancy body mass index and the presence of maternal diabetes, adjusting the determinations for potential confounding factors strengthened the inverse relationship between birth weight and GDM development. These findings are in line with the theory that a susceptibility to diabetes and related conditions may occur during fetal life, with the specific example of GDM.

▶ This is an ingenuous use of matched live birth registry data and the New York state records of hospital discharges to explore the relationship between a woman's birth weight and her subsequent risk of GDM and, presumably, ultimately frank diabetes during her first pregnancy. Women were selected for study who were born between 1970 and 1985 and for whom a first delivery occurring between 1994 and 1998 was fully documented. Pregnancies from 1970 to 1985 marked by significant chronic or acute disorders, multiple pregnancies, or illegal drug use were discarded. GDM was inferred from entries in the 1994 to 1998 newborn record or evidence in the mother's chart of GDM or abnormal glucose tolerance.

The 444 women who qualified for entry had a mean age at delivery of 21.1 years, with a range from 12 to 28 years of age. Controls were chosen from women with uncomplicated first pregnancies delivered in the same time span. Initial analysis of risk ratios for GDM as a function of the mother's birth weight were made by univariant statistics, and logistic regression was used to test the impact of the mother's body mass index, age, height, and other possible confounders.

As the mothers' birth weight increased from less than 2 kg to 4 kg, the risk of GDM with their first pregnancy declined from a value of 2.2-fold increase to 0. That is no increased risk at 4 kg. Women with birth weights greater than 4 kg showed an increased risk of GDM on univariant analysis, but correcting for mothers with high body mass index and maternal diabetes ablated the significance of the apparently increased risk ratio at high birth weights.

Both increases in the mother's age and body mass index at the time of the 1994 to 1998 deliveries increased the risk of GDM during that pregnancy, especially if she was relatively short with a relatively small body mass index. Women born of diabetic mothers prior to 1970 had a 4-fold greater chance of showing GDM with the first pregnancy compared to nondiabetics. It is useful to contrast the clarity of these results with an earlier study from Southhampton based on arguable diagnostic entities from data collected 60 to 75 years ago.[1]

One may argue whether these relationships stem from fetal conditioning in utero or from the joint inheritance of genes resulting in insulin resistance and a predisposition for diabetes expressed mutually to mothers born 30 years earlier than their later first-born infants. The data, however, have intrinsic value in counseling and preventative measures as well as case detection of diabetes in children and young adults born at low birth weights close to term.

T. H. Kirschbaum, MD

Reference

1. 2002 YEAR BOOK OF OBSTETRICS, GYNECOLOGY, AND WOMEN'S HEALTH, pp 11-13.

Intra-Hepatic Cholestasis of Pregnancy in Hepatitis C Virus Infection
Paternoster DM, Fabris F, Palù G, et al (Univ of Padua, Italy)
Acta Obstet Gynecol Scand 81:99-103, 2002   4–26

Background.—Hepatitis C virus (HCV) infects 0.14% to 6% of pregnant women. A liver disease that may occur in pregnancy, intrahepatic cholestasis of pregnancy (ICP), develops in response to environmental and hormonal factors in genetically predisposed women. The presence of HCV infection may be associated with a higher incidence of ICP. Whether HCV infection actually affects the natural history and incidence of ICP and produces different characteristics in HCV-positive versus HCV-negative women with ICP was assessed prospectively.

Methods.—From January 1996 to January 1999, 5840 pregnant women were assessed at the University of Padua, Italy, Prenatal Department. ICP was diagnosed on clinical grounds, specifically the occurrence of pruritus that began during pregnancy, persisted until delivery, and disappeared after delivery, and was not accompanied by skin or medical conditions that normally accompany pruritus. In addition, elevated serum alanine amino transferase (ALT) and total serum bile acid levels were noted. HCV was assessed using the enzyme-linked immunosorbent assay, recombinant immuno blot assay, and polymerase chain reaction. Statistical analyses were then conducted.

Results.—Of 105 women who tested positive for anti-HCV, 59 tested positive for HCV RNA. Of the 56 in whom ICP developed, 12 were HCV RNA–positive and 2 were co-infected with HIV. Two HCV RNA–positive women and 4 HCV RNA–negative women had recurrent gestational cholestasis. ICP was found in 20.33% of HCV RNA–positive women and in 0.76% of HCV RNA–negative women. A significantly earlier gestational week at the onset of symptoms as well as lower ALT and serum aspartate amino trans-

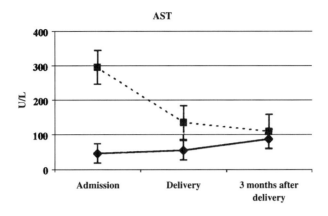

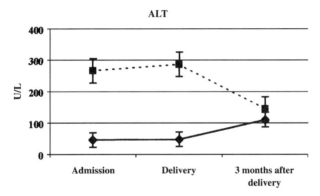

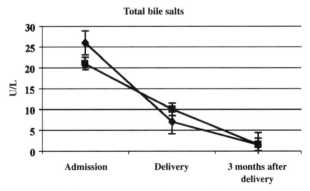

FIGURE 1.—Serum levels of aspartate aminotransferase (*AST*), alanine aminotransferase (*ALT*) and total bile acids at admission, at delivery, and after delivery in intrahepatic cholestasis of pregnancy (ICP) hepatitis C virus (HCV) RNA–positive (*black diamond*) and ICP HCV RNA–negative women (*black square*). (Courtesy of Paternoster DM, Fabris F, Palù G, et al: Intra-hepatic cholestasis of pregnancy in hepatitis C virus infection. *Acta Obstet Gynecol Scand* 81:99-103, 2002. Publisher Munksgaard International Publishers Ltd.)

ferase (AST) levels were found among women with ICP who were HCV RNA–positive compared with those who were negative.

In the women with ICP who were HCV RNA–positive, ALT and AST levels were significantly higher 3 months after delivery than during pregnancy and delivery, and bile salt levels were significantly lower after delivery than on admission. The mean viral load showed a significant decline after delivery. The symptoms and laboratory findings of those with ICP who were HCV RNA–negative resolved completely by the time of the first postpartum visit, whereas those women who were HCV RNA–positive maintained higher AST and ALT levels for 3 months after delivery (Fig 1). All of the infants born to the mothers studied were HCV RNA–negative by age 12 months.

Conclusion.—Women in whom ICP develops during their third trimester should be tested for the presence of HCV. It appears that there is a higher risk of HCV infection in this population, although the impact of the infection is as yet undetermined.

▶ ICP is a not uncommon pregnancy complication, particularly in Scandinavia and parts of South America. Its association with increased perinatal mortality in some regions is puzzling, and since an early outbreak in North Africa was confused with an epidemic of viral hepatitis, it becomes important in making the diagnosis to rule out HCV.

This 3-year study in Italy where ICP is uncommon (0.96% of 5840 women here) is aimed at confirming an earlier retrospective report of an increased incidence of ICP among HCV-infected gravidas.[1] The incidence of HCV-positive antibody by enzyme-linked immunoassay was 1.8% in this population, and 1% showed active viremia based on quantitative HCV RNA assay. Each woman with HCV antibody was followed up monthly with determinations of serum ALT and AST, and hepatic US was done to rule out biliary stones. The presence of HIV antibody was also sought. The diagnosis of ICP was based on maternal clinical findings, blood ALT, and bile salt concentration.

Of the 59 women HCV RNA–positive, 12 or 20.3% had ICP compared with 0.8% of those who were HCV negative. Women positive for HCV maintained high concentrations of ALT and AST throughout pregnancy and as long as 3 months post partum, whereas bile salt concentration in blood decreased promptly with delivery in both HCV-positive and HCV-negative women. The presence of ICP did not appear to increase the presence or quantity of HCV RNA among positive women. There was no apparent perinatal mortality or morbidity associated with ICP in this study. Because of the inordinate incidence of ICP among HCV-infected women, it is important that HCV studies be done in women either with HCV antibody or with circulating HCV RNA.

T. H. Kirschbaum, MD

Reference

1. Locatelli A, Roncaglia N, Arreghini A, et al: Hepatitis C virus infection is associated with a higher incidence of cholestasis of pregnancy. *Br J Obstet Gynaecol* 106:498-500, 1999.

Viral Load in HCV RNA–Positive Pregnant Women

Paternoster DM, Santarossa C, Grella P, et al (Inst of Hygiene, Padua, Italy; Univ of Padua, Italy)
Am J Gastroenterol 96:2751-2754, 2001   4–27

Background.—Newborns have an estimated 5% risk of hepatitis C virus (HCV) infection. However, in the presence of HIV infection, this risk is greatly increased. Viral load is one of the major factors associated with the vertical transmission of HCV. The behavior of HCV viral load during pregnancy was investigated in relation to HIV co-infection, liver enzymes, and vertical transmission.

Methods and Findings.—Three thousand seven hundred forty-eight consecutive women in their first trimester of pregnancy underwent HCV infection screening. Sixty-five were anti-HCV+/HCV RNA+. These women were followed up clinically and serologically throughout their pregnancy and for 6 months post partum. None of the women tested positive for anti-HIV or hepatitis B surface antigen. The mean HCV RNA was 12×10^6 copies/mL in the first trimester and 10.9×10^6 in the second, increasing to 19.5×10^6 in the third trimester.

Viral load returned to baseline 6 months after delivery. Changes in viral load were nonsignificant. Transaminases tended to decrease from baseline in the second and third trimesters. Increased AST and ALT levels were noted 6 months after delivery. However, when women with abnormal AST and ALT levels on the first test were considered, no significant changes occurred during follow-up (Fig 1). Overall, the rate of vertical transmission was 4.6%.

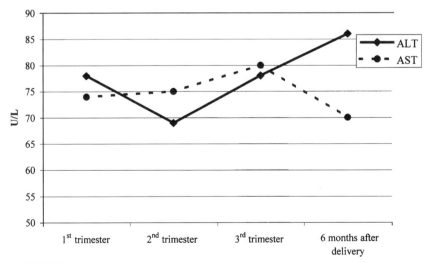

FIGURE 1.—Behavior of transaminases in the group of pregnant women with abnormal liver enzymes. AST normal value is 10 to 45 U/L. AST normal value is 5 to 55 U/L. Data are median values. (Reprinted by permission of the publisher from Paternoster DM, Santasrossa C, Grella P, et al: Viral load in HCV RNA–positive pregnant women. *Am J Gastroenterol* 96:2751-2754, 2001. Copyright 2001 with permission from Elsevier Science.)

Conclusion.—Monitoring transaminases in HCV-positive women during pregnancy is not necessary. Assessing liver enzymes at the beginning of pregnancy is sufficient. Qualitative polymerase chain reaction should be performed once during pregnancy. However, any liver disease staging should be done after delivery.

▶ HCV infection is important because of its relationship to chronic hepatitis, cirrhosis, and hepatic cancer, but its fetal transmission rate is far smaller than is the case for maternal hepatitis B. Maternal evidence of HCV infection (presence of HCV antibody and HCV RNA in maternal blood) occurs in 1% to 2.4% of gravidas, and fetal infection occurs in roughly 5% of those women. Though IV drug abuse and sexually transmitted diseases, especially HIV, are risk factors for maternal infection and constitute indications to screen women for HCV, screening of gravidas is generally not indicated because of the low transmission rate and the absence of effective prophylaxis and therapy for carriers of the virus.[1] Presence of a prior pregnancy marked by fetal infection does not significantly increase the risk of transmission for subsequent fetuses,[2] while co-infection with HIV significantly increases the risk of fetal infection.[3]

Here the question posed is whether the copy numbers of HCV RNA in infected women might be useful in predicting fetal transmission and thereby justifying screening. The authors find it does not and that neither HCV RNA copy numbers nor hepatic transaminase concentrations change significantly during pregnancy in such women. They recommend qualitative HCV polymerase chain reaction and serum transaminase concentrations be determined in women with HCV-antibody but that quantitative polymerase chain reaction and repeated transaminase determinations are not useful through the course of the subsequent pregnancy.

T. H. Kirschbaum, MD

References

1. 1994 YEAR BOOK OF OBSTETRICS, GYNECOLOGY, AND WOMEN'S HEALTH, pp 97-98; pp 115-116.
2. 2001 YEAR BOOK OF OBSTETRICS, GYNECOLOGY, AND WOMEN'S HEALTH, pp 138-139.
3. 1999 YEAR BOOK OF OBSTETRICS, GYNECOLOGY, AND WOMEN'S HEALTH, pp 271-273.

Epitope Mapping of TSH Receptor-Blocking Antibodies in Graves' Disease That Appear During Pregnancy
Kung AWC, Lau KS, Kohn LD (Univ of Hong Kong, China; Natl Inst of Diabetes and Digestive and Kidney Diseases, Bethesda, Md)
J Clin Endocrinol Metab 86:3647-3653, 2001   4–28

Introduction.—Spontaneous remission of Graves' disease during pregnancy is considered to be caused by a decrease in thyroid-stimulating antibody activity. It is possible that a broader change in thyroid-stimulating hormone (TSH) receptor antibody characteristics may have an important role in modulating disease activity during pregnancy. To define the epitopes and clinical significance of thyroid stimulating-blocking antibodies (TBAbs) that are present during pregnancy, the following variables were measured in 13 pregnant patients with Graves' disease at the first, second, and third trimesters and 4 months post partum: TSH binding inhibitory Ig, thyroid-stimulating antibody, and TBAbs.

Methods.—To measure and epitope-map thyroid-stimulating antibody and TBAb activities, CHO cells transfected with wild-type human TSH receptor or with several TSH receptor–luteinizing hormone/human chorionic gonadotropin (LH/hCG) receptor chimeras were used. They were Mcl+2, Mc2, and Mc4. These chimeric cells have their respective TSH receptor residues 9-165, 90-165, and 261-370 substituted with comparable residues of the LH/hCG receptor.

Results.—Overall thyroid-stimulating antibody was diminished, whereas TBAb rose progressively during pregnancy. The TSH binding inhibitory Ig fluctuated in individual patients, yet the overall activities remained statistically unchanged. The TBAb was observed in patients who either tested negative for thyroid-stimulating antibody or whose thyroid-stimulating antibody activity rose or decreased during pregnancy. Epitope mapping revealed that the thyroid-stimulating antibodies were primarily directed against residues 9-165 of the N-terminus of the TSH receptor extracellular domain. All TBAbs demonstrated blocking activities against residues 261-370 of the C-terminus of the ectodomain. Most of the TBAbs also had a hybrid conformational epitope directed against N-terminal residues 9-89 or 90-165. In spite of a change in the activity level, no change was observed in the epitope of either the stimulating or blocking Abs as pregnancy advanced.

Conclusion.—A change in the specificity of TSH receptor antibody from stimulating to blocking activity was seen during pregnancy. The appearance of TBAbs may contribute to the remission of Graves' disease during pregnancy.

▶ Over the past 10 years, investigators have expanded the knowledge available of the impact of heterogeneity and autoantibodies directed at the TSH receptor during Graves' disease in pregnancy, and the clinical implications of those changes. The fundamental disturbance in Graves' disease results from the production of a stimulatory autoimmune globulin (TSAb) which reacts with TSH receptor to generate increased thyroid cyclic adenosine monophosphate (cAMP) and symptoms of thyrotoxicosis. The variety of antibodies directed at reactive antigenic segments of the TSH receptor (epitopes) includes thyroid blocking antibodies (TBAb) and TSH binding inhibitory immunoglobulins (TBII) which are capable of inhibiting TSH or TSAb binding to the TSH receptor and/or of blocking the production cAMP in response. Further, case studies have shown that blocking antibodies may serve either as agonists or antagonists to TSH receptor stimulation, that TSAb may produce either neonatal Grave's disease or hyperthyroidism, and that maternal and fetal thyroid status may differ as the pattern of blocking antibodies produced by the mother changes with time in pregnancy. TSAb tends to complex with epitopes near the N-terminal or variable region of the antibody within 9 to 165 amnioacids from the N terminus. On the other hand, blocking antibodies react to segments of the immunoglobulin molecule adjoining the C terminus, usually in the range of 260 to 370 amino acids. This makes it easy to understand the unpredictable variation in thyroid function that occurs in the puerperium in many women[1] and the hypothyroid phase of Hashimoto's thyroiditis marked by the production of large amounts of TBAb.

These authors report longitudinal thyroid antibody assays in 13 women with mild Graves' disease requiring less than 100 mg of PTU per day. They found that TSAb decreased in most as pregnancy advances but was accompanied by an increase in TBAb unrelated apparently to the presence or absence of TSAb or symptoms of thyrotoxicosis. TBII fluctuated unpredictably during pregnancy independent of TBAb or TSAb. In general, the more heterogeneity in the distribution of epitopes exhibited by the gravidas blocking antibody repertoire, the greater the likelihood that the patient would undergo remission of thyroxicosis in later pregnancy. The converse is true for women with homogeneous blocking antibody production during pregnancy. These findings help explain the variations in response to Graves' disease in the course of otherwise normal pregnancy.[1]

T. H. Kirschbaum, MD

Reference

1. 2001 YEAR BOOK OF OBSTETRICS, GYNECOLOGY, AND WOMEN'S HEALTH, pp 204-207.

Presentation, Etiology, and Outcome of Stroke in Pregnancy and Puerperium
Skidmore FM, Williams LS, Fradkin KD, et al (Indiana Univ, Indianapolis; Regenstrief Inst, Indianapolis, Ind; Hoosier Neurology, Indianapolis, Ind)
J Stroke Cerebrovasc Dis 10:1-10, 2001   4–29

Introduction.—Earlier trials have indicated that there is an increased incidence of strokes in the puerperium period. The primary focus of these trials has been incidence and risk factors, not details of presentation, management, and stroke outcome. Stroke and cerebral venous thrombosis (CVT) in pregnancy and the puerperium were examined retrospectively to determine the causes, presentation, and outcome of pregnancy-related stroke.

Methods.—International Classification of Diseases (ICD 9) codes and a computerized records database were used to identify medical records of women with stroke during pregnancy and the puerperium. The records from 1992 to 1999 were available at 2 hospitals and from 1994 to 1999 at a third hospital. Medical records of all patients with ischemic stroke (IS), hemorrhagic stroke (HS), or CVT occurring during pregnancy and including events up to 12 weeks postpartum were examined.

Results.—Of 36 patients identified, 21 had IS, 11 had HS, and 4 had CVT. Most events (89%) occurred in the third trimester and postpartum period. Sixteen (44%) events occurred in postpartum week 1 (Fig 3). Of the 8 African-American patients evaluated, 5 had HS (63%); 18 of 25 white pa-

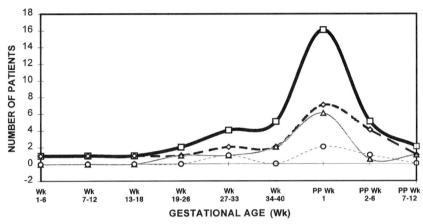

FIGURE 3.—The distribution of events by gestational age. A number of events increased in the third trimester and clustered in postpartum (*PP*) week 1, after which numbers rapidly declined. *Squares* indicate total events; *diamonds*, ischemic stroke; *triangles*, hemorrhagic stroke; and *circles*, cerebral venous thrombosis. (Courtesy of Skidmore FM, Williams LS, Fradkin KD, et al: Presentation, etiology, and outcome of stroke in pregnancy and puerperium. *J Stroke Cerebrovas Dis* 10:1-10, 2001.)

tients (72%) had IS. A definable cause was determined in 72% of IS and 82% of HS cases. Some causes of IS include preeclampsia or eclampsia (13%), cardioembolism (23%), and a number of other causes, including hypercoagulable states, thrombotic thrombocytopenic purpura, cerebral vasculitis, cerebrovascular mucormycosis, and migrainous infarction (Fig 5). Preeclampsia/eclampsia (37%) and ruptured atrioenous malformation (36%) were the major causes of HS. None of the CVT cases demonstrated a clear etiology other than the pregnant or puerperal state. Risk factors included systemic lupus erythematosus (negative antiphospholipid antibodies and lupus anticoagulant) in 1 patient and dehydration in another patient. Hypertensive disorders of pregnancy were the most frequently seen comorbid conditions for both IS and HS, affecting 45% of those with IS and 64% of those with HS. The presentation with IS tended to be focal deficits (76%); with HS, it tended to be an altered level of consciousness (73%) and headache (64%). All 4 patients with CVT were first seen with headache; 2 had an altered level of consciousness. Most patients with HS were discharged to nursing homes or rehabilitation centers (63%); 73% of patients with IS and 3 patients with CVT were discharged home. There was 1 death caused by a brain herniation after a massive hemispheric IS.

Conclusion.—The etiology of stroke in pregnancy and the puerperium is varied. Strokes are most likely to occur in the third trimester of pregnancy and postpartum period, with clustering in the first postpartum week.

▶ Stroke, acute acquired cerebral deficit, is an uncommon complication of pregnancy and, despite its diverse etiology, this account of 36 case reports collected from data held by 3 Indianapolis hospitals over 7 years provides some useful generalities. On the basis of inpatient evaluation, strokes are characterized as ischemic, hemorrhagic, and venous thrombotic. Nearly 60% of report-

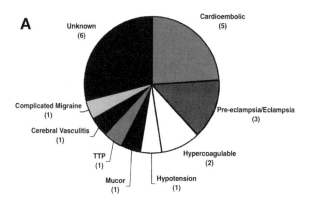

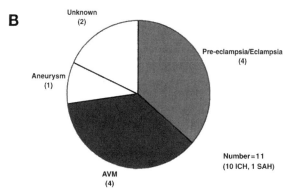

FIGURE 5.—**A**, Ischemic stroke had a diverse array of etiologies. Preeclampsia/eclampsia was the cause of relatively few events (3 of 21). Cardioembolism caused more ischemic stroke than any other 1 factor (5 of 21). Other causes included hypoxia/hypotension, thrombotic thrombocytopenic purpura, hypercoagulable state, cerebral vasculitis, migrainous infarction, and cerebrovascular mucormycosis. **B**, The etiology of hemorrhagic stroke was more restricted, with preeclampsia/eclampsia and intracranial vascular malformations (*[AVMs]* and aneurysms) causing the vast majority of events. (Courtesy of Skidmore FM, Williams LS, Fradkin KD, et al: Presentation, etiology, and outcome of stroke in pregnancy and puerperium. *J Stroke Cerebrovas Dis* 10:1-10, 2001.)

ed cases were judged ischemic and 30% hemorrhagic. African-Americans accounted for 22% of the stroke patients and were somewhat disproportionally distributed in the HS category, probably a consequence of the increased likelihood of the development of hypertension and pregnancy-induced hypertension.

Only 14% of strokes appeared in the first and second trimesters of pregnancy; the remaining 86 occurred in the third trimester and the postpartum period. The first week post partum provided the largest fraction of cases per unit time. IS, caused most commonly by embolic events or pregnancy-induced hypertension, was seen most commonly with focal neurologic deficits. The embolic events were usually cardiac in origin. With HS arising from pregnancy-induced hypertension, arteriovenous malformations or aneurysms, headaches, and decreased levels of consciousness were most common.

Only 4 cases of CVT were seen; clearly CVT is of more consequence to the fetus and placenta than it is to the maternal brain. Many of these cases arose prior to current knowledge and concern about the impact of thrombogenic clotting factor disturbances. Of the women receiving medical therapy, two thirds had residual chronic neurologic deficits and acute mortality was infrequent (1 out of 36 of these reported patients).

T. H. Kirschbaum, MD

Placental Characteristics and Reduced Risk of Maternal Breast Cancer
Cohn BA, Cirillo PM, Christianson RE, et al (Public Health Inst, Berkeley, Calif; Univ of California San Francisco)
J Natl Cancer Inst 93:1133-1140, 2001   4–30

Introduction.—There is considerable evidence that pregnancy exerts a powerful influence on a woman's subsequent risk of breast cancer. Evidence

FIGURE 1

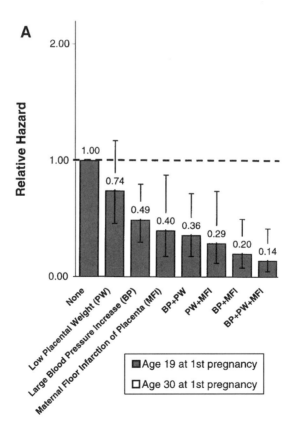

(*Continued*)

FIGURE 1 (cont.)

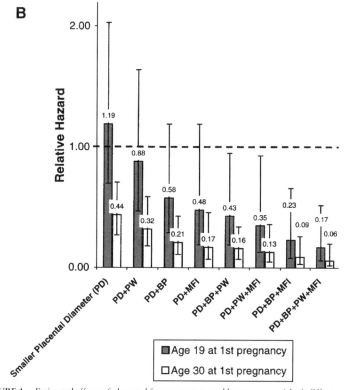

FIGURE 1.—Estimated effects of placental factors on maternal breast cancer risk. **A,** Effects considered one at a time and in combination. Relative hazards were estimated from a single Cox proportional hazards model adjusted for all placental risk factors shown, as well as for mother's birth year, age at first pregnancy, age at index pregnancy, parity, weight gain, and an interaction between age at first pregnancy and placental diameter. There were no other interactions between any other variables in this model. In this model, age variables are represented as continuous variables, parity is dichotomized as 3 or more versus all others, weight gain is represented as a continuous variable, blood pressure increase is represented as 3 indicator variables (quartile 2, quartile 3, and quartile 4) with the lowest quartile as the reference group, placental weight is dichotomized as the first quartile versus all others, and placental diameter is dichotomized as the lower 3 quartiles versus the highest. Maternal floor infarction of the placenta is coded as present versus absent, lower placental weight is defined as the first quartile versus all others, higher blood pressure increase is defined as the fourth quartile versus the first quartile, and smaller placental diameter is defined as the lower 3 quartiles versus the first quartile. **B,** Effects on risk of placental factor combinations that involve placental diameter. Because of the interaction between placental diameter and age at first pregnancy (P for interaction, .008), risk factor combinations that involve placental diameter are shown for 2 specific ages. Age 19 years is the mean for the first quartile of age at first pregnancy for the study sample, and age 30 years is the mean for the fourth quartile. *Error bars* in both graphs reflect boundaries for upper and lower 95% confidence limits. (Courtesy of Cohn BA, Cirillo PM, Christianson RE, et al: Placental characteristics and reduced risk of maternal breast cancer. *J Natl Cancer Inst* 93:1133-1140, 2001. By permission of Oxford University Press.)

suggests that immune, hormonal, or genetic mechanisms that induce hypertension or preeclampsia during pregnancy diminish the risk of breast cancer in both the mother and her female offspring. Possible markers of compromised placental function other than preeclampsia were examined

TABLE 2.—Association of Placental Factors with Breast Cancer

Factor	Relative Hazard (95% Confidence Interval)	
	Age, Parity and Weight Adjusted*	Fully Adjusted†
Systolic blood pressure change between trimesters 2 and 3		
Quartile		
1, <0 mmHg/wk	1.00 (referent)	1.00 (referent)
2, 0-0.37 mmHg/wk	0.89 (0.58 to 1.35)	0.92 (0.60 to 1.40)
3, 0.38-0.80 mmHg/wk	0.64 (0.40 to 1.02)	0.64 (0.40 to 1.02)
4, ≥0.81 mmHg/wk	0.50 (0.31 to 0.82)	0.49 (0.30 to 0.80)
P for trend‡	P = .0001	P = .0001
Maternal floor infarction of the placenta: present/absent	0.49 (0.23 to 1.05)	0.40 (0.18 to 0.88)
Lower placental weight,§ <400 g	0.66 (0.42 to 1.02)	0.74 (0.46 to 1.17)
Smaller placental diameter,‖ <21 cm		
Age 19 yr at first pregnancy	1.01 (0.60 to 1.69)	1.19 (0.70 to 2.04)
Age 30 y at first pregnancy	0.44 (0.28 to 0.71)	0.44 (0.27 to 0.71)
P for intereaction¶	P = .03	P = .008

*All associations were estimated by a Cox model that included variable with adjustment for birth year (continuous), age at index pregnancy (continuous), age at first pregnancy (continuous), maternal weight gain (continuous), and parity (dichotomized as 3 or more vs all others).

†The fully adjusted model includes systolic blood pressure increase (quartile 2, quartile 3, and quartile 4, with quartile 1 as the reference group), maternal floor infarction of the placenta (present vs absent), adjustment variables, birth year, age at first pregnancy, age at index pregnancy, maternal weight gain (continuous variables), and parity (dichotomized as 3 or more vs all others).

‡To test for trend, blood pressure was entered as a continuous variable into the designated Cox models.

§Placental weight classification is first quartile versus all others.

‖Placental diameter classification is lower 3 quartiles versus fourth quartile. The interaction term was constructed as the product of smaller placental diameter (first, second, and third quartiles vs fourth quartile) by age at first full-term pregnancy (continuous variable).

¶To test for interaction, the Wald test was used to test the statistical significance of the product term between age at first pregnancy (continuous) and smaller placental diameter (lower three quartiles vs all other).

(Courtesy of Cohn BA, Cirillo PM, Christianson RE, et al: Placental characteristics and reduced risk of maternal breast cancer. *J Natl Cancer Inst* 93:1133-1140, 2001. By permission of Oxford University Press.)

to determine whether they were also related to decreased risk of maternal breast cancer.

Methods.—A subset of 3804 white women for whom data were available from the Child Health and Development Studies—a pregnancy cohort that has been followed for 40 years to evaluate the prenatal determinants of pregnancy outcome and child health and development—was evaluated. As of 1997, invasive breast cancer had developed in 146 women in the subset. Proportional hazards models were used to estimate correlations of breast cancer with markers of placental function.

Results.—A blood pressure rise between the second and third trimesters demonstrated a linear relationship with breast cancer rate. The highest quartile showed a 51% decrease (95% CI, 20%-70%) that was not explained by preeclampsia. A smaller placental diameter was independently correlated with a decreased breast cancer rate. This correlation rose with age at first pregnancy (P = .008). Maternal floor infarction of the placenta was correlated with a 60% decrease in breast cancer rate (95% CI, 12%-82%). Combined, placental risk factors were correlated with a decrease in the breast cancer rate of as high as 94% (95% CI, 80%-98%) (Fig 1 and Table 2).

Conclusion.—Smaller placentas, maternal floor infarction of the placenta, and increasing blood pressure during pregnancy were correlated with a decreased maternal breast cancer rate. With smaller placental diameter, the greater decrease seen with older age at first pregnancy indicates a process in which promotion of an existing lesion is blocked. Determining the mechanisms for these associations could offer clues to breast cancer prevention and treatment.

▶ This study together with the authors' references[1-5] represent the entire epidemiologic support for the contention that preeclampsia is inversely related to the risk of breast cancer in later life. Prior studies, performed on data from the Centers for Disease Control, upstate New York, California, and Sweden all support the hypothesis with varying levels of certainty. This analysis done on the Child Health and Development Data collected by the NICHD and NINDS from 1959 to 1966[6,7] approaches the relationship from the perspective of the detailed placental examination protocol produced by Dr Kurt Bernirchke for that study, based on his contention that the placental pathology of preeclampsia consists of decidual arteriolopathy, infarcts, placental abruption, and syncytiotrophoblast nuclear degeneration and hyalinization.

These findings are not always present, nor are they confined to women with the clinical diagnosis of preeclampsia.[8] The placenta is necessary for the presence of preeclampsia. Since the syndrome disappears after the third stage of labor and a fetus is not required for the development of this syndrome, placental study was an appropriate approach during the original child development study.

Maternal floor infarction consisting of fibrinous diffuse deposition at the site of placental attachment apparently reflects abnormal maternal and fetal vascular interrelationships and was included as an independent variable of particular interest. Placental examinations were complete in 3804 women who were then followed up using the California Cancer Registry and Department of Motor Vehicle records to determine a possible relationship with breast cancer over a mean duration of 40 years. The incidence of preeclampsia was 2.3% and of maternal floor infarction, 7.6%.

As anticipated, age at study entry, age at first pregnancy, and parity were all significantly increased risk factors for the development of cancer of the breast. Although small placental weight and diameter, an increase in blood pressure in the first three quartiles of gestation, and maternal placental floor infarction were also associated with significant decreases in the risk of diagnosis of breast cancer and since the placental associations were independent and without interaction, the reductions in cancer risk were additive and as much as 94% (see Fig 1). These are the largest environmental reductions in relative hazards for breast cancer reported.

If one accepts that this relationship exists, it means that the placental lesions are fundamental in the impact of the preeclampsia and that hypertension and other clinical findings are secondary and perhaps a consequence of the placental pathology. The mechanism is by no means clear, but it may represent a genetic, immunologic, or hormonal effect, or some combination of all 3.

T. H. Kirschbaum, MD

References

1. Polednak AP, Janerich DT: Characteristics of first pregnancy in relation to early breast cancer: A case-control study. *J Reprod Med* 28:314-318, 1983.
2. Thompson WD, Jacobson HI, Negrini B, et al: Hypertension, pregnancy, and risk of breast cancer. *J Natl Cancer Inst* 81:1571-1574, 1989.
3. Troisi R, Weiss HA, Hoover RN, et al: Pregnancy characteristics and maternal risk of breast cancer. *Epidemiology* 9:641-647, 1998.
4. Ekbom A, Hsieh CC, Lipworth L, et al: Intrauterine environment and breast cancer risk in women: A population-based study. *J Natl Cancer Inst* 89:71-76, 1997.
5. Ekbom A, Trichopoulos D, Adami HO, et al: Evidence of prenatal influences on breast cancer risk. Lancet 340:1015-1018, 1992.
6. 1987 YEARBOOK OF OBSTETRICS AND GYNECOLOGY, pp 243-245.
7. 1988 YEARBOOK OF OBSTETRICS AND GYNECOLOGY, pp 116-118.
8. Benirschke K, Kaufmann P: Pathology of the human placenta.New York, Springer-Verlag, 1955, pp 351-366, 406-412, 500-501.

5 Surveillance

Frequency of Uterine Contractions and the Risk of Spontaneous Preterm Delivery
Iams JD, for the National Institute of Child Health and Human Development Network of Maternal-Fetal Medicine Units (Ohio State Univ, Columbus; et al)
N Engl J Med 346:250-255, 2002   5–1

Background.—It has been suggested that assessment of the frequency of uterine contractions could be used as a screening method to identify pregnant women who are at an increased risk of preterm delivery (before 35 weeks of gestation) and also as a diagnostic test for detecting preterm labor in its earlier stages. However, the clinical value of this measurement is not clear. Ambulatory monitoring of uterine contractions continues to be used, even though several randomized trials have indicated that measurement of the frequency of contractions as a screening or diagnostic test has not been useful for reducing the rate of preterm delivery. This observational study assessed the frequency of uterine contractions as a predictor of spontaneous preterm delivery. The study also included other variables that could affect the frequency of contractions, such as the duration of gestation, the time of day, and the woman's history with regard to preterm delivery. Other proposed markers of the risk of preterm delivery were also evaluated.

Methods.—A total of 306 women were enrolled, all of whom had singleton pregnancies between 22 and 24 weeks of gestation. The women monitored the frequency of their contractions twice daily on 2 or more days per week with a home contraction monitor to delivery or 37 weeks' gestation.

Results.—A total of 34,908 hours of successful monitoring were obtained. More contractions were experienced by women who delivered before 35 weeks than by women who delivered at 35 weeks or later, but there was no identifiable threshold frequency that effectively identified women who delivered preterm infants. Other proposed screening tests, including digital and US evaluations of the cervix and assays for fetal fibronectin in cervicovaginal secretions, also demonstrated low sensitivity and positive predictive value for preterm labor (Table 3).

Conclusions.—The likelihood of preterm delivery is increased with increasing frequency of uterine contractions. However, it does not appear that this measurement is clinically useful for the prediction of preterm delivery.

TABLE 3.—Value of Tests in Predicting Spontaneous Delivery at Less Than 35 Weeks

Test	Week of Gestation at Time of Testing		
	22-24	27-28	31-32
		percent	
Maximal nighttime contraction frequency ≥4/hr			
Sensitivity	8.6	28.1	27.3
Specificity	96.4	88.7	82.0
Positive predictive value	25.0	23.1	11.3
Negative predictive value	88.3	91.1	93.0
Maximal daytime contraction frequency ≥4/hr			
Sensitivity	0	12.9	13.6
Specificity	98.4	93.9	84.9
Positive predictive value	0	20.0	7.1
Negative predictive value	87.0	90.2	92.1
Cervicovaginal fibronectin ≥50 ng/ml			
Sensitivity	18.9	21.4	41.2
Specificity	95.1	94.5	92.5
Positive predictive value	35.0	30.0	30.4
Negative predictive value	89.4	91.6	95.2
Cervical length ≤25 mm			
Sensitivity	47.2	53.6	82.4
Specificity	89.2	82.2	74.9
Positive predictive value	37.0	25.0	20.9
Negative predictive value	92.6	94.1	98.1
Bishop score ≥4*			
Sensitivity	35.1	46.4	82.4
Specificity	91.0	77.9	61.8
Positive predictive value	35.1	18.8	14.7
Negative predictive value	91.0	92.9	97.8

*The Bishop score is a composite measure of cervical length, dilatation, position, consistency, and the degree of descent (station) of the presenting part of the fetus. The results indicate the degree of readiness for labor; values from 0 to 4 indicate not ready for labor, and values from 9 to 13 indicate ready for labor.
(Reprinted by permission of *The New England Journal of Medicine* from Iams JD, for the National Institute of Child Health and Human Development Network of Maternal-Fetal Medicine Units: Frequency of uterine contractions and the risk of spontaneous preterm delivery. *N Engl J Med* 346:250-255. Copyright 2002, Massachusetts Medical Society. All rights reserved.)

▶ Although the title of this study directs attention to home monitoring of uterine contractions for the detection of incipient preterm labor, for which it should surely sound the death knell, there is further evidence for the failure of use of cervical vaginal fibronectin[1-5] and cervical shortening at 22 to 32 weeks' gestational age[6-9] to affect a change in the occurrence of preterm labor. This product of the NICHD Maternal Fetal Medicine Network enrolled 306 women with prior histories of preterm delivery from 20 to 36 weeks or with second trimester bleeding into an observational study of the usefulness of home monitoring of uterine contractions for 1 hour twice a day, morning and evening, between 22 to 36 weeks' gestation. Contraction data were transmitted to a central data coordinating center where they were collected and analyzed. Women were seen at 2- to 3-week intervals where cervical length was measured digitally and by ultrasound and cervical vaginal fibronectin samples obtained. One hundred six women (35%) experienced preterm delivery. Although the frequency of uterine contractions tended to be greater in women destined for preterm delivery, the low sensitivity of a contraction frequency 4 or more times per hour and the false-positive findings ranging from 75% to 100% indicate its uselessness as a predictive finding. The same result was reported here earlier.[10] Once again, using new patient data aggregates and a high prevalence of preterm delivery, vaginal fibronectin concentration greater than 15 µg/mL and cervical length less than 2.5 cm were associated both with false-positive rates of 60% to 80% and poor sensitivities for detection. Surely it is time to give up hope for this as a means of preterm labor detection.

T. H. Kirschbaum, MD

References

1. 1995 Year Book of Obstetrics, Gynecology, and Women's Health, pp 66-67.
2. 1996 Year Book of Obstetrics, Gynecology, and Women's Health, pp 36-39.
3. 1997 Year Book of Obstetrics, Gynecology, and Women's Health, pp 29-31.
4. 1998 Year Book of Obstetrics, Gynecology, and Women's Health, pp 53-54.
5. 1999 Year Book of Obstetrics, Gynecology, and Women's Health, pp 35-37.
6. 2000 Year Book of Obstetrics, Gynecology, and Women's Health, pp 47-49.
7. 1997 Year Book of Obstetrics, Gynecology, and Women's Health, pp 27-28.
8. 1998 Year Book of Obstetrics, Gynecology, and Women's Health, pp 54-56.
9. 2001 Year Book of Obstetrics, Gynecology, and Women's Health, pp 45-47.
10. 1993 Year Book of Obstetrics, Gynecology, and Women's Health, pp 156-157.

Metabolic Information From the Human Fetal Brain Obtained With Proton Magnetic Resonance Spectroscopy

Kok RD, van den Bergh AJ, Heerschap A, et al (Univ Med Ctr, Nijmegen, The Netherlands)
Am J Obstet Gynecol 185:1011-1015, 2001   5–2

Background.—In a previous pilot study, the authors showed that metabolic information could be acquired from the human fetal brain in vivo by using proton MR spectroscopy (^{1}H MRS). ^{1}H MRS was further investigated as a diagnostic tool for assessing fetal brain metabolism.

Methods.—Twenty-one normal, singleton fetuses were studied at 36 to 41 weeks' gestation. ^{1}H MRS was done from a selected volume of brain tissue. By using brain water content as an internal reference, the absolute brain metabolite tissue concentrations were estimated.

Findings.—^{1}H MR spectra demonstrated resonances for 4 dominating brain metabolites: inositol, choline, creatine, and N-acetylaspartate. These metabolites were detected with mean tissue levels of 7.42 mmol/L, 3,31 mmol/L, 4.16 mmol/L, and 5.03 mmol/L, respectively. At times, the resonance for N-acetylaspartate could not be resolved from contaminating lipid signals.

Conclusions.—¹H MRS of the human fetal brain can provide useful data on the condition of the fetus. The metabolite tissue levels for the fetal brain were in the range reported for neonates of similar gestational age.

▶ MRS can be used for quantitative estimates of some atoms whose nuclear proton and neutron number is odd, allowing them to function as magnetic dipoles. The most commonly used isotopes are ³¹P and ¹H; examples of the former have been reviewed here earlier.[1-4] MRS for ³¹P allows estimates of adenosine triphosphate (ATP), phosphocreatine, and pyrophosphates from which intracellular energetics and pH can be measured and calculated. ¹H MRS is more technically difficult because of the ubiquity of protons in intracellular water and fat tissue. As these authors demonstrate, ¹H MRS when performed satisfactorily, in 18 of 24 attempts in this case, can be performed without side effects on fetuses in utero.

This is a work in progress, and more development is needed. Preliminary filtering for water and fat tissue without access to direct brain measurements was made before processing quantitative data, and specific signals were excluded if they failed to correspond to known signal frequencies. Signals for water and choline were processed by a computer-based interface, and other concentrations were measured in a relationship to this derived choline concentration. The sequence is not entirely satisfactory since resulting estimates of brain creatinine and choline differed from known concentration measurements in vivo. But the important matter is the proof that an approach to evaluating brain function biochemically can be carried out on the human fetus in utero with some level of adequacy.

T. H. Kirschbaum, MD

References

1. 2001 YEAR BOOK OF OBSTETRICS, GYNECOLOGY, AND WOMEN'S HEALTH, pp 245-248.
2. 1998 YEAR BOOK OF OBSTETRICS, GYNECOLOGY, AND WOMEN'S HEALTH, pp 241-243.
3. 1992 YEAR BOOK OF OBSTETRICS, GYNECOLOGY, AND WOMEN'S HEALTH, pp 189-191.
4. 1990 YEAR BOOK OF OBSTETRICS, GYNECOLOGY, AND WOMEN'S HEALTH, pp 123-124, 206-207.

Decreased Amniotic Fluid Index in Low-Risk Pregnancy
Kreiser D, El-Sayed YY, Sorem KA, et al (Stanford Univ, Calif)
J Reprod Med 46:743-746, 2001   5–3

Introduction.—A finding of diminished amniotic fluid volume at antepartum US may indicate impaired placental function. The perinatal outcomes of pregnancies complicated by isolated decreased amniotic fluid index (AFI) after 30 weeks' gestation were examined retrospectively.

Methods.—Included in the analysis were 150 singleton, nonanomalous pregnancies with decreased AFI (≤5 cm or >5 cm but <2.5th percentile) and intact membranes. Previous perinatal loss, previous cesarean section, suspected fetal growth restriction, and decreased fetal movement were among

TABLE 3.—Neonatal Outcomes

Outcome	Study Group (Total) (n = 150) (%)	AFI ≤5 (n = 57) (%)	AFI >5 But <2.5th Percentile (n = 93) (%)
Gestational age (wk) at delivery	38.9 ± 1.8	39.2 ± 2.2	38.8 ± 1.6
Birth weight (g)	3174 ± 536	3111 ± 585	3213 ± 503
Apgar score <7	1 (0.66)	0	1 (1.1)
Perinatal mortality	0	0	0
Admissions to neonatal intensive care unit	0	0	0

Data presented as mean ± SD, number, and %.
No statistically significant differences between groups.
(Courtesy of Kreiser D, El-Sayed YY, Sorem KA, et al: Decreased amniotic fluid index in low-risk pregnancy. *J Reprod Med* 46:743-746, 2001.)

the indications for fetal surveillance. Seven pregnancy outcomes were assessed: fetal heart rate abnormalities before labor, induction of labor because of an abnormal nonstress test (NST), emergency cesarean section because of fetal heart rate abnormalities, the presence of meconium, Apgar score <7 at 5 minutes, admission to neonatal ICU, and perinatal mortality.

Results.—Fifty-seven pregnancies had an AFI ≤5 cm, and 93 had an AFI >5 but <2.5th percentile. On average, the women remained undelivered for more than 2 weeks from diagnosis. The 2 groups did not differ significantly in mean maternal age, parity, gestational age at the start of testing, or number of antenatal NSTs performed. Antepartum fetal heart rate changes, intrapartum outcomes, and neonatal outcomes (Table 3) were also similar in the 2 groups, except that variable decelerations on NST were significantly more common among patients in the AFI ≤5 cm group.

Discussion.—The association between low AFI and poor pregnancy outcome is uncertain, and opinions vary regarding the actual threshold for defining a low AFI. But in otherwise-uncomplicated pregnancies, intensive antepartum monitoring is an alternative to immediate delivery in cases of low or borderline AFI.

▶ It is not clear that more data regarding the innocuous nature of uncomplicated oligohydramnios diagnosed by US are needed, but since the condition appears persistently to be a frequent indication for labor induction and the increased risk of cesarean section that ensues, it may be worth citing another.[1,2] This is a report of 150 such patients collected over 2 years at Stanford University. All represent singlet pregnancies past 30 weeks of gestational age with low amniotic fluid indices and intact membranes. Two criteria for the diagnosis of oligohydramnios by US are used. In 57 cases, Phalens definition of AFI (≤5 cm is used). In 93 cases, a more-liberal definition based on the study of amniotic fluid index in pregnancies followed for acardiac monochorionic twins is used.[3] Generally, those deemed to have oligohydramnios by virtue of an amniotic fluid index at or below the 2.5th percentile for gestational age by the Moore criteria have AFIs in the range of 6 to 9 cm. Exclusions from this study, an important item to remember, are premature preterm rupture of membranes, diabetes, preeclampsia, growth retardation, or maternal medical disease. There is no control group here, and management varied among cases, but this becomes of less concern when one rates that there was no perinatal morbidity as reflected in low birth weight notes, reduced Apgar scores, perinatal mortality, or neonatal ICU admission. Granted the exclusionary criteria, oligohydramnios defined by contemporary US criteria in otherwise-normal pregnancies, lacking other risk factors for perinatal mortality, appears to be of no obstetrical consequence whatsoever.

T. H. Kirschbaum, MD

References

1. 2001 YEAR BOOK OF OBSTETRICS, GYNECOLOGY, AND WOMEN'S HEALTH, pp 35-38.
2. 2002 YEAR BOOK OF OBSTETRICS, GYNECOLOGY, AND WOMEN'S HEALTH, pp 252-254.
3. Moore TR, Gale S, Benirschke K: Perinatal outcome of 49 pregnancies complicated by acardiac twinning. *Am J Obstet Gynecol* 163:907, 1990.

Neonatal Screening for Medium-Chain Acyl-CoA Dehydrogenase Deficiency
Pourfarzam M, Morris A, Appleton M, et al (Univ of Newcastle Upon Tyne, England)
Lancet 358:1063-1064, 2001   5–4

Background.—Neonatal screening for medium-chain acyl-CoA dehydrogenase (MCAD) deficiency is not yet available in the United Kingdom. Concerns have been raised about the specificity of the screening test and the uncertainty of the natural history of this disorder. These issues were further explored.

Methods.—Concentrations of acylcamitines in stored neonatal blood spots were studied retrospectively. Patients with high octanoylcamitine levels at 7 to 9 years of age were also studied.

Findings.—The specificity of screening for MCAD deficiency was found to be 100% (Figure). The sensitivity of the test was difficult to determine. In most of the patients with MCAD deficiency symptoms developed in early childhood. The morbidity and mortality rates associated with MCAD deficiency were high.

Conclusions.—These data support the introduction of MCAD deficiency screening to the United Kingdom. The test had a 100% specificity, and the morbidity and mortality rates associated with this deficiency were high.

▶ This is a retrospective study employing archival neonatal blood spots obtained between 1991 and 1993 at the Royal Victoria Infirmary at Newcastle on Tyne. Samples were subjected to extraction and aqueous dissolution; experimental storage at 4°C in sealed containers led to an estimate of 15% to 17% analyte loss over the average storage time of up to 5 years. Samples were then subjected to tandem mass spectrometry.[1] In brief, the technique allows organ-

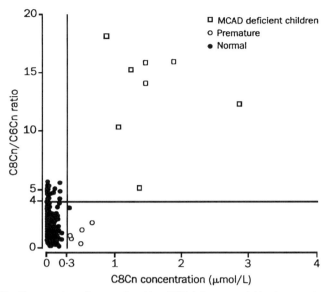

FIGURE.—Concentration of octanoylcamitine (C8Cn) in neonatal blood spots plotted against octanoylcamitine/hexanoylcamitine concentration ratio (C8Cn/C6Cn). *Abbreviation: MCAD*, Medium-chain acyl-CoA dehydrogenase deficiency. (Courtesy of Pourfarzam M, Morris A, Appleton M, et al: Neonatal screening for medium-chain acyl-CoA dehydrogenase deficiency. *Lancet* 358:1063-1064, 2001. Reprinted with permission from Elsevier Science.)

ic assays to be done quickly at low unit cost, enabling routine universal screening for neonatal genetic metabolic defects. Here the method is applied to detect abnormalities in mitochondrial DNA, which may in turn lead to defects in fatty acid metabolism in later life. What then results is an accumulation of unmetabolized fatty acids, conjugated as carnitates, which facilitates mitochondrial penetration. The clinical picture is of severe metabolic acidosis, glycogenolysis to compensate for deficient lipid energy metabolism, hypoglycemia, encephalopathy, and multiple organ failure. Obstetricians are most familiar with this syndrome in the form of acute fatty liver of pregnancy.[2-6] The diagnosis of a gene defect was confirmed in 3 samples obtained from children known to have the dehydrogenase deficiency, 14 cases with elevated acyl carnitate concentrations were found, and 8 with confirmation of either homozygous or heterozygous gene mutations. The resultant dehydrogenase deficiency incidence of 1 per 7000 births is somewhat above the range of incidence figures reported for the United Kingdom. Since false-negative findings are unknowable in a retrospective cohort study, sensitivity or predictive strength cannot be calculated from this experience. This is, however, a nice example of the use of this screening method easily adapted to multiple protein and organic analytes, for routine neonatal screening for genetic abnormalities.

T. H. Kirschbaum, MD

References

1. 2001 YEAR BOOK OF OBSTETRICS, GYNECOLOGY, AND WOMEN'S HEALTH, pp 236-238.
2. 1992 YEAR BOOK OF OBSTETRICS, GYNECOLOGY, AND WOMEN'S HEALTH, pp 69-73.
3. 1994 YEAR BOOK OF OBSTETRICS, GYNECOLOGY, AND WOMEN'S HEALTH, pp 109-110.
4. 1995 YEAR BOOK OF OBSTETRICS, GYNECOLOGY, AND WOMEN'S HEALTH, pp 116-117.
5. 1996 YEAR BOOK OF OBSTETRICS, GYNECOLOGY, AND WOMEN'S HEALTH, pp 68-69.
6. 1997 YEAR BOOK OF OBSTETRICS, GYNECOLOGY, AND WOMEN'S HEALTH, pp 198-199.

A Critical Appraisal of the Use of Umbilical Artery Doppler Ultrasound in High-Risk Pregnancies: Use of Meta-analyses in Evidence-based Obstetrics

Westergaard HB, Langhoff-Roos J, Lingman G, et al (Copenhagen Univ; Univ Hosp, Lund, Sweden)
Ultrasound Obstet Gynecol 17:466-476, 2001   5–5

Background.—The efficacy of Doppler velocimetry in high-risk pregnancies has been evaluated in randomized, controlled trials and several systematic reviews since 1992. However, recent reports have questioned its benefits. Randomized, controlled trials on the use of umbilical Doppler velocimetry in high-risk pregnancies were reanalyzed to determine which of these pregnancies can benefit from the use of Doppler velocimetry.

Methods.—A search of the Medline, Cochrane Library, and Embase databases was used to identify 13 randomized, controlled trials of Doppler velocimetry in high-risk pregnancies. Six of these trials included pregnancies with strictly defined suspected intrauterine growth restriction and hypertensive disease of pregnancies; these were classified as "well-defined studies." The rest of the trials included a wide variety of high-risk pregnancies and were classified as "general risk studies." All of the studies were analyzed in terms of heterogeneity and outcome. A panel of 32 international experts audited the perinatal deaths reported in the trials.

Results.—A more uniform study design was noted for the well-defined studies in comparison with the general risk studies, and the well-defined studies demonstrated a significant reduction in antenatal admissions, inductions of labor, elective deliveries, and cesarean sections. Audits showed that more of the perinatal deaths in the "well-defined studies" were potentially avoidable with the use of Doppler velocimetry. The rate of avoidable perinatal deaths was higher among control subjects than among case subjects (50% vs 20%) in the well-defined studies (Table 4).

Conclusion.—There were significant differences in study design and technical and clinical issues in the randomized, controlled trials of umbilical artery Doppler velocimetry, and these differences indicate that the trials should not be pooled in a simple meta-analysis. Stratification indicated that umbilical artery Doppler velocimetry reduced the number of perinatal deaths and unnecessary obstetric interventions only in pregnancies with suspected intrauterine growth restriction or hypertensive disease of pregnancy.

TABLE 4.—The Results of the Meta-analysis of the Analyzed High-Risk Studies

Outcome	Odds Ratio (95% Confidence Interval)		
	'Well-Defined Studies' (n = 6)	'General Risk Studies' (n = 8)	All High-Risk Studies
Perinatal mortality*	0.66 (0.36-1.22)	0.68 (0.43-1.08)	0.67 (0.47-0.97)
Antenatal admission	0.56 (0.43-0.72)	—	—
Induction of labor	0.78 (0.63-0.96)	0.95 (0.84-1.07)	0.90 (0.81-1.00)
Elective delivery	0.73 (0.61-0.88)	1.00 (0.90-1.12)	0.92 (0.84-1.01)
Cesarean sections	0.78 (0.65-0.94)	0.96 (0.84-1.11)	0.91 (0.81-1.01)
elective	0.99 (0.76-1.29)	1.15 (0.94-1.40)	1.09 (0.93-1.28)
emergency	0.78 (0.61-1.00)	0.88 (0.74-1.03)	0.85 (0.74-0.97)
Low Apgar score at 5 min	0.72 (0.45-1.15)	0.98 (0.71-1.15)	0.89 (0.68-1.16)
Admission to NICU	0.87 (0.70-1.07)	0.98 (0.83-1.15)	0.93 (0.82-1.06)

*Singletons, non-malformed.
Abbreviation: NICU, Neonatal intensive care unit.
(Courtesy of Westergaard HB, Langhoff-Roos J, Lingman G, et al: A critical appraisal of the use of umbilical artery Doppler ultrasound in high-risk pregnancies: Use of meta-analyses in evidence-based obstetrics. *Ultrasound Obstet Gynecol* 17:466-476, 2001. Reprinted by permission of Blackwell Science, Inc.)

▶ Over the past 9 years, a series of 13 randomized, clinical trials designed to evaluate the clinical usefulness of this procedure have appeared. There is general agreement that trials conducted on low-risk or unselected populations showed no benefits from Doppler velocimetry.[1] Although a 1994 meta-analysis of the Cochrane Pregnancy and Childbirth data reported a 49% decrease in perinatal mortality attributed to the use of umbilical artery Doppler,[2] several subsequent studies—including a 1996 repeat Cochrane analysis—have failed to demonstrate a significant benefit, including meta-analyses of the later, larger data aggregates. This detailed report by the Department of Biostatistics at Copenhagen University makes it clear that the analyses are compromised by data heterogeneity and other inadequacies. A nonparametric test for significant data heterogeneity in this analysis resulted in a probability estimate of 80% likelihood.

In an effort to deal with these problems, the authors segregate 6 "well-defined studies" of relatively high quality, all dealing with women with suspected fetal growth retardation and/or pregnancy hypertension. The other 7 are "general risk studies" with more widely ranging indications for US and less inclusive data. For both, criteria for diagnoses of pregnancy hypertension were largely absent and varied considerably among investigators when present. It is uncertain in most cases whether multiple pregnancies were or were not included.

Exclusion criteria were very different among studies; gestational age was not specified in 7 of 13 studies and was totally absent in 5 others. The nature of antenatal testing varied widely among investigators, and action plans given an abnormal Doppler result were undefined in 6 studies and only present in part in 4 of 6 of the "well-defined" subset. US equipment, training, and examiner experience differed considerably and absent end-diastolic flow velocity was reported in only 9 of 13 studies.

In calculating odds ratios between those exposed to Doppler evaluation and control subjects, significant differences were associated only with decreased perinatal mortality, induction of labor, or antenatal admission and only among the "well-defined" studies. No trace of benefit was attributable in the "general risk" category. Mean perinatal mortality rates were lower in the well-defined studies (16/1000 live births) than in the controls (23/1000 live births) and neonatal ICU admissions were similarly different (21.6/1000 and 23.6/1000 live births respectively). Labor inductions were less common with Doppler evaluation (28.2%) versus controls (33.4%). No other differences were noted among the general risk categories with respect to those variables or to Apgar scores, cesarean section, or emergency delivery occurrences.

Since measures of variance cannot be accurately calculated, there is no way to test statistical significance for any of these differences. The authors conclude that there is hope for continued study of women with growth-retarded fetuses or pregnancy hypertension but that Doppler need not be used in pregnancies marked by decreased fetal movement, postdatism, antepartum hemorrhage, and a few other clinical problems. The data heterogeneity comes ultimately from poorly designed studies and a lack of familiarity with the work of others in the field, from whom new experiences might be structured to allow comparability. The past 9 years have shown decreasing objective reason for enthusiasm for this mode of fetal surveillance.

T. H. Kirschbaum, MD

References

1. Beattie RB, Hannah ME, Dornan JC: Compound analysis of umbilical artery velocimetry in low risk pregnancy. *J Matern Fetal Investig* 2:269-276, 1992.
2. Neilson JP: Doppler ultrasound in high risk pregnancies, in *Cochrane Database of Systematic Reviews*. Review No. 03889. Oxford, UK, Update Software (Cochrane Updates on Disc), 1994.

Doppler Assessment of Umbilical Artery, Thoracic Aorta and Middle Cerebral Artery in the Management of Pregnancies With Growth Restriction
Madazli R, Uludağ S, Ocak V (Univ of Istanbul, Turkey)
Acta Obstet Gynecol Scand 80:702-707, 2001   5–6

Background.—Antepartum fetal surveillance is done to prevent perinatal mortality, morbidity, and long-term neurologic complications by enabling timely delivery of the fetus. The best use of information acquired from Doppler studies of umbilical artery, thoracic aorta, and middle cerebral artery in the management of growth-restricted pregnancies was investigated.

Methods.—One hundred pregnant women with intrauterine growth-restricted fetuses were studied. Doppler flow velocity waveforms were obtained from the umbilical and middle cerebral arteries as well as from the thoracic aorta, and groups were formed on the basis of results. Twenty-nine fetuses had a normal pulsatility index (PI); 30 had a high PI; and 41 had absent end-diastolic velocity (AEDV) in the umbilical artery.

Findings.—Worsening of the diastolic flow in the umbilical artery was associated with significantly decreasing birth weight and umbilical vein pH at birth and a significantly increasing perinatal mortality rate. Increased umbilical artery PI correlated significantly with increased thoracic aorta PI and reduced middle cerebral artery PI. Perinatal mortality rate resulting from fetal asphyxia in fetuses with AEDV in the umbilical artery was 39.5%, and in those with AEDV in both the umbilical artery and thoracic aorta it was 50%. The detection of AEDV in the thoracic aorta was the strongest predictor of perinatal death.

Conclusions.—The extent of Doppler abnormalities parallels the severity of fetal compromise in women with growth-restricted pregnancies. Such fetuses with AEDV in both the umbilical artery and the thoracic aorta are severely compromised. Gaining time for these fetuses in utero is of no benefit.

▶ This is an attempt to evaluate the value of Doppler indices in predicting perinatal asphyxia. One hundred women with fetal growth retardation excluding aneuploidies and other anomalies, were evaluated by Doppler PI from fetal umbilical arteries, middle cerebral arteries, and the thoracic aorta. It is not clear whether both umbilical arteries were scanned, and the duration of gestation varied considerably among subjects. Of the 100, there were 29 with normal Doppler indices, 30 with umbilical artery PI greater than 2 standard deviations from the mean for gestational age, and 40 with umbilical artery absent end diastolic velocity. Management was uncontrolled and left to physician discretion. Simple linear correlation coefficients were used to show covariance between increased umbilical artery PI and thoracic aortic PI together with decreased middle cerebral artery PI, assumed to be signs of fetal jeopardy. Increasing thoracic PI had a significant inverse correlation with decreased middle cerebral artery PI. Nothing can be said about predictability from these findings because of the absence of controlled observations and the inability to estimate false-positive and false-negative rates for any of the 3 independent variables. When logistic regression was performed against perinatal death, only thoracic aortic PI, a partial measure of fetal cardiac output, was significantly correlated. In 11 fetal and 7 neonatal deaths, with time intervals between Doppler evaluations to death ranging from 2 to 40 days, the Doppler estimates were clearly useless in the prevention of perinatal death. This study fails to provide evidence supporting the clinical utility of the Doppler measurements which these investigators performed.

T. H. Kirschbaum, MD

Arterial Doppler Ultrasound in 115 Second- and Third-Trimester Fetuses With Congenital Heart Disease
Meise C, Germer U, Gembruch U (Med Univ of Lübeck, Germany)
Ultrasound Obstet Gynecol 17:398-402, 2001   5–7

Background.—Fetal arterial Doppler US is especially used as a diagnostic and prognostic tool in pregnancies complicated by uteroplacental insufficiency leading to intrauterine growth retardation in the fetus. However, the value of fetal arterial Doppler US in the diagnosis of congenital heart disease (CHD) is still controversial. The influence of isolated CHD on fetal arterial Doppler blood flow velocity waveforms was evaluated.

Methods.—A total of 115 consecutive fetuses with anatomically diagnosed CHD underwent Doppler flow velocimetry in the umbilical and middle cerebral arteries. The gestational age of the fetuses ranged from 19 to 41 weeks. Group A consisted of 55 fetuses with isolated CHD, with cardiogenic hydrops fetalis in 6 fetuses. Group B consisted of 60 fetuses in whom there were complications of chromosomal or nonchromosomal extracardiac malformation, uteroplacental dysfunction, or noncardiogenic nonimmune hydrops fetalis. A control was formed, consisting of 100 healthy fetuses of uncomplicated pregnancies. For statistical analysis, individual pulsatility index measurements were converted to their Z-scores.

Results.—The 115 fetuses with CHD demonstrated a significantly greater difference from the normal mean for gestation on the umbilical artery pulsatility index than did the control group. However, of 33 fetuses with indexes above the 95% reference interval, 29 fetuses were associated with extracardiac malformations, uteroplacental dysfunction, or noncardiogenic nonimmune hydrops fetalis. Fetuses with isolated CHD still demonstrated significantly higher values than healthy fetuses, but the umbilical artery pulsatility index exceeded the 95% reference interval in only 4 of 55 (7%) fetuses (Fig 1). This finding was not significantly different from that of the control group, in which only 4 of 100 fetuses had an umbilical artery pulsatility index above the 95% reference interval.

The only fetuses in which elevated umbilical artery pulsatility indexes were seen were 4 in which there was severe obstruction of the outflow tracts, leading to reverse perfusion of the affected great artery and, in 1 case, Eb-

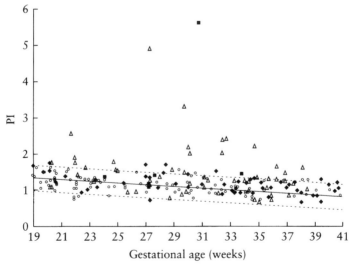

FIGURE 1.—Umbilical artery pulsatility indexes (*PI*) of 49 fetuses with isolated congenital heart disease (*black diamonds*), 6 with cardiogenic nonimmune hydrops fetalis (*black squares*), 60 with nonisolated congenital heart disease (*white triangles*), and 100 healthy fetuses of the control group (*white circles*). The *solid line* is the regression line, and *broken lines* show the 95% reference intervals. (Courtesy of Meise C, Germer U, Gembruch U: Arterial Doppler ultrasound in 115 second- and third-trimester fetuses with congenital heart disease. *Ultrasound Obstet Gynecol* 17:398-402, 2001. Reprinted by permission of Blackwell Science, Inc.)

steins's anomaly with pulmonary insufficiency. All 4 fetuses with isolated CHD and an elevated umbilical artery pulsatility index died. Fourteen of the 18 fetuses with lethal outcome had normal pulsatility index values in the umbilical artery. There were no significant differences between fetuses with and without CHD or in any subgroups in investigations of blood flow in the middle cerebral artery.

Conclusion.—The alterations seen in arterial blood flow velocity waveforms in fetuses with isolated CHD are not of diagnostic value. In most patients with CHD, the increase in the pulsatility index of umbilical arterial blood flow velocity waveforms is the result of extracardiac anomalies, particularly uteroplacental dysfunction and chromosomal abnormalities. Umbilical artery Doppler US is not clinically helpful in predicting fetal outcome.

▶ Fetal US fails to diagnose CHD more often than it succeeds, but this study is aimed at the converse problem; given an elevated pulsatility index in umbilical arteries, is this sufficient to justify fetal echocardiographic study if no other possible reason exists? The authors' negative view is based on the analysis of umbilical artery Doppler studies done on 115 fetuses varying from 19 to 41 weeks' gestational age, all instances of the antenatal diagnosis of CHD and compared with 100 normal fetuses. An attempt was made to separate fetuses with CHD and associated extracardiac abnormalities or uteroplacental insufficiency, by which the authors mean birth weight less than the 10th percentile, growth retardation, or abnormal uterine artery Doppler signals. It is not clear how many exhibited this latter finding with its uncertain relationship to pregnancy outcome. Control subjects showed normal estimated fetal weight and no evidence of placental insufficiency as defined above.

The mean percentage of deviation of the pulsatility index from normal is greater among the 55 singlet pregnancies with no extracardiac abnormalities, but this was the impact of 4 cases, or 3.5%, of the fetuses studied. Two of these had pulmonary and tricuspid atresia with retrograde pulmonary artery perfusion through the ductus arteriosus, another had hypoplastic left ventricle and aorta, and a fourth had Epstein's anomaly compromising the left ventricle and umbilical artery flow characteristic. In all of the cases, the pulsatility index was normal for gestational age as was the pulsatility index done simultaneously on middle–cerebral artery vessels.

The authors conclude that isolated CHD yields normal umbilical artery Doppler signals, except when modified by associated genetic or developmental defects that should be discernible by other techniques. The number of such cases (4 out of 55) was not significantly different from instances of an elevated umbilical artery pulsatility index in normal control subjects (4 out of 100). Neither is an elevated pulsatility index in CHD a reliable index of the severity of the anomaly nor of the likelihood of fetal and neonatal death in such infants.

T. H. Kirschbaum, MD

Multicenter Screening for Pre-eclampsia and Fetal Growth Restriction by Transvaginal Uterine Artery Doppler at 23 Weeks of Gestation

Nicolaides KH, for The Fetal Medicine Foundation Second Trimester Screening Group (King's College, London)
Ultrasound Obstet Gynecol 18:441-449, 2001   5–8

Introduction.—Several Doppler US investigations of the uteroplacental circulation have verified that increased impedance to flow in these vessels is correlated with an increased risk for subsequent development of preeclampsia, fetal growth restriction (FGR), or both. The value of transvaginal color Doppler examination of the uterine arteries at 23 weeks' gestation in predicting the subsequent development of preeclampsia and FGR was examined in a multicenter screening investigation in approximately 8000 singleton pregnancies.

Methods.—Females with singleton pregnancies attending routine ultrasound examination at 23 weeks' gestation in 7 participating hospitals underwent Doppler assessment of the uterine arteries. The presence of an early diastolic notch in the waveform was recorded, and the mean pulsatility index of the 2 arteries was determined. Screening characteristics in the prediction of preeclampsia and the delivery of a low birth weight infant were ascertained.

Results.—Doppler assessment of the uterine arteries was attempted in 8335 consecutive singleton pregnancies. Of these, adequate waveforms were obtained from both vessels in 8202 (98.4%) cases. Complete outcome data were available from 7851 (95.7%). The mean gestational age was 23 weeks (range, 22-24 weeks). The mean uterine artery pulsatility index was not significantly altered with gestation ($r = -0.0078; P = .483$). The median value was 1.04; the 95th percentile was 1.63. In 9.3% of patients, the early diastolic notches in the waveform from both uterine arteries were present. In an additional 11.1% of patients, there were notches unilaterally. Preeclampsia with FGR was observed in 42 (0.5%) patients, preeclampsia without FGR in 71 (0.9%), and FGR without preeclampsia in 698 (8.9%) patients. The sensitivity of an increased pulsatility index above the 95th percentile (1.63) for preeclampsia with FGR was 69%, for preeclampsia without FGR was 24%, for FGR without preeclampsia was 13%, for preeclampsia irrespective of FGR was 41%, and for FGR irrespective of preeclampsia was 16%. The sensitivity of FGR defined by the 5th versus the 10th percentile was higher (19% vs 16%). The sensitivity for both preeclampsia and FGR was inversely associated with gestational age at delivery. When delivery occurred before 32 weeks' gestation, the sensitivity for all cases of preeclampsia with FGR, preeclampsia without FGR, and FGR without preeclampsia rose to 93%, 80%, and 56%, respectively. The sensitivity of bilateral notches in predicting preeclampsia, FGR, or both was similar to that of increased pulsatility index; the screen-positive rate with notches (9.3%) was considerably higher than that with increased pulsatility index (5.1%).

Conclusion.—A one-stage color Doppler screening program at 23 weeks can identify most females who subsequently develop severe preeclampsia, FGR, or both.

▶ Here is yet another attempt to demonstrate the usefulness of uterine artery Doppler measurements in the second trimester in screening for preeclampsia and growth retardation. This study stemmed from 7 hospitals largely in and surrounding London and was performed by different investigators with different equipment. Congenital anomalies were excluded on the basis of detection at a routine scan at 11 to 14 weeks' gestational age. All ultrasonographers had been certified by the Fetal Medicine Foundation housed at King's College Hospital. Of the 8202 women described, the prevalence of preeclampsia was 1.4%, of growth retardation 8.9%, and of both coexisting 0.5%. The incidence of growth retardation is inevitably determined by the arbitrary identification of growth retardation at the 10th percentile for birth weight at gestational age. Results are reported for cases with a uterine artery pulsativity index (PI) greater than 1.63 (such cases exceed the 90% probability of occurrence), bilateral diastolic notching, and both increased PI and notching together. The authors feel notching without an increase in pulsativity index doubles the positive screen incidence without influencing sensitivity. False-positive rates were all prohibitively high. For preeclamspia, false-positive rates are 92.8%, 96.3%, and 96.2% for each of the 3 predictors above. For growth retardation, they are 95.8%, 97.5%, and 96.9%. For preeclampsia with growth retardation, corresponding false-positive rates were 77.1%, 80.9%, and 81.8%. The likelihood ratios cited represent ratios of ratios and are very sensitive to errors stemming from the presence of small denominators. It's hard to tell how the receiver operating curves were drawn for the values of false-positive rates less than 75% since none were observed. All in all, this is another disappointing effort in an attempt to justify uterine artery Doppler measurements as an obstetric screening procedure in the second trimester.

T. H. Kirschbaum, MD

Aspirin for the Prevention of Preeclampsia in Women With Abnormal Uterine Artery Doppler: A Meta-analysis
Coomarasamy A, Papaioannou S, Gee H, et al (Birmingham Women's Hosp, England)
Obstet Gynecol 98:861-866, 2001   5–9

Background.—Several randomized studies have assessed the efficacy of aspirin in preventing preeclampsia in women with abnormal uterine Doppler findings. However, these studies generally lacked the statistical power to yield conclusive findings. A meta-analysis was done to further define the efficacy of aspirin in preventing preeclampsia in women identified as high risk by abnormal second-trimester uterine artery Doppler assessment.

Methods.—All randomized trials comparing the efficacy of aspirin with that of placebo or no treatment in women with an abnormal uterine artery

Doppler finding were included in the meta-analysis. Five relevant studies were identified.

Findings.—When the findings of the trials were pooled, it was found that aspirin significantly reduced preeclampsia, with an odds ratio of 0.55. In women with abnormal uterine artery Doppler findings, the baseline risk of preeclampsia was 16%. To prevent 1 case of preeclampsia, 16 women needed aspirin treatment. The infants of women receiving aspirin were a mean 82 g heavier than those of control subjects, although this finding was not significant statistically.

Conclusion.—Uterine artery Doppler assessment identifies women at high risk for preeclampsia in whom aspirin treatment would be beneficial. Aspirin therapy in such women significantly reduces preeclampsia.

▶ This is an attempt, through meta-analysis of data from 5 individual studies, to gain a claim of statistical significance by aggregating case studies, any 1 of which has insufficient case numbers to justify that claim. Curiously, the authors feel justified in ignoring a series of earlier studies,[1,2] including the CLAST study in which 9364 gravidas were randomly exposed to low-dose aspirin as prophylaxis for preeclampsia. All but 1 of these failed to support the use of aspirin for that purpose.

The authors seem less than discriminating in accepting the data they employ in this new analysis. McParland et al[3] find that the uterine artery resistance index suffices in the 24th week of pregnancy to identify a population of patients with a 25% risk of term pregnancy hypertension.[4] In an accompanying article in the same issue,[5] the same authors indicate both the Kappa index and the false-positive rate render the uterine artery Doppler value clinically useless.

The study by Bower et al [6,7] suffers from the unblinded subjective diagnosis of preeclampsia and discriminatory recruiting practices identified by the journal's editor. The study by Zimmerman et al[8] uses bilateral Doppler notching as the sole criterion for US abnormality, a criterion that makes the data different from all others. Morris et al[9] uses uterine US evaluation at 18 weeks of pregnancy and finds no impact of aspirin on any outcome variable.

Finally, in Harrington,[10,11] test subjects subdivided into 4 subsets and test control groups differed with respect to antepartum testing and the intense antepartum surveillance afforded women with abnormal Doppler findings but not the controls. These problems in experimental design and data heterogeneity render the odds ratio for the risk of occurrence of preeclampsia in 498 aspirin users versus control patients of 0.55 meaningless.

T. H. Kirschbaum, MD

References

1. 1994 YEAR BOOK OF OBSTETRICS, GYNECOLOGY, AND WOMEN'S HEALTH, pp 57-58; pp 61-63.
2. 1995 YEAR BOOK OF OBSTETRICS, GYNECOLOGY, AND WOMEN'S HEALTH, pp 58-60; pp 71-74.
3. McParland P, Pearce JM, Chamberlain GV: Doppler ultrasound and aspirin in recognition and prevention of pregnancy-induced hypertension. *Lancet* 335:1552-1555, 1990.

4. 1992 YEAR BOOK OF OBSTETRICS AND GYNECOLOGY, pp 53-54.
5. 1992 YEAR BOOK OF OBSTETRICS AND GYNECOLOGY, pp 54-56.
6. Bower SJ, Harrington KF, Schuchter K, et al: Prediction of pre-eclampsia by abnormal uterine Doppler ultrasound and modification by aspirin. *Br J Obstet Gynaecol* 103:625-629, 1996.
7. 1998 YEAR BOOK OF OBSTETRICS, GYNECOLOGY, AND WOMEN'S HEALTH, pp 51-53.
8. Zimmermann P, Eirio V, Koskinen J, et al: Effect of low-dose aspirin treatment on vascular resistance in the uterine, uteroplacental, renal and umbilical arteries—A prospective longitudinal study on a high risk population with persistent notch in the uterine arteries. *Eur J Ultrasound* 5:17-30, 1997.
9. Morris JM, Fay RA, Ellwood DA, et al: A randomized controlled trial of aspirin in patients with abnormal uterine artery blood flow. *Obstet Gynecol* 87:74-78, 1996.
10. Harrington K, Kurdi W, Aquilina J, et al: A prospective management study of slow-release aspirin in the palliation of uteroplacental insufficiency predicted by uterine artery Doppler at 20 weeks. *Ultrasound Obstet Gynecol* 15:13-18, 2000.
11. 2001 YEAR BOOK OF OBSTETRICS, GYNECOLOGY, AND WOMEN'S HEALTH, pp 165-167.

Screening for Down Syndrome Using First-Trimester Ultrasound and Second-Trimester Maternal Serum Markers in a Low-Risk Population: A Prospective Longitudinal Study

Audibert F, Dommergues M, Benattar C, et al (Université Paris XI; Université Paris V)
Ultrasound Obstet Gynecol 18:26-31, 2001   5–10

Background.—Alternative techniques for Down syndrome screening have been studied in the past 10 years. Nuchal translucency and second-trimester maternal serum measures were compared.

Methods.—A total of 4130 consecutive women younger than 38 years with a singleton pregnancy were included in the study. The women were considered at low risk. Nuchal translucency was measured at 10 to 14 weeks, and maternal serum screening by human chorionic gonadotrophin and α-fetoprotein was performed at 14 to 18 weeks. Amniocentesis was recommended for women with a nuchal translucency measure of 3 mm or greater and for those with a maternal serum screening-derived risk of 1 in 250 or greater. In addition, all women had a detailed, second-semester US scan. Pregnancy outcomes were documented prospectively.

Findings.—Twelve cases of Down syndrome occurred in the 4130 pregnancies followed up, for an incidence of 0.28%. All cases were detected prenatally. In 7 cases (58%), the nuchal translucency measure was 3 mm or greater. Six of 10 cases with available maternal serum screening (60%) had a calculated risk of 1 in 250 or greater. Subsequent maternal serum screening detected 4 of the 5 cases with a nuchal translucency measure of less than 3 mm. At a 5% positive test threshold, the sensitivity of nuchal translucency was 75%; of maternal serum screening, 60%; and of combined risk screening, 90% (Table 5).

Conclusion.—An approach that combines the findings of first-trimester nuchal translucency and second-trimester biochemistry is effective in screening for Down syndrome. This combined approach improves the detection

TABLE 5.—Screen-positive Rate, Sensitivity, and Positive Predictive Value for Down Syndrome With Different Modes of Screening

Mode of Screening	Screen-Positive Rate (n (%))	Sensitivity for Down Syndrome (n (%))	PPV for Down Syndrome (% (Proportion))
NT ≥ 3 mm	83/4130 (2.0)	7/12 (58)	8.4 (1 : 12)
NT risk ≥ 1/250	186/4130 (4.5)	8/12 (67)	3.9 (1 : 25)
NT ≥ 95th percentile	210/4130 (5.0)	9/12 (75)	4.3 (1 : 23)
MSS ≥ 1/250	130/3790 (3.4)	6/10 (60)	4.6 (1 : 22)
NT ≥ 3 or MSS ≥ 1/250	191/3790 (5.0)	9/10 (90)	4.7 (1 : 21)
Combined risk ≥ 1/250	106/3790 (2.8)	9/10 (90)	8.5 (1 : 12)

Abbreviations: PPV, Positive predictive value; NT, nuchal translucency; MSS, risk estimated by maternal age and second-trimester serum markers.
(Courtesy of Audibert F, Dommergues M, Benattar C, et al: Screening for Down syndrome using first-trimester ultrasound and second-trimester maternal serum markers in a low-risk population: A prospective longitudinal study. *Ultrasound Obstet Gynecol* 18:26-31, 2001. Reprinted by permission of Blackwell Science, Inc.)

rate, compared with the use of any single test. However, the false-positive rate is likely to be higher with this strategy. Interpretation of maternal serum screening-derived risk should be combined with the first-trimester nuchal translucency measure.

▶ These authors use a retrospective cohort approach to evaluate the impact of adding US evaluation of nuchal translucency (NT) in the first trimester to second trimester maternal serum alpha fetoprotein testing and human chorionic gonadotropin, for the detection of Down syndrome. What is involved is the need to balance test sensitivity (the fraction of positive cases detected by screening) against the false-positive rate of screening and the need to minimize the number of amniocenteses needed to clarify equivocal results. Specifically, the authors hope to determine whether adding US NT determination to maternal serum screening increases the number of false positives as reported by others. They confirm that it does. The results are complicated, however, by the use of several different criteria for evaluating the patients.

There were 4130 women who had primary US evaluation and 3790 who had the second trimester maternal serum screen. The incidence of Down syndrome was 0.3% in these women with a mean age of 30.1 years. The incidence of amniocentesis for karyotype determination was 7.6%, but this included a 4.7% incidence of amniocentesis in the 87% of women who were negative to both screens. Though NT detected 75% of fetuses with Down syndrome and serum testing detected 60%, the difference was not statistically significant because of small case numbers.

Comparing results of NT at least 3 mm in thickness alone in women with combined risks for Down syndrome greater than 1:256 for both screens, sensitivity is enhanced, though fewer cases were identified because 8% of women screened by US did not receive maternal serum screening. This had the effect of excluding 2 women with Down infants and reduced the size of the denominator in the sensitivity calculation, one sixth. The false-positive rate is slightly larger for the combined screen but is nearly 91% for both methods.

Though there is not much improvement in objective results through adding NT as a screen, many argue that there is benefit from the US evaluation of fetal dating, the diagnosis of twins, and early detection of anomalies when the US procedure is well done. Overall, that seems a fair assessment.

T. H. Kirschbaum, MD

The Prediction and Prevention of Intrapartum Fetal Asphyxia in Preterm Pregnancies
Low JA, Killen H, Derrick EJ (Queen's Univ, Kingston, Ont, Canada)
Am J Obstet Gynecol 186:279-282, 2002   5–11

Background.—Intrapartum fetal asphyxia in preterm pregnancy contributes to CNS and other organ system complications, brain damage, and fetal and early neonatal death. The value of electronic fetal heart rate (FHR) monitoring in predicting and preventing intrapartum fetal asphyxia in preterm pregnancy was investigated.

Methods.—Forty pregnancies with biochemically verified intrapartum fetal asphyxia were studied. Twenty women delivered abdominally were matched to 20 delivered vaginally.

Findings.—Fetal asphyxia was categorized as mild in 21 pregnancies and moderate or severe in 19. In 27 pregnancies, the FHR record was predictive of fetal asphyxia. Predictive FHR records were the main indication for intervention in 21 of the 24 women delivered by cesarean in the first stage or by operative vaginal delivery in the second stage of labor. In 10 pregnancies with mild fetal asphyxia and 9 with moderate or severe fetal asphyxia, newborn outcomes may have been influenced by intervention and delivery because of predictive FHR records.

Conclusions.—Electronic fetal monitoring is useful for predicting intrapartum fetal asphyxia in preterm pregnancies. A prediction of fetal asphyxia that results in intervention and delivery may prevent or ameliorate neonatal morbidity.

► Dr Low and his colleagues have produced findings that are important in evaluating the role of FHR monitoring in predicting birth asphxia in term fetuses.[1,2] Here they deal with a matched case-control study of 40 births associated with asphyxiated newborns exhibiting umbilical artery blood base excess less than 12 mmol/L, half delivered by cesarean section and half matched for gestational age and cord blood base excess delivered vaginally. Predictive FHR tracings before births were said to exist if they showed absent or minimal beat-to-beat baseline variability and later, prolonged decelerations. Such tracings were seen in 60% of 21 fetuses with mild asphyxia (ie, without encephalopathy or multisystem pathology) and in 83% of 19 fetuses with moderate asphyxia (ie, with both encephalopathy and multisystem disorders). From this they conclude that FHR monitoring is useful in predicting fetal asphyxia in preterm fetuses, whether associated with preeclampsia, antepartum bleeding, preterm premature rupture of membranes, or preterm labor.

The problem, of course, is the absence of controls for FHR monitoring in this experience. An unproven assumption is that intervention on behalf of the fetus cannot be conducted without FHR monitoring. The design of the study is to construct controls for abdominal versus vaginal births, but the number of cases is too small to allow conclusions in that dimension. To construct indices of predictability, the presence of FHR monitoring must be controlled, and the outcomes of women not monitored must be compared with those who received monitoring. Only in this way can false-positive and false-negative rates be compared. Only then can it be concluded that FHR monitoring reduces the number of asphyxiated fetuses born to women with preeclampsia or other complications. Without that data the authors' conclusions are questionable.

T. H. Kirschbaum, MD

References

1. 1994 YEAR BOOK OF OBSTETRICS, GYNECOLOGY, AND WOMEN'S HEALTH, pp 226-227.
2. 2000 YEAR BOOK OF OBSTETRICS, GYNECOLOGY, AND WOMEN'S HEALTH, pp 153-155.

Reproductive Risk Factors of Fetal Asphyxia at Delivery: A Population Based Analysis

Heinonen S, Saarikoski S (Kuopio Univ, Finland)
J Clin Epidemiol 54:407-410, 2001   5–12

Background.—It would appear that there is less neurologic damage associated with intrapartum fetal asphyxia than was previously thought; however, the early identification of fetal hypoxia at delivery is crucial to prevent neurologic damage. Early recognition of events related to intrapartum asphyxia on the basis of known reproductive risk factors is difficult, presenting a dilemma for obstetricians. The development of any strategy to prevent fetal asphyxia at delivery depends on developing an understanding of the underlying pathophysiologic mechanisms and etiologic factors involved in this complication. The reproductive risk factors involved in intrapartum fetal asphyxia were investigated.

Methods.—The total population giving birth at 1 Finnish hospital between January 1990 and December 1998 was reviewed with logistic regression and maternal and obstetric risk factors of intrapartum asphyxia.

Results.—From a total of 22,302 structurally normal singleton pregnancies, intrapartum asphyxia occurred in 556 births, for an incidence of 2.5%. Of these asphyxiated newborns, 98 (17.6%) required admission to a neonatal ICU for more than 24 hours compared with 1549 (6.7%) infants in the general population. Multivariate logistic regression revealed that independent risk factors of intrapartum asphyxia (and their adjusted relative risks) were placental abruption (3.74), primiparity (3.10), alcohol use during pregnancy (1.75), low birth weight (1.57), preeclampsia (1.49), male fetuses (1.48), and small for gestational age births (1.33) (Table 3). Women with intrapartum asphyxia had operative deliveries and meconium passage significantly more often than did the reference group.

Conclusions.—Risk screening cannot provide accurate prediction of women who will eventually need emergency care for fetal asphyxia because

TABLE 3.—Multivariate Regression Analysis

Risk Factor	OR	95% CI
Placental abruption	3.74	2.15-6.51
Primiparity	3.10	2.57-3.74
Alcohol consumption	1.75	1.18-2.59
Low birth weight	1.57	1.18-2.09
Preeclampsia	1.49	1.06-2.08
Male fetus	1.48	1.24-1.77
Small-for-gestational age (<10th centile)	1.33	1.04-1.70
Elevated liver enzyme	1.66	0.799-3.46
Postdates	1.34	0.942-1.91
Infertility	1.26	0.942-1.68
Amniotic infection	1.15	0.273-4.81
Second pregnancy in 12 months	1.12	0.721-1.75
Unmarried	1.01	0.833-1.22
Prematurity (<37 weeks)	0.926	0.633-1.36
Previous miscarriage	0.835	0.637-1.09

(Courtesy of Heinonen S, Saarikoski S: Reproductive risk factors of fetal asphyxia at delivery: A population-based analysis. *J Clin Epidemiol* 54:407-410, 2001. Copyright 2001 with permission from Elsevier Science.)

most cases of intrapartum fetal asphyxia occur in women with low-risk pregnancies.

▶ It is important in evaluating this retrospective case-control cohort study to remember the nature of prenatal care in Finland. The data represent the experience in a tertiary care unit for the Eastern Finnish region. Up to 95% of Finnish gravidas enroll for free, readily accessible prenatal care at the hands of midwives and physicians. Primigravidas average 8 to 10 visits, whereas multiparas average about 6 through the course of pregnancy. Antenatal surveillance consists of non-stress tests; measurements of amniotic fluid index and contraction stress tests or biophysical profiles are used for backup of equivocal non-stress tests. If either backup exam is not reassuring, labor induction is used. The diagnosis of intrapartum fetal asphyxia was made on the basis of umbilical artery base excess of minus 12/mEq per liter or less. Its incidence was 2.5%, 550 cases among 22,302 births, averaging 2540 births per year. The incidence of birth asphyxia has been relatively constant in Finland for many years. Univariant comparisons with controls show primiparity, but not age, and a history of prior reproductive failures to be disproportionately common among mothers of fetuses with acidosis at birth. Multivariate analysis yielded the usual increased risk ratios for abruption, primiparity, low birth weight, preeclampsia, but not postdatism or amnionitis. Prematurity was not significantly related to an increased risk of fetal asphyxia in this experience. Labor induction was equally common, about 16%, in both groups. What is most noteworthy is that fetal asphyxia occurred most often in low-risk women not receiving special care for high-risk pregnancy. Specifically, in only 5% of cases of preeclampsia or growth retardation was "asphyxia" noted; that is, fetal acidosis was not noted in 95% of patients with those diagnoses.

Ultimately the data suggest the failure of antenatal surveillance to alter the likelihood of development of newborn asphyxia and that concerns for post-datism, preeclampsia, and growth retardation in this population were not borne out by newborn outcomes.

T. H. Kirschbaum, MD

Computerised Analysis of Fetal Heart Rate Recordings in Maternal Type I Diabetes Mellitus
Tincello D, White S, Walkinshaw S (Univ of Liverpool, England; Univ Hosp Aintree, Liverpool, England; Liverpool Women's Hosp, England)
Br J Obstet Gynaecol 108:853-857, 2001   5–13

Background.—Many clinicians implement some form of fetal surveillance in women with maternal insulin-dependent diabetes mellitus (type I), including ultrasonography and cardiotocography (CTG). Computerized CTG parameters from women with type I diabetes were studied, and the significance of observed differences from the expected normal values was determined.

Methods.—Twenty-six women with type I diabetes carrying a single fetus were enrolled in the prospective, observational study. Computerized CTG recordings were obtained every week from 28 to 39 weeks. Parameters were compared with those from uncomplicated singleton pregnancies published in the literature.

Findings.—One hundred thirty-one recordings were obtained, a median of 5 per patient. Compared with the expected value of 0.8%, 11.3% showed absent episodes of high variation. In addition, there were differences in short-term variation, basal heart rate, frequency of fetal movements, and heart rate accelerations, which changed the gestation. Overall, the parameters indicated a more immature form of fetal heart rate than expected. These changes did not appear to be associated with adverse fetal outcomes.

Conclusions.—Parameters on CTGs in women with maternal type I diabetes differed significantly from parameters for normal fetuses. The changes observed may indicate a delay in fetal maturation. However, there is no evidence that these changes are pathologic. Computerized analysis is not recommended for assessing pregnancies complicated by maternal type I diabetes mellitus.

▶ In 1992, the Liverpool Women's Hospital adopted use of the computerized approach to fetal heart rate analysis first proposed by Dawes and Redman in 1982.[1-3] In 1998, these authors published a retrospective study of 38 gravidas with type I insulin-deficient diabetes mellitus with respect to the prevalence of absent intervals of high heart rate beat to beat variability over a 60-minute recording period in comparison with the internal database consisting of 20,000 recordings in normal pregnancies. In that analysis, they have found that 30.5% of type I diabetics had such potentially ominous intervals on analysis, compared with 0.8% of normals, but the difference was not reflected in adverse outcome measurements for the diabetic pregnancies.[4] Since they recognize several sources of bias in the earlier study, which hampered comparison with Dawes and Redman, they carried out this prospective observational analysis for 1½ years beginning in 1996, in order to ensure data comparability. The medical staff was blinded to fetal heart rate assessments, and the investigators performed simultaneous capillary blood sugar measurements in mother and fetus and used an analytic model which compensates for variability in gestational age and the number of patients at each age interval under study. Twenty-six such type I diabetics were studied with a median of five 60-minute heart rate variability recordings each. Twenty-one percent of the roughly 131 recordings failed to meet criteria for normal heart rate variability responses, an incidence figure of 10.7%. This compared with 0.8% incidence of such findings in normals. There was no significant difference between maternal blood glucose concentration, gestational age at delivery, cord blood gases, birth weight, or NICU admission between the resulting infants. The authors' position, reasonably enough, is that the comparative fetal heart rate difference in diabetic women exists but is neither indicative nor predictive of abnormal neonatal outcome in insulin-deficient diabetic pregnancies.

T. H. Kirschbaum, MD

References

1. 1990 YEAR BOOK OF OBSTETRICS, GYNECOLOGY, AND WOMEN'S HEALTH, pp 131-133.
2. 1993 YEAR BOOK OF OBSTETRICS, GYNECOLOGY, AND WOMEN'S HEALTH, pp 149-152.
3. 1994 YEAR BOOK OF OBSTETRICS, GYNECOLOGY, AND WOMEN'S HEALTH, pp 160-161.
4. Tincello DG, El-Sapagh KM, Walkinshaw SA: Computerized analysis of fetal heart rate recordings in patients with diabetes mellitus. *J Perinat Med* 26:102, 1998.

6 Fetal Therapy

Sustained Correction of X-Linked Severe Combined Immunodeficiency by Ex Vivo Gene Therapy

Hacein-Bey-Abina S, Le Deist F, Carlier F, et al (Hôpital Necker Enfants Malades, Paris; Institut Pasteur, Paris; Inst of Child Health, London; et al)

N Engl J Med 346:1185-1193, 2002   6–1

Introduction.—Deficiency of the common γ (γc) chain, an X-linked disorder, causes the most frequent manifestation of severe combined immunodeficiency disease. This lethal condition can be cured by allogeneic stem-cell transplantation. Infusion of autologous hematopoietic stem cells that had been transduced in vitro with the γc gene were examined for their ability to restore the immune system in patients with severe combined immunodeficiency.

Methods.—Five consecutive male children without HLA-identical donors whose diagnosis was X-linked severe combined immunodeficiency were evaluated. The CD34+ bone marrow cells from these patients were transduced ex vivo by using a defective retroviral vector. Integration and expression of the γc transgene and the development of lymphocyte subgroups and their functions were sequentially analyzed for up to 2.5 years after gene transfer.

Results.—There were no adverse events. Four patients had clear-cut clinical improvement (Table 1). Transduced T cells and natural killer cells were observed in the blood of 4 patients within 4 months. In 3 patients, the number of T cells reached normal values 3 to 4 months after therapy (Fig 1). The number and phenotypes of T cells, the repertoire of T-cell receptors, and the in vitro proliferative responses of T cells to several antigens after immunization were almost normal up to 2 years after treatment. Thymopoiesis was verified by the presence of naive T cells and T-cell antigen-receptor episomes and the development of a normal-sized thymus gland. The frequency of transduced B cells was low. Serum immunoglobulin levels and antibody production after immunization were adequate, thus eliminating the need for IV immunoglobulin. Correction of the immunodeficiency obliterated established infections and permitted patients to experience a normal life.

Conclusion.—Ex vivo gene therapy with γc can safely correct the immune deficiency of patients who have X-linked severe combined immunodeficiency.

TABLE 1.—Characteristics of the Patients

Patient No.	Age at Treatment	Clinical Status Before Treatment	Engraftment of Maternal T-Cells	Mutation	γc Expression Before Treatment	Infused Cells			Clinical Status After Treatment	Follow-Up
							CD34+	CD34γc+		
								cells/kg		
	mo		cells/mm^3							yr
1	11	*Pneumocystis carinii* pneumonitis Protracted diarrhea Failure to thrive	0	Arg 289→stop	Yes		15 million	7 million - 14 million	Well Normal growth	2.5
2	8	*Pneumocystis carinii* pneumonitis Protracted diarrhea Graft-versus-host disease–like lesions Failure to thrive	<10	Deletion of exon 6	No		16 million	5 million	Well Normal growth	23
3	10	Disseminated bacille Calmette–Guérin infection Adenovirus and respiratory syncytial virus infections in the lungs Protracted diarrhea Failure to thrive	0	Deletion of exon 4	No		14 million	5 million	Improving*	0.7
4	1	Well Free of infection	0	Tyr 219→stop	No		27 million	14 million	Well Normal growth	1.8
5	3	Graft-versus-host disease–like lesions	2000	Gln 285→Ala	No		38 million	20 million	Well Normal growth	1.6

*Eight months after gene therapy; patient 3 underwent allogeneic stem cell transplantation.

(Reprinted by permission of Hacein-Bey-Abina S, Le Deist F, Carlier F, et al: Sustained correction of X-linked severe combined immunodeficiency by ex vivo gene therapy. *N Engl J Med* 346:1185-1193, 2002. Copyright 2002, Massachusetts Medical Society. All rights reserved.)

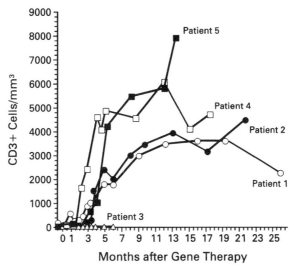

FIGURE 1.—Absolute numbers of CD3+ cells after gene transfer in patients 1 through 5. (Reprinted by permission of Hacein-Bey-Abina S, Le Deist F, Carlier F, et al: Sustained correction of X-linked severe combined immunodeficiency by ex vivo gene therapy. *N Engl J Med* 346:1185-1193, 2002. Copyright 2002, Massachusetts Medical Society. All rights reserved.)

▶ This study of 5 infants with severe X-linked immunodeficiency due to an inactivating mutation of the γc gene on the X chromosome in male infants is an extension of preliminary data reported earlier by the same group[1] and a signal contribution to successful human gene therapy. The γc gene encodes messages essential to expression of 5 cytokine receptors, which are in turn essential for the development of normal T and natural killer (NK) cells, vital parts of natural and acquired immunity. Without therapy, such infants experience recurrent severe infections which result in death, usually in the first year of infancy. Transplantation with HLA identical hematopoetic stem cells—from an identical twin, perhaps, for example—increases short-term survival to 90%. With HLA haploidentical stem cells, survival is 70% to 78%. For those without satisfactory donors, this procedure of ex vivo transfer of autologous hematopoietic stem cells into which a normal γc chain has been transduced is applicable.

This report concerns 5 infants, aged 1 to 11 months, who lacked HLA identical donors and for whom the diagnosis rests on clinical findings, γc mutation analysis, and peripheral blood studies. Autologous bone marrow was used to provide CD34 cells, a clonal designator for stem cells. Transduction using a γc chain previously described was carried out in vitro, confirmatory tests for transgene incorporation performed, and reconstituted stem cells infused. Results were followed over the next 1 to 2 years and were based on the identification of T-cell and T-antigen receptor assay, NK cytotoxicity assays, and the analysis of DNA extracted from circulating blood from the infants.

Four of 5 infants showed marked clinical improvement, with disappearance of skin lesions due to secondary graft-host disease. T cells identified by CD3 markers were seen in all cases. γc transgene and T-cell antigen receptors, as well as the development of normal patterns of clonal designated immune cells were seen. Four of the individuals showed normal thymus development on MRI. NK activity became normal 150 days after transfusion or less.

Because the γc insert does not correct B-cell deficiency in these infants, immunoglobulin (Ig) G replacement is often needed for life. In 3 infants, IgG, IgM, and IgA concentrations reached normal limits within 15 to 20 months. Three of the infants required nutrient supplement for severe diarrhea and case No. 3, followed for only 8 months at the time of this report, is improving clinically if not immunologically.

With all the travails of vector formation and transduction inefficiency in human gene transfer experience, these cases represent confirmation of the feasibility of the approach so important to the future of gene therapy.

T. H. Kirschbaum, MD

Reference

1. 2001 YEAR BOOK OF OBSTETRICS, GYNECOLOGY, AND WOMEN'S HEALTH, pp 223-225.

Prenatal Diagnosis for Congenital Adrenal Hyperplasia in 532 Pregnancies
New MI, Carlson A, Obeid J, et al (New York Presbyterian Hosp)
J Clin Endocrinol Metab 86:5651-5657, 2001   6–2

Background.—The classic form of congenital adrenal hyperplasia results from a deficiency of 21-hydroxylase (21-OHD) and accounts for more than 90% of cases of congenital adrenal hyperplasia. In this classic form there is simple virilizing and salt wasting, and androgen excess causes external genital ambiguity in female newborns and progressive postnatal virilization in both males and female newborns. For more than a decade, dexamethasone has been used successfully for prenatal treatment of congenital adrenal hyperplasia. An update on a group of pregnancies prenatally diagnosed at one hospital between 1978 and 2001 is presented.

Methods.—A total of 532 pregnancies were prenatally diagnosed by amniocentesis or chorionic villous sampling from 1978 to 2001. Of these, 281 were treated prenatally for congenital adrenal hyperplasia because of the risk of 21-OHD deficiency. For this study, all the cases received follow-up telephone interviews with mothers, genetic counselors, endocrinologists, pediatricians, and obstetricians.

Results.—A total of 116 babies were affected with classic 21-OHD (Fig 3). There were 61 girls affected, of whom 49 were treated prenatally with dexamethasone. Dexamethasone was effective in reducing virilization when it was administered at or before 9 weeks' gestation (Fig 6). The only statistical differences in the symptoms during pregnancy between mothers treated with dexamethasone and those not treated with dexamethasone were in weight gain, edema, and striae, which were greater among mothers treated with dexamethasone. There were no significant or long-lasting side effects in

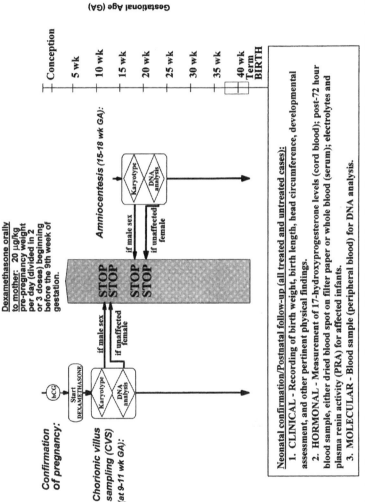

FIGURE 3.—Algorithm depicting prenatal management of pregnancy in families at risk for a fetus affected with 21-OHD. (Courtesy of New MI, Carlson A, Obeid J, et al: Prenatal diagnosis for congenital adrenal hyperplasia in 532 pregnancies. *J Clin Endocrinol Metab* 86:5651-5657, 2001. Copyright The Endocrine Society.)

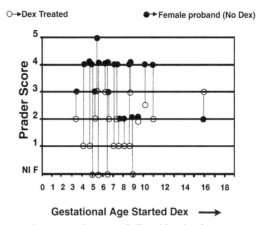

FIGURE 6.—Diagram depicting Prader stages of affected female infants in monitored, dexamethasone prenatally treated pregnancies in relation to gestational age when dexamethasone was started. Affected untreated siblings are shown attached by a *dotted line*. (Courtesy of New MI, Carlson A, Obeid J, et al: Prenatal diagnosis for congenital adrenal hyperplasia in 532 pregnancies. *J Clin Endocrinol Metab* 86:5651-5657, 2001. Copyright The Endocrine Society.)

the fetuses in the treatment group, and prenatally treated newborns did not differ in weight from untreated, unaffected newborns.

Conclusions.—These results indicated that prenatal diagnosis and proper prenatal treatment of 21-OHD can reduce or eliminate virilization in the newborn female, sparing her the adverse consequences of genital ambiguity and surgery and possible sex misassignment.

▶ The extensive experience of the Cornell Medical Center in the prenatal diagnosis of congenital adrenal hyperplasia is important because of the evidence they provide for the value of fetal therapy with dexamethasone. The gene defect is well known. The gene for 3 beta hydroxysteroid dehydrogenase (21 OHD here) in the microsomal fraction of the fetal zone of the adrenal cortex interferes with the conversion of pregnenolone to 17 hydroxy progesterone, the latter essential to fetal cortisol production. The fetal syndrome consists of some degree of salt losing in three fourths of cases and genital malformation in female infants. Other nonclassical forms occur, presumably representing various atypical mutations at the gene site at 6p. The authors make the diagnosis in 522 antepartum cases at 9 to 11 weeks by using measurements of 17 hydroxy progesterone and 4 androstenedione in amniotic fluid obtained by amniocentesis at 15 to 18 weeks in two thirds of cases and DNA analysis of fetal cells obtained by chorion villous biopsy at 9 to 11 weeks in one third. It has been clear since 1984 that dexamethasone, 20 μg/kg per day given to pregnant women with a fetus affected with congenital adrenal hyperplasia prevents the phenotypic abnormalities if begun before 9 weeks' gestational age. Because that date precedes the definitive diagnosis of sex and identifiable effects in female fetuses, the authors' practice since 1992 has been to give maternal dexamethasone to all women with potentially affected infants based on chorionic villous biopsy at 9 to 11 weeks (105 of 532 candidates) and stop administration of dexamethasone on evidence of male fetal sex or unaffected females based on amniocentesis and steroid analysis at 15 to 18 weeks. Of the 105 who began therapy, 34 proved to have male fetuses, and 36 in addition were unaffected fetuses based on amniotic fluid analysis. Of the 25 affected females, 22 showed normal or marginally abnormal phenotypes. In viewing the 70 fetuses whose exposure to dexamethasone was retrospectively unnecessary, the authors found they ultimately differed in no significant way from untreated fetuses with respect to birth weight and length, head dimensions, and rates of perinatal morbidity and mortality. Long-term studies of possible developmental and behavioral effects are underway. The benefit of this fetal therapy program is that it avoids the psychological consequences of genital deformity and surgery and uncertainty in newborn sex assignment. The immediate neonatal consequences of newborn hypocorticism are avoided as well. Although this is an approach that warrants careful follow-up studies, it is worth consideration by all of us.

T. H. Kirschbaum, MD

The Ex Utero Intrapartum Treatment (EXIT) Procedure in Fetal Neck Masses: A Case Report and Review of the Literature
Stevens GH, Schoot BC, Smets MJW, et al (Univ Hosp Maastricht, The Netherlands; Catharina Hosp, Eindhoven, The Netherlands)
Eur J Obstet Gynecol Reprod Biol 100:246-250, 2002   6–3

Background.—The prenatal diagnosis of fetal anatomic malformations has been improved by modern technology such as ultrasonography and MRI. The improved diagnosis of fetal anatomic malformations may improve the perinatal management for children with a life-threatening airway obstruction such as occurs with large fetal neck masses such as cervical teratoma, cystic hygroma, hemangioma, neuroblastoma, or congenital goiter. These masses may result in neonatal hypoxia caused by airway obstruction. The ex utero intrapartum treatment (EXIT) can be used to obtain a fetal airway while feto-maternal circulation is preserved. Uterine relaxation, which is achieved with high-dose inhalation anesthetics during cesarean section, is vital to the maintenance of feto-maternal circulation. For delivery by cesarean section, a well-documented protocol is required to create an optimal situation for the procedure. A case was reported that demonstrates the importance of multidisciplinary management in a patient with a prenatally diagnosed large fetal neck mass.

Case Report.—Woman, 33, who was gravida 2 para 1, was referred at 27 weeks' gestation because of polyhydramnion and a fetal neck mass. US examination revealed a fetal neck mass of 4 cm in diameter located ventrally to the spinal cord, and polyhydramnion with an amniotic pool of more than 11 cm. There were no other anatomic abnormalities. Her first pregnancy ended with the spontaneous birth of a healthy boy with a birth weight of 4100 g. The patient was hospitalized at 27 weeks 2 days of gestation because of preterm labor with frequent, regular uterine contractions. The contractions were successfully treated with IV fenoterol, 2.5 μg/min. Beta-methasondinatriumfosfate-acetate, 12 mg IM, was given for 2 days at 27 and 28 weeks' gestation to improve lung development in the fetus. Amniocentesis was performed at 28, 30, 31, and 32 weeks' gestation, and a total amount of 10.5 L of amniotic fluid was drained. Serial US examinations showed an increase in the size of the tumor up to 9 cm at 33 weeks' gestation. An MR scan showed a neck mass at sagittal acquisition (Fig 1). A successful EXIT procedure was performed. Repeat MRI showed a large multicystic neck tumor. The infant underwent surgery 11 days after birth, and an encapsulated tumor weighing 190 g and measuring 10 cm × 7.5 cm × 4 cm was resected. Its origin was the thyroid gland, which was almost totally removed. Histopathologic examination showed an immature thyroid teratoma grade II with 30% immature neuroglia. This type of teratoma is benign and has no additional therapeutic consequences other than thyroid hormone suppletion. After a complicated postoperative course, the patient was discharged to home at 6 weeks of age in good condition. At 3 years of age, the child is doing well.

Conclusions.—Large fetal neck masses may cause airway obstruction and potential fetal demise after delivery. The relationship of the neck mass to airway structures can be defined prenatally with ultrasound and with MRI. The EXIT procedure can be used to obtain a fetal airway while feto-maternal cir-

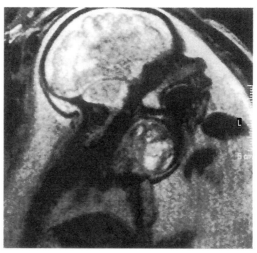

FIGURE 1.—MRI at 33 weeks' gestation, sagittal acquisition. (Courtesy of Stevens GH, Schoot BC, Smets MJW, et al: The ex utero intrapartum treatment (EXIT) procedure in fetal neck masses: A case report and review of the literature. *Eur J Obstet Gynecol Reprod Biol* 100:246-250. Copyright 2002 from Elsevier Science.)

culation is preserved to optimize fetal outcome. A literature review is included in the discussion.

▶ Although simple in concept, this approach demands a great deal of planning, multidisciplinary collaboration, superb anesthesiology, and early fetal detection. A large fetal neck mass left unattended until birth may so distort the oral pharynx that respiration and intubation may be impossible when the transition from fetal to infant life takes place. If after hysterotomy the umbilical circulation is maintained intact, it may be possible to maneuver the fetal head and neck to effect tracheal intubation surgically, prior to delivery, and to resect part of the tumor and complete its excision after delivery in the hands of an otorhinolaryngologist and a pediatric surgeon. The authors describe a new case and summarize 27 others previously recorded. The procedures have commonly involved teratomas and cystic hygromas. One of the cases reported in 1998 originated from UAB and resulted in a successful birth and reconstruction.[1] This is a reference useful to those confronted with this uncommon problem.

T. H. Kirschbaum, MD

Reference

1. Shih GH, Boyd GL, Vincent RD Jr, et al: The EXIT procedure facilitates delivery of an infant with a pretracheal teratoma. *Anesthesiology* 89:1573-1575, 1998.

Parthenogenetic Stem Cells in Nonhuman Primates
Cibelli JB, Grant KA, Chapman KB, et al (Advanced Cell Technology, Worcester, Mass; Wake Forest Univ, Winston-Salem, NC; Sloan Kettering Cancer Ctr, New York; et al)
Science 295:819, 2002   6–4

Introduction.—Parthenogenesis is the ability of an egg to develop into an embryo in the absence of sperm. This process has been characterized to some degree in nonhuman primates, although no primate parthenogenetic embryonic stem (ES) cell lines have been derived to date. Chimeras of parthenogenetic cells with biparentally derived embryonic tissues have produced apparently normal offspring. Reported are broad differentiation capabilities of primate pluripotent stem cells derived by parthenogenesis.

Findings.—After in vitro maturation for 36 hours with media supplemented with pregnant mare serum and hCG, 28 of 77 primate eggs (*Macaca fascicularis*) achieved metaphase II. Eggs were parthenogenetically activated by previously described protocols. Four (14%) eggs developed to blastocyte stage. Inner cell masses (ICM) were isolated by immunosurgery. One week after plating, cell proliferation was seen in 3 ICMs, and 1 stable cell line (Cyno-1) was obtained. These cells had a small cytoplasmic/nuclear ratio and numerous and prominent nucleoli and cytoplasmic lipid bodies and could be extensively propagated in vitro (10 months) while maintaining their undifferentiated state. They were positive for markers of primate ES cells (excluding SSEA-3). High telomerase activity observed in the undifferentiated cells was lost after 2 weeks of differentiation, indicating that telomerase activity is regulated in Cyno-1 cells. Karyotyping showed 40 + 2 chromosomes, which is expected for *Macaca fascicularis*. Neural differentiation of Cyno-1 cells was induced by a multistep culture procedure; astrocytes and neurons were obtained. As much as 25% of dopaminergic neurons were able to be obtained by using immunocytochemical criteria. Neuronal identity and function were verified by high-performance liquid chromatography analysis. A large variety of specialized cell types were generated in vitro by modifying culture conditions. The capacity of Cyno-1 cells to differentiate was tested in vivo by injecting them into the peritoneal cavity of immunocompromised severe combined immunodeficiency disease mice. Teratomas were isolated at 8 and 15 weeks postinjection and underwent histologic analysis. Derivations of all 3 germ layers were seen, including cartilage, muscles, and bone (mesoderm); neurons; melanocytes, skin, and hair follicles (ectoderm); and intestinal and respiratory epithelia (endoderm). The presence of mitotic figures in these tumors suggested they had a benign nature.

Conclusion.—The in vitro differentiation of these cells to well-characterized dopaminergic neurons is of interest, especially their potential to replace lost neurons in Parkinson's disease. These findings suggest an alternative to human therapeutic cloning.

▶ The fertilization of an ovum and its subsequent conversion into an embryo in the absence of sperm is parthenogenesis. Although this may seem a matter of little interest to clinicians, the process may provide a vital alternative to the current ethical and political barriers to human therapeutic cloning erected by the Bush administration and increase the potential prospects for achieving the benefits of stem cell transfusion in human beings[1] in prophylaxis and therapy for fetuses, infants, and adults. Human stem cells usually are obtained from cells derived from the blastocyst inner cell mass and are propagated by nuclear transfer into enucleated differentiated human somatic cells. This is a first account of successful isolation and characterization of stem cells from nonhuman primate embryos generated by parthenogenesis. A collection of 77 primate ova were matured for 36 hours in medium supplemented by pregnant mare serum and hCG. Twenty-eight ova underwent maturation to the point of meiotic developmental arrest in metaphase II. To reverse the meiosis arrest requires 2 successive steps. The first injects calcium ion into the cell with ionomycin, a calcium ionophore, or electrophoresis in vitro. These steps were followed by exposure to an inhibitor of protein synthesis (cyclohexamine) and/or of phosphorylation (2 dimethyl aminopurine). After these exposures, 4 of the 28 ova developed to the blastocyst stage sufficient to allow isolation and culture of the cells of the inner cell mass. After 1 week in culture, growth was noted in 3 preparations and a stable cell line was isolated and propagated for 10 months. The cells had the morphology and surface cell markers of primate embryonic stem cells (ESC). They possessed a normal Macaca karyotype and showed the same class II histocompatability markers on lymphocytes as the parent animals. Environmental culture manipulation led to differentiation into astrocytes and neurones, up to 25% demonstrating dopaminergia, potentially useful for cell replacement in Parkinson's disease. Cardiomyocytes, serotonin secreting cells, smooth muscle cells, adipocytes, and ciliated epithelia were also noted. Transplantation of ESC into genetically immunocompromised mice resulted in teratomas, exhibiting all 3 term layers, an essential step for ESC identity. This approach avoids the use of normal potentially viable embryos as a cell source and negates any concern based on the well-being of the cell donor, an embryo with no conceivable prospects for growth and development. It's an important step in the emerging science of human specific stem cell therapy.

T. H. Kirschbaum, MD

Reference

1. 2000 YEAR BOOK OF OBSTETRICS, GYNECOLOGY, AND WOMEN'S HEALTH, pp 171-172.

A Case of Successful Fetal Therapy for Congenital Chylothorax by Intrapleural Injection of OK-432
Tanemura M, Nishikawa N, Kojima K, et al (Nagoya City Univ, Japan)
Ultrasound Obstet Gynecol 18:371-375, 2001   6–5

Introduction.—The first successful fetal treatment of severe congenital chylothorax with hydrops fetalis by intrapleural injection of OK-432 was described.

Case Report.—Woman, 38, gravida 4 para 3, with an unremarkable family history, was referred at 19 weeks and 6 days' gestation because of severe hydrops fetalis. Sonography revealed severe pleural effusion, ascites, skin edema, and polyhydraminos (Fig 1). Doppler analysis revealed circulatory failure. The karyotype was normal. Intrathoracic fluid was aspirated, and 95% of the cells were lymph cells. There was no sign of infection. The diagnosis was congenital fetal chylothorax. Therapeutic thoracocentesis was performed at 21 and 22 weeks, but pleural infusion returned rapidly.

The parents decided to try sonographically-guided, intrapleural injection of OK-432, a lyophilized incubation mixture of group A streptococcus. Thoracocentesis followed by bilateral, intrapleural OK-432 injection was performed at 23 and 23 weeks' gestation. US was performed at 1 week intervals. After injection, an adhesion-like echo was observed between pleural membrane and lung surface. Pleural diffusion decreased and disappeared by 34 weeks. Amniotic fluid was removed 4 times between 25 and 32 weeks but began to taper off and remained at normal volume. Fetal skin edema and ascites decreased and disappeared by week 36. Fetal breathing movements then resumed.

A male neonate was delivered vaginally at 37 weeks and 3 days, with a 1-minute Apgar score of 8. Respiration was stabilized with oxygen, and the infant was admitted to the neonatal ICU. There was

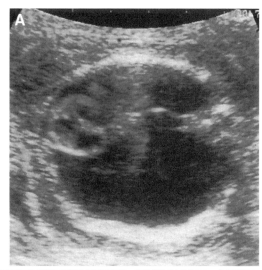

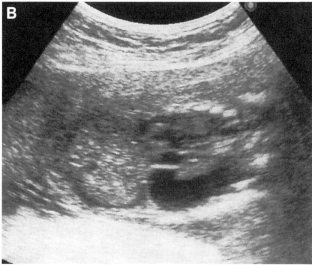

FIGURE 1.—Sonographic findings at 20 weeks and 1 day of gestation. Severe bilateral pleural effusion (**A** and **B**), skin edema, and slight ascites (**B**) were observed. (Courtesy of Tanemura M, Nishikawa N, Kojima K, et al: A case of successful fetal therapy for congenital chylothorax by intrapleural injection of OK-432.*Ultrasound Obstet Gynecol* 18:371-375, 2001. Reprinted by permission of Blackwell Science, Inc.)

no sign of infection. Oxygen was administered for only 8 days. US revealed an enlarged right kidney. Right kidney function was poor, but left kidney function was normal (Fig 6). The infant was discharged on the 34th postnatal day and the subsequent course was favorable.

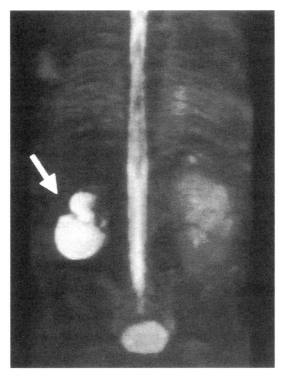

FIGURE 6.—The result of an MR pyelogram at 10 days revealed right pyelectasis (*arrow*) caused by urinary tract stenosis and extremely low excretory function of the right kidney. (Courtesy of Tanemura M, Nishikawa N, Kojima K, et al: A case of successful fetal therapy for congenital chylothorax by intrapleural injection of OK-432.*Ultrasound Obstet Gynecol* 18:371-375, 2001. Reprinted by permission of Blackwell Science, Inc.)

Conclusion.—Adhesion induced by intrapleural injection of OK-432 appeared to reduce the pleural effusion and prevented pulmonary hypoplasia. The neonate was healthy except for right renal dysfunction. This method should only be considered in cases that are detected early, when hydrothorax is the major manifestation, and when shunt insertion is difficult or ineffective. Further follow-up studies are required to determine the usefulness of this procedure for the treatment of congenital chylothorax.

▶ This is, I believe, a first report of the successful use of a pleural sclerotic agent in this uncommon situation. After the development of severe bilateral hydrothorax, mild ascites, and apparent left and right ventricular failure, the diagnosis of nonimmune hydrops fetalis was made by maternal antibody analysis, cordocentesis, and amniocentesis. The failure of demonstration of congenital or acquired cardiac abnormalities then followed. After 2 sets of thoracenteses at 21 and 22 weeks yielding about 40 mm of pleural fluid each, an escharotic derived from a streptococcus cell product was injected into each pleural cavity at 23, 24, and 25 weeks of gestational age. Over 2 to 4 weeks, edema formation began to resolve and the cardiac Doppler signals were encouraging. The infant was born normally at 37 weeks and showed evidence of pleural scarring but required no pulmonary assistance beyond oxygen administration for the first 8 days of life.

T. H. Kirschbaum, MD

7   Surgery, Anesthesia, and Delivery

Outcomes at 3 Months After Planned Cesarean vs Planned Vaginal Delivery for Breech Presentation at Term: The International Randomized Term Breech Trial
Hannah ME, for the Term Breech Trial 3-Month Follow-up Collaborative Group (Univ of Toronto; et al)
JAMA 287:1822-1831, 2002   7–1

Introduction.—The Term Breech Trial, a large, multicenter, international, randomized, controlled trial, reported a significant decrease in adverse perinatal outcomes without an increased risk of immediate maternal morbidity with planned cesarean delivery, compared with planned vaginal birth. No randomized, controlled trials of planned cesarean delivery have assessed benefits and risks of postpartum outcomes months after birth. Maternal outcomes of planned cesarean delivery and planned vaginal birth at 3 months postpartum were examined in a follow-up investigation of the Term Breech Trial.

Methods.—A total of 1596 females from 110 centers worldwide with a singleton fetus in breech presentation at term completed a follow-up questionnaire at 3 months postpartum. The primary outcome measures were breast-feeding; infant health; ease of caring for infant and adjusting to being a new mother; sexual relations and relationship with husband/partner; pain; urinary, flatal, and fecal incontinence; depression; and views regarding the childbirth experience and study participation.

Results.—Baseline data were similar for both groups. Women in the planned cesarean delivery group were less likely to report urinary incontinence compared with those in the planned vaginal birth group (4.5% vs 7.3%; relative risk, 0.62; 95% CI, 0.41-0.93). Incontinence of flatus was similar between groups; it was less of a problem in the planned cesarean than in the planned vaginal group when it occurred ($P = .006$). There were no between-group differences in any other outcomes.

Conclusion.—Planned cesarean delivery for pregnancies with breech presentation at term may be associated with a lower risk of incontinence and is not correlated with an increased risk of other problems for women at 3 months postpartum. Long-term outcome has yet to be determined.

▶ As vaginal delivery of term infants presenting by the breech has become so infrequent as to be rare, it has become important to know whether its increasingly prevalent alternative, scheduled elective cesarean section, exposes women and their infants to increased risks compared with the older alternative. This group from the Centre for Research and Women's Health at the University of Toronto has experience with these issues in an earlier publication.[1] That earlier study showed fewer adverse perinatal outcomes with planned cesarean section. However, a subsequent metaanalysis[2] showed the cost to be increased risk ratios for maternal complications. This multinational, collaborative, randomized controlled study of 1596 women with term singletons presenting by the frank or full breech was designed to attempt to settle the issue and explore other matters as well. Of 798 women randomly assigned to scheduled repeat cesarean section, 90.9% carried out that intent, whereas only 57.1% of those randomly assigned to vaginal birth did so. The rest of the latter developed obstetric contraindications during or before labor. Crucially, since the lost cases may have altered data interpretations, 21.5% of the 1596 women originally enrolled were lost at follow-up 3 months postpartum.

In general, the results of scheduled cesarean sections failed to show much evidence of increased morbidity to mother or infant. Urinary incontinence postpartum was more common in the multiparous patients regardless of the route of the delivery, and cesarean section decreased the rate of appearance of incontinence postpartum independent of parity. Those delivered abdominally, reasonably enough, had an increased likelihood of abdominal pain and a decreased incidence of perineal pain postpartum. Route of delivery had no discernible effect on the successful return of sexual function, nursing, retrospective satisfaction, or depression. It's important that follow-up was limited to 3 months postpartum. Women who underwent cesarean sections for obstetric emergencies whose postpartum courses were marked both by delivery and the trauma of the emergency that motivated it were omitted from the intent to treat–based analysis. This has the effect of decreasing the number of negative afterthoughts. Nonetheless, there is little evidence here that we do women with breech presentations at term much harm by electively sectioning them.

T. H. Kirschbaum, MD

References

1. 2002 YEAR BOOK OF OBSTETRICS, GYNECOLOGY, AND WOMEN'S HEALTH, pp 81-85.
2. Hofmeyr GJ, Hannah ME: Planned caesarean section for term breech delivery, in *The Cochrane Library, Issue 1*. Oxford, England, Update Software, 2001.

Risk of Uterine Rupture During Labor Among Women With a Prior Cesarean Delivery

Lydon-Rochelle M, Holt VL, Easterling TR, et al (Univ of Washington, Seattle)
N Engl J Med 345:3-8, 2001   7–2

Introduction.—Every year in the United States, nearly 60% of women with a prior cesarean delivery who become pregnant again attempt labor. There are concerns that a trial of labor may increase the risk of uterine rupture. Statewide linked birth certificate and hospital discharge data were used to evaluate the risk of uterine rupture associated with spontaneous onset of labor, induction of labor not involving prostaglandins, induction of labor with prostaglandins, and repeated cesarean delivery without labor among women with 1 prior cesarean delivery.

Methods.—A population-based, retrospective analysis was performed using data from all primiparous women who gave birth to live singletons by cesarean section in civilian hospitals in Washington state between 1987 and 1996 and who delivered a second singleton child during the same period. A total of 20,095 women were assessed for the risk of uterine rupture from deliveries with spontaneous onset of labor, those with labor induced by prostaglandins, and those in whom labor was induced by other means. These 3 groups of deliveries were compared with those of women who had repeated cesarean delivery without labor.

Results.—The rate of uterine rupture was 1.6/1000 among women with repeated cesarean delivery without labor (11), 5.2/1000 among women with spontaneous onset of labor (56), 7.7/1000 among women whose labor was induced without prostaglandins (15), and 24.5/1000 among women with prostaglandin-induced labor (9). Compared with the risk for women with repeated cesarean delivery without labor, uterine rupture was more likely among women with spontaneous onset of labor (relative risk, 3.3; 95% CI, 2.4-9.7) and induction with prostaglandins (relative risk, 15.6; 95% CI, 8.1-30.0) (Table 3).

TABLE 3.—Incidence and Relative Risk of Uterine Rupture During a Second Delivery Among Women With a Prior Cesarean Delivery

Type of Delivery	No. of Women	Incidence (per 1000)	Relative Risk (95% Confidence Interval)
Repeated cesarean delivery without labor	6,980	1.6	1.0
Spontaneous onset of labor	10,789	5.2	3.3 (1.8-6.0)
Induction of labor without prostaglandins	1,960	7.7	4.9 (2.4-9.7)
Induction of labor with prostaglandins	366	24.5	15.6 (8.1-30.0)

Note: Incidence is expressed as the number of cases of uterine rupture per 1000 women who delivered a second singleton infant after a prior cesarean delivery. Women who had repeated cesarean delivery without labor served as the reference group.
(Reprinted by permission of *The New England Journal of Medicine*. Courtesy of Lydon-Rochelle M, Holt VL, Easterling TR, et al: Risk of uterine rupture during labor among women with a prior cesarean delivery. *N Engl J Med* 345:3-8, 2001. Copyright 2001, Massachusetts Medical Society. All rights reserved.)

Conclusion.—For women with 1 prior cesarean delivery, the risk of uterine rupture is higher among those whose delivery is induced versus those with repeated delivery without labor. The highest risk is among women whose labor is induced with prostaglandins.

▶ The introduction of the low transverse cesarean section incision by Kerr in 1926[1] dramatically changed the implications of uterine rupture in subsequent pregnancies, although possibly not its frequency, at least until the last 6 to 8 years. As the Kerr incision gained in popularity, A. L. Wilson was first to provide a comprehensive report of the differences from the classic fundal incision in subsequent pregnancies.[2] Of 498 women pregnant after a prior cesarean section, 56% with the prior classical fundal incision, rupture of the uterus occurred in 3%: half ruptured prior to labor, 6 with classical scars, and half ruptured during labor. All of the latter had lower segment incisions. The fetal mortality rate was 1.4%: no deaths occurred as a result of the ruptured low transverse incisions. Hellegers and Eastman reported again that rupture was as likely to occur before the onset of labor as it was after labor began.[3]

A subsequent report of 115 uterine ruptures in 7595 women in whom those with prior classic scars were excluded from an attempt at vaginal birth yielded an incidence of uterine rupture of 1.5%. Half of these were noted to be dehiscences, the defect being found only on postpartum uterine exploration or as an incidental finding at repeat cesarean section. The sole perinatal death in this series—0.8% of women with ruptured uteri— was caused by operative delay. It would follow of necessity that women who undergo an elective cesarean section prior to the onset of labor for pregnancy following a prior cesarean section would have the risk of uterine disruption roughly halved.

Disruption of a prior lower segment incision has much different clinical implications than does rupture of a fundal incision. Because the site of placenta attachment is not involved, except in placenta previa, the quantity of bleeding and loss of placental exchange surface is far less with the separation of the lower incision. Since the fetus is far less likely to be extruded through a lower segment defect, fetal jeopardy from umbilical cord occlusion is very uncommon. Indeed, separation of the Kerr incision is so different from the disrupted fundal scar that a new term, "dehiscence," was coined to distinguish it from classical uterine rupture.

Regrettably, these authors did not identify the differentiation between dehiscence and uterine rupture, apparently because dehiscence was not a codable option in the birth certificate–hospital discharge data they extracted. Neither is the distinction between prior classical and lower segment incisions reported, apparently since the location of the prior incision is not included in documents available to these investigators. The site of the prior scar is, however, an important determinant of outcome and remains an unknown and uncontrolled variable in this study. It seems likely that if, among 191 cases of intrauterine rupture, the fetal mortality rate was 5.5%, many, if not all, of those cases resulting in fetal death must have been the results of fundal ruptures of prior classic incision—to most of us a contraindication to an attempt at vaginal birth. From the perspective of record reviews, the rupture of classical scars is identified by emergency laparotomy, need for blood transfusion, fetal injury or death. Any such information is lacking here.

The relative benignity of uterine dehiscence after a prior lower cervical incision makes the increased risk of relatively bloodless separation in 0.6% to 1.0% of women attempting vaginal birth after cesarean section an acceptable risk balanced against the 80% acceptance rate and 80% to 85% success rate of a trial of labor in such women. Confined to women with known prior lower transverse cesarean sections, two thirds may be successfully delivered vaginally. The failure to identify the location of the prior scar and differentiate rupture from dehiscence reduces the value of the observations which these authors provide. They do, however, provide new data in support of the incremental hazard of induction of labor and the hazards of combining prostaglandins with oxytocin for induction in patients with a prior cesarean section scar. These are clearly the most important observations here.

T. H. Kirschbaum, MD

References

1. Kerr JMM: The technique of cesarean section with special reference to the lower uterine segment incision. *Am J Obstet Gynecol* 12:729, 1926.
2. Wilson AL: Labor and delivery after cesarean section. *Am J Obstet Gynecol* 62:1225, 1951.
3. Hellegers AE, Eastmen NJ: The problem of prematurity in gravidas with cesarean section scars. *Am J Obstet Gynecol* 82:679, 1961.

WHO Multicentre Randomised Trial of Misoprostol in the Management of the Third Stage of Labour

Villar J, for the WHO Collaborative Group to Evaluate Misoprostol in the Management of the Third State of Labour (WHO, Geneva; et al)
Lancet 358:689-695, 2001   7–3

Introduction.—Postpartum hemorrhage remains a leading cause of severe maternal morbidity and death, particularly in less developed countries. Uterotonic agents administered during the third stage of labor can reduce the amount of bleeding and the need for transfusion. Misoprostol, a prostaglandin E1 analogue used to treat peptic ulcer disease, has strong uterotonic effects and can be administered orally. The efficacy of misoprostol was compared with that of oxytocin in a multicenter, double-blind, randomized trial.

Methods.—Women eligible for the study were about to deliver vaginally at hospitals in Argentina, China, Egypt, Ireland, Nigeria, South Africa, Switzerland, Thailand, and Vietnam. Each woman received 600 µg misoprostol orally or 10 IU oxytocin IV or IM, plus corresponding identical placebos. The drugs were administered immediately after delivery. Primary outcomes were a postpartum blood loss of 100 mL or more and the need for additional uterotonics. Blood loss was measured from the time of delivery until transfer of the mother to postnatal care.

TABLE 2.—Primary and Secondary Outcomes According to Treatment Group

	Misoprostol	Oxytocin	Relative Risk (95% CI)	p
Primary outcomes				
Blood loss ≥1000 mL *	366/9214 (4%)	263/9228 (3%)	1·39 (1·19-1·63)	<0·0001
Use of additional uterotonics*	1398/9225 (15%)	1002/9228 (11%)	1·40 (1·29-1·51)	<0·0001
Secondary outcomes				
Blood loss ≥500 mL	1793/9213 (20%)	1248/9227 (14%)	1·44 (1·35-1·54)	<0·0001
Need for blood transfusion	72/9221 (0·8%)	97/9226 (1%)	0·74 (0·55-1·01)	0·06
Manual removal of placenta	219/9225 (2%)	215/9228 (2%)	1·02 (0·85-1·23)	0·88
Delayed postpartum haemorrhage	37/9226 (0·4%)	31/9229 (0·3%)	1·19 (0·74-1·92)	0·54
Bimanual compression	84/9224 (0·9%)	80/9231 (0·9%)	1·05 (0·77-1·43)	0·81
Exploration under general anaesthesia	70/9224 (0·8%)	61/9231 (0·7%)	1·15 (0·82-1·62)	0·48
Hysterectomy	4/9224 (0·04%)	8/9231 (0·09%)	0·50 (0·15-1·66)	0·39
Admission to intensive care	4/9224 (0·04%)	5/9231 (0·05%)	0·80 (0·22-2·98)	1·00†
Maternal death	2/9225 (0·02%)	2/9230 (0·02%)	1·00 (0·14-7·10)	1·00†

*Excluding 37 and 34 women with emergency cesarean section and 13 and 4 women lost to follow-up in misoprostol and oxytocin groups, respectively, for blood loss of more than or equal to 1000 mL, and 2 and 4 women without information on the need for additional uterotonics.
†Fisher's exact test used.
(Courtesy of Villar J, for the WHO Collaborative Group to Evaluate Misoprostol in the Management of the Third Stage of Labour: WHO multicentre randomised trial of misoprostol in the management of the third stage of labour. Lancet 358:689-695, 2001. Reprinted by permission from Elsevier Science.)

Results.—Between April 1998 and November 1999, 29,295 women were screened for eligibility, 19,025 (65%) were eligible, and 18,530 (97%) were enrolled. Excluded from analysis were 71 women who underwent emergency cesarean section and 23 with missing data. Blood loss of more than or equal to 1000 mL and the use of additional uterotonics occurred in a higher proportion of women in the misoprostol group than in the oxytocin group (4% vs 3% and 15% vs 11%, respectively) (Table 2). Oxytocin was the most commonly used additional uterotonic in both misoprostol (77%) and oxytocin (80%) groups. Misoprostol was associated with a significantly higher incidence of shivering and raised body temperature in the first hour after delivery. The relative risk of shivering with misoprostol was higher among women with epidural analgesia.

Conclusion.—Although misoprostol is inexpensive, can be given orally, and does not need refrigeration for storage, oxytocin proved more effective in reducing blood loss when administered in the third stage of labor. Women who received oxytocin were also less likely to require additional uterotonics.

▶ This large multicenter, randomised, and double-blinded prospective study sponsored by the World Health Organization is aimed at the reduction of maternal deaths caused by postpartum hemorrhage in developing nations. It involves centers in South America, Asia, Western Europe, and Africa, including countries where maternal mortality rates from postpartum hemorrhage range as high as 0.2 to 2.2%. Comparisons are drawn between the use of oxytocin, 10 units IV or IM versus misoprostol 600 µg PO administered at the beginning of the third stage of labor. Gravidas with asthma, abortion, fever or other allergic disorders were excluded. The primary outcome measurements were blood loss, both more than 0.5 and more than 1.0 L measured by volume, and the need for additional oxytocic dosage. Because no comparisons with placebos were included, nothing should be inferred about the absolute value of misoprostol nor the relative merits of the 2 agents in treatment, not prevention, of postpartum hemorrhage. Oxytocin yielded better results in preventing blood loss at both of the 2 levels measured, and in not requiring use of supplementary oxytocic agents. No significant differences were noted in a series of secondary outcome measurements, including manual placental removal, hysterectomy, delayed hemorrhage, or maternal death. At a 95% CI, oxytocin was judged to be 20% to 60% better in preventing hemorrhage and 30% to 50% better as sole oxytocic agent than was misprostol. Significant heterogeneity was noted among the centers, with, for instance, risk ratios for misoprostol and postpartum bleeding ranging from 0.5 to 2.37. Multivariant analysis failed to explain the differences, but it likely stems from differences in execution of care between Ireland and Switzerland on the one hand and Nigeria and South Africa on the other. In any event, although misoprostol is cheaper than oxytocin and doesn't require parenteral administration or refrigerated storage, oxytocin is the preferred drug in the prevention of postpartum hemorrhage administered at the completion of the second stage of labor.

T. H. Kirschbaum, MD

Active Phase Labor Arrest: Revisiting the 2-Hour Minimum

Rouse DJ, Owen J, Savage KG, et al (Univ of Alabama, Birmingham)
Obstet Gynecol 98:550-554, 2001   7–4

Introduction.—In a previously described labor management protocol developed before the widespread use of epidural analgesia, objective criteria for duration of labor arrest requiring cesarean delivery were a minimum of 4 hours (if uterine activity was >200 Montevideo units) or 6 hours (if >200 Montevideo units could not be sustained). Earlier guidelines had recommended cesarean after a labor arrest of 2 hours. The 2-hour minimum was examined in a cohort of spontaneously laboring women receiving oxytocin for abnormally progressive labor.

Methods.—The 501 women studied were at or beyond 36 weeks' gestation with regular uterine contractions. Excluded were women with a nonvertex presentation, previous cesarean, multiple gestation, or a nonreassuring fetal heart rate tracing or chorioamnionitis before the start of oxytocin. Management included an intrauterine pressure catheter with an intent to sustain at least 200 Montevideo units for 4 hours or more before cesarean for labor arrest. Maternal and neonatal outcomes were examined according to parity and uterine contraction pattern.

Results.—Nulliparous women made up 57% of the study group. The mean gestational age at delivery was 40 weeks for both nulliparous and parous groups, and mean birth weights were similar. Cesarean rates were 18% for nulliparas and 5% for parous women. In both groups, women who underwent cesarean delivery had received oxytocin for a significantly longer time than those who delivered vaginally (Table 1). Women who were delivered by cesarean dilated much more slowly. After initiation of oxytocin, 54% of women achieved a sustained uterine contraction pattern (Table 2) of at least 200 Montevideo units. Twenty-three of 38 women with labor arrest for >2 hours despite at least 200 sustained Montevideo units achieved a vaginal delivery (Table 3). The rates of chorioamnionitis and endometritis for these 38 women were 26%, but no infant sustained a serious complication.

Conclusion.—Because oxytocin-augmented labor proceeds far more slowly than spontaneous labor, the criterion of labor arrest for 2 hours despite at least 200 sustained Montevideo units should not be the sole reason for cesarean delivery. Most women in this category will achieve vaginal delivery with continued oxytocin augmentation.

▶ Hellman and Prystowski have reviewed the interesting history of the 2-hour rule for the duration of a normal second stage of labor.[1] They cite Dennam's rule that forceps should not be used for delivery until 6 hours of the second stage have elapsed and other means of delivery have failed.[2] Later, Dennam's disciple S. Merrinau, in an unverifiable reference, indicated that Dennam's rule was too stringent and recommended 2 hours as a reasonable duration for the normal second stage. Hellman and Prystowski found surplus fetal mortality when the second stage exceeded 150 minutes. The authors of this study, persuaded that epidural analgesia and oxytocin stimulation of labor may well have

TABLE 1.—Labor Characteristics of 501 Women Who Underwent Oxytocin Augmentation for Active Phase Arrest or Protraction

	Nulliparas (n = 286)		Parous women (n = 215)	
	Vaginal Delivery (n = 235)	Cesarean Delivery (n = 51)	Vaginal Delivery (n = 204)	Cesarean Delivery (n = 11)
Montevideo units after oxytocin*	175 (38-272)	175 (70-272)	166 (49-289)	188 (98-277)
P	.62†		.36†	
Maximum oxytocin infusion (mu/min)	8 (1-45)	10 (2-30)	6 (1-60)	8 (2-30)
P	.07†		.81†	
Oxytocin duration (hr)	3.9 (0.5-14.2)	7.4 (1.7-21.1)	2.3 (0.2-11.1)	6.9 (1.5-10.0)
P	<.001†		<.001†	
Cervical dilation with oxytocin (cm/hr)	1.4 (0.2-4.5)	0.3 (0-1.4)	1.8 (0.3-12.0)	0.4 (0-0.8)
10th percentile	0.6	0.04	0.6	0
5th percentile	0.5	0	0.5	0
P	<.001†		<.001†	

Note: Unless otherwise noted, results are reported as median (range).
*Average of all recorded 10-minute windows for individual women.
†P values for the comparison of vaginal and cesarean delivery groups.
(Courtesy of Rouse DJ, Owen J, Savage KG, et al: Active phase labor arrest: Revisiting the 2-hour minimum. *Obstet Gynecol* 98:550-554, 2001. Reprinted with permission from the American College of Obstetricians and Gynecologists.)

TABLE 2.—Labor Outcome Versus Uterine Contraction Pattern: Nulliparas

Type of Delivery	Never Achieved 200 Montevideo Units (n = 59)	Nonsustained 200 Montevideo Units (n = 70)	Sustained 200 Montevideo Units (n = 157)
Vaginal (%)	83	74	85
Cesarean (%)	17	26	15
Indication (%)			
Dystocia arrest	12	16	11
Fetal intolerance	3	3	3
Both	2	7	1

(Courtesy of Rouse DJ, Owen J, Savage KG, et al: Active phase labor arrest: Revisiting the 2-hour minimum. *Obstet Gynecol* 98:550-554, 2001. Reprinted with permission from the American College of Obstetricians and Gynecologists.)

altered the management of the second stage, take a small step in Dennam's direction and support this with data from a well-structured protocol but one lacking controls and blinded observations. Nonetheless, the results are interesting.

They studied 501 gravidas, 57% nulliparous, at or beyond 36 weeks' gestational age with spontaneous onset of labor and uterine contractions at least every 5 minutes but requiring oxytocin supplementation for slow or arrested labor. Women with malpresentations, multiple pregnancies, prior cesarean sections, clinical amnionitis, or nonreassuring fetal heart rate patterns were excluded. Labor inductions were also excluded. Oxytocin was given by a protocol that aimed at producing at least 200 Montevideo units, and the researchers found, comparing women by parity and successful vaginal births, with 95% of parous women and 81.8% of primigravidas delivered vaginally. Mean cervical dilatation rates were 1.8 cm/h for parous and 1.4 cm/h for primigravid women. Fifty-four percent of all women sustained a level of uterine contractility greater than 200 Montevideo units on oxytocin supplementation, and nulliparas able to do so had an 83% vaginal delivery rate versus 74% for those who failed to reach that level. Vaginal delivery rates from multiparas were independent of the measured level of uterine contractile activity. In a second subset of 38 women with the arrest of cervical dilatation for 2 hours despite uterine contractions greater than 200 Montevideo units, 79% of them primigravid, about 60% subsequently delivered vaginally, albeit with a 13% incidence of shoulder

TABLE 3.—Labor Outcome Versus Uterine Contraction Pattern: Parous Women

Type of Delivery	Never Achieved 200 Montevideo Units (n = 66)	Nonsustained 200 Montevideo Units (n = 33)	Sustained 200 Montevideo Units (n = 116)
Vaginal (%)	97	94	94
Cesarean (%)	3	6	6
Indication (%)			
Dystocia Arrest	1.5	0	4
Fetal intolerance	0	0	1
Both	1.5	6	1

(Courtesy of Rouse DJ, Owen J, Savage KG, et al: Active phase labor arrest: Revisiting the 2-hour minimum. *Obstet Gynecol* 98:550-554, 2001. Reprinted with permission from the American College of Obstetricians and Gynecologists.)

dystocia and 26% incidence of endometriosis and chorioamnionitis, significantly greater than in those without labor arrest. No other differences in perinatal morbidity or mortality were noted as a result of this approach, probably attributable to the skill of the attending obstetricians. Those who adopt this approach must be reasonably certain that they are equally deft.

T. H. Kirschbaum, MD

References

1. Hellman LM, Prystowski H: The duration of the second stage of labor. *Am J Obstet Gynecol* 63:1223, 1952.
2. Dennam CT: *Aphorisms on the Application and Use of Forceps*, ed 6. London, J Collum Ed, 1817.

Risk of Perinatal Death Associated With Labor After Previous Cesarean Delivery in Uncomplicated Term Pregnancies

Smith GCS, Pell JP, Cameron AD, et al (Cambridge Univ, England; Greater Glasgow Health Board, Scotland; Queen Mother's Hosp, Glasgow, Scotland; et al)
JAMA 287:2684-2690, 2002   7–5

Background.—A trial of labor after a previous cesarean section has been used to reduce the overall proportion of cesarean deliveries, yet it presents a significantly increased risk of uterine rupture. Women who previously had a cesarean delivery may choose to deliver an uncomplicated pregnancy vaginally. The relative and absolute risks of perinatal death that women run with a trial of labor in an otherwise uncomplicated term pregnancy were evaluated. Comparisons were made between women with uncomplicated term pregnancies who had a trial of labor after previous cesarean delivery, those having a planned repeat cesarean delivery, and nulliparous or multiparous women who had not delivered by planned cesarean method at term.

Methods.—The 313,238 singleton births were assessed retrospectively. Data were obtained from the Scottish Morbidity Record and the Stillbirth and Neonatal Death Enquiry. Delivery-related perinatal death were compared among the 4 groups of women.

Results.—A total of 15,515 women had previously delivered by cesarean method but now underwent a trial of labor; 9014 women had had cesarean delivery and planned a second; 137,160 women had not delivered previously but planned to use cesarean delivery; and 151,549 women had had no previous cesarean delivery and did not undergo planned cesarean delivery currently.

Women having a trial of labor had the highest rate of perinatal death, more than 11 times over that of women having a planned repeat cesarean delivery. Risk of death with a trial of labor resembled that of nulliparous women in labor but exceeded that of other multiparous women by 100%. Approximately 91% of the deaths related to delivery among women who had had a previous cesarean delivery was attributable to the trial of labor's increased risk of death. When compared with elective repeat cesarean delivery, adjustments made for maternal age, smoking status, height, deprivation quintile, gestational age at birth, and birth weight decile produced a stronger relationship between trial of labor and perinatal death.

The risk of a perinatal death for women having a trial of labor was over 8 times greater than the risk for having a mechanical failure that caused death or the risk associated with intrapartum anoxia. Women who had a trial of labor had an increased risk of dying from a mechanical cause also. No relationship was found between these increased risks of perinatal death and maternal height, smoking status, socioeconomic status, age, fetal growth, or week of gestation when delivery was accomplished.

Conclusion.—The risk of perinatal death was significantly higher for women who had a trial of labor than for those having a planned repeat cesarean delivery. In addition, uterine rupture was noted to cause an excess number of deaths among women undergoing a trial of labor when compared with other women in labor.

▶ This analysis of the impact of trial of labor after at least 1 prior cesarean section on perinatal mortality is derived from data collected in the Scottish Morbidity Record and the Stillbirth and Neonatal Death inquiry begun in 1983. It is an important contribution. Its interpretation, however, suffers mightily from the failure to discriminate the results of vaginal birth after cesarean section following prior classical and prior low-segment transverse uterine incisions.

This is a crucial matter since obstetricians recognize that the risks to mother and fetus in labor with a prior classical incision are prohibitive and, for the most part, a contraindication to trial of labor. Rupture of a fundal scar risks hemorrhage and placental disruption if the tear involves the placental attachment site. Further, the risk of cord prolapse and occlusion through the fundal defect further compromises the fetus.

This omission in data evaluation has been noted before, and the rationale for treating women candidates with a trial of labor with a prior lower-segment incision given at some length (see Abstract 7–2). This difference seems not to be a concern by biostaticians, but one would have expected better of the first author, an obstetrician.

In a series of 24529 women pregnant with singlets presenting by the vertex with living fetuses without anomaly at 37 to 43 weeks' gestation, 15,515, or 63%, underwent a trial of labor. In 25.4% of cases, emergency cesarean section was carried out for a success rate of trial or labor of 74.6%, at the low range of reported success rates for most centers. Among those with a trial of labor, there were 7 cases of intrapartum fetal death and 13 neonatal deaths (through 28 days of life) for a perinatal mortality rate of 12.9/10,000 live births, compared with a remarkably low neonatal death rate of 1.1/10,000 live births for those sectioned electively.

This should be compared to the total US neonatal death rate for 1998 of 4.8/10,000 live births. Sixty percent of deaths during a trial of labor occurred during cesarean section for a failed trial of labor. Perinatal deaths associated with uterine rupture and fetal hypoxia accounted for 70% of the total. An average incidence figure for the observed occurrence of uterine rupture during a trial of labor (0.5%) would yield an expected 77 cases of rupture for which 20 neonatal deaths (26%) is extremely high for lower-segment ruptures as reported by others, but about what one would expect for rupture of classical scars. Since the authors don't provide data regarding the incidence of classical scar rupture, it seems appropriate to use the data of other investigators.

Correspondingly, perinatal mortality figures for Scottish women laboring without prior cesarean section were 9.8/10,000 live births for primigravidas and 5.9/10,000 for multiparas. Only for the latter is the mortality rate significantly less than that reported here for women undergoing a trial of labor. Regrettably, we are left with the conclusion that if one ignores the location of the prior cesarean section uterine incision during vaginal birth after cesarean section, one can expect an outcome less favorable than with elective cesarean sections. No possible implication can be drawn here for the hazard of vaginal birth after cesarean section done on women with a prior low transverse cesarean section.

T. H. Kirschbaum, MD

Does Epidural Analgesia Prolong Labor and Increase Risk of Cesarean Delivery? A Natural Experiment

Zhang J, Yancey MK, Klebanoff MA, et al (Natl Inst of Child Health and Human Development, Bethesda, Md; Tripler Army Med Ctr, Honolulu, Hawaii)
Am J Obstet Gynecol 185:128-134, 2001   7–6

Objective.—More than 50% of pregnant women in the United States are using epidural analgesia for labor pain. However, whether epidural analgesia prolongs labor and increases the risk of cesarean delivery remains controversial.

Study Design.—We examined this question in a community-based, tertiary military medical center where the rate of continuous epidural analgesia in labor increased from 1% to 84% in a 1-year period while other conditions remained unchanged—a natural experiment. We systematically selected 507 and 581 singleton, nulliparous, term pregnancies with spontaneous onset of labor and vertex presentation from the respective periods before and after the times that epidural analgesia was available on request during labor. We compared duration of labor, rate of cesarean delivery, instrumental delivery, and oxytocin use between these 2 groups.

Results.—Despite a rapid and dramatic increase in epidural analgesia during labor (from 1% to 84% in 1 year), rates of cesarean delivery overall and for dystocia remained the same (Fig 1) (for overall cesarean delivery: adjusted relative risk, 0.8; 95% CI, 0.6-1.2; for dystocia: adjusted relative risk, 1.0; 95% CI, 0.7-1.6). Overall instrumental delivery did not increase (adjusted relative risk, 1.0; 95% CI, 0.8-1.4); nor did the duration of the first stage and the active phase of labor (multivariate analysis; $P > .1$). However, the second stage of labor was significantly longer by about 25 minutes ($P < .001$).

Conclusion.—Epidural analgesia during labor does not increase the risk of cesarean delivery; nor does it necessarily increase oxytocin use or instru-

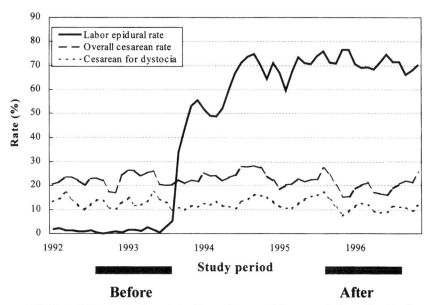

FIGURE 1.—Epidural analgesia use during labor and cesarean delivery rates, both overall and for dystocia among nulliparous women, 1992-1996. (Courtesy of Zhang J, Yancey MK, Klebanoff MA, et al: Does epidural analgesia prolong labor and increase risk of cesarean delivery? A natural experiment. *Am J Obstet Gynecol* 185:128-134, 2001.)

mental delivery because of dystocia. The duration of the active phase of labor appears unchanged, but the second stage of labor is likely prolonged.

▶ The use of historical controls in evaluating the impact of a new approach to patient management is fraught with problems. If the change in management takes place over a long period of physician training and experience, the chances of changes in the patient composition or in provider identities, attitudes, and abilities arise as potential confounding variables with time. To the extent that the change in management is not universally acceptable to medical staff, notorious for resisting change, the impact of the change on outcome variables is diminished or altered by the differing characteristics of physicians who embrace changes or don't. This study, in which Defense Department policy mandated the availability of epidural analgesia for women in labor at Tripler Army Medical Center in 1993, brought the epidural rates from 1% to approximately 70% in a period of 1 year. During that time, the military dependent obstetric population changed little, although the mean age of the women increased by 1 year and primigravidity decreased from 77% to 68%. Midwives and physician attendants appeared to change little because staffing was defined more by military orders than by socioeconomic factors. Data analysis was based on the preexisting data collection system in place during the 2 12-month intervals chosen before and after the anesthesia policy changed. Defects in that system prevented detailed analysis of the length of labor or separation of spontaneous from induced labor, but no impacts of epidural employment on the overall duration of the first stage of labor, oxytocin use, incidence of cesarean section or incidence of dystocia and operative birth were seen. The incidence of a second stage of labor longer than 2 hours and the use of outlet procedures for delivery was significantly increased among women delivered from 1995 to 1996. This is a strong vote for the lack of significant effects on labor of the use of epidural analgesia.

T. H. Kirschbaum, MD

A Randomized Trial of Intrapartum Analgesia in Women With Severe Preeclampsia

Head BB, Owen J, Vincent RD, Jr, et al (Univ of Alabama at Birmingham)
Obstet Gynecol 99:452-457, 2002   7–7

Background.—Controversy still exists around the choice of intrapartum pain relief for women with severe preeclampsia. Retrospective studies have recommended both epidural analgesia and systemic opioids, but it appears that no published comparative trials on laboring women with severe preeclampsia. Epidural analgesia is considered by most obstetric anesthesiologists to be the preferred method of intrapartum pain relief. However, this method can result in maternal sympathetic blockade and cause hypotension, decreased uteroplacental perfusion, and nonreassuring fetal heart rate patterns. Systemic opioids are easily administered and unlikely to cause maternal hypotension and nonreassuring fetal heart patterns. However, systemic opioids cross the placenta easily and may cause neonatal respiratory depression. Whether the rate of cesarean delivery differs between women with severe preeclampsia who receive intrapartum epidural analgesia and those with patient-controlled IV opioid analgesia was investigated.

Methods.—A group of 116 women who were at least 24 weeks' gestation with severe preeclampsia were randomly assigned to receive either intrapartum epidural (56 patients) or patient-controlled IV opioid analgesia (60 patients) (Table 4). Data were analyzed by intention to treat.

Results.—Maternal characteristics and neonatal outcomes were similar for the 2 groups. The groups had similar rates of cesarean delivery (18% for the epidural group and 12% for the patient-controlled analgesia group). Women who received epidural analgesia were more likely to need ephedrine to treat hypotension (9% vs 0%); however, their infants were less likely to require naloxone at delivery (9% vs 54%). The patients' responses to a visual analogue intrapartum pain assessment and a postpartum pain management survey showed that epidural analgesia provided significantly better pain relief.

Conclusion.—Intrapartum epidural analgesia did not significantly increase the rate of cesarean delivery in women with severe preeclampsia compared with patient-controlled IV opioid analgesia at 1 level III center. Intra-

TABLE 4.—Mode of Delivery and Indications for Cesarean Delivery in
Women With Severe Preeclampsia Who Received Either Intrapartum
Epidural or Patient-Controlled IV Opioid Analgesia

	Epidural Analgesia (n = 56)	Patient-controlled Analgesia (n = 60)
Vaginal delivery, n (%)		
Spontaneous	43 (77)	50 (83)
Operative	3 (5)	3 (5)
Cesarean delivery, n (%)	10 (18)	7 (12)
Cesarean indications, n (%)		
Nonreassuring FHR	4 (40)	5 (71)
Active phase labor arrest	5 (50)	0 (0)
Failed induction (dilatation ≤4 cm)	1 (10)	2 (29)

Abbreviation: FHR, Fetal heart rate.
(Reprinted with permission from The American College of Obstetricians and Gynecologists, courtesy
of Head BB, Owen J, Vincent RD, Jr, et al: A randomized trial of intrapartum analgesia in women with
severe preeclampsia. *Obstet Gynecol* 99:452-457, 2002.)

partum epidural analgesia also provided more effective pain relief than
intrapartum epidural analgesia.

▶ Apart from general concerns regarding the role of epidural analgesia in cesarean section incidence,[1-3] there is some special concern for its use in women
with severe preeclampsia. Pre-anesthetic fluid and electrolyte loading may introduce complications in women with abnormal body fluid distribution, and the
use of hypertensive agents such as ephedrine to treat incidental hypotension
introduces additional hazards. On the other hand, the alternative use of opioids
is associated with newborn depression and potential problems in cardiovascular and respiratory adjustments to neonatal life. For these reasons, this study
of 116 women with severe preeclampsia prospectively randomized between
epidural analgesia and opioids for pain relief in labor is of interest.

Women with singlet pregnancies and severe preeclampsia at a mean gestational age of 33 weeks were randomized to receive bupivicaine epidural
analgesia if the cervix was 5-cm dilated or less. The diagnosis of severe preeclampsia was based on the presence of marked albuminuria with severe
hypertension, thrombopenia, and abnormal aspartate aminotransferase or
eclampsia. Opioid analgesia was available by patient-controlled administration, and the adequacy of analgesia was reported both by patients and attending nurses. Seventy-five percent of women had cervical ripening performed prior to induction, using laminaria or extra-amniotic saline injection.
The primary outcome measurement—the incidence of cesarean section—
showed no significant difference between those receiving epidural analgesia
(18%) and opioids (12%).

Ephedrine was employed for hypotension in 9% of epidural recipients.
There were no maternal deaths, and pulmonary edema occurred once in each
group. The incidences of postpartum hemorrhage and endometritis showed
no significant differences between the groups. Those receiving epidural analgesia indicated better pain relief and satisfaction than opioid recipients. There
were 3 remote neonatal deaths at the 14th, 10th, and 10th days of life in the

epidural group, the infants weighing anywhere from 500 to 800 g at birth with normal umbilical blood gases at delivery. Two of the deaths were associated with intestinal perforation.

It will take many more cases, of course, to prove the absence of a negative outcome associated with this form of treatment. Since good outcomes reflect both the intrinsic risks of epidural analgesia and the skill with which it is executed, the latter is an essential requisite. This work does, however, provide some support for those who share in its employment in severe hypertensive disease in pregnancy.

T. H. Kirschbaum, MD

References

1. 1999 YEAR BOOK OF OBSTETRICS, GYNECOLOGY, AND WOMEN'S HEALTH, pp 173-174 and 182-183.
2. 2000 YEAR BOOK OF OBSTETRICS, GYNECOLOGY, AND WOMEN'S HEALTH, pp 183-187.
3. 2001 YEAR BOOK OF OBSTETRICS, GYNECOLOGY, AND WOMEN'S HEALTH, pp 193-195.

Increased Risk of Cesarean Delivery With Advancing Maternal Age: Indications and Associated Factors in Nulliparous Women

Ecker JL, Chen KT, Cohen AP, et al (Harvard Medical School, Boston)
Am J Obstet Gynecol 185:883-887, 2001   7–8

Background.—The childbearing American population is aging. The risk of cesarean delivery increases with maternal age. To understand the factors that contribute to the increased risk of cesarean delivery with maternal age, a large database was reviewed for variables that might affect delivery.

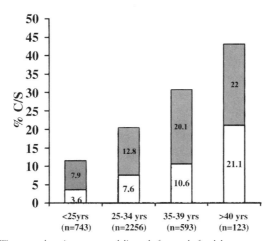

FIGURE 1.—Women undergoing cesarean delivery before and after labor as a percentage of all term, nulliparous women delivering in each age group; *P* = .001 for trend for overall cesarean delivery rates and for trends of cesarean delivery rates with (*shaded bars*) and without labor (*open bars*). (Courtesy of Ecker JL, Chen KT, Cohen AP, et al: Increased risk of cesarean delivery with advancing maternal age: Indications and associated factors in nulliparous women. *Am J Obstet Gynecol* 185: 883-887, 2001.)

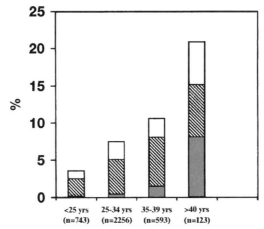

FIGURE 2.—Indications for cesarean delivery without labor as a percentage of all term, nulliparous vaginal deliveries analyzed according to maternal age. Previous myomectomy (*shaded bars*), malpresentation (*hatched bars*), other (*open bars*). (Courtesy of Ecker JL, Chen KT, Cohen AP, et al: Increased risk of cesarean delivery with advancing maternal age: Indications and associated factors in nulliparous women. *Am J Obstet Gynecol* 185: 883-887, 2001.)

Study Design.—A database containing information on all births at the Brigham and Women's Hospital during 1998 was reviewed. This database contains information on 3710 term nulliparous deliveries. Demographic variables, preexisting maternal conditions, antepartum complications, intrapartum data, indications for induction and cesarean delivery were obtained from the database. Inductions were considered to be elective if no indication was noted in the record. If gestational age was greater than 40 ⁶/₇ weeks, induction was considered to be the result of post-date. Women were classified by age as follows: 743 were less than 25 years, 2256 were 25 to 34

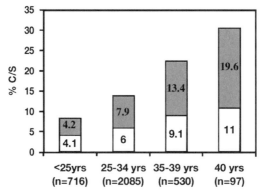

FIGURE 3.—Women undergoing cesarean delivery after labor as a percentage of all women delivering in each age group after labor; *P* = .001 for trends of overall rate as well as for trends of rates following spontaneous and induced labors. Cesarean delivery after induced labor (*shaded bars*), cesarean delivery after spontaneous labor (*open bars*).(Courtesy of Ecker JL, Chen KT, Cohen AP, et al: Increased risk of cesarean delivery with advancing maternal age: Indications and associated factors in nulliparous women. *Am J Obstet Gynecol* 185: 883-887, 2001.)

TABLE 2.—Percentage of Women Induced According to Indication and
Maternal Age

	Age (y)			
	<25 (n = 149)	25-34 (n = 727)	35-39 (n = 231)	≥40 (n = 49)
Percentage induced				
Elective	2.9	5.9	6.2	11.3
Post-dates	7.3	6.3	9.1	11.3
Medical indications	5.5	6.5	8.5	7.2
Fetal indications	4.3	2.9	4.9	3.1
Other indications	7.8	13.3	14.7	17.5
Total*	27.8	34.9	43.6	50.5

*P = .001 for trend.
(Courtesy of Ecker JL, Chen KT, Cohen AP, et al: Increased risk of cesarean delivery with advancing maternal age: Indications and associated factors in nulliparous women. *Am J Obstet Gynecol* 185: 883-887, 2001.)

years, 593 were 35 to 39 years, and 123 were at least 40 years of age. The rate of cesarean section was calculated for each age group and for those with and without labor.

Findings.—Cesarean delivery rates increased with increasing maternal age (Fig 1). Older women were also more likely to have a cesarean delivery without labor. Malpresentation and prior myomectomy were the most common indications for cesarean section without labor and were more prevalent among the older mothers (Fig 2). Even among those women with either spontaneous or induced labor, cesarean delivery rates increased with maternal age (Fig 3). Cesarean delivery increased with induced labor and rates of induction increased with maternal age, especially rates of elective induction (Table 2). Cesarean delivery for failure to progress or fetal distress was more common among older mothers. Among those women who had a cesarean section because of failure to progress, treatment and length of labor did not vary with age.

Conclusion.—Older women are at higher risk for cesarean delivery. This analysis of a large database suggests that both biological and behavioral factors play a role in the increase in cesarean deliveries with maternal age. Although the intrinsic contractility of older myometrium and other factors such as prior uterine surgery cannot be changed, the use of elective induction—which is more common among older mothers—might be targeted to reduce the rate of cesarean delivery.

▶ These authors explore the experience at the Brigham and Women's Hospital for calendar year 1998 with the hope of understanding the possible impact of an aging obstetrical population on the increase in the incidence of cesarean section at that institution. Though their approach is to use univariate statistics, their data analysis is logical and provides some fresh insights. To avoid confounding impacts on the relationship between age and cesarean section, only nulliparous women delivering at term were included. Since post datism is variously defined by obstetricians, the authors designate labor induction at less than 40 6/7 weeks as elective and past that time as motivated by post datism.

Three-thousand seven hundred fifteen women were divided into 4 age intervals of unequal length.

Clearly, cesarean section rates increased with maternal age both at delivery, prior to, and after labor onset. In the former category, prior myomectomy and especially malpresentation, largely breech presentations, were the most likely indications. Both the incidence of breech presentation and the likelihood of cesarean section for that diagnosis increased with age. Though only 40% to 45% of women had a trial of version, none of the 7 women 40 years or older had a version attempt made.

Cesarean section after labor was preceded by an increased incidence of elective inductions and post datism, both increasing with patient age from about 16% to 30% of sections at stated maternal age. Failures of induction were attributed to fetal distress, usually a subjective diagnosis, and failure to progress, possibly reflecting uterine age–related biology. What is most impressive is the contribution of induction, both elective and for post datism, to the increase in cesarean section incidence. So too is the rarity with which women with malpresentations were allowed a trial of labor. Clearly, both physician and patient behavioral events are a remediable part of the age-related increase in cesarean section in the data reviewed. Inductions of labor, which increased from 15.7% to 29.8% as one looks at women aging from 25 to more than 40 years, seems to be the principal factor in additional cesarean section rates related to maternal age.

T. H. Kirschbaum, MD

Perineal Massage in Labour and Prevention of Perineal Trauma: Randomised Controlled Trial

Stamp G, Kruzins G, Crowther C (Univ of South Australia, Adelaide; Women's and Children's Hosp, North Adelaide, Australia; Univ of Adelaide, North Adelaide, Australia)
BMJ 322:1277-1280, 2001   7–9

Background.—Morbidity in the short and long term is associated with perineal trauma during and after childbirth. Urinary and fecal incontinence, painful intercourse, and persistent perineal pain may result. The effects of perineal massage in the second stage of labor on perineal outcomes were investigated.

Methods.—The randomized controlled trial included 1340 women expecting normal birth of a singleton. During the second stage of labor, the perineum was treated with massage and stretching with a water soluble lubricant. Primary outcomes were rates of intact perineum; episiotomies; and first, second, third, and fourth degree tears. Secondary outcomes were pain 3 and 10 days after birth and pain, dyspareunia, resumption of sexual intercourse, and urinary and fecal incontinence and urgency 3 months after birth.

Findings.—The massage and control groups had similar rates of intact perineum, first and second degree tears, and episiotomies. The incidence of third degree tears was 1.7% in the massage group and 3.6% in the control group. None of the secondary outcomes differed between groups.

Conclusion.—Perineal massage in labor does not increase the likelihood of an intact perineum. This intervention also does not reduce the risk of pain, dyspareunia, or urinary and fecal problems.

▶ This is the third of 3 randomized, controlled trials in appraising the value of massage and stretching of the perineum during the second stage of labor, "ironing out" to many, in reducing the incidence of episiotomy, perineal laceration, and perineal pain post partum. The time of resumption of coitus and urinary and fecal incontinence were outcome measures at 3 months post partum. The 2 prior studies failed to demonstrate a significant decrease in the incidence of a perineal trauma as a result. This is the largest and in many ways the best structured of the 3 trials. Research midwives were in charge of experimental design, recruitment, randomization, and execution of the study.

During the second stage of labor, 2 lubricated fingers inside the vagina were used to gently stretch the perineum short of patient discomfort. The power calculation was based on the requirement of 80% power to detect an increase in intact perineum post partum from 32.5% (a figure derived from midwives in 7 Australian delivery sites) to 40% or more. Of 1340 women with randomized singlet pregnancies, 49% were multiparous. No significant difference was observed compared with controls of the incidence of intact perineum post partum, nor in the incidence of perineal and vaginal pain and dyspareunia 3 to 10 days post partum or incontinence at 3 months. Although one could argue that skill in performance of massage is important and was uncontrolled here, the cumulative evidence of these 3 studies suggest that if any benefit accrues, it is very small.

T. H. Kirschbaum, MD

Effect of Low-Dose Mobile Versus Traditional Epidural Techniques on Mode of Delivery: A Randomised Controlled Trial
Shennan AH, for the Comparative Obstetric Mobile Epidural Trial (COMET) Study Group UK (Univ of Birmingham, England; et al)
Lancet 358:19-23, 2001   7–10

Background.—The most effective relief of labor pain is obtained from epidural analgesia, but it is associated with increased rates of instrumental vaginal delivery, prolonged labor, and oxytocin augmentation. However, the likelihood of cesarean section delivery does not appear to be affected by epidural analgesia. The effects may be related to the poor motor function associated with traditional epidural techniques. Newer forms of epidural analgesia have been developed by using combinations of opioid and less concentrated local anesthetic. This approach has been shown to preserve motor function and allow ambulation for the patient. However, these low-dose epidurals are not in wide use. A randomized trial was conducted to

TABLE 3.—Mode of Delivery

Delivery	Traditional Epidural (n = 353)	Combined Spinal Epidural (n = 351)	Low-dose Infusion Epidural (n = 350)
Normal vaginal	124 (35%)	150 (43%)	150 (43%)
Instrumental vaginal	131 (37%)	102 (29%)	98 (28%)
Caesarean section	98 (28%)	99 (28%)	102 (29%)

Note: P = .04, 1DF for normal versus other deliveries.
(Courtesy of Shennan AH, for the Comparative Obstetric Mobile Epidural Trial [COMET] Study Group UK: Effect of low-dose mobile versus traditional epidural techniques on mode of delivery: A randomised controlled trial. *Lancet* 358:19-23, 2001. Reprinted with permission from Elsevier Science.)

compare the use of low-dose combined spinal epidural and low-dose infusion (mobile) techniques with traditional epidural technique.

Methods.—In a 14-month trial, 1054 nulliparous women requesting epidural pain relief were randomly assigned to traditional (353 patients), low-dose combined spinal epidural (351 patients), or low-dose infusion epidural analgesia (350 patients). The primary outcome was mode of delivery, and the secondary outcomes were progress of labor, efficacy of procedure, and effect on neonates. Data were obtained during labor, and women were interviewed postnatally.

Results.—In the traditional epidural group, the normal vaginal delivery rate was 35.1%; the rate was 42.7% in the low-dose combined spinal group and 42.9% in the low-dose infusion group (Table 3). A reduction in instrumental vaginal delivery was responsible for these differences. Apgar scores of 7 or less at 5 minutes were more frequent with the low-dose technique. The low-dose infusion group had a higher rate of high-level resuscitation.

Conclusion.—These findings indicate the benefits for delivery outcome with the use of low-dose epidural techniques for labor analgesia. The continued use of traditional epidurals may not be justified.

▶ Despite the popularity of epidural conductance and anesthetic techniques for labor analgesia, there is widespread interest in alternative techniques that might employ lesser doses of conduction blockers combined with opioids to allow patients to maintain motor function, pelvic tone, and uncompromised Valsalva efforts. Here a traditional epidural technique (2% lidocaine, 60 mg test dose, plus 25 mg of 0.25% bupivacaine with repeat 25 mg boluses) was compared with 2 "mobile" methods. The low-dose method uses a combination of 10 mg of bupivicaine supplemented with 2 μg of fentanyl injected into the epidural space with boluses as needed. The low-dose infusion method uses a "needle through needle" technique employing 2.5 mg of bupivacaine and 25 μg of fentanyl in the subarachnoid space.

When the spinal anesthetic wore off, bipuvicaine, 15 mg, and fentanyl, 30 μg, was given through the epidural catheter. Bolus repeats were given no oftener than every 30 minutes, and failed intrathecal entry led to epidural dosage of the low-dose mixture. A total of 1054 nulliparous women were randomly allocated to the 3 groups.

The low-dose techniques were associated with an average 7.6% increase in the incidence of normal vaginal delivery, with the low-dose infusion technique somewhat more effective. There were no differences in delay in the second stage of labor necessitating operative delivery techniques nor any evidence of fetal distress, neonatal ICU admission, or the efficacy of pain relief. There was, as a reflection of opioid, a significantly increased incidence of APGAR scores at 5 minutes of 7 or less among those receiving the low-dose combination, but this had no impact on newborn outcome. The authors feel that use of the low-dose method prevents the 1 of every 4 operative deliveries that took place with traditional epidural techniques. This is a convincing demonstration of the use of these methods. It would have been more convincing had the incidence of normal, spontaneous vaginal birth been greater than the 40% the authors note.

T. H. Kirschbaum, MD

Labor Epidural Analgesia and Intrapartum Maternal Hyperthermia
Yancey MK, Zhang J, Schwarz J, et al (Tripler Army Med Ctr, Honolulu, Hawaii; Natl Inst of Child Health and Human Development, Bethesda, Md)
Obstet Gynecol 98:763-770, 2001   7–11

Introduction.—Previous studies have found labor epidural analgesia to be associated with an increased incidence of maternal intrapartum fever, but

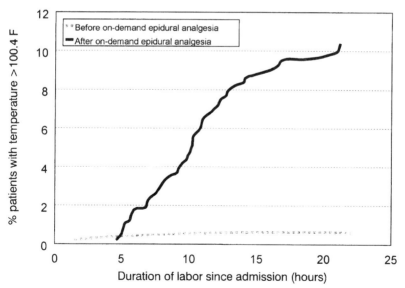

FIGURE 1.—Plot of the percentage of undelivered women with maximal intrapartum temperature of at least 100.4°F relative to hours since admission to labor unit for the two study periods. *P* < .001 by log rank test. (Courtesy of Yancey MK, Zhang J, Schwarz J, et al: Labor epidural analgesia and intrapartum maternal hyperthermia. *Obstet Gynecol* 98:763-770, 2001. Reprinted with permission from The American College of Obstetricians and Gynecologists.)

TABLE 4.—Incidence of Maternal Febrile Morbidity Relative to Study Period

Characteristics	Before On-Demand Epidural Analgesia (N = 498)	After On-Demand Epidural Analgesia (N = 572)	RR (95% CI)
Intrapartum temperature ≥99.5F*	41 (8.2%)	150 (26.2%)	3.2 (2.3, 4.4)
Intrapartum temperature ≥100.4F*	3 (0.6%)	63 (11.0%)	18.3 (5.8, 57.8)
Chorioamnionitis*	2 (0.4%)	50 (8.7%)	21.8 (5.3, 89.0)
Intrapartum fever of undetermined origin*†	5 (1.0%)	31 (5.9%)	5.9 (2.3, 15.0)
Endometritis‡	33 (6.6%)	23 (4.7%)	0.69 (0.42, 1.2)

Data presented as *n* (%). Analysis by χ^2 test or Fisher exact test, as appropriate.
*$P < .01$.
†Excluded women diagnosed with chorioamnionitis.
‡Excluded women with chorioamnionitis or intrapartum fever.
Abbreviation: RR, Relative risk.
(Courtesy of Yancey MK, Zhang J, Schwarz J, et al: Labor epidural analgesia and intrapartum maternal hyperthermia. *Obstet Gynecol* 98:763-770, 2001. Reprinted with permission from The American College of Obstetricians and Gynecologists.)

patient crossover and self-selection bias may have affected outcomes. In a retrospective cohort analysis, women eligible for on-request labor epidural analgesia were compared for intrapartum fever with women who did not have this option.

Methods.—Before October 1993, epidural analgesia in laboring women was available at the study institution only to those with a medical indication. After this date, round-the-clock on-demand labor epidural analgesia was provided. Women eligible for the study were nulliparous with term gestations and in spontaneous labor. During the year before the policy change, 498 eligible women delivered (Before group); 572 delivered in the first year of on-demand epidural analgesia (After group). The techniques and dosing used for labor epidural analgesia were similar in the 2 periods. Excluded from analysis were women admitted with a temperature of at least 99.5° F.

Results.—Labor epidural analgesia was used by 5 (1.0%) women in the Before group and by 475 (83.0%) in the After group. The mean maximal intrapartum temperature was higher in women who had labor epidural analgesia than in those who did not (99.1° F vs 98.4° F). A maximal temperature of at least 99.5° F was recorded in 30% of women with epidural analgesia, but in only 8.7% of those who did not receive epidural analgesia. In multivariable analysis, on-request labor epidural analgesia was significantly associated with an intrapartum temperature of at least 99.5° F and an intrapartum temperature of at least 100.4° F (Fig 1). The relative incidence of maternal febrile morbidity is shown in Table 4. In the After group, there were statistically significant increases in the frequency of neonatal screening complete blood cell counts and blood cultures, and in the median length of stay. No cases of culture-proven neonatal sepsis occurred, and the proportion of infants who received antibiotic therapy was similar in the Before (4.6%) and After (5.8%) groups.

Conclusion.—Labor epidural analgesia is associated with a clinically significant increase in the incidence of intrapartum fever. The precise etiology of this effect is unknown, but it may be related to alteration in maternal thermoregulatory physiology.

▶ Studies of the clinical application of epidural analgesia for labor are almost inevitably complicated by uncertain patient and physician selection variables. It's clear that women with past histories of prolonged labors tend to opt disproportionately for conduction anesthesia techniques, which in turn influences comparative outcomes. Crossover phenomena, when women who initially choose or are randomized to one analgesic approach opt for another during labor, are difficult to deal with in evaluating outcome measurements.

In January 1994, the Tripler Army Medical Center in Oahu instituted an administrative policy change making epidural analgesia administration by certified nurse anesthetists or anesthesiologists available on round-the-clock basis for all patients. Epidural analgesia acceptance rates jumped from 1% to 83% as a result of this change. There were no changes in the population of military medical staff or dependents who used the facility, and patient management, housing, income, and universal access to health care remained unchanged. This same population has been used to study the impact of epidural analgesia on labor duration reported here (see Abstract 7–10).

Only primigravidas with singlet uncomplicated pregnancies were accepted for comparison. Epidural analgesia was begun with a cervix at least 4 cm dilated; 18 women with temperature elevations greater than 99.5° F on entry were rejected. Chorioamnionitis was diagnosed on the basis of a temperature greater than 100.4° F and maternal or fetal tachycardia with or without uterine tenderness. Univariant analysis showed a significant monotonic increase in the incidence of temperature greater than 100.4° F during labor as a function of time since admission, in comparing patients before and after the policy change. When logistic regression was used to test for confounding variables (labor, ruptured membrane, duration, number of pelvic examinations, prepregnancy weight and temperature elevation on admission) the epidural recipients had a 20.2-fold greater likelihood of temperature elevation during labor than did the nonepidural group. It is important that no increased incidence of postpartum endometritis occurred in these women and, though laboratory evaluation of the babies whose mothers received epidural analgesia were common, there were no differences in antibiotic use or median neonatal length of stay between the 2 groups. Although this study used historical controls, there is little suggestion that management prescribed by physicians changed with time, a primary strength of this study. The mechanism of temperature elevation is still obscure. The principal lesson here is that extended and expensive laboratory evaluation of mothers or neonates does not seem warranted with findings other than the transient temperature elevation noted during analgesic administration.

T. H. Kirschbaum, MD

8 Puerperium

Group A Streptococcal Puerperal Sepsis Preceded by Positive Surveillance Cultures
Stefonek KR, Maerz LL, Nielsen MP, et al (Oregon Health Division, Portland; Willamette Falls Hosp, Oregon City, Ore; Ctrs for Disease Control and Prevention, Atlanta, Ga)
Obstet Gynecol 98:846-848, 2001   8–1

Background.—Carriers of group A streptococci may be identified during screening of pregnant women for vaginal and rectal carriage of group B streptococci. The clinical significance of group A streptococcal carriage during pregnancy has not been established. Two cases were reported.

> *Case Reports.*—Group A streptococcal puerperal sepsis developed in 2 women who gave birth 15 months apart at 1 hospital. Hysterectomy was indicated for the first patient. Complications during surgery included subcapsular hepatic hematoma, pleural effusion, and prolonged ileus. This patient was finally discharged from the hospital after 35 days. In the second patient, endometritis developed. This patient subsequently recovered. Both had had isolation of group A streptococci from vaginal and rectal cultures obtained at prenatal group B streptococcal screening. The acute sepsis isolates were both M-type 28. However, the 2 strains were unrelated on pulsed-field gel electrophoresis.

Conclusion.—Detecting group A streptococci on prenatal culture should alert clinicians to the possibility of serious postpartum infection. Further research is needed.

▶ In reporting 2 women with group B puerperal streptococcal sepsis, these authors raise an interesting issue about which too little is known. Both patients were multiparas, the first developing purulent endometritis with uterine and adnexal abscesses and peritonitis on the fourth postpartum day. The second developed a less intense endometritis on postpartum day 1, was afebrile by postpartum day 3 with a penicillin-sensitive organism. Both had group A streptococci reported 3 weeks and 11 days, respectively, ante partum as findings incidental for group B streptococcus. On pages 721-723 of the issue in which this article appears, Dr Philip Mead provides a useful comment.

Group A streptococcus is present in the vagina at delivery in about 1 in 3500 women; the attack rate for postpartum streptococcal infection is unknown but, fortunately, is very small. Routine screening for an anticipated positive finding in 1 of 3500 gravidas seems inappropriate, especially since its management is uncertain and unproven. Prophylactic therapy as per group B streptococcus (GBS) using 10 days of either penicillin or rafampin seems an extreme measure in view of the rarity of reported group A strep sepsis and the failure of prophylaxis to prevent GBS under such circumstances. Dr Mead comments that intrapartum therapy with penicillin may be a reasonable step but is unproven by the experience of others. Perhaps conversation with a laboratory screening for vaginal GBS with respect to cost benefit considerations for group A streptococcus may be a reasonable step for those who worry about this admittedly small hazard.

T. H. Kirschbaum, MD

Differences in Postpartum Morbidity in Women Who Are Infected With the Human Immunodeficiency Virus After Elective Cesarean Delivery, Emergency Cesarean Delivery, or Vaginal Delivery
Marcollet A, Goffinet F, Firtion G, et al (Hôpital Cochin, Paris)
Am J Obstet Gynecol 186:784-789, 2002   8–2

Background.—Elective cesarean delivery has been used, with some controversy, to prevent the transmission of HIV from mother to child. However, the morbidity and mortality risks for the mother are increased with cesarean delivery, with the risk of death directly attributable to this procedure reported to be as high as 6-fold over that with vaginal delivery. The impact that the type of delivery exerts on postpartum morbidity among women who are HIV seropositive was assessed.

Methods.—The charts of 401 women with HIV infections that occurred over a period of 10 years and who subsequently delivered children were reviewed retrospectively. Cesarean deliveries (201 women, with 109 elective and 92 emergency deliveries) were compared with vaginal deliveries (200 women) in terms of outcome.

Results.—The median values for the mothers were age, 30 years; parity, 1; weight at delivery, 72 kg; CD4 lymphocyte count, 459/mm^3; and plasma HIV RNA, 250 copies/mL. Serious complications occurred in 8 women who had vaginal delivery, 7 who had elective cesarean delivery, and 11 who had emergency cesarean delivery. Postpartum fever was the most frequent morbidity. Factors found to be significantly associated with complications were antepartum or intrapartum hemorrhage or fever, uterine scarring, and use of forceps in the delivery. On multivariate analysis adjusted for maternal CD4 lymphocyte count and antepartum hemorrhage, the relative risk of any complication occurring after delivery was increased by 1.85 for elective cesarean delivery and 4.17 after emergency cesarean when compared with vaginal delivery.

Conclusion.—The women who were infected with HIV and underwent emergency cesarean delivery had the highest incidence of postpartum morbidity, exceeding that found in HIV seropositive women having elective cesarean procedures.

▶ At least in Europe, use of cesarean section for HIV-1 positive gravidas, designed to reduce maternal-to-fetal viral transmission rates, has raised the question of whether—given the increased risk of maternal morbidity and mortality for abdominal versus vaginal birth—it adds to the intrinsic maternal hazard. As in this case, the answer is clouded a bit by heterogeneity in drug therapy afforded the women.

This is a retrospective chart review study of 401 HIV-1–positive women, part of the French Perinatal HIV Study, all delivered at a Parisian hospital during the years 1989 to 1999. During the first 5 years, no antiretroviral therapy was available to the gravidas. From 1994 to 1997, azidothymidine was routinely used during pregnancy and in the early neonatal period. From 1997 to 1999, cesarean section for HIV-1–positive women with intact membranes not in labor was offered. Only 9% of the women reported here received protease inhibitors.

Immunologic data disclosed somewhere between 6% and 14% of women had fewer than 200,000 CD4 cells/L and 3% to 14% had greater than 10,000 HIV-1 RNA copies/mL of blood. Those delivered by emergency cesarean section had a 2.8% incidence of HIV-1 copies greater than 10,000/mL. Elective cesarean section was done most often, in 64% of such cases to reduce maternal-to-fetal transmission rates. Emergency cesarean sections were done usually for failure of labor progression or fetal heart rate irregularity. The most prevalent postpartum morbidity was fever, significantly more common among women with emergency cesarean sections and inversely related to the size of their CD4 counts. Beyond that, morbidity was not much different when comparing vaginal to cesarean section births.

Bear in mind that cesarean section after rupture of membranes or the onset of labor has not been demonstrated to result in reduced maternal-to-fetal transmission rates of the HIV-1 infection. Multivariate analysis yields risk ratios for postpartum complications, compared with vaginal births, of 1.85 for elective cesarean section and 4.17 for emergency section. It therefore seems important to minimize the number of emergency procedures for such women in the interest of preventing newborn infection. As data reflecting the care of HIV-1–positive women treated with protease inhibitors—which decrease the number of HIV-1 RNA copies in plasma—become available, the role of cesarean section in their treatment will need to be reappraised.

T. H. Kirschbaum, MD

9 Genetics and Teratology

Quantitative Analysis of the Bidirectional Fetomaternal Transfer of Nucleated Cells and Plasma DNA
Lo YMD, Lau TK, Chan LYS, et al (Chinese Univ of Hong Kong)
Clin Chem 46:1301-1309, 2000   9–1

Background.—The fetomaternal transfer of nucleated cells and plasma DNA has been of much interest recently. However, no systematic quantitative comparisons of these 2 directions and 2 modalities of trafficking have been published.

Methods.—Fetus-to-mother transfer of nucleated cells and plasma DNA was studied in pregnant women carrying male fetuses. Real-time quantitative polymerase chain reaction assay was used to study the SRY gene. To study mother-to-fetus transfer, real-time quantitative polymerase chain reaction assays for the insertion/deletion polymorphisms involving the gutathione S-transferase M1 and angiotensin-converting enzyme genes were used.

Findings.—Data on 50 informative mother-baby pairs were analyzed. Maternal DNA was found in the cellular fraction of umbilical cord blood in 24%. The median fractional concentration was 2.6×10^{-4}. In the plasma fraction of cord blood, maternal DNA was detected in 30% of cases, the median fractional level being 3×10^{-3}. Fetus-to-mother transfer of nucleated cells was found in 26% of cases, the median fractional concentration being 3.2×10^{-4}. In the plasma fraction, fetal DNA was found in 100% of maternal plasma. The median fractional concentration was 3×10^{-2} (Table 3).

Conclusion.—Significantly more fetal DNA is found in the plasma of pregnant women than DNA from the cellular fraction of maternal blood. Maternal DNA was also seen in the cellular and plasma fractions of cord blood after delivery.

▶ Fetal cells have been demonstrated in maternal blood repeatedly and in increasing amounts after the first trimester,[1] and enhanced fetal-to-maternal transfer has been noted in aneuploidies[2] and preeclampsia.[3] Fetal cells have been demonstrated to have prolonged chimeric presence in maternal tissues[4] and apparently form the basis for chronic autoimmune disturbances in some

TABLE 3.—Number of Cases Tabulated With Regard to the Cellular and Plasma DNA Transfer Status

A. Mother-to-fetus transfer.

		Cellular DNA transfer*	
		+	−
Plasma DNA transfer*	+	6	9
	−	6	29

B. Fetus-to-mother transfer.

		Cellular DNA transfer*	
		+	−
Plasma DNA Transfer*	+	13	37
	−	0	0

* + and − denote cases with detectable and undetectable trafficking, respectively.
(Courtesy of Lo YMD, Lau TK, Chan LYS, et al: Quantitative analysis of the bidirectional fetomaternal transfer of nucleated cells and plasma DNA. *Clin Chem* 46:1301-1309, 2000. Copyright 2000, The American Association for Clinical Chemistry [1-800-892-1400].)

cases.[5,6] Maternal-to–fetal cell transfers have been well studied, but maternal hematopoietic stem cells in cord blood establish the fact that the converse occurs as well.[7] Further, fetal-to-maternal trafficking of fetal DNA has been established,[8] exhibiting very rapid DNA clearance from maternal blood[9] and showing increased concentrations in preeclampsia[10] and Down syndrome.[11]

This important study simultaneously estimates the quantities of transfer of cells and plasma DNA between mothers and fetuses in a series of 50 informative term pregnancies. Fetal-to-maternal cellular transfer was estimated from conventional polymerase chain reaction done on maternal blood buffy coat DNA preparations using primers for the SRY gene present in male fetuses. Maternal-to-fetal cell transfers were estimated from polymorphisms in a GESTM 1 gene observed in only half of individuals and from insertion-deletion polymorphisms in the ACE gene. Cases were informative of transfer in which mothers bear the GSTM 1 gene and fetuses do not. For ACE insertion deletion polymorphism, pregnancies were informative of transfer when fetuses were homozygous for the mutation and mothers were heterozygous. Real time quantitative polymerase chain reaction using the Taq Man polymerase system[12] with primers appropriate to SRY, GSTM1, and ACE genes was used to track cell and plasma DNA between mother and fetus. One hundred six women whose maternal and fetal genomes were not informative were excluded from this study.

Fetus-to–maternal plasma DNA transfers were seen in all pregnancies, but in only 30% were transfers of maternal-to-fetal DNA noted. Maternal nucleate cells and plasma DNA transfers occur in 24% of fetal samples, compared with 26% of fetal-to-maternal cellular transfer. Maternal cellular and plasma DNA were seen in median concentrations of 56 genomic equivalents/mL and in fetal blood in a relative concentration of 0.3%. For fetal cells and DNA in maternal blood, the relative concentration was 0.032% of total DNA.

The study shows that bidirectional cellular and DNA transfers between mother and fetus are common and that fetal DNA occurs with 10 times the prevalence of fetal cells and in 100% of fetal cases in maternal blood, making it a readily accessible source for fetal genetic analysis. The lack of correlation between fetal-to-maternal transfers of cellular and plasma DNA probably means that trophoblastic epithelial cells, not fetal blood cells, are its dominant origin. This study should properly mark the beginnings of extensive efforts in the use of fetal DNA in maternal blood for fetal diagnosis and, because of the rapid clearance rates in maternal blood, offers a near real time opportunity at fetal diagnosis.

T. H. Kirschbaum, MD

References

1. Lo YMD, Lo ESF, Watson N, et al: Two-way cell traffic between mother and fetus: Biologic and clinical implications. *Blood* 88:4390-4395, 1996.
2. 1999 YEAR BOOK OF OBSTETRICS, GYNECOLOGY, AND WOMEN'S HEALTH, pp 191-193.
3. 2000 YEAR BOOK OF OBSTETRICS, GYNECOLOGY, AND WOMEN'S HEALTH, pp 103-104.
4. 1997 YEAR BOOK OF OBSTETRICS, GYNECOLOGY, AND WOMEN'S HEALTH, pp 202-203.
5. 1999 YEAR BOOK OF OBSTETRICS, GYNECOLOGY, AND WOMEN'S HEALTH, pp 89-91.
6. 2002 YEAR BOOK OF OBSTETRICS, GYNECOLOGY, AND WOMEN'S HEALTH, pp 158-159 and 221-222.
7. Cairo MS, Wagner JE: Placenta and/or umbilical cord blood: An alternative source of hematopoietic stem cells for transplantation. *Blood* 90:4665-4678, 1997.
8. 1999 YEAR BOOK OF OBSTETRICS, GYNECOLOGY, AND WOMEN'S HEALTH, pp 193-196.
9. 2000 YEAR BOOK OF OBSTETRICS, GYNECOLOGY, AND WOMEN'S HEALTH, pp 207-208 and pp 218-224.
10. 2000 YEAR BOOK OF OBSTETRICS, GYNECOLOGY, AND WOMEN'S HEALTH, pp 184-188.
11. 2001 YEAR BOOK OF OBSTETRICS, GYNECOLOGY, AND WOMEN'S HEALTH, pp 217-219.
12. 1999 YEAR BOOK OF OBSTETRICS, GYNECOLOGY, AND WOMEN'S HEALTH, pp 193-196.

Kinetics of Fetal Cellular and Cell-Free DNA in the Maternal Circulation During and After Pregnancy: Implications for Noninvasive Prenatal Diagnosis

Ariga H, Ohto H, Busch MP, et al (Blood Ctrs of the Pacific, San Francisco; Univ of California, San Francisco; Fukushima Med Univ, Japan; et al)
Transfusion 41:1524-1530, 2001   9–2

Background.—Many studies have supported the concept of a physical and immunologic barrier at the maternal-fetal interface, but little is known about how the semi-allogeneic fetus is protected from attack by the maternal immune system. It is thought that bidirectional cell trafficking across the maternal-fetal interface may play a role in this process. Fetal genetic material is detectable in the maternal circulation, but there are few data available concerning its quantity and natural history during gestation. The kinetics and natural history of fetal DNA in the maternal circulation were investigated.

Methods.—The kinetics of cellular and cell-free fetal DNA were characterized in the circulation of 25 healthy women during and after uncomplicated pregnancy. Human Y-chromosome sequences were quantitated with real-time kinetic polymerase chain reaction (PCR), and liquid oligomer hybridization with ^{32}P-labeled probes was used in the verification of amplified products.

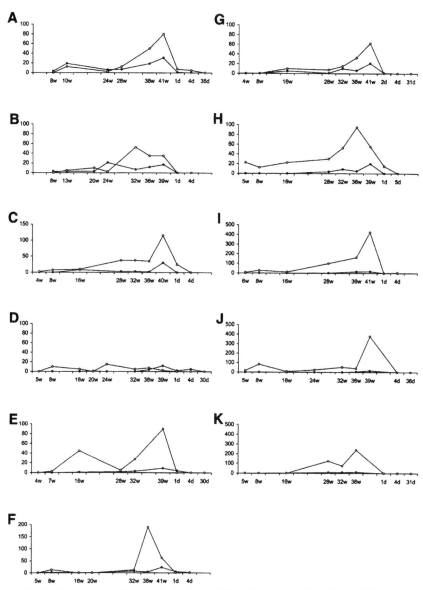

FIGURE 2.—Comparison between fetal cellular DNA (*solid circles*) and fetal cell-free DNA (*open circles*) throughout pregnancy for 11 women (**A-K**) carrying a male fetus. The y-axis represents the copy number of SRY + DNA per 0.5 mL of maternal blood, and the x-axis represents time. *Abbreviations: SRY,* Sex-determining region of the Y chromosome; *w,* weeks; *d,* days. (Courtesy of Ariga H, Ohto H, Busch MP, et al: Kinetics of fetal cellular and cell-free DNA in the maternal circulation during and after pregnancy: Implications for noninvasive prenatal diagnosis. *Transfusion* 41:1524-1530, 2001. Reprinted by permission of Blackwell Science, Inc.)

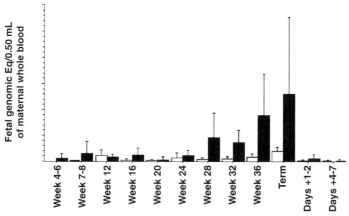

FIGURE 3.—Direct comparison is shown between fetal cell–associated (*open bars*) and cell-free (*solid bars*) DNA in maternal blood during and after pregnancy for 11 women carrying a male fetus. The y-axis represents the copy number of SRY + DNA per 0.5 mL of maternal blood, and the x-axis represents gestational age. A transient low-level increase in fetal DNA during 7 to 16 weeks of gestation is followed by a steady increase in concentration, which is most marked in the cell-free compartment (maternal plasma) and which reaches a maximum at term. Clearance of all fetal DNA is extremely rapid after parturition. *Error bars* indicate ± 1 SD. *Abbreviation: SRY*, Sex-determining region of the Y chromosome. (Courtesy of Ariga H, Ohto H, Busch MP, et al: Kinetics of fetal cellular and cell-free DNA in the maternal circulation during and after pregnancy: Implications for noninvasive prenatal diagnosis. *Transfusion* 41:1524-1530, 2001. Reprinted by permission of Blackwell Science, Inc.)

Results.—Low-level fetal Y-chromosome DNA was detected in both cellular and cell-free compartments in all male pregnancies but in no female pregnancies, in both cellular and cell-free compartments, beginning at 7 to 16 weeks and increasing steadily after 24 weeks, peaking at parturition (Fig 2). There was a rapid decline in fetal DNA after birth (Fig 3).

Conclusions.—The quantity of fetal genetic material detectable throughout pregnancy is a function of gestational age and of whether the plasma or cellular compartment is examined. The absolute quantity of fetal DNA and its ratio to total DNA are greater in the plasma than in the cellular compartment. Fetal DNA is cleared rapidly from both compartments after parturition (Table 2), suggesting that turnover of fetal DNA is dynamic. These findings and kinetic PCR methods may have implications for noninvasive prenatal diagnosis, since they provide prospective and quantitative data concerning fetal DNA levels.

▶ This article is an important contribution in the compelling development of fetal genetic analysis using fetal cells transferred passively to the maternal circulation. Twenty normal gravidas provided blood samples every 4 to 8 weeks between 4 and 34½ weeks' gestational age. By centrifugation, the cellular fraction was separated from plasma, and quantities of cellular and cell-free DNA were estimated by using real-time PCR employment of Taq polymerase.[1] In all, 11 gravid subjects were known to bear male fetuses, and fetal blood was identified by using primers chosen to delimit the sex-determining region of the Y chromosome (SRY) to prove fetal origin. The sensitivity of the method was proven by serial deletions of DNA specimens, and the specificity by failure

TABLE 2.—Fetal Cell–Associated DNA in Genomic Equivalents (gEq) per 0.50 mL Maternal Whole Blood by Week of Gestation and Postpartum Among 20 Women Carrying Male Infants

Gestation or Postpartum	SRY + Cell Number (Geq/0.50 mL)	Range	Proportion of Total Samples Positive
4-6 w	0.12	0-2	2/17 (12)
7-8 w	1.05	0-4	9/20 (45)
12 w	8.00	2-19	3/3 (100)
16 w	2.47	0-8	13/17 (77)
20 w	2.00	0-5	4/5 (80)
24 w	7.00	0-20	6/8 (75)
28 w	5.80	0-15	14/15 (93)
32 w	7.86	0-30	12/14 (86)
36 w	15.12	2-56	17/17 (100)
parturition	31.84	6-144	19/19 (100)
1-2d	1.56	0-5	11/18 (61)
4-7d	0.53	0-5	4/19 (11)
25-36d	0.36	0-4	2/14 (14)

Abbreviations: SRY, Sex-determining region of the Y chromosome; *w*, weeks; *d*, days.

(Courtesy of Ariga H, Ohto H, Busch MP, et al: Kinetics of fetal cellular and cell-free DNA in the maternal circulation during and after pregnancy: Implications for noninvasive prenatal diagnosis. *Transfusion* 41:1524-1530, 2001. Reprinted by permission of Blackwell Science, Inc.)

to yield amplification products in 16 women bearing female fetuses. The identification of amplification products after more than 40 cycles of PCR was proven by failure of hybridization of a ^{32}P-labeled probe to a Y chromosome DNA fragment.

Fetal cells could be identified from 4 weeks' gestational age to delivery in amounts shown in Table 2. Please note these are cell counts per 0.5 mL and must be doubled to compare with other studies. Fetal cells increased transiently at 8 to 12 weeks' gestational age but reached a peak at 36 weeks (30 cells/mL of maternal blood) and during parturition (63.5 cells/mL in maternal blood). At 1 to 2 days' postpartum, an average of 3 cells/mL persist. Cell-free DNA is much more abundant in plasma, anywhere from 3.3 to 9.5 times greater than in the cellular fraction. These longitudinal data are superior to the cross-sectional data available elsewhere, though there are no conflicts with the data either of Lo[2,3] or Bianchi[4] previously reviewed.

T. H. Kirschbaum, MD

References

1. 1999 YEAR BOOK OF OBSTETRICS, GYNECOLOGY, AND WOMEN'S HEALTH, pp 193-196.
2. 2001 YEAR BOOK OF OBSTETRICS, GYNECOLOGY, AND WOMEN'S HEALTH, pp 217-219.
3. 2000 YEAR BOOK OF OBSTETRICS, GYNECOLOGY, AND WOMEN'S HEALTH, pp 103-104.
4. 1999 YEAR BOOK OF OBSTETRICS, GYNECOLOGY, AND WOMEN'S HEALTH, pp 191-193.

Accuracy of Fetal Gender Determination by Analysis of DNA in Maternal Plasma
Sekizawa A, Kondo T, Iwasaki M, et al (Showa Univ, Tokyo)
Clin Chem 47:1856-1858, 2001   9–3

Background.—Researchers have reported the potential of fetal cell-free DNA analysis for the prenatal diagnosis of fetal gender and rhesus D status. However, the accuracy of prenatal diagnosis has not been established. The diagnostic accuracy of fetal gender determination using cell-free DNA from maternal plasma obtained at early gestation was investigated.

Methods and Findings.—Three hundred two maternal plasma samples were analyzed in a blinded fashion. One hundred forty-three women were carrying male fetuses, and 159 were carrying females. In 97.2% of women carrying male fetuses, polymerase chain reaction detected the DYS14 sequence. Results were false-negative in 4 women at 9, 11, or 13 weeks. Overall, the positive and negative predictive values for determining male gender from maternal plasma were 100% and 97.5%, respectively.

Conclusion.—This is the first report of the diagnostic accuracy of fetal gender determination from a large number of maternal plasma samples acquired early in gestation. This noninvasive, highly accurate test can be used as a first step in various clinical settings.

▶ Stimulated by the demonstration by oncologists of tumor DNA in the plasma of some of their patients, several perinatal investigators have demonstrated fetal DNA present in maternal plasma during pregnancy.[1-4] Further work has demonstrated that some plasma DNA is contained in intact fetal cells in the maternal circulation, thus opening the door to recombinant DNA techniques in fetal cells obtained without entering the conceptus per se. This is the first large-scale effort in 302 patient samples to assay the accuracy of such determinations on fetal cells obtained in this way.

Gender is determined genetically by polymerase chain reaction using primers for the Y chromosome marker DYS-14. Identification of this sequence means that the gravida bears a male fetus, exempting a small chance of maternal chimerism.[5,6] In a population 47% of which contained male fetuses, sensitivity of male gender identification was 97.2 and specificity 100%. There were 2.5% false-negatives and no false-positive results obtained from pregnancies dating from 7 to 16 weeks' gestational age. These are generally excellent results and provide a firm basis for clinical genetic analysis of fetal cells obtained solely through the maternal circulation.

T. H. Kirschbaum, MD

References

1. 1999 YEAR BOOK OF OBSTETRICS, GYNECOLOGY, AND WOMEN'S HEALTH, pp 193-196.
2. 2000 YEAR BOOK OF OBSTETRICS, GYNECOLOGY, AND WOMEN'S HEALTH, pp 207-208.
3. 2001 YEAR BOOK OF OBSTETRICS, GYNECOLOGY, AND WOMEN'S HEALTH, pp 317-318.
4. 2002 YEAR BOOK OF OBSTETRICS, GYNECOLOGY, AND WOMEN'S HEALTH, pp 219-221.
5. 2000 YEAR BOOK OF OBSTETRICS, GYNECOLOGY, AND WOMEN'S HEALTH, pp 99-100.

6. 2002 YEAR BOOK OF OBSTETRICS, GYNECOLOGY, AND WOMEN'S HEALTH, pp 221-222 and pp 158-159.

Detection of Maternal Deoxyribonucleic Acid in Umbilical Cord Plasma by Using Fluorescent Polymerase Chain Reaction Amplification of Short Tandem Repeat Sequences

Bauer M, Orescovic I, Schoell WM, et al (Karl Franzens Univ of Graz, Austria; Tufts Univ, Boston)

Am J Obstet Gynecol 186:117-120, 2002   9–4

Background.—A transfer of blood cells between the fetal and maternal circulations has been observed despite the physical separation of both systems by villous trophoblast layers of the placenta. The passage of fetal cells into the maternal circulation is a well-known phenomenon; the transmission of intact maternal cells to the fetus was first described more than 30 years ago. Now there is some evidence that fetal cells may persist for decades after birth and may be involved in the pathogenesis of connective tissue disease. Umbilical cord blood is a source of hematopoietic stem cells for transplantation, but there have been concerns about the contamination of umbilical blood by maternal cells, which theoretically could present a risk of graft-versus-host disease. The frequency of maternal DNA contamination in umbilical cord plasma was assessed.

Methods.—The presence of maternal DNA sequences in cord plasma was evaluated in 57 mother/child pairs using fluorescent polymerase chain reac-

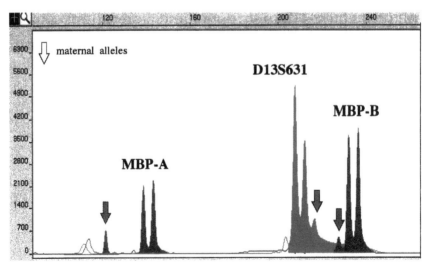

FIGURE.—Electrophoretogram of amplification products from an umbilical plasma sample using 3 short tandem repeat markers (*MBP-A, MBP-B,* and *D13S631*). The *arrows* indicate the maternal specific amplified alleles. (Courtesy of Bauer M, Orescovic I, Schoell WM, et al: Detection of maternal deoxyribonucleic acid in umbilical cord plasma by using fluorescent polymerase chain reaction amplification of short tandem repeat sequences. *Am J Obstet Gynecol* 186:117-120, 2002.)

tion (PCR) amplification of highly polymorphic short tandem repeat DNA markers. The markers included D21S11, D21S1411, D21S1412, D18S386, D18S535, MBP-A, MBP-B, D13S631, and D13S634.

Results.—All 57 pairs were informative for the identification of uniquely maternal alleles in at least 2 of the 9 repeat markers (Figure). Forty-three (75%) of the cord plasma samples were found to have uniquely maternal DNA sequences.

Conclusions.—These findings show that maternal DNA is present in the majority of umbilical cord plasma samples. The technique described in this report might be applicable to the screening of cord blood samples for the presence of contaminating maternal genetic material.

▶ Though maternal cells have been reported in umbilical cord blood before, the finding rests with the recognition of ^{51}Cr for maternal tagged red cells and female cell sex chromosomes found transiently in the blood of male newborns. Further, those reports are nearly 40 years old. This study uses recombinant DNA techniques to explore the question of maternal transfers in cord blood samples of 57 newborns. The basis for maternal identification is DNA fingerprinting,[1] which is based on the characteristics of multiple tandem DNA repeat sequences. Several thousand such DNA sequences exist in the human genome, where they compromise 3% to 6% of all DNA. Within them clusters of 3 to 4 base identical sequences are repeated in the range of 100 to 300 times; the number of repeats is a highly individual characteristic and differs regularly among them. When restriction endonucleases are used to break bonds between specific base pairs, yielding differing parts of a repeat sequence, gel electrophoresis produces patterns of DNA segments which are as unique to an individual as are their tandem repeat sequences. In this case, 9 separate maternal and fetal alleles existing on chromosomes 13, 18, and 21 were employed and PCR carried out using primers which flanked the tandem repeat segments. PCR was then carried out on the amplification products, and the results were deemed informative if at least 2 of the 9 amplified sequences sufficed to show fragments of the unique maternal alleles present in fetal DNA fragments of the tandem repeat sequences obtained from cord blood. In that sense, all maternal-fetal paired samples were informative and maternal DNA was found in 43 of 57 cord blood samples or 75%. One other investigator[2] used similar techniques using 6 tandem repeat sites and material derived from the cellular components of cord blood samples. They found maternal cell derived DNA in only 1.26% of the 79 maternal and fetal pairs.

There is then evidence of both cellular and plasma DNA transfers from mother to fetus during pregnancy, the plasma transfers being much more common. The mechanism of transfer is uncertain, as is its biological significance. The observation does raise the possibility of producing microchimeras in stem cell recipients following stem cell transfusion based on cells isolated from cord blood.[3]

T. H. Kirschbaum, MD

References

1. 1990 YEAR BOOK OF OBSTETRICS, GYNECOLOGY, AND WOMEN'S HEALTH, pp 171-172.
2. Petit T, Gluckman E, Carosella E, et al: A highly sensitive polymerase chain reaction method reveals the ubiquitous presence of maternal cells in human umbilical cord blood. *Exp Hematol* 23:1601-1605, 1995.
3. 2001 YEAR BOOK OF OBSTETRICS, GYNECOLOGY, AND WOMEN'S HEALTH, pp 219-220.

Enrichment, Immunomorphological, and Genetic Characterization of Fetal Cells Circulating in Maternal Blood

Vona G, Béroud C, Benachi A, et al (Unité INSERM 370, Paris; Hôpital Necker-Enfant Malades, Paris)
Am J Pathol 160:51-58, 2002   9–5

Background.—Fetal cells such as epithelial cells circulating in the peripheral blood of pregnant women may be a target for noninvasive genetic analyses. Trophoblastic cells are larger than peipheral blood leukocytes. Circulating trophoblastic cells were enriched with use of the isolation by size of epithelial tumor cells (ISET) method.

Methods.—Thirteen women were studied at 11 to 12 weeks of gestation. All were carrying fetuses at risk of a genetic disorder. Seven fetuses were female, and 6 were male. Peripheral blood cells isolated by ISET were stained with hematoxylin and eosin or by immunohistochemistry. Large epithelial cells were microdissected. Fetal cell identification was obtained by polymerase chain reaction, with short tandem repeats or Y-specific primers.

Findings.—In only 2 mL of blood, 1 to 7 Y-positive cells were identified in all 6 women carrying a male fetus. None of the cells isolated from the women carrying a female fetus tested positive. Six of 11 cells analyzed by short tandem repeat-specific markers showed a fetal profile and 5 showed a maternal profile consistent with Y-specific findings (Fig 2).

Conclusions.—The current approach is effective for enriching circulating fetal cells and proving their fetal origin. The ISET approach permits fluorescence in situ hybridization analyses to be performed and DNA point mutations to be detected in single microdissected cells. These data may have implications for noninvasive prenatal diagnosis of genetic disorders.

▶ These authors demonstrate a method for isolation of fetal cells for genetic analysis from maternal blood based on cell morphology and the large size of trophoblastic epithelial cells which offers simplicity and large yields at a cost of requiring their demonstrable sophistication in single cell dissection, DNA extraction, and PCR. Their method avoids the losses in numbers of cells and cell injury associated with cell sorters in the hands of others. Five-milliliter blood samples for each of 13 gravidas at risk of genetic disease were obtained, and buffered diluted blood was filtered through polycarbamate filters with pore size 8 μm retained cells were stained and 2 fetal cell patterns were seen. Multinucleated syncytiotrophoblast cells were identified, as were larger mononucleated cells, usually but not always cytotrophoblasts. Maternal lymphocytes

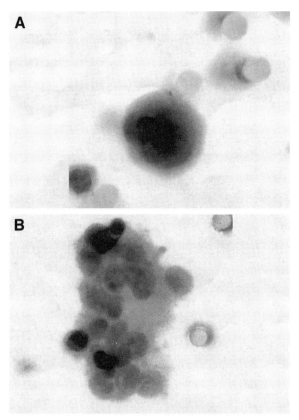

FIGURE 2.—Morphological and immunohistochemical characterization of circulating cells isolated by ISET and proved to be fetal by Y-specific single-cell PCR testing. **A,** Mononucleated cell (diameter, 27.5 μm) with cytotrophoblastic-like morphology lying on a filter pore (round mark in the nucleus). Three empty pores are visible on the top right and a neutrophil on the bottom left of the picture (hematoxylin-eosin staining). **B,** Polynucleated, syncytiotrophoblastic cell (hematoxylin-eosin). (Courtesy of Vona G, Béroud C, Benachi A, et al: Enrichment, immunomorphological, and genetic characterization of fetal cells circulating in maternal blood. *Am J Pathol* 160:51-58, 2002. Permission granted: Copyright American Society for Investigative Pathology.)

and myeloid cells had to be excluded in this group using immunohistochemistry. On average, 5 fetal cells could be obtained from the 5-mL blood samples drawn from pregnant women. Microdissection was used to manipulate single cells, and DNA was isolated for PCR using primers appropriate to DNA fingerprinting for female fetuses and Y chromosomal identification for 4 male fetuses. On average, 5 PCR runs using the Taq polymerase system could be performed on DNA from each sample. Specificity was proven using 20 samples of known male and female DNA. Fluorescent in situ hybridization was carried out using an X-chromosome specific probe and a cell line known to carry a glycine to valine point mutation needed to prove the capacity of the system to discern mutational events in 5 independent trials. All 6 male fetuses and 7 female fetuses were correctly identified by this technique and a wide range of recombinant DNA techniques successfully carried out on single cell DNA aggregates.

This is a further somewhat remarkable step in the pursuit of the goal of noninvasive fetal genetic diagnosis from maternal blood.

T. H. Kirschbaum, MD

Diagnosis of Trisomy 21 in Fetal Nucleated Erythrocytes from Maternal Blood by Use of Short Tandem Repeat Sequences
Samura O, Sohda S, Johnson KL, et al (Tufts Univ, Boston; Univ of Graz, Austria; Womens Health Services, Chestnut Hill, Mass; et al)
Clin Chem 47:1622-1626, 2001   9–6

Background.—Previous researchers have reported the isolation of intact nucleated fetal cells from maternal blood and subsequent prenatal diagnosis of human aneuploidies. This study determined whether aneuploid fetal nucleated erythrocytes (NRBCs) could be identified in maternal blood through the use of fluorescent polymerase chain reaction (PCR) amplification with polymorphic short tandem repeat (STR) markers as an alternative or to complement fluorescent in situ hybridization (FISH) analysis.

Methods and Findings.—Peripheral blood samples from 7 women who had recently undergone pregnancy termination because of fetal trisomy 21 were analyzed. To isolate candidate fetal cells, antibodies to the γ chain of fetal hemoglobin and Hoechst 33342 were flow sorted. In FISH analysis, chromosome-specific probes for X, Y, and 21 were used. Fetal NRBCs were micromanipulated separately and subjected to fluorescent PCR amplification of chromosome 21 STR markers. In 5 of the 7 cases analyzed, fetal NRBCs were aneuploid, evidenced by the presence of triallelic or diallelic peaks of chromosome 21 sequences compared with sequences from the maternal leukocytes.

Conclusion.—Fluorescent PCR amplification of STRs can identify fetal aneuploidy. This method may be useful when hybridization efficiency with FISH analysis is poor. In the near future, combined fetal aneuploidy and single-gene diagnoses using DNA microassays may be possible.

▶ This study of 7 gravidas bearing infants with trisomy 21—3 males and 4 females—explores and supports a technical advance in fetal diagnosis from fetal NRBCs isolated from maternal blood samples. Cells were identified using fluorescent tagged antibody to fetal hemoglobin γ chains and the Hoechst antigen and collected by fluoroscent-driven cell sorting.[1] FISH using differentially colored fluorescent probes specific to chromosomes X, Y, and 21 was performed and the results compared in the same fetal cell with the fluoroscent PCR technique, using 3 STR DNA sequences specific to chromosome 21, each with known primers.

The technique yields confirmation of the FISH data and has greatly enhanced sensitivity appropriate to single cell studies. Further, it would facilitate use of DNA micro-arrays, an important step in high pass-through rate multichannel DNA screening, a certain desirable in clinical genetics. The authors success in demonstrating equivalence to FISH in 5 of 7 cases represents an advance in the progress toward increased accuracy and use of multiple STR segments from recombination hot spots in exploring a wide range of potential gene defects in the future.

T. H. Kirschbaum, MD

Reference

1. DeMaria MA, Zheng YL, Zhen D, et al: Improved fetal nucleated erythrocyte sorting purity using intracellular antifetal hemoglobin and Hoechst 33342. *Cytometry* 25:37, 1996.

Fetal Nucleated Red Blood Cells From CVS Washings: An Aid to Development of First Trimester Non-Invasive Prenatal Diagnosis
Voullaire L, Ioannou P, Nouri S, et al (Royal Children's Hosp, Parkville, Victoria, Australia)
Prenat Diagn 21:827-834, 2001   9–7

Background.—Fetal nucleated red blood cells (n-rbc) are a potential source of fetal cells for noninvasive prenatal diagnosis. However, their low incidence has made the development of reliable techniques for their isolation difficult. This study describes a technique for the collection of fetal n-rbc from chorionic villous sampling washings that allows a recovery rate of more than 70% for both ϵ- and γ-globin–producing n-rbc when spiked into normal adult female blood at 1 or 10 cells/mL.

Methods.—Chorionic villous sampling washings were obtained from women of 10 to 13 weeks' gestation who previously had a chorionic villous sampling taken for prenatal diagnosis. The sampling was collected into 10 to 15 mL of phosphate-buffered saline with the addition of antibiotics. The washings were coded and only the gestational age was obtained. Blood samples were also obtained from nonpregnant female volunteers. After immunocytochemical staining, the identification of male fetal n-rbc was carried out using fluorescent in situ hybridization and a probe to the Y long arm heterochromatic region (PtRS14). The washings were then used to model first trimester noninvasive prenatal diagnosis.

Results.—There was a rapid decline in the ratio of ϵ- to γ-globin–producing cells from 10 to 13 weeks, along with a decline in the ratio of nucleated to nonnucleated rbc. The vast majority of cells containing ϵ- or γ-globin are anucleate by 13 weeks. The fetal n-rbc were highly variable in size and density and sedimented over a wide density range, and a high proportion of fetal n-rbc (more than 80%) were at a density overlapping with that of maternal rbc. The enrichment procedure devised as part of this study used Orskoff lysis to differentially lyse the maternal cells. After this enrichment procedure, the maternal cells were subjected to density centrifugation and separation with magnetic beads, which allowed recovery of 70% of fetal cells when added at approximately 10 fetal cells/mL maternal blood. The addition of 1 fetal cell/mL maternal blood to a total volume of

10 mL resulted in more variable recovery, but the recovery remained at about 70% and in all cases at least 1 fetal cell was recovered.

Conclusions.—The protocol described here should allow for effective first trimester noninvasive prenatal diagnosis.

▶ This study provides another option for obtaining fetal cells for prenatal diagnosis without invading the amniotic cavity. When chorion villous samples are suspended in phosphate-buffered saline to allow dissection, the saline washings contain fetal red cells, both nucleated and nonnucleated, resulting from loss of integrity of umbilical capillaries. Because anucleate cells contain little or no DNA, it is important to use biopsies obtained as close to the end of the first trimester as possible since the relative number of nonnucleated fetal red cells diminishes 10-fold from 10 to 13 weeks' gestation. Fetal cells may be identified by using antibody to γ-globin sequences and collecting them visually, noting staining characteristics, or by labeling the anti-γ chain antibodies to enable use of a cell sorter. Fluorescent in situ hybridization can be used to identify male fetal cells using oligonucleotide probes to sequences on the Y chromosome. The authors have devised a system in which mixed adult human blood, mixed with nucleated fetal red cells, is differentially lysed by using an aqueous solution of ammonium chloride and bicarbonate that, because of the low carbonic anhydrase content of fetal red cells, lyses them more slowly than it does adult red cells. What results is a great deal of time saving in processing. Intact fetal cells may then be separated from the adult ghost red cells by density gradient centrifugation. Using this approach, the authors demonstrate 70% efficiency in recovering fetal red cells added to known amounts of adult red cells. This approach allows access to fetal nucleated cells without cordocentesis or fetal liver biopsy. It adds to maternal plasma and amniotic fluid soluble DNA as well as maternal serum as potential sources.[1,2] However, the cost is that much less abundant fetal DNA material is available for analysis from chorion villous biopsy compared with amniotic fluid in which fetal DNA concentrations may be as much as 100 to 200 times higher than in the maternal plasma.

T. H. Kirschbaum, MD

References

1. 1999 Year Book of Obstetrics, Gynecology, and Women's Health, pp 191-193.
2. 2000 Year Book of Obstetrics, Gynecology, and Women's Health, pp 211-212.

Differential DNA Methylation Between Fetus and Mother as a Strategy for Detecting Fetal DNA in Maternal Plasma
Poon LLM, Leung TN, Lau TK, et al (Chinese Univ, Hong Kong)
Clin Chem 48:35-41, 2002   9–8

Background.—There has been much interest recently in the biology and diagnostic applications of circulating nucleic acids. The discovery that fetal DNA circulates in maternal plasma has opened new possibilities for nonin-

A

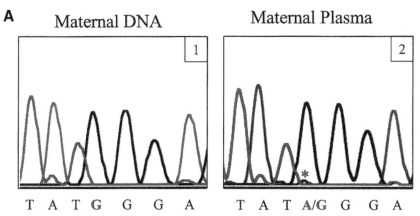

FIGURE 4A.—Detection of unmethylated (maternally inherited) fetal DNA in maternal plasma. Unmethylated DNA sequences were detected in maternal buffy coat (**panel 1**) and a third trimester maternal sample (**panel 2**) with direct sequencing. The presence of unmethylated fetal DNA in maternal plasma is indicated by *asterisk*. (Courtesy of Poon LLM, Leung TN, Lau TK, et al: Differential DNA methylation between fetus and mother as a strategy for detecting fetal DNA in maternal plasma. *Clin Chem* 48:35-41. Copyright 2002, The American Association for Clinical Chemistry [1-800-892-1400].)

vasive prenatal diagnosis. The noninvasive prenatal detection of several conditions has been achieved, including fetal rhesus D status, myotonic dystrophy, achondroplasia, and some chromosomal translocations. However, in these situations, only genes or mutations inherited from the father have been detected, since they are genetically distinguishable from the mother. The reason for this limitation is that fetal DNA in maternal plasma and serum is present in an excess background of maternal DNA. The possibility of using epigenetic markers for the specific detection of fetal DNA in maternal plasma was investigated.

Methods.—A differentially methylated region in the human *IGF2-H19* locus and a single-nucleotide polymorphism in this region were selected for study. The single-nucleotide polymorphism was typed by direct sequencing of polymerase chain reaction (PCR) products, and the methylation status of this region was determined by bisulfite conversion and methylation-specific PCR. Direct sequencing and a primer-extension assay were used to detect differentially methylated fetal alleles. A total of 16 women in the second and third trimesters of pregnancy who were heterozygous for the single-nucleotide polymorphism were recruited.

Results.—In 11 of the 16 women, paternally inherited methylated fetal alleles were different from the methylated alleles of the respective mothers. Direct sequencing detected paternally inherited methylated fetal DNA in 6 of 11 women (55%). In 8 of the 16 heterozygous women, the fetuses were found to have an unmethylated maternally inherited allele that was different from the unmethylated allele of the mother (Fig 4A). A primer-extension assay detected fetal-derived maternally inherited alleles in maternal plasma in 4 (50%) of 8 cases.

Conclusions.—These study findings demonstrated the first use of fetal epigenetic markers in noninvasive prenatal analysis and could have implications for the evaluation of other forms of chimerism.

▶ This proof of concept study, though admittedly not easy to understand, offers an important new step in the process of fetal DNA analysis obtainable from maternal blood sampled during pregnancy.[1,2] The basic problem is that because of the vast surplus of maternal plasma DNA over fetal DNA in maternal blood during pregnancy, fetal DNA bearing a mutant gene polymorphism cannot be identified if the mother shares the same polymorphism. Nor can an allele inherited by the fetus from the mother be identified unquestionably. The problem has usually been handled by searching for polymorphisms coexisting with Y-chromosome markers in pregnancies bearing male fetuses. This leaves proof of maternal origin of gene mutations expressed in fetal cells in maternal blood unattainable.

This work relies on the ability of phenotype to be determined in part by nongenetic or epigenetic phenomena. The most important of these appears to be methylation, a chemical process that plays a role in gene activation and inactivation as well as in gender imprinting in which expression of a fetal gene inherited from paternal DNA differs from that inherited from the mother.[3,4] The method depends on a marker gene segment (*IGF2-H19*) that is methylated when paternally derived (PAT) and unmethylated when maternally derived (MA). The gene contains an adenine/guanine polymorphism that can be detected by gene sequencing. With the TaqMan procedure,[5] PCR is carried out on maternal serum or plasma containing maternal and fetal DNA with primers designed to span the A to G polymorphism in *IGF2-H19*. The products are treated with bisulfate, which changes unmethylated maternally derived cytosine to uracil, a base identifiable by gene sequencing. Those products are treated with methylation-specific PCR (MSP) that uses 2 sets of primers, which in turn yield products of differing nucleotide lengths identifiable on gel electrophoresis. This enables location of fetal DNA contained in maternal plasma consisting of DNA for which the mother is heterozygous for a suspect gene. The identification is carried out by the combination of demonstration of the A to C polymorphism and the lack of methylation present in the marker gene *IGF2-H19*. Not only is the approach important in improving the identification of maternally inherited fetal DNA, but also in dealing with the analysis of such gender-imprinted inheritance as occurs in the Prater Willi and Ascherman syndromes. It is a very major contribution to this field.

T. H. Kirschbaum, MD

References

1. 2001 YEAR BOOK OF OBSTETRICS, GYNECOLOGY, AND WOMEN'S HEALTH, pp 217-219.
2. 2002 YEAR BOOK OF OBSTETRICS, GYNECOLOGY, AND WOMEN'S HEALTH, pp 218-220.
3. 1999 YEAR BOOK OF OBSTETRICS, GYNECOLOGY, AND WOMEN'S HEALTH, pp 199-200.
4. 1998 YEAR BOOK OF OBSTETRICS, GYNECOLOGY, AND WOMEN'S HEALTH, pp 205-207.
5. 1999 YEAR BOOK OF OBSTETRICS, GYNECOLOGY, AND WOMEN'S HEALTH, pp 193-196.

The Risk of Major Birth Defects After Intracytoplasmic Sperm Injection and In Vitro Fertilization

Hansen M, Kurinczuk JJ, Bower C, et al (Univ of Western Australia, Perth; Health Dept of Western Australia, Perth; Western Australian Birth Defects Registry, Perth; et al)
N Engl J Med 346:725-730, 2002   9–9

Introduction.—Most trials have not reported an increased risk of major birth defects in children conceived with either intracytoplasmic sperm injection or standard in vitro fertilization. Most of this research has been compromised by methodologic problems. The prevalence of major birth defects among infants conceived by fertility procedures was compared with that of a random sample of naturally conceived infants by using the same classification system for all birth defects.

Methods.—Data were obtained from 3 registries in Western Australia concerning births, births after assisted conception, and major birth defects in infants born between 1993 and 1997. The prevalence of major birth defects diagnosed by 1 year of age was evaluated in infants conceived naturally or with the use of intracytoplasmic sperm injection or in vitro fertilization.

Results.—Twenty-six of 301 infants conceived with intracytoplasmic sperm injection (8.6%) and 75 of 837 infants conceived with in vitro fertilization (9.0%) had a major birth defect diagnosed by 1 year of age versus 168 of the 4000 naturally conceived infants (4.2%; $P < .001$) for the comparison between either type of technology and natural conception (Fig 1). Compared with that for natural conception, the odds ratios for a major birth defect by the age of 1 year were 2.0 (95% CI, 1.3-3.2) for intracytoplasmic sperm injection and 2.0 (95% CI, 1.5-2.9) for in vitro fertilization, after adjusting for maternal age and parity, infant gender, and correlation between siblings. Infants conceived with either of the assisted reproductive technologies were more likely than naturally conceived infants to experience multiple

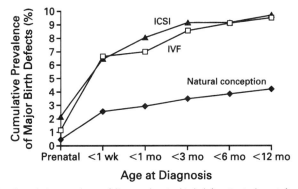

FIGURE 1.—Cumulative prevalence of diagnosed major birth defects in singleton infants, according to age at diagnosis. *Abbreviations*: *ICSI*, Intracytoplasmic sperm injection; *IVF*, in vitro fertilization. (Reprinted by permission of *The New England Journal of Medicine*, courtesy of Hansen M, Kurinczuk JJ, Bower C, et al: The risk of major birth defects after intracytoplasmic sperm injection and in vitro fertilization. *N Engl J Med* 346:725-730, 2002. Copyright 2002, Massachusetts Medical Society. All rights reserved.)

TABLE 2.—Mode of Delivery and Characteristics of Infants Conceived With Intracytoplasmic Sperm Injection, With In Vitro Fertilization, or Naturally*

	All Infants					Singletons Only				
Variable	ICSI (n=301)	P Value	IVF (n=837)	P Value	Natural Conception (n=4000)	ICSI (n=186)	P Value	IVF (n=527)	P Value	Natural Conception (n=3906)
Delivered by cesarean section—no. (%)	95 (32)	<0.001	365 (44)	<0.001	816 (20)	48 (26)	0.05	183 (35)	<0.001	776 (20)
Male sex—no. (%)	165 (55)		454 (54)	<0.001	2048 (51)	102 (55)		286 (54)		2000 (51)
Stillborn—no. (%)	2 (1)		17 (2)		26 (1)	0		6 (1)		25 (1)
Birth weight—g	2847±799	0.02	2806±844	0.005	3345±592	3271±552	0.02	3182±686	<0.001	3368±571
Preterm delivery (<37 wk)—no. (%)	93 (31)	<0.001	265 (32)	<0.001	273 (7)	16 (9)		73 (14)	0.001	225 (6)
Multiple birth—no. (%)	115 (38)	<0.001	310 (37)	<0.001	94 (2)	—		—		—
Low birth weight—no. (%)										
<1500 g	18 (6)	<0.001	65 (8)	<0.001	51 (1)	2 (1)	<0.001	19 (4)	<0.001	41 (1)
<2500 g	75 (25)	<0.001	188 (22)	<0.001	196 (5)	12 (6)	0.002	38 (7)	0.002	163 (4)
Gestational age—wk	37.0±3.3	0.004	36.7±3.8	0.002	39.0±2.1	38.6±2.2	0.03	38.0±3.0	0.03	39.1±2.0

*Plus-minus values are means ±SD. P values are for the comparisons with the natural-conception group and are not significant if not shown.

Abbreviations: ICSI, Intracytoplasmic sperm injection; IVF, in vitro fertilization.

(Reprinted by permission of The New England Journal of Medicine, courtesy of Hansen M, Kurinczuk JJ, Bower C, et al: The risk of major birth defects after intracytoplasmic sperm injection and in vitro fertilization. N Engl J Med 346:725-730, 2002. Copyright 2002, Massachusetts Medical Society. All rights reserved.)

major defects and to have chromosomal and musculoskeletal defects. They were also more likely to be delivered by cesarean section, to have low birth weight, and to be born before term (Table 2).

Conclusion.—Infants conceived by intracytoplasmic sperm injection or in vitro fertilization are at twice the risk of having a major birth defect by 1 year of age compared with naturally conceived infants.

▶ In vitro fertilization (IVF) in Western Australia, a region recognized for expertise and data management in clinical research, is carried out in 3 private clinics. A 1991 legislative enactment mandated data reporting of all instances of assisted reproductive technology (ART) to the Reproductive Technology Registry, and this is a report based on 1138 women participants and the 4141 cycles of embryo transfer they experienced since April 1993. Intracytoplasmic sperm injection, introduced in 1992, was a special concern, and those 301 cases were reported separately, whereas classic IVF, including both cervical and intratubal transfers, were aggregated. Probabilistic-based software was used to construct a group of 4000 women naturally conceiving for comparisons. Data organization and numbers as well as the definition of birth defects described in the *International Classification of Diseases, Ninth Revision (ICD-9)* were used to respond to critiques of earlier studies on this topic. Birth defect information is obtained from the Australian Birth Registry, and prevalences were calculated based on the reported presence at 1 year of age, with singlet pregnancies studied separate from the rest. Women using ART were on average older, more often married, white urban dwellers and had the high rates of cesarean section, low birth weight, and preterm deliveries commonly seen in such populations. As shown in Figure 1, the prevalence of birth defects at 1 year was 8.6% for sperm injection and 9.0% for classic IVF, compared with 4.2% for normal conceptions. Most birth defects were diagnosed by 1 month of age, with karyotypic abnormalities, and cardiovascular, urologic, and musculoskeletal defects predominating. The exclusion of multiple births and data corrections for differences in maternal age, parity, and infant gender did not alter the results, nor did inclusion of data from pregnancies terminated once malformation was noted. Although maternal age and parity or multiple pregnancy differences did not appear to explain the differences noted, it seems likely that the presence of underlying maternal/paternal defects, which help determine infertility and preclude normal pregnancy development, as well as environmental artificialities of ART, likely each play a role.

As the dominant approach to studying the early reproductive process changes from descriptive anatomy to molecular biology, the vast number of important contributing elements, the complexity of their timing and interaction, the evidence of evanescent intervals when simultaneous interactions must occur, and the largely unknown staggeringly complex methods needed for appropriate control of gene expression seem almost unimaginable. The changes in expression of surface adhesion molecules in trophoblast cells invading decidua and implantation are a nice example.[1-3] The progressive trophoblast gene expression with increased depth of its invasion from simple integrins in the decidua to vascular cadherins which convey connective tissue like properties need for deeper blood vessel invasion and incorporation into their trophoblast and collagen receptors as anchoring trophoblastic columns form are truly extraordinary. Further, the repertoire of maternal leukocytes with properties seemingly designed both for allograft immune tolerance and selective and focal remodeling of connective tissue, cellular and extracellular decidual matrices necessary to allow for the expansion and revision of the relationships and placentation are equally impressive (see Abstract 1–7). Our ability to describe human embryonic development in molecular genetic terms is still rudimentary, but animal experimentation suggests it is amazingly complex even for simple systems.[4] For many of these as yet largely undefined elements, there is a chance for DNA nucleotide deletions, replacements, inversions, and translations that might impede normal fertility, fetal development, or both. Clearly, ART operates with wonderful but crude technology in an enormous sea of as yet unknown cell biology.

T. H. Kirschbaum, MD

References

1. 1994 YEAR BOOK OF OBSTETRICS, GYNECOLOGY, AND WOMEN'S HEALTH, pp 59-60.
2. 1998 YEAR BOOK OF OBSTETRICS, GYNECOLOGY, AND WOMEN'S HEALTH, pp 18-21.
3. 1998 YEAR BOOK OF OBSTETRICS, GYNECOLOGY, AND WOMEN'S HEALTH, pp 50-51.
4. Davidson EH, Rast JP, Olivari P, et al: A genomic regulatory network for development. *Science* 295:1669, 2002.

Low and Very Low Birth Weight in Infants Conceived With Use of Assisted Reproductive Technology
Schieve LA, Meikle SF, Ferre C, et al (Ctrs for Disease Control and Prevention, Atlanta, Ga)
N Engl J Med 346:731-737, 2002   9–10

Background.—One important contributor to the rate of low birth weight in the United States is the use of assisted reproductive technology, because it is associated with a higher rate of multiple births, which is in turn associated with low birth weight. The use of assisted reproduction accounted for more than 40% of triplets born in the United States by 1997. Studies have suggested that there is a higher rate of low birth weight among singleton infants conceived with assisted reproductive technology than among naturally conceived singleton infants or among all infants in the general population. However, it is unclear whether infants conceived with the use of assisted reproductive technology have a higher risk of low birth weight than infants who are conceived spontaneously.

Methods.—Population-based data were used to compare the rates of low birth weight ($\leq$2500 g) and very low birth weight (<1500 g) among infants who were conceived with assisted reproductive technology, with the rates in the general population.

Results.—A total of 42,463 infants born in 1996 and 1997 and conceived with assisted reproductive technology were compared with 3,389,098 infants born in the United States in 1997. Among singleton infants born at 37

TABLE 3.—Observed and Expected Cases of Low Birth Weight and Very Low Birth Weight Among Singleton Infants Conceived With Assisted Reproductive Technology in 1996 and 1997*

Variable	Total No.	No. of Cases Observed	No. of Cases Expected†	Standardized Risk Ratio (95% CI)
Low birth weight				
All infants	18,398	2423	1339.4	1.8 (1.7-1.9)
Pregnancies with one fetal heart	16,730	2104	1197.1	1.8 (1.7-1.8)
Use of donor oocytes, no diagnosis of male-factor infertility	1,397	190	119.3	1.6 (1.4-1.8)
Diagnosis of male-factor infertility	2,759	329	195.9	1.7 (1.5-1.9)
Use of gestational carrier	180	16	13.3	1.2 (0.6-1.8)
Very low birth weight				
All infants	18,398	480	263.4	1.8 (1.7-2.0)
Pregnancies with one fetal heart	16,730	408	239.2	1.7 (1.5-1.9)
Use of donor oocytes, no diagnosis of male-factor infertility	1,397	49	23.5	2.1 (1.5-2.7)
Diagnosis of male-factor infertility	2,759	78	38.5	2.0 (1.6-2.5)
Use of gestational carrier	180	0	2.6	—

*Ten infants with missing data on parity were not included in these analyses.

†The number of expected cases was calculated by applying the rates of low birth weight from the 1997 US birth-certificate data to the population of infants conceived with assisted reproductive technology. The values were adjusted to account for differences in the distributions of age (in the following categories: 20 to 29 years, 30 to 34 years, 35 to 39 years, 40 to 44 years, and ≥45 years) and parity (0, 1, or ≥2) between the 2 populations.

(Reprinted by permission of *The New England Journal of Medicine*, courtesy of Schieve LA, Meikle SF, Ferre C, et al: Low and very low birth weight in infants conceived with use of assisted reproductive technology. *N Engl J Med* 346:731-737, 2002. Copyright 2002, Massachusetts Medical Society. All rights reserved.)

weeks' gestation or later, the risk of low birth weight was 2.6 times higher among infants conceived with assisted reproductive technology than among the general population (Table 3). Although the use of assisted reproductive technology was associated with an increased rate of multiple gestations, it was not associated with an additional increase in the risk of low birth weight in multiple births. Among twin births, the ratio of the rate of low birth weight after the use of assisted reproductive technology to the rate in the general population was 1.0. In 1997, infants conceived with assisted reproductive technology accounted for 0.6% of all infants born to mothers aged 20 years or older, but they accounted for 3.5% of low birth weight and 4.3% of very low birth weight infants.

Conclusions.—A disproportionate number of low birth weight and very low birth weight infants in the United States are attributed to the use of assisted reproductive technology. This is caused in part by the absolute increases in multiple gestations, and in part by the higher rates of low birth weight among singleton infants born to women who make use of this technology.

► Each year, the Society for Assisted Reproductive Technology collects data on the use of assisted reproductive technology (ART) throughout the country and reports it to the Centers for Disease Control and Prevention. This is a report and analysis for data from 1996 to 1997 inclusive for women aged 20 to 60 years. Of 136,972 procedures, 23% resulted in live births. The complex data matrices include demographics, medical history, and diagnostic procedures and are stratified with respect to ART technology (fresh or frozen embryos, donor or autologous ova, surrogate carriers, and intracytoplasmic sperm injection or not). Birth order in multiple pregnancies are provided, and fetal deaths (0.4%) were excluded. Although prevalence rates were available from birth certificate data reported for approximately 3,400,000 births in 1997, the principal intent here is to explore the relative merits with various options in ART.

Clearly, the findings of this study are somewhat different than those presented in the previous Australian study (Abstract 9–9). The incidence of multiple births in this study was 43% versus 37% in the latter study, and low birth weight occurred in 13.2% of singlets in this study versus 9.9% in the latter. The incidence of low birth weight in single pregnancies was larger than in the general population, unexplainable by the effects of maternal age, parity, and gestational age, just as was the case in the Australian series. This points to the impact of environmental deterrents in in vitro fertilization, such as ovum aging, endometrial timing, asynchronisms, abnormalities attributable to culture media, artificial ovulation, and physical trauma to the conceptus during the procedures. The incidence of both low birth weight and preterm birth was not increased in ART with surrogate carriers, suggesting maternal constitutional variables among infertile women are important to successful pregnancy. Similarly, the increase in low birth weight is not seen in twin pregnancies carried to term. By using the 1997 data with an overall incidence of low birth weight of 0.6%, ART accounted for 3.5% of all low birth weight infants and 4.3% of very low birth weight infants. For obstetricians not performing ART, the principal contribution here is the evidence that both maternal variables and those related to the procedure are independently and apparently separately reflected in growth impairment in children conceived in that way.

T. H. Kirschbaum, MD

Birth of a Healthy Infant After Preimplantation Confirmation of Euploidy by Comparative Genomic Hybridization
Wilton L, Williamson R, McBain J, et al (Melbourne IVF, East Melbourne, Australia; Royal Children's Hosp, Parkville, Victoria, Australia)
N Engl J Med 345:1537-1541, 2001   9–11

Introduction.—Even in experienced centers, the implantation rate during in vitro fertilization is 15% to 20%. Comparative genomic hybridization is a molecular cytogenic technique that can be used with single cells in interphase to permit simultaneous enumeration of every chromosome (Fig 1). Reported is the birth of a healthy infant to a woman with a history of implantation failure after the use of comparative genomic hybridization to ascertain that the karyotype of a single embryo was normal.

Case Report.—Woman, 38, had a 7-year history of unexplained primary infertility. She underwent a cycle of ovarian stimulation, oocyte collection, in vitro fertilization, and embryo transfer with cryopreservation of excess embryos. Eight embryos were transferred in 4 separate procedures with no resultant pregnancy. A second transfer

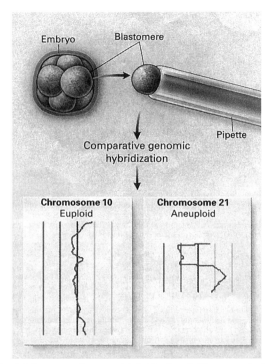

FIGURE 1.—Analysis by comparative genomic hybridization of a blastomere obtained by biopsy of a 6- to 8-cell embryo. Comparative genomic hybridization simultaneously evaluates all chromosomes from a single cell for aneuploidy. Selected results from chromosome 10, which is euploid, and chromosome 21, which is aneuploid, are shown in the *boxes.* See figure 2 of Wilton L, Williamson R, McBain J, et al: Birth of a healthy infant after preimplantation confirmation of euploidy by comparative genomic hybridization. *N Engl J Med* 345:1537-1541, 2001 for an explanation of the chromosomal diagram. (Reprinted by permission of *The New England Journal of Medicine*, courtesy of Elias S: Preimplantation genetic diagnosis by comparative genomic hybridization. *N Engl J Med* 345:1569-1571, 2001. Copyright 2001, Massachusetts Medical Society. All rights reserved.)

of 2 embryos during a second cycle also resulted in no pregnancy. During a third cycle, comparative genomic hybridization was used to obtain a complete embryonic karyotype before transfer of the embryo through in vitro fertilization. The transfer of a single embryo identified as normal with the use of this approach resulted in the birth of a normal, full-term infant.

Conclusion.—The use of comparative genomic hybridization to obtain a complete karyotype of all chromosomes can make it possible to detect karyotypically normal embryos with greater certainty and may be useful in increasing the number of live births per embryo transfer.

▶ Although this report adds nothing conceptionally to the use of preimplantation diagnosis in in vitro fertilization (IVF), it introduces a new analytic technique that offers to improve implantation efficiency through recognition of abnormalities in chromosome number and mosaicism previously missed in conventional fluorescent in situ hybridization (FISH) of preimplantation blastomeres. Successful implantation rates for IVF embryos approximates 15% to 20%, and FISH done conventionally with fluor-labeled oligonucleotides for chromosomes 13, 16, 18, 21, 22, X, and Y yields abnormalities in chromosome number in cultured embryos at a rate of 50% to 70%. Most of these fail normal development, fail to implant, or both. This technique uses full genome polymerase chain reaction amplification by using a large number of random primers. The resulting test DNA is hybridized to oligonucleotides conjugated to a fluor, in this case green. By using the same procedure on lymphocyte DNA from a normal male, a red fluorescent marker is hybridized to provide a normal reference. Both test and reference DNA were simultaneously hybridized to a metaphase spread of normal male chromosomes, and the relative intensity of red and green colors was used to detect aneuploidies. In some cases, monosomies of chromosomes 4, 8, 9, trisomic chromosomes 15, 16, and 6P were found, all undetected with conventional FISH done on amniocentesis or CVS material in the early second trimester. Because the procedure requires 5 days, prospective transplant embryos must be frozen and thawed after the completion of the analysis before attempting embryo transplantation. This exciting new technique offers the prospect of improving the detection of aneuploidy and mosaicism preimplantation, thereby improving the rate of successful embryo transfer.

T. H. Kirschbaum, MD

Neuronal Target Genes of the Neuron-restrictive Silencer Factor in Neurospheres Derived From Fetuses With Down's Syndrome: A Gene Expression Study
Bahn S, Mimmack M, Ryan M, et al (Babraham Inst, Cambridge, England; Genome Campus Hinxton, Cambridge, England; Univ of Cambridge, England; et al)
Lancet 359:310-315, 2002   9–12

Background.—Identifying genes and characterizing their function are important in increasing understanding of the complex pathophysiologic abnormalities in Down's syndrome. Gene expression abnormalities were studied in human neuronal stem cells and progenitor cells from Down's syndrome and non-Down's syndrome postmortem human fetal tissue.

Methods.—Postmortem fetal tissue 8 to 18 weeks after conception was analyzed. Indexing-based differential display polymerase chain reaction (PCR) was performed on neuronal precursor cells derived from the cortex of a fetus with Down's syndrome. Findings were compared with those of 2 control samples. Results were then validated using real-time quantitative PCR on neurosphere preparations from 3 independent fetuses with Down's syndrome features and 5 unaffected fetuses.

Findings.—Differential display PCR analysis demonstrated that SCG10, a neuron-specific growth-associated protein regulated by the neuron-restrictive silencer factor REST, was barely detectable in the Down's samples

(Fig 1). Real-time PCR validated this finding (Fig 2). Other genes regulated by the REST transcription factor were repressed selectively, whereas non-REST-regulated genes with similar characteristics were not affected. Changes in the expression of several key developmental genes in Down's syndrome stem-cell and progenitor-cell pool were associated with notable changes in neuron morphology after differentiation.

Conclusions.—Dysregulation of the REST transcription factor may be associated with some of the neurologic deficits in Down's syndrome. Experimental REST downregulation appears to trigger apoptosis, which may account for the striking, selective loss of neurons in differentiated Down's syndrome cell preparations.

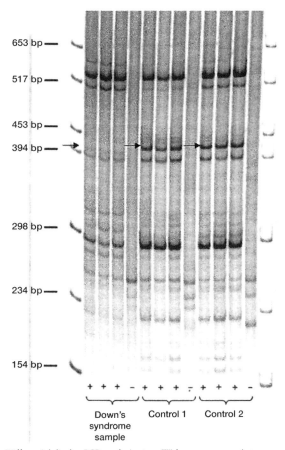

FIGURE 1.—Differential display PCR analysis. + = With reverse transcriptase; − = without reverse transcriptase. *Arrows* show the expected position of SCG10. (Courtesy of Bahn S, Mimmack M, Ryan M, et al: Neuronal target genes of the neuron-restrictive silencer factor in neurospheres derived from fetuses with Down's syndrome: A gene expression study. *Lancet* 359:310-315, 2002. Reprinted with permission from Elsevier Science.)

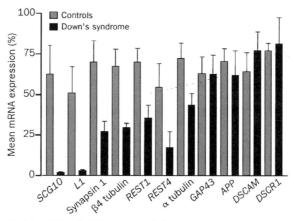

FIGURE 2.—Real-time PCR with SYBR green. α-tubulin gene, *GAP43, AOO, DSCAM,* and *DSCR1* are not regulated by REST. mRNA expression levels are nromalized against GAPDH. Data represent absolute RNA levels of every gene. *Bars* = Mean; *lines* = SE. (Courtesy of Bahn S, Mimmack M, Ryan M, et al: Neuronal target genes of the neuron-restrictive silencer factor in neurospheres derived from fetuses with Down's syndrome: A gene expression study. *Lancet* 359:310-315, 2002. Reprinted with permission from Elsevier Science.)

▶ The cerebral cortex in individuals with Down syndrome shows defective cortical lamination, decreased neuronal density, malformed dendrites, and abnormal synapses. Further, the histopathology shows progression over 3 to 4 decades of life to something closely resembling Alzheimer's disease. This remarkable example of modern molecular biology sheds considerable light on the genetic mechanisms of these changes, long a puzzle. The authors make use of neurospheres, clusters of pluripotent neural precursor cells, capable of extended in vitro propagation, whose differentiation is limited to neurons and glial cells. Neurospheres are free of epithelial and hematogenous precursors, have the potential for organ repair, and contain the genetic changes of Down syndrome. Here they are grown from cultures of cerebral cortex from a fetus with Down syndrome and postmortem normal control fetuses. Neurospheres are grown with the assistance of growth factors, RNA extracted and DNA removed with DNA-ase. Using ^{33}P label, molecular indexing was done using a complex system of adaptors which allowed differential displays of cDNAs in gel electrophoresis following PCR amplification and quantitation of mRNA using the Taq DNA system.[1] A band present in normals but absent in the Down's specimens was isolated, sequenced, and found in the database for the Cambridge human genome mapping project to represent gene SCG 10 (Fig 1), which facilitates a series of other genes important to the normal differentiation, plasticity, and synaptic development of neurons. Real time PCR demonstrated near total absence of nerve adhesive molecules and striking downregulation of synapsin and β-4 tubulin in the presence of the mutant gene form. The specificity of downregulation of SCG10 was confirmed by demonstrating normal expression of similar genes not regulated by the repressor element silencing transcript (REST) and of a series of cellular expression factors located on chromosome 21. Finally, neurosphere culture from Down syndrome showed reduction of neurone numbers, a 57% reduction of neurite links, and excessive side branching and disordered cell body shape compared to normals.

This study needs to be confirmed by measurements of protein corresponding to the mRNAs studied here. It does raise the possibility that gene manipulation or drug therapy might alter the neuropathology related to the expression of the REST mutation in Down syndrome which these workers demonstrate.

T. H. Kirschbaum, MD

Reference

1. 1999 YEAR BOOK OF OBSTETRICS, GYNECOLOGY, AND WOMEN'S HEALTH, pp 193-196.

The Impact of Prenatal Alcohol Exposure on Frontal Cortex Development in Utero
Wass TS, Persutte WH, Hobbins JC (Univ of Denver; Univ of Colorado, Denver)
Am J Obstet Gynecol 185:737-742, 2001   9–13

Objective.—Whether prenatal alcohol exposure was associated with a reduction in the frontal cortex was examined.

Study Design.—Pregnant women (n = 167) received multiple ultrasonographic assessments. During the assessment, brain structures were visualized and measured, including the distance from the posterior margin of the cavum to the calvarium, the distance from the posterior margin of the thalamus to the calvarium, the transcerebellar diameter, and the biparietal diameter.

Results.—Regression analyses and odds ratios demonstrated that alcohol exposure was associated with a reduction in the frontal cortex, but not other brain structures. Strikingly, the percent of fetuses with a frontal cortex below the 10th percentile increased from 4% for nonexposed fetuses to 23% for heavily exposed fetuses (Table 7).

TABLE 7.—Descriptive Statistics for the Percent of Cases With FL
Below 25th or 10th Percentiles

Critieria	Alcohol Group	Cases Below Criteria (%)	Odds Ratio*	χ^2
25th Percentile	FL_{25}			$\chi^2(2, n = 143) = 7.52, P < .03$
	Abstainer/low	19.77		
	Moderate	22.58	1.18	
	Heavy	46.15	3.48	
10th Percentile	FL_{10}			$\chi^2(2, n = 143) = 8.11, P < .02$
	Abstainer/low	4.65		
	Moderate	12.90	3.04	
	Heavy	23.08	6.15	

* Odds ratios were calculated by comparing the moderate and heavy exposure groups individually to the abstainer/low group.
Abbreviation: FL, Frontal lobe.
(Courtesy of Wass TR, Persutte WH, Hobbins JC: The impact of prenatal alcohol exposure on frontal cortex development in utero. *Am J Obstet Gynecol* 185:737-742, 2001.)

Conclusion.—There was a relationship between frontal brain size and maternal alcohol consumption, suggesting that ultrasonography may be a sensitive tool for detecting alcohol-induced changes in the fetal brain.

▶ This study provides strong direct evidence that ethanol is a teratogen to the human fetal brain if one accepts delayed development of the frontal lobes as sufficient evidence. In 155 gravidas selected from prenatal care facilities with or without a history of alcohol use in pregnancy, together with participants in rural and outpatient substance abuse facilities, alcohol use was estimated by interview and converted to ounces of absolute alcohol consumed per day. Alcohol use was categorized as absent to low if women reported consuming less than 1 ounce per day, moderate if women reported consuming 2 to 3 ounces per day, and heavy if women reported consuming more than 3 ounces per day; the latter amount represents more than 6 drinks per day. Particular attention was paid to intake estimates during the first 4 weeks of pregnancy because these were strongly predictive of ethanol use throughout pregnancy and into the puerperium. Fetal cerebral US measurements were done as often as 6 times through the course of pregnancy, and, of the 5 measurements taken, including head circumference, only those reflecting frontal lobe size proved to be useful outcome measurements. Significant correlations between ethanol and cigarette, marijuana, and cocaine use were evident. Therefore, stepwise regression analysis was used to prove impaired frontal lobe dimensions were related predominantly to ethanol use; about 75% of variance in that measurement was attributable to alcohol. When the 10th and 25th percentiles from derived frequency distributions of fetal lobe size were used, both moderate and heavy drinkers showed risk ratios significantly greater than 1.

What is unresolved here is whether this level of decreased development of the frontal lobes is sufficient to account for functional brain impairment noted in, for instance, the fetal alcohol syndrome. Certainly, this evidence is strong justification for the interdiction on ethanol use during pregnancy.

T. H. Kirschbaum, MD

10 Newborn

Outcomes in Young Adulthood for Very-Low-Birth-Weight Infants
Hack M, Flannery DJ, Schluchter M, et al (Case Western Reserve Univ, Cleveland, Ohio; Cleveland State Univ, Ohio; Kent State Univ, Ohio)
N Engl J Med 346:149-157, 2002   10–1

Background.—At school age, very low birth weight children have poorer academic performance and cognitive function compared with normal birth weight control subjects. The learning problems observed in these children persist into adolescence and have been seen even in very low birth weight children who have normal intelligence and no neurologic impairment. Whether these adverse effects of very low birth weight persist into adulthood was studied.

Methods.—The study group was composed of a cohort of 242 young adults who were very low birth weight infants born between 1977 and 1979 and 233 control subjects from the same population in Cleveland who had normal weights at birth. Those born at very low birth weight had a mean weight at birth of 1179 g and a mean gestational age at birth of 29.7 weeks. For both of these groups investigators assessed the level of education, cognitive and academic achievement, as well as the rates of chronic illness and risk-taking behavior at 20 years of age. The outcomes were adjusted for sex and sociodemographic status.

Results.—Rates of graduation from high school were lower among very low birth weight young adults than among control subjects (74% vs 83%). The very low birth weight adults had rates of chronic conditions that were significantly higher than rates for the control subjects (Table 2). Very low birth weight men were significantly less likely than male control subjects to be enrolled in postsecondary education (30% vs 53%); however, this was not true of very low birth weight women (Table 3). Young adults in the very low birth weight group also had a lower mean IQ than the normal control group (87 vs 92) and lower academic achievement scores as well as higher rates of neurosensory impairment (10% vs 1%). Subnormal height was also more prevalent among the very low birth weight young adults compared with normal control subjects (10% vs 5%). Adults in the very low birth weight group reported less used of alcohol and drugs and had lower rates of pregnancy than normal control subjects; these differences remained when only participants without neurosensory impairment were compared (Table 5).

TABLE 2.—Chronic Conditions at 20 Years of Age Among Very Low Birth Weight and Normal Birth Weight Participants*

Variable	Men		Women	
	Very Low Birth Weight (N=116)	Normal Birth Weight (N=108)	Very Low Birth Weight (N=126)	Normal Birth Weight (N=125)
	No. of Participants (%)			
Neurosensory condition	11 (9)	1 (1)†	14 (11)	0‡
Cerebral palsy§	6 (5)	0	9 (7)	0
Hydrocephalus necessitating the placement of a shunt	1 (1)	0	4 (3)	0
Blindness¶	3 (3)	0	1 (1)	0
Deafness‖	1 (1)	1 (1)	2 (2)	0
Medical or psychiatric illness	22 (19)	17 (16)	29 (23)	20 (16)
Asthma**	8 (7)	6 (6)	11 (9)	7 (6)
Diabetes	0	0	1 (1)	1 (1)
Sickle cell anemia	0	1 (1)	1 (1)	1 (1)
Epilepsy	1 (1)	1 (1)	3 (2)	0
Arthritis	3 (3)	2 (2)	10 (8)	6 (5)
Bone or muscle disorder	10 (9)	7 (6)	5 (4)	7 (6)
Bipolar disorder	3 (3)	2 (2)	2 (2)	0
Other††	0	0	1 (1)	2 (2)
Height <3rd percentile‡‡	9 (8)	5 (5)	14 (11)	6 (5)
Total with at least one condition	36 (31)	23 (21)	45 (36)	25 (20)§§

*Chronic conditions were defined as those with a duration of ≥12 months. Data for the general categories of neurosensory condition and medical or psychiatric illness are the numbers and percentages of participants with at least 1 condition in that category.

†P = .004 for the comparison with the men in the very low birth weight group.

‡P = .005 for the comparison with the women in the very low birth weight group.

§Nine of the participants had spastic diplegia, 2 had spastic hemiplegia, and 4 had spastic quadriplegia.

¶One participant had bilateral blindness and 3 had unilateral blindness.

‖Data are for participants who required a hearing aid.

**Data are for participants who had had an asthma attack in the previous 12 months, were taking asthma medication, or both.

††One participant in the very low birth weight group had hypertension caused by Liddle's syndrome (pseudoaldosteronism); 1 participant in the control group had endometriosis, and 1 had narcolepsy.

‡‡Height percentiles from the Centers for Disease Control and Prevention growth charts were used. The analysis includes 11 participants who were not measured but reported their own height.

§§P = .006 for the comparison with the women in the very low birth weight group.

(Courtesy of Hack M, Flannery DJ, Schluchter M, et al: Outcomes in young adulthood for very-low-birth-weight infants. N Engl J Med 346:149-157, 2002. Copyright Massachusetts Medical Society.)

Conclusions.—The neurodevelopmental and growth-related sequelae of very low birth weight and the poor academic achievement reported in these children appears to persist into adulthood. However, these adverse effects were not associated with increased risk-taking behavior or criminal activity in this cohort.

▶ With this publication Dr Hack extends her many studies of the consequences of very low birth weight (that is, <1.5 kg) into the range of young adulthood.[1,2] The 242 subjects of this case-control study born in 1977 to 1979 were successfully followed up to the age of 20 years. They were then compared with a control group with mean birth weight of 3279 g identified by a retrospective population sampling procedure at age 8 years and compared with the very low birth weight group with respect to a number of sociodemographic, medical, educational, cognitive, and sociobehavioral variables. One of my respect-

TABLE 3.—Level of Education at 20 Years of Age Among Very Low Birth Weight and Normal Birth Weight Participants*

Variable	Men			Women			Total Population
	Very Low Birth Weight (N=116) No. (%)	Normal Birth Weight (N=108) No. (%)	Odds Ratio (95% CI)	Very Low Birth Weight (N=126) No. (%)	Normal Birth Weight (N=125) No. (%)	Odds Ratio (95% CI)	Odds Ratio (95% CI)
High-school graduation†	77 (66)	81 (75)	0.7 (0.4-1.3)	102 (81)	112 (90)	0.5 (0.2-1.1)	0.6 (0.4-1.0)‡
Current study							
None	70 (60)	44 (41)	2.1 (1.2-3.7)§	56 (44)	53 (42)	1.1 (0.6-1.8)	
High school or GED¶	11 (9)	8 (7)	1.2 (0.5-3.2)	6 (5)	4 (3)	1.4 (0.4-5.3)	1.5 (1.0-2.1)‡
Postsecondary study‖	35 (30)	57 (53)	0.4 (0.2-0.7)**	64 (51)	68 (54)	0.9 (0.5-1.5)	1.3 (0.6-2.8)
Community college††	17 (15)	9 (8)	1.9 (0.8-4.5)	22 (17)	21 (17)	1.0 (0.5-2.0)	
Four-year college‡‡	18 (16)	47 (44)	0.2 (0.1-0.4)§§	42 (33)	47 (38)	0.8 (0.5-1.5)	1.3 (0.8-2.2)

*ORs for men and women were adjusted for sociodemographic status; ORs for the population were adjusted for sociodemographic status and sex.
†Data include 12 participants in the very low birth weight group and 17 controls who had obtained a GED.
‡P = .04 for the comparison between groups.
§P = .007 for the comparison between groups.
¶Twelve very low birth weight participants and 7 controls were in high school, and 5 very low birth weight participants and 5 controls were in a GED program.
‖P = .04 for the interaction between birth weight and sex. Because this interaction was significant, the adjusted difference from the pooled analysis is not presented.
**P = .002 for the comparison between groups.
††Data include 2 very low birth weight participants and 4 controls who were in business school and 15 very low birth weight participants and 7 controls who were in technical school.
‡‡P = .004 for the interaction between birth weight and sex. Because this interaction was significant, the adjusted difference from the pooled analysis is not presented.
§§P <.001 for the comparison between groups.
Abbreviation: GED, General equivalency diploma.
(Courtesy of Hack M, Flannery DJ, Schluchter M, et al: Outcomes in young adulthood for very-low-birth-weight infants. *N Engl J Med* 346:149-157, 2002. Copyright Massachusetts Medical Society.)

TABLE 5.—Self-Reported Substance Use, Criminal Activity, and Sexual Activity at 20 Years of Age Among Very Low Birth Weight Participants*

Variable	Men				Women				Total Population	
	Very Low Birth Weight (N=116) No. (%)	Normal Birth Weight (N=108) No. (%)	Odds Ratio (95% CI)	P Value	Very Low Birth Weight (N=126) No. (%)	Normal Birth Weight (N=124) No. (%)	Odds Ratio (95% CI)	P Value	Odds Ratio (95% CI)	P Value
Substance use during the previous year										
Tobacco	66 (57)	64 (59)	0.9 (0.5-1.6)		50 (40)	59 (48)	0.7 (0.4-1.2)		0.8 (0.6-1.2)	
Alcohol	84 (72)	89 (82)	0.6 (0.3-1.1)		77 (61)	103 (83)	0.3 (0.2-0.6)	<0.001	0.4 (0.3-0.6)	<0.001
Illicit drugs	49 (42)	57 (53)	0.6 (0.4-1.1)		38 (30)	54 (44)	0.6 (0.3-0.9)	0.03	0.6 (0.4-0.9)	0.007
Marijuana	49 (42)	56 (52)	0.7 (0.4-1.1)		37 (29)	52 (42)	0.6 (0.3-1.0)	0.04	0.6 (0.4-0.9)	0.01
Other†	10 (9)	9 (8)	1.1 (0.4-2.9)		5 (4)	9 (7)	0.5 (0.2-1.7)		0.8 (0.4-1.7)	
Contact with the police										
Violation of law (excluding traffic laws)	43 (37)	56 (52)	0.5 (0.3-0.9)	0.03	30 (24)	29 (23)	1.0 (0.6-1.8)		0.7 (0.5-1.1)	
Convicted of crime‡	23 (20)	29 (27)	0.7 (0.4-1.2)		3 (2)	4 (3)	0.7 (0.1-3.2)		0.7 (0.4-1.2)	
Incarcerated§	30 (26)	28 (26)	0.9 (0.5-1.7)		8 (6)	7 (6)	1.1 (0.4-3.2)		0.9 (0.6-1.6)	
Sexual activity¶										
Intercourse	96 (83)	88 (81)	0.8 (0.4-1.7)		82 (65)	97 (78)	0.5 (0.2-0.8)	0.01	0.6 (0.4-0.9)	0.02
Pregnancy||	30 (26)	25 (23)	1.1 (0.6-2.0)		36 (29)	51 (41)	0.5 (0.3-0.9)	0.02	0.7 (0.5-1.1)	
Live birth**	17 (15)	19 (18)	0.7 (0.4-1.5)		17 (13)	30 (24)	0.4 (0.2-0.9)	0.02	0.6 (0.3-0.9)	0.02

*ORs for men and for women were adjusted for sociodemographic status; ORs for the total population were adjusted for sociodemographic status and sex.

†Data include the use of inhalants (by 4 very low birth weight men, 1 male control, and 1 female control), amphetamines (by 5 very low birth weight women, 3 male controls, and 5 female controls), cocaine (by 2 very low birth weight men, 1 very low birth weight woman, 2 male controls, and 3 female controls), and hallucinogens (by 3 very low birth weight men, 3 very low birth weight women, 7 male controls, and 7 female controls).

‡Data include convictions for driving under the influence of alcohol.

§Incarceration was defined as ever being held in jail, including for several hours or overnight, or in juvenile detention.

¶For men, the data for pregnancy or live birth indicate pregnancy in the man's partner or live birth of a child fathered by the man.

||Data include 13 very low birth weight women and 9 female controls who were pregnant at the time of the interview.

**Data include 3 very low birth weight women and 5 female controls who had more than 1 live birth.

(Courtesy of Hack M, Flannery DJ, Schluchter M, et al: Outcomes in young adulthood for very-low-birth-weight infants. *N Engl J Med* 346:149-157, 2002. Copyright Massachusetts Medical Society.)

ed teachers taught me that the impairments associated with immature birth or birth trauma tend to be obliterated by the transcendent impact of environmental variables by age 3 to 4 years, except for early neonatal physical limitations discernable before that time. The demographic variables are therefore very important. Fifty percent of both very low birth weight and control infants were born to black women, 50% to 55% of them high school graduates with comparable sociodemographic scores. The very low birth weight group has significantly more chronic neurosensory conditions, cerebral palsy accounting for half or more. Mean IQ scores and measures of academic achievement were perhaps understandably less among very low birth weight infants, though most of the IQs in that group at age 20 were within the normal range. Postsecondary study and enrollment in 4-year colleges were significantly less common among premature males. Use of alcohol and illicit drugs was less common in very low birth weight females compared with controls, and contact with police and the judicial system less common in male very low birth weight individuals than controls; these rates showed no significant difference for either sex compared with the control group. What emerges is that past the implications of neurosensory disturbances and infant losses (36% of very low birth weight infants failed to survive to 2 years), most at age 20 were almost as successful citizens as their normal control counterparts. Inevitably, studies using such long follow-up periods leave one wondering whether the possible impact of improvements in antenatal and neonatal care might affect these relatively comforting 20-year findings. Then, too, the impact of differences in community environment other than those in the Cleveland area are items for curiosity. We can only look hopefully for the continued efforts of Dr Hack and her colleagues for more understanding in these important concerns.

T. H. Kirschbaum, MD

References

1. 1996 YEAR BOOK OF OBSTETRICS, GYNECOLOGY, AND WOMEN'S HEALTH, pp 243-245.
2. 1998 YEAR BOOK OF OBSTETRICS, GYNECOLOGY, AND WOMEN'S HEALTH, pp 239-241.

Pregnancy Complications and Maternal Risk of Ischaemic Heart Disease: A Retrospective Cohort Study of 129 290 Births
Smith GCS, Pell JP, Walsh D (Univ of Glasgow, Scotland; Common Services Agency Edinburgh, Scotland)
Lancet 357:2002-2006, 2001   10–2

Background.—The risk of ischemic heart disease (IHD) in later life is increased in individuals who are small at birth. One proposed explanation of this increased risk is the hypothesis of fetal adaptation to a suboptimum intrauterine environment. As a result, individuals are physiologically programmed for a "thrifty phenotype" in which the risk of hypertension and IHD in later life would be increased. An alternative theory is that common genetic factors create a predisposition to intrauterine growth restriction, preterm birth, and IHD. If this alternative hypothesis is correct, then moth-

FIGURE 1

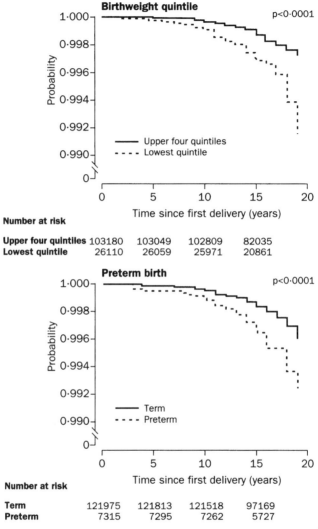

(*Continued*)

ers whose pregnancies are complicated by intrauterine growth restriction or preterm delivery should also be at increased risk for development of IHD. In this study, a possible association between pregnancy complications related to low birth weight and risk of subsequent IHD was investigated.

Methods.—The singleton first births in Scotland between 1981 and 1985 were identified by means of routine discharge data. Linkage of the mothers' subsequent admissions and deaths yielded 15 to 19 years of follow-up data. The mothers' risks of death from any cause or from IHD and admission for

FIGURE 1 (cont.)

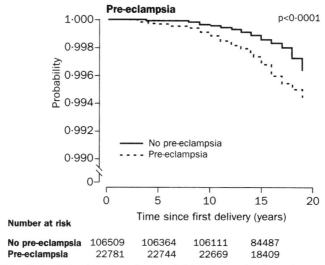

FIGURE 1.—Kaplan-Meier plots of cumulative probability of survival without admission for IHD or death from IHD after first pregnancy in relation to birth weight quintile, preterm delivery, and diagnosis of preeclampsia during pregnancy. (Courtesy of Smith GCS, Pell JP, Walsh D: Pregnancy complications and maternal risk of ischaemic heart disease: A retrospective cohort study of 129 290 births. *Lancet* 357:2002-2006, 2001. Reprinted with permission from Elsevier Science.)

or death from IHD were related to adverse obstetric outcomes in the first pregnancy. Hazard ratios were then adjusted for several variables, including socioeconomic deprivation, maternal height and age, and essential hypertension.

Results.—Data were obtained for a total of 129,290 eligible deliveries. The maternal risk of IHD admission or death was found to be associated with delivery of a baby in the lowest birth weight quintile for gestational age, preterm delivery, and preeclampsia. There was an additive nature to the associations, with women with all 3 characteristics demonstrating a risk of IHD admission or death 7 times greater than that in the reference category (Fig 1).

Conclusions.—There is an association between the complications of pregnancy linked to low birth weight and an increased risk of subsequent IHD in the mother. The link between birth weight and risk of IHD in both the individual and the mother might be explained by common genetic risk factors.

▶ There is a well-established association between low birth weight and the risk of subsequent cardiovascular disease in the later life of the infant. Those who accept Barker's hypothesis feel that inadequate fetal nutrition associated with low birth weight physiologically programs the infant to an increased risk of hypertension and ischemic heart disease as an adult. This is a study of 129,290 births of singlet living firstborn infants past the 24th week of gestation delivered over a 5-year period and includes the subsequent records of maternal contacts with the Scottish National Health Service over the 15 to 19 years after delivery. It offers support for an alternative explanation, that common maternal factors are responsible both for fetal growth retardation, preterm birth, and ischemic heart disease in themselves and ultimately in their offspring. When arrayed by birth weights specific to gestational age, mothers in the lowest quintile at the time of their birth (26,110 infants) were compared with those in the upper 4 quintiles. Multivariant analysis demonstrated a significant association of low birth weight, preterm delivery, and preeclampsia exhibited by pregnant women with an increased likelihood of subsequent episodes of ischemic heart disease, death secondary to ischemic heart disease, and mortality in general. Among the mothers over the ensuing 15 to 19 years, multivariant analysis adjusting for possible confounding relationships with maternal age, height, socioeconomic status, and incidence of essential hypertension failed to change the prior conclusion. If only fetal programming was responsible, no such commonality between maternal hypertension and ischemic heart disease and fetal hypertension and ischemic heart disease would be expected to occur except as a reflection of random chance. Clearly maternal increase in the risk of ischemic heart disease and that in their growing infants occurs more often than would be expected by chance and likely represents genetic determinants which both mother and fetus share. This is a strong argument against the Barker hypotheseis.

T. H. Kirschbaum, MD

Birthweight, Early Environment, and Genetics: A Study of Twins Discordant for Acute Myocardial Infarction
Hübinette A, Cnattingius S, Ekbom A, et al (Karolinska Institutet, Stockholm; Karolinska Hosp, Stockholm; McGill Univ, Montreal)
Lancet 357:1997-2001, 2001   10–3

Background.—Twin studies help to overcome the genetic and socioeconomic factors that may influence a perceived association between restricted fetal growth and increased risk of coronary heart disease in adult life. The population-based Swedish Twin Registry and cause of death registries were used for data comparing birth characteristics and the development of acute myocardial infarction (AMI) in same-sexed twin pairs. It was hypothesized that if birth characteristics and AMI were related in external control twins and among within-pair co-twin controls, then birth characteristics could be the reason for increased AMI risk. Alternatively, if a relationship was only found in external controls but not in co-twin controls, genetic, maternal, or environmental effects may have intervened.

Methods.—The two control groups for this study consisted of unaffected unrelated twins and unaffected co-twins; there were 132 same-sexed twin pairs discordant for AMI as well as 118 individually matched control twin pairs. Records were evaluated for information on birth and maternal characteristics.

TABLE 1.—Birth and Maternal Characteristics in Twins With AMI and
External Control Twins

Characteristic	Cases (n=118)	Controls (n=118)	P
Anthropometry			
Mean (SD) birthweight in g	2556 (500)	2699 (530)	0·04*
Mean (SD) birth length in cm†	47·1 (2·8)	47·9 (2·7)	0·04*
Mean (SD) head circumference in cm†	33·0 (1·8)	33·5 (2·0)	0·03*
Mean (SD) ponderal index	2·43 (0·27)	2·43 (0·26)	0·93*
Mean (SD) gestational age in weeks	37·6 (2·8)	38·0 (2·9)	0·27*
Maternal age (years)			
≤19	2 (2%)	2 (2%)	
20-29	52 (44%)	60 (51%)	
≥30	64 (54%)	56 (47%)	0·58‡
Parity†			
1	32 (28%)	39 (33%)	
≥2	84 (72%)	78 (67%)	0·34‡
Marital status			
Married	93 (79%)	105 (89%)	
Unmarried/separated	25 (21%)	13 (11%)	0·03‡
Occupational status†			
Manual worker	86 (79%)	71 (63%)	
Non-manual worker	15 (14%)	28 (25%)	
Self-employed	8 (7%)	13 (12%)	0·04‡
Area of residence			
Country	5 (4%)	7 (6%)	
Village	57 (48%)	54 (46%)	
City	56 (47%)	57 (48%)	0·81‡

Note: Data are number of individuals unless otherwise stated.
*Paired *t* test.
†Birth length was missing for 2 cases and 2 external controls. Head circumference was missing for 26 cases and 26 external controls. Numbers for cases and controls do not add up to total study size because of missing information on some variables. Some percentages do not add up to 100 because of rounding.
‡Test for homogeneity.
(Courtesy of Hübinette A, Cnattingius S, Ekborn A, et al: Birthweight, early environment, and genetics: A study of twins discordant for acute myocardial infarction. *Lancet* 357:1997-2001, 2001. Reprinted with permission from Elsevier Science.)

Results.—External controls were noted to have significantly higher mean birth weights (2699 g compared to 2556 g), lengths (47.9 cm compared to 47.1 cm), and head circumferences (33.5 cm compared to 33.0 cm) than the cases being studied (Table 1). Ponderal index was similar, and mean gestational age was lower in cases than in controls, but this did not reach significance. Unmarried mothers and parents with manual occupations were seen significantly more frequently among the histories of cases than among those of controls. No significant differences were noted between birth measurements when AMI cases and healthy co-twins were compared within the pairs (Table 3).

Conclusions.—Because there were no significant differences found when within-pair comparisons were done regarding birth characteristics and AMI, genetic, maternal, and environmental factors may be the reason for an increased risk of AMI in those with restricted fetal growth.

TABLE 3.—Differences in Birth Characteristics in Twins With AMI and Their Co-Twin Controls

Variable	All Twins (n=132)			Monozygotic Twins (n=40)			Dizygotic Twins (n=72)		
	Cases	Controls	P*	Cases	Controls	P*	Cases	Controls	P*
Birthweight (g)	2548 (510)	2534 (530)	0·73	2373 (470)	2417 (560)	0·54	2676 (510)	2620 (490)	0·29
Birth length (cm)†	47·1 (2·8)	47·2 (2·8)	0·91	45·9 (3·0)	46·6 (3·1)	0·09	47·9 (2·6)	47·6 (2·6)	0·30
Head circumference in cm†	33·0 (1·7)	33·0 (1·8)	0·92	32·3 (1·8)	32·3 (2·0)	0·72	33·4 (1·6)	33·3 (1·7)	0·73
Ponderal index	2·43 (0·28)	2·41 (0·27)	0·32	2·46 (0·32)	2·38 (0·27)	0·27	2·45 (0·27)	2·43 (0·27)	0·55

Note: Data are mean (SD).

*Paired *t* test.

†Birth length was missing for 9 cases and co-twin controls. Head circumference was missing for 30 pairs.

(Courtesy of Hübinette A, Cnattingius S, Ekborn A, et al: Birthweight, early environment, and genetics: A study of twins discordant for acute myocardial infarction. *Lancet* 357:1997-2001, 2001. Reprinted with permission from Elsevier Science.)

▶ The controversy over the meaning of the relationship between low birth weight and the risk of arteriosclerotic heart disease in later life continues to occupy investigators over the question of whether intrauterine nutrition programs the low birth weight infant's cardiovascular system to that end (the Barker hypothesis), or whether confounding maternal genetic and familial socioeconomic factors were operative. The former hypothesis has been discussed here[1-5] previously. In this study, data from the Swedish Twin Registry and Cause of Death Registry are used to explore the incidence of myocardial infarction as an index of arteriosclerotic heart disease in monochorionic dizygotic twins as a possible correlate of low birth weight. In one study, 118 twins with an episode of myocardial infarction were compared with an equal size control group alive at the time of analysis with no history of myocardial infarction, and matched for gender and years at risk of infarction. Confirming earlier investigators, those twin pairs with a history of myocardial infarction had lesser mean weight, length, and head circumference but had the same mean ponderal indices as twins without the myocardial infarction history. In a second portion of the study, 132 twins failed to show any differences between birth weight and size in twins discordant for myocardial infarction. The work will be criticized for failing to control for maternal smoking and the relatively small number of cases upon which to base a negative conclusion. However, the lack of significant difference in newborn size at birth in intratwin comparisons is a failure to demonstrate a direct relationship between birth weight and myocardial infarction in later life. Furthermore, these data suggest the apparent relationship may be affected by genetic or environmental differences underlying the observation of reduced birthweight.

T. H. Kirschbaum, MD

References

1. 1998 Year Book of Obstetrics, Gynecology, and Women's Health, pp 39-41.
2. 2000 Year Book, pp 11-13.
3. 2002 Year Book, pp 71-73.
4. 2002 Year Book, pp 73-77.
5. 2002 Year Book, pp 254-256.

Long-Term Effects of Indomethacin Prophylaxis in Extremely-Low-Birth-Weight Infants
Schmidt B, for the Trial of Indomethacin Prophylaxis in Preterms Investigators (McMaster Univ, Hamilton, Ont, Canada; et al)
N Engl J Med 344:1966-1972, 2001 10–4

Introduction.—The prophylactic administration of indomethacin decreases the rate of patent ductus arteriosus and severe intraventricular hemorrhage in very low birth weight infants (birth weight below 1500 g). It is not known whether prophylaxis with indomethacin offers any long-term benefits that outweigh the risk of drug-induced decreases in renal, intestinal, and cerebral blood flow. This was evaluated in 1202 infants with birth weights of 500 to 999 g (extremely low birth weight).

Methods.—Soon after birth, infants were randomly allotted to receive either indomethacin (0.1 mg/kg body weight) or placebo IV once daily for 3 days. The major outcome was a composite of death, cerebral palsy, cognitive delay, deafness, and blindness at a corrected age of 18 months. Secondary long-term outcomes included hydrocephalus requiring the placement of a shunt, seizure disorder, and microcephaly, all within the same time frame. Secondary short-term outcomes were patent ductus arteriosus, pulmonary hemorrhage, chronic lung disease, US evidence of intracranial abnormalities, necrotizing enterocolitis, and retinopathy.

Results.—Of 574 infants in the indomethacin group, 271 (47%) died or survived with impairments, compared with 261 of 569 infants (46%) in the placebo group (odds ratio [OR], 1.1; 95% CI, 0.8-1.4; *P* = 0.61). The incidence of patent ductus arteriosus was lower in the indomethacin group than in the placebo group (24% vs 50%; OR, 0.3; *P* < .001); for severe periventricular hemorrhage and intraventricular hemorrhage, rates were 9% and 13%, respectively; OR, 0.6; *P* = .02. No other outcomes were changed by the prophylactic administration of indomethacin (Fig 2 and Table 3).

Conclusion.—For extremely low birth weight infants, prophylaxis with indomethacin does not enhance survival without neurosensory impairment

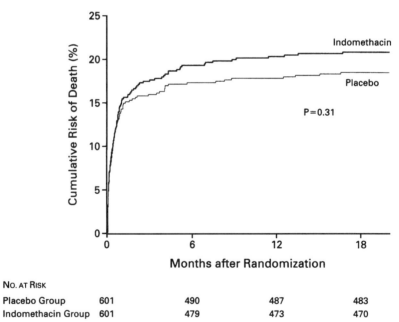

FIGURE 2.—Kaplan-Meier estimates of the cumulative risk of death in the indomethacin and placebo groups. For infants with unknown status at 18 months, these estimates include information on the last dates on which the infants were known to be alive. (Reprinted by permission of *The New England Journal of Medicine* courtesy of Schmidt B, for the Trial of Indomethacin Prophylaxis in Preterms Investigators: Long-term effects of indomethacin prophylaxis in extremely-low-birth-weight infants. *N Engl J Med* 344:1966-1972, 2001. Copyright 2001, Massachusetts Medical Society. All rights reserved.)

TABLE 3.—Primary Outcome of Death or Neurosensory Impairment

Outcome	Event Rate no./Total no. (%)		Odds Ratio		P Value
	Indomethacin Group	Placebo Group	Unadjusted	Adjusted (95% CI)	
Composite					
Death or impairment	271/574 (47)	261/569 (46)	1.1	1.1 (0.8-1.4)	0.61
Components					
Death before 18 mo corrected age*	125/595 (21)	111/594 (19)	1.2	1.2 (0.9-1.6)	0.27
Cerebral palsy†	58/467 (12)	55/477 (12)	1.1	1.1 (0.7-1.6)	0.64
Cognitive delay (MDI <70)†	118/444 (27)	117/457 (26)	1.1	1.0 (0.8-1.4)	0.86
Hearing loss requiring amplification†	10/456 (2)	10/466 (2)	1.0	1.0 (0.4-2.5)	0.93
Bilateral blindness†	9/465 (2)	7/472 (1)	1.3	1.3 (0.5-3.6)	0.58

Note: Odds ratios have been adjusted for the birth weight stratum and center, except for the odds ratios for hearing loss and bilateral blindness, which were adjusted only for the birth weight stratum. *P* values are for the adjusted odds ratios.

*These data do not include the 13 infants who were lost to follow-up at 18 months.

†Data for this outcome exclude infants who died before scheduled tests and those who were alive but were not tested or were lost to follow-up.

Abbreviation: MDI, Mental development index.

(Reprinted by permission of *The New England Journal of Medicine* courtesy of Schmidt B, for the Trial of Indomethacin Prophylaxis in Preterms Investigators: Long-term effects of indomethacin prophylaxis in extremely-low-birth-weight infants. *N Engl J Med* 344:1966-1972, 2001. Copyright 2001, Massachusetts Medical Society. All rights reserved.)

at 18 months despite the fact that it decreases the rate of patent ductus arteriosus and severe periventricular and intraventricular hemorrhage.

▶ The tocolytic use of indomethacin exposes the fetus to a series of risks reflecting the vital role of prostaglandin production in normal fetal life. The resulting closure of the ductus arteriosus reduces fetal cardiac output from the sum of the outputs of its 2 ventricles minus pulmonary blood flow and, to the extent that the ductus is fully closed, to the output of the lesser of the 2 ventricular chambers. This appears to expose the fetus to risks for necrotizing enterocolitis and intraventricular hemorrhage and, through direct affects on fetal kidneys, to oliguria and oligohydramnios.[1,2] Failure of controlled observations to prove effectiveness as a tocolytic makes this drug a poor choice for threatened or active preterm labor.[3,4]

This collaborative study, supported by the Canadian Medical Research Council, is in response to the work of Ment et al who have provided evidence of the effect of low-dose indomethacin treatment in the prevention of intraventricular hemorrhage in newborns.[5] From a series of neonatal centers in Australia, New Zealand, Canada and the United States, 1202 infants weighing 0.5 to 1.0 kg at birth were randomly assigned to receive indomethacin 0.1 mg/kg every day for 3 days or placebo. This birth weight range was chosen because of the high rate of neonatal complications to which it is subject. Primary outcome measurements were mortality or severe sensoromotor defects—cerebral palsy, blindness, deafness, or cognitive delay. Evidence of patent ductus arteriosus, hydrocephaly or microcephaly were also noted.

Clearly, ductus arteriosus closure results from inhibition of local endothelial prostaglandin synthesis, and a decreased incidence of intraventricular hemorrhage might possibly reflect decreased cerebral blood flow caused by the same decrease in cardiac outflow seen in the fetus centrally. Tissue oxygen supply depends upon both blood flow and blood oxygen content. If closing the ductus improves the oxygen concentration of arterial blood by abolishing cardiac shunting and at the same time decreases organ blood flow, organ oxygen supply may increase or decrease, depending upon the relative sizes of those 2 opposing effects. This means that brain or gastrointestinal ischemia might result in necrotizing enterocolitis, pulmonary hemorrhage, and chronic lung dysfunction, retinapathy, or neurologic abnormalities.

The results show no benefits in terms of mortality nor in the incidence of any of the primary or secondary outcome measurements at 18 month of age. Ductus arteriosus closure clearly results from the therapy, and neonatal surgery is seldom needed. Although severe intraventricular or periventricular hemorrhage—Papile class III or IV—occurs with a significantly decreased incidence in association with indomethacin use compared with controls, the difference in occurrence rate (4%) is so small as to have little effect on overall morbidity. This study makes clear that all one can expect for certain from prophylactic indomethacin in very low birth weight infants is closure of the dutus arteriosus.

T. H. Kirschbaum, MD

References

1. 1995 YEAR BOOK OF OBSTETRICS, GYNECOLOGY, AND WOMEN'S HEALTH, pp 246-248.
2. 1999 YEAR BOOK OF OBSTETRICS, GYNECOLOGY, AND WOMEN'S HEALTH, pp 115-117 and 221-223.
3. 2000 YEAR BOOK OF OBSTETRICS, GYNECOLOGY, AND WOMEN'S HEALTH, pp 63-65.
4. 2002 YEAR BOOK OF OBSTETRICS, GYNECOLOGY, AND WOMEN'S HEALTH, pp 68-70.
5. Ment LR, Oh WO, Elwenkranz RA, et al: Low dose indomethacin and prevention of intraventricular hemorrhage: A multicenter randomized trial. *Pediatrics* 105:45, 2000.

Proton Spectroscopy and Diffusion Imaging on the First Day of Life After Perinatal Asphyxia: Preliminary Report
Barkovich AJ, Westmark KD, Bedi HS, et al (Univ of California, San Francisco; Clear Lake Regional Med Ctr, Webster, Tex)
AJNR Am J Neuroradiol 22:1786-1794, 2001   10–5

Background.—The development and improvement of MR techniques have significantly affected the diagnosis of brain injury in the neonate. The improvement of techniques has led to a change in the goal of imaging studies, from identification of damage to identification of it at an early stage, when medical intervention might be useful. MRI has proved helpful in the assessment of brain injury from perinatal asphyxia when the injury is subacute or chronic, underscoring the need for MR assessment of the brain within the first few hours of life. The results of early (first 24 hours after birth) MRI in 7 patients, including proton MR spectroscopy in 6 patients, are described.

Methods.—Seven consecutive patients underwent MR studies within the first 24 hours of life. All of the patients were encephalopathic after complicated deliveries. Standard T1-, T2-, and diffusion-weighted sequences were performed in all of the patients, and 6 patients also underwent single-voxel MR spectroscopy in 2 locations. Follow-up MR studies were performed in 4 patients at the ages of 7, 8, 9, and 15 days, respectively.

Results.—All 7 patients had normal T1-weighted images. T2-weighted images were normal in 3 of the 7 patients, whereas in the other 4 these images revealed T2 prolongation in the basal ganglia or white matter. Diffusion images in all 7 patients showed small abnormalities in the lateral thalami or internal capsules, and follow-up studies in 4 patients showed that the diffusion images had underestimated the extent of injury to the brain (Fig 3). A significant elevation of lactate was shown in all 6 patients who underwent proton MR spectroscopy. Two patients died during the neonatal period, and the remaining 5 patients experienced significant neurologic impairment.

Conclusions.—MR spectroscopy in the first 24 hours of life can demonstrate the presence of hypoxic-ischemic brain injury; however, diffusion im-

FIGURE 3

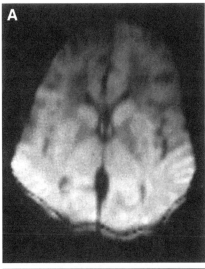

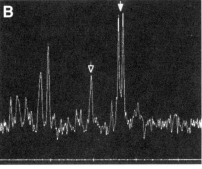

(*Continued*)

aging may identify but also underestimate the extent of damage. This finding will be explored in further studies.

▶ Data from animal experimentation in acute fetal ischemia provides strong support for the premise that the first 24 to 36 hours after ischemia results in relatively little injury, but that the subsequent time interval is marked by irreversible neuronal and glial injury.[1-3] Further, it's apparent that some forms of therapy during that early interval may diminish later brain injury.[4] For those reasons, early objective evidence of significant brain injury has become very important to pediatric neurologists. This small series of 6 brain-injured neonates compares the result of NMR proton spectroscopy (see Abstract 9–11), and MRI technique is important. All 6 infants were born at term with 10-minute Apgars less than 5 and buffer base excess values from −11 to −27. Two infants expired in the NICU, and the others had profound persistent neurologic impair-

FIGURE 3 (cont.)

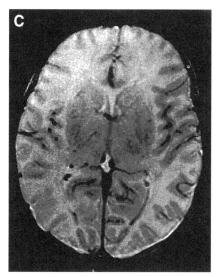

FIGURE 3.—Patient 2. **A,** Diffusion-weighted image (b = 700 s/mm2) at the level of the basal ganglia performed at age 16 hours shows diffusely reduced diffusion in cortex and deep gray nuclei. On initial evaluation, this image was thought to be normal; however, subsequent analysis revealed a reduction in the ADC of about 15% throughout the brain. The distortion and hyperintensity of the back of the head results from chemical blankets used to keep the body temperature at 37°C. **B,** Proton MR spectrum (2000/288) from the thalami and basal ganglia at age 16 hours shows marked reduction of NAA (singlet at 2.01 ppm, indicated by *open arrow*) and marked elevation of lactate (doublet at 1.33 ppm, indicated by *solid arrow*). **C,** Axial SE (3000/120) image at age 18 hours shows some mildly diffuse T2 prolongation. (Courtesy of Barkovich AJ, Westmark KD, Bedi HS, et al: Proton spectroscopy and diffusion imaging on the first day of life after perinatal asphyxia: Preliminary report. *AJNR Am J Neuroradiol* 22:1786-1794, 2001, copyright by American Society of Neuroradiology. [www.ajnr.org])

ment. On NMR spectroscopy done in the first 24 hours of life, particularly that directed at the basal ganglia and deep thalamus, lactate tissue concentration was strikingly elevated and N-acetylaspartate concentration decreased, suggesting ischemic hypoxic interference with ATP production and decreased cellular metabolic energy availability in the brain. NMR-weighted fusion imaging done at the same time interval was not clearly abnormal, showing only an area of reduced diffusion in the posterior internal capsule in 1 of 6 cases. Subsequent NMR imaging done at 7 to 15 days of life was distinctly abnormal, and normal lactate concentration was present in 3 out of 4 infants at that time. There seems little question that NMR spectroscopy is more sensitive in providing evidence of early ischemic hypoxic neonatal brain injury than is the imaging technique.

T. H. Kirschbaum, MD

References

1. 1990 Year Book of Obstetrics, Gynecology, and Women's Health, pp 206-207.
2. 1992 Year Book of Obstetrics, Gynecology, and Women's Health, pp 189-191.

3. 1993 YEAR BOOK OF OBSTETRICS, GYNECOLOGY, AND WOMEN'S HEALTH, pp 123-124.
4. 1998 YEAR BOOK OF OBSTETRICS, GYNECOLOGY, AND WOMEN'S HEALTH, pp 231-235.

Early Increases in Brain *myo*-Inositol Measured by Proton Magnetic Resonance Spectroscopy in Term Infants With Neonatal Encephalopathy

Robertson NJ, Lewis RH, Cowan FM, et al (Imperial College of Science, Technology and Medicine, London)
Pediatr Res 50:692-700, 2001   10–6

Background.—Cellular adaptation to osmotic stress is a vital process that protects cells from the effects of dehydration or edema. Osmolytes are particularly important in the brain because alterations in ion composition would affect excitability. *myo*-Inositol is a major osmolyte in the CNS. Brain *myo*-inositol/creatine plus phosphocreatine (Cr) was assessed in the first

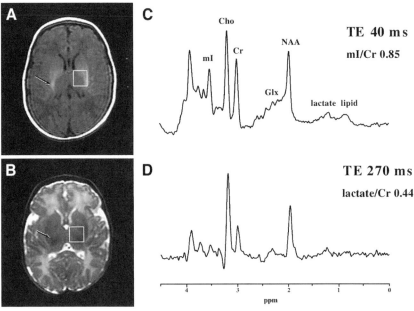

FIGURE 1.—Infant born at 41 weeks gestational age by emergency cesarean section with Apgar scores of 1 at 1 minute and 5 at 5 minutes (patient 4). The infant was examined by MRI and MR spectroscopy (MRS) on day 4. This infant had normal MRI and a normal neurodevelopmental outcome at 1 year of age. A, T$_1$-weighted (conventional spin echo 500/15) transverse MR image illustrating bilateral high signal intensity (SI) from myelin in the posterior half of the posterior limb of the internal capsule (PLIC) (*arrow*). The position of the 8-cm³ voxel from which the ¹H MRS data were obtained is shown. B, T$_2$-weighted (fast spin echo 4200/15/210) transverse MR image demonstrating bilateral regions of low SI representing myelin in the PLIC (*arrow*). C, ¹H MR spectrum acquired from the voxel shown in A and B using point-resolved spectroscopy localization sequence, echo time (TE) 40 milliseconds. *myo*-Inositol (*mI*)/Cr was 0.85. D, Localized ¹H MR spectrum acquired using TE 270 milliseconds. Lactate/Cr was 0.44. *Abbreviations: Cho*, Choline-containing compounds; *Glx*, glutamine; *NAA*, N-acetyl-aspartate. (Courtesy of Robertson NJ, Lewis RH, Cowan FM, et al: Early increases in brain *myo*-inositol measured by proton magnetic resonance spectroscopy in term infants with neonatal encephalopathy. *Pediatr Res* 50(6):692-700, 2001.)

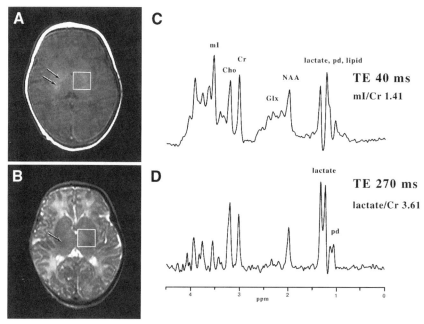

FIGURE 2.—Infant born at 39 weeks gestational age by assisted breech delivery with Apgar scores of 0 at 1 minute and 0 at 5 minute (patient 13). This infant was enrolled at less than 6 hours of age into the pilot study of treatment with whole-body hypothermia for neonatal encephalopathy. MRI and MR spectroscopy (MRS) studies were undertaken on day 1 while the patient was being cooled. This infant had abnormal MRI and died on day 2 of age. **A,** T_1-weighted (conventional spin echo 500/15) transverse MR image illustrating loss of the signal intensity (SI) from the posterior limb of the internal capsule (PLIC) *(arrow)*. There is evidence of brain swelling. There are some small abnormal SIs in the basal ganglia and thalami *(arrows)*. The position of the 8-cm³ voxel from which the ¹H MRS data were obtained is shown. **B,** T_2-weighted (fast spin echo 4200/15/210) transverse MR image. There is no obvious low signal attributable to myelin in the PLIC but an exaggeration of the low SI in the lateral thalamus *(arrow)*. **C,** ¹H MR spectrum acquired from the voxel shown in **A** and **B** using point-resolved spectroscopy localization sequence, echo time (TE) 40 milliseconds. Relative *myo*-Inositol *(ml)* levels were increased, as illustrated by the mI/Cr metabolite ratio of 1.41. **D,** Localized ¹H MR spectrum acquired using TE 270 milliseconds, illustrating markedly elevated lactate/Cr of 3.61. *Abbreviations: Cho,* Choline-containing compounds; *Glx,* glutamine; *NAA,* N-acetyl-aspartate. (Courtesy of Robertson NJ, Lewis RH, Cowan FM, et al: Early increases in brain *myo*-inositol measured by proton magnetic resonance spectroscopy in term infants with neonatal encephalopathy. *Pediatr Res* 50(6):692-700, 2001.)

week in term infants with neonatal encephalopathy by using localized short echo time proton MR spectroscopy, and these findings were related to measurements of brain injury, specifically lactate/Cr in the first week, changes in the basal ganglia on MRI, and neurodevelopmental outcome at 1 year.

Methods.—MRI and MR spectroscopy were performed at 3.5 ± 2.1 days on 14 term infants with neonatal encephalopathy. The infants had a mean age 39.6 ± 1.6 weeks and a mean birth weight of 3270 ± 490 g. In addition, 5 infants were enrolled in a pilot study of treatment with moderate whole-body hypothermia for neonatal encephalopathy. Two of these infants were being cooled at the time of the scan. T_1- and T_2-weighted transverse MR images were graded as normal or abnormal based on the presence or absence of the normal signal intensity of the internal capsule and signal intensity changes in the basal ganglia. Local proton MR spectroscopy data were obtained at echo times of 40 and 270 milliseconds, and the peak area rates of *myo*-inositol/Cr and lactate/Cr were measured. Outcome was scored with Griffith's development scales and a neurodevelopmental examination at 1 year.

Results.—Six infants had normal MRI findings and outcomes, and 8 infants had abnormal MRI findings and outcomes (Fig 1). *myo*-Inositol/Cr and lactate/Cr were higher in the 8 infants with abnormal MRIs and outcomes (Fig 2). A correlation was identified between *myo*-inositol and lactate/Cr, and both were correlated with the Griffith's developmental scales.

Conclusions.—These preliminary findings suggest that early increases in *myo*-inositol/Cr in the brain basal ganglia of infants with neonatal encephalopathy are associated with increased lactate/Cr, MRI changes of severe injury, and a poor neurodevelopmental outcome at 1 year.

▶ This experience based on proton MR spectroscopy and imaging of 14 term newborns with at least clinical evidence of birth asphyxia provides some further support to earlier studies reported here that chart the events in brain chemistry within the first week of life.[1-4] The cord blood analyses on samples obtained within 30 minutes of birth are somewhat heterogeneous with respect to biochemical indices of hypoxic injury. Cases 3, 7, 8, 10, 12, and 14 failed to show metabolic acidosis, and cord blood data are lacking in case 1. Use of proton MR spectroscopy provides indirect evidence of changes in cell energetics and here, *myo*-inositol, which increases in intercellular content in hypoxic-ischemic injury of the brain, is a principal outcome variable. Simultaneously, its concentration reflects sodium intracellular flux with which it shares a cotransfer system (SMIT). Five infants were treated with hypothermia (cases 7, 9, 12, 13, 14) to 33°C to 34°C rectally for 48 hours, but the equivocal effects of that treatment were not large.

In general, but with some exclusions, newborns with biochemical acidosis in cord blood show reduced serum osmolality and serum sodium concentrations, reflecting intracellular fluxes of sodium and water. Since power spectrum analysis cannot yield absolute quantitative results, creatine and phosphocreatine, said to be unchanged during acute hypoxic-ischemic brain injury, are used as reference values. This introduces some statistical noise since phosphocreatine is known to decrease with acute hypoxic-ischemic brain injury. Nevertheless, the qualitative observations seem sound, and *myo*-inositol/Cr ratios correlate with lactate/Cr ratios, the latter reflecting inadequate adenosine triphosphate (ATP) to carry out mitochondrial oxidative glycolysis. Clinical studies at age 1 year confirm that infants 1 through 5 and infant 8 to be neurologically normal, but the rest were grossly abnormal. Nothing here conflicts with what has been written before about the pathophysiology of acute brain asphyxia, but some new supportive data are added.

T. H. Kirschbaum, MD

References

1. 1990 YEAR BOOK OF OBSTETRICS, GYNECOLOGY, AND WOMEN'S HEALTH, pp 206-207.
2. 1992 YEAR BOOK OF OBSTETRICS, GYNECOLOGY, AND WOMEN'S HEALTH, pp 89-91.

3. 1998 YEAR BOOK OF OBSTETRICS, GYNECOLOGY, AND WOMEN'S HEALTH, pp 231-235.
4. 2002 YEAR BOOK OF OBSTETRICS, GYNECOLOGY, AND WOMEN'S HEALTH, pp 241-244.

Long-Chain 3-Hydroxyacyl-CoA Dehydrogenase Deficiency: Clinical Presentation and Follow-up of 50 Patients

den Boer MEJ, Wanders RJA, Morris AAM, et al (Univ of Amsterdam; Univ of Newcastle Upon Tyne, England)
Pediatrics 109:99-104, 2002   10–7

Background.—Long-chain 3-hydroxyacyl-CoA dehydrogenase (LC-HAD) deficiency, an autosomal recessive inborn error of fatty acid oxidation, is a rare and potentially fatal disorder. A large cohort of LCHAD-deficient patients was reviewed to improve early recognition and management.

Methods.—The referring physicians of 61 patients with LCHAD deficiency diagnosed at 1 center were sent a questionnaire. The return rate was 82%. Thus, data on 50 patients were analyzed.

Findings.—Patient age at initial assessment ranged from 1 day to 26 months. Fifteen percent were investigated initially in the neonatal period. Seventy-eight percent presented with hypoketotic hypoglycemia, which is characteristic of a fatty acid oxidation disorder. Twenty-two percent of the patients were seen initially with chronic problems, such as failure to thrive, feeding difficulties, cholestatic liver disease, or hypotonia. On retrospective analysis, 82% of the patients initially seen with an acute metabolic derangement also had a combination of chronic nonspecific symptoms before the metabolic crises. The mortality rate was 38%. All the children who died did so within 3 months after diagnosis. Among surviving patients, morbidity was high, including recurrent metabolic crises and muscle problems, despite treatment.

Conclusions.—Children with LCHAD deficiency commonly have a combination of chronic, nonspecific symptoms. In the absence of the classic metabolic derangement, early diagnosis is difficult. Although prompt diagnosis can improve survival, morbidity is alarmingly high, even with current therapeutic regimens.

▶ Mitochondria are subcellular organelles, primarily responsible for aerobic metabolism of carbohydrates and lipids, unique in that their enzymatic contents are encoded in mitrochondrial DNA, transmitted only from maternal DNA to offspring. This Dutch study deals with a deficiency in 1 of the enzymes responsible for oxidation of fatty acids, present usually as a missense point mutation in gravidas and their offspring. The resulting pathology is uncommon and most often seen by obstetricians in the form of acute fatty liver of pregnancy and by pediatricians in the form of Reye's syndrome and several other disturbances. Included among the latter are cardiomyopathy, liver disease, central nervous system disturbances, feeding disorders, and death due to hypoglycemia. The defective gene impedes or blocks fatty acid metabolism, resulting in accumulation of free fatty acids in blood, which produce severe metabolic acidosis, liver deposition of free fatty acids, hepatic dysfunction, and episodes of stupor and coma. Carbohydrate stores are metabolized to replace the deficit of activated electrons derived from fat metabolism, and when glycogen is depleted hypoglycemia ensues.[1-3] This report discloses 50 cases from 45 families with a total of 47 pregnancies expressing deficient mitochondrial function of this type. The diagnosis may be made by identification of surplus urinary 3-hydroxyacyl dicarboxylic acid or of the corresponding 3-hydroxyacyl carnitine in plasma, the latter by tandem mass spectrometry.[4] More recently the diagnosis has been made by mutational analysis aimed at the dominant point mutation, present in 86% of cases studied here. Though the potential for clinical pathology exists throughout life, symptoms are often expressed only with coexistent infectious disease, trauma, or pregnancy. Pediatric pathology becomes manifest in the first 26 months of life in the 45 infants reported and infant mortality is 38%, often due to hypoglycemia and metabolic acidosis. Of 47 pregnancies reported in women with the mutation, acute fatty liver of pregnancy occurred in 2 women and HELLP syndrome was diagnosed in 7, probably as a reflection of pregnancy-induced hypertension coupled with the hepatic dysfunction of acute fatty liver of pregnancy. What is important here is, given a woman with acute fatty liver of pregnancy, particular attention must be directed to current and future offspring to prevent the high potential infant mortality rates remediable by early newborn diagnosis and treatment. If this group of women is representative, for every woman who develops acute fatty liver of pregnancy, there are somewhere between 7 and, at most, 24 others, depending upon the precision of the diagnosis, who carry the missense mutation and the capacity for episodic metabolic disorders in themselves and their infants.

T. H. Kirschbaum, MD

References

1. 1995 YEAR BOOK OF OBSTETRICS, GYNECOLOGY, AND WOMEN'S HEALTH, pp 116-117.
2. 1996 YEAR BOOK OF OBSTETRICS, GYNECOLOGY, AND WOMEN'S HEALTH, pp 68-69.
3. 1997 YEAR BOOK OF OBSTETRICS, GYNECOLOGY, AND WOMEN'S HEALTH, pp 198-199.
4. 2001 YEAR BOOK OF OBSTETRICS, GYNECOLOGY, AND WOMEN'S HEALTH, pp 236-238.

Low Prevalence of Large Intraventricular Haemorrhage in Very Low Birthweight Infants Carrying the Factor V Leiden or Prothrombin G20210A Mutation
Göpel W, Gortner L, Kohlmann T, et al (Univ of Lübeck, Germany; Univ of Giessen, Germany)
Acta Paediatr 90:1021-1024, 2001   10–8

Background.—The effects of coagulation-increasing genetic factors on the extension of intraventricular hemorrhage (IVH) in infants with very low birth weight are unclear. The frequency and effect of the factor V Leiden and

TABLE 2.—Prevalence of Intraventricular Hemorrhage (IVH) in Very Low Birth Weight (VLBW) Infants With and Without Factor V Leiden and/or Prothrombin G20210A Mutation

	No IVH	IVH Grade I	IVH Grade II	IVH Grade III	IVH Grade IV	p^*
VLBW with factor V Leiden (n = 29)	24 (82.8)	4 (13.8)	0	0	1 (3.4)	0.05
VLBW with prothrombin G20210A (n = 15)	12 (80)	2 (13.3)	0	0	1 (6.6)	0.37
VLBW with factor V Leiden and/or prothrombin G20210A mutation (n = 43)	35 (81.4)	6 (14)	0	0	2 (4.6)	0.02
VLBW without factor V Leiden or prothrombin G20210A mutation (n = 262)	219 (83.6)	11 (4.2)	10 (3.8)	11 (4.2)	11 (4.2)	
All VLBW infants (n = 305)	254 (83.3)	17 (5.6)	10 (3.3)	11 (3.6)	13 (4.3)	

Data are given as n (%).
*IVH grade I versus IVH grade II-IV, compared with VLBW infants without prothrombotic mutations (Fisher's exact test, 2-sided).
(Courtesy of Göpel W, Gortner L, Kohlmann T, et al: Low prevalence of large intraventricular haemorrhage in very low birthweight infants carrying the factor V Leiden or prothrombin G20210A mutation. *Acta Paediatr* 90:1021-1024, 2001. Published by Taylor & Francis, Ltd. at http://www.tandf.cc.uk/journals/jsp.htm.)

prothrombin G20210A mutations in 1 population-based cohort were investigated.

Methods and Findings.—Three hundred five preterm infants weighing less than 1500 g were included. Forty-three had prothrombotic mutations, and 262 did not. The overall prevalence of IVH in these 2 groups was 18.6% and 16.4%, respectively, a nonsignificant difference. However, the risk of developing extension to IVH grade II or higher was significantly reduced in infants with prothrombotic mutations. In a multivariate regression model including potential confounders, being a carrier of factor V Leiden or prothrombin G20210A mutation predicted a low rate of IVH grade II to IV (Table 2).

Conclusions.—Factor V Leiden and prothrombin G20210A mutations appear to be associated with improved control of intraventricular bleeding in very low birth weight infants. The current findings may have implications for future research and treatment.

▶ Obstetricians have, over the past 8 years, come to recognize a series of autosomal dominant inherited gene mutations which render gravidas relatively hypercoagulable. The Leiden factor V and the prothrombin G20210A mutations tip the delicate maternal balance between blood coagulation versus liquidity in the direction of the former, manifest by differences in the prevalence of phlebothrombosis and pulmonary embolus during pregnancy and the puerperium.[1,2] The effects are most marked in the maternal intervillous space, where the absence of vascular endothelium, the heterogeneity of maternal blood flow patterns, the slow subchorionic blood flow rates, and the relative commonality of villous trophoblastic degenerative changes set the stage for fetal injury and death due to intervillous thrombosis and placenta bed infarction. This study of the relationship between the presence of procoagulant mutations and the incidence and extent of IVH in 305 VLBW infants cared for at the University of Lübeck suggests a positive role for procoagulant mutations in modifying the 51 cases of IVH (16.7%) seen among the patients studied. The overall incidence of IVH was the same with (8.6%) or without (6.4%) the factor V Leiden and prothrombin G2021A mutations seen in 14.1% of the pregnancies. This relatively high prevalence reflects the general relative frequency of procoagulant mutations among Caucasians. The difference here lies in the incidence of IVH Papille classes II to IV present in 4.6% of babies born of women with procoagulant mutations compared with 14.6% born of those without. The incidence of stage I IVH blood confined to the periventricular germinal matrix but neither present in nor distending the ventricles, was the same in procoagulant neonates as in normals. The frequency of stage 4 lesions with parenchymal brain involvement was the same in both groups.

These data suggest but fail to prove that stage I lesions had a different etiology than more extensive intraventricular hemorrhages and that the procoagulant mutations aid in preventing extension of IVH into the brain tissue by facilitating coagulation. It is also tempting to consider the possible value of therapeutic procoagulants in the presence of VLBW neonates with Papille class I hemorrhagic lesions.

T. H. Kirschbaum, MD

References

1. 1999 YEAR BOOK OF OBSTETRICS, GYNECOLOGY, AND WOMEN'S HEALTH, pp 71-74.
2. 2001 YEAR BOOK OF OBSTETRICS, GYNECOLOGY, AND WOMEN'S HEALTH, pp 135-137.

Cytomegalovirus Infection of Extremely Low–Birth Weight Infants via Breast Milk

Maschmann J, Hamprecht K, Dietz K, et al (Univ of Tübingen, Germany; Univ of Würzburg, Germany)
Clin Infect Dis 33:1998-2003, 2001   10–9

Introduction.—Human breast milk is a potential source of cytomegalovirus (CMV) infection. Various rates of virus transmission from mother to child have been reported. Detailed clinical data on primary CMV infection of premature infants during a 3-year observational period were reported.

Methods.—Between July 1, 1995 and June 30, 1998, all mother-infant pairs of inborn premature infants with a birth weight of less than 1500 g or born before the completed 32nd week of gestation were evaluated and prospectively screened for CMV infection. All mother-infant pairs underwent initial serologic testing; virus culture and polymerase chain reaction (PCR) of breast milk and urine samples obtained at biweekly intervals until discharge were examined. At the corrected age of 3 months, 1 last urine specimen was collected from each child. Strict donation of the infant's mother's breast milk was required. For infants with clinical deterioration, infection, or cholestasis, a small blood sample was taken for CMV PCR analysis of leukocytes and plasma. Any abnormal findings were monitored until the findings returned to normal or the infant was discharged.

Results.—Of 170 infants evaluated, no CMV transmission was observed in the 80 infants of seronegative mothers and in the 3 infants of seropositive mothers who did not shed CMV DNA into the breast milk. Transmission was identified in 33 (38%) of the 87 CMV-exposed infants, 16 of whom were seen with symptoms that included hepatopathy, neutropenia, thrombocytopenia, and sepsis-like deterioration. Both low birth weight and early postnatal virus transmission were risk factors for symptomatic infection.

Conclusion.—The rate of CMV transmission to preterm infants by breast milk was 38%. To prevent postnatal CMV transmission to preterm infants, it is recommended that noninfectious breast milk be given to babies younger than 30 weeks' gestation or whose birth weight is less than 1000 g.

▶ This is a reminder that, with respect to neonatal CMV infection, very low birth weight infants are at exceptional risk. In this 3-year prospective cohort study, 176 infants who weighed less than 1500 g at birth, were less than 32 weeks of gestational age, or both were identified in 151 mothers, 145 (52%) of whom were of known CMV status and also carried out breast-feeding. Newborn screening was conducted at birth and at 3 months of age. Maternal-infant serology, CMV culture, and PCR done on milk samples were carried out. An infant urinalysis for megalocytes was done at 3 months of age, and careful clinical observations done on the 38% of infants where CMV positive women exhibited virus in milk. Infant infection was not noted in infants of CMV-negative mothers, or in the 3 infants of CMV-positive mothers who had no discernable virus in their milk. Clinical findings were noted in most newly infected infants (apnea/bradycardia, petechiae, hepatomegaly, altered liver function tests, and neutropenia). One infant with a birth weight of 630 g was severely involved. Given this as an unavoidable newborn infection risk, the authors recommend that nursing CMV-positive women use CMV sterile milk for their infant feedings. A method for easy sterilization of infected milk is clearly needed to prevent neonatal infection and maternal-to-fetal transmission.

T. H. Kirschbaum, MD

Circulating Adrenomedullin Is Increased in Preterm Newborns Developing Intraventricular Hemorrhage

Gazzolo D, Marinoni E, Giovannini L, et al ("G Gaslini" Univ, Genoa, Italy; Univ "La Sapienza," Rome)
Pediatr Res 50:544-547, 2001   10–10

Background.—Intraventricular hemorrhage (IVH) is the most common type of cerebral hemorrhage in preterm infants. Andrenomedullin is a recently discovered vasoactive peptide involved in the regulation of fetal hemodynamic modifications and cardiovascular adaptation. Whether plasma

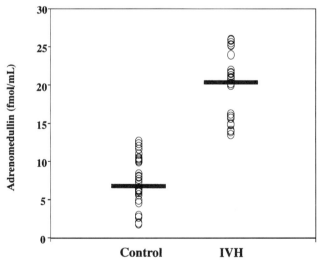

FIGURE 1.—Individual values of adrenomedullin concentrations in plasma of newborns in whom intraventricular hemorrhage (*IVH*) did not develop (*Control*) and in those in whom IVH developed. Horizontal bars represent the mean values. Values for IVH were higher than those for controls (*P* < .01, Mann-Whitney U 2-sided test). (Courtesy of Gazzolo D, Marinoni E, Giovannini L, et al: Circulating adrenomedullin is increased in preterm newborns developing intraventricular hemorrhage. *Pediatr Res* 50(4):544-547, 2001.)

adrenomedullin levels sampled within a few hours of birth could be used to identify preterm infants at risk for IVH was investigated.

Study Design.—All newborns admitted to the neonatal ICU were routinely sampled for evaluation of clinical parameters. In this case-control study, after IVH was diagnosed in 24 preterm neonates, clinical parameters were reassessed, including plasma adrenomedullin concentration, and compared with those obtained from 48 preterm infants matched for gestational age in whom IVH did not develop. The Mann-Whitney U 2-sided test was used to compare adrenomedullin concentrations between these 2 groups. Multiple linear regression analyses were performed to examine the influence of clinical parameters on adrenomedullin levels.

Findings.—Blood adrenomedullin levels and middle–cerebral artery pulsatility index values were significantly higher in neonates with IVH than in the control neonates (Fig 1). Blood adrenomedullin levels were correlated with both middle–cerebral artery pulsatility index and grade of IVH extension. Other laboratory and clinical parameters were similar between the 2 groups.

Conclusion.—Assessment of plasma adrenomedullin levels in preterm infants in the early postnatal period might be useful for detection of infants at increased risk for IVH. The mechanism of the increase in adrenomedullin and its relevance to the pathophysiology of IVH remain to be elucidated.

▶ Adrenomedullin is a vasoactive peptide recently isolated from pheochromocytoma tissue, which appears to act by inducing vasodilatation through increasing cAMP in tissues of origin. Cultured endothelial and smooth muscle cells bear that capacity and adrenomedullin is found in CNS tissue and CSF, where it appears to play a role in the cardiovascular readjustments after fetal brain injury, particularly in IVH. The diagnosis of IVH is conventionally made by observing changes in the CNS sonolucency, which appear 72 to 96 hours after birth in such cases. The possibility of earlier detection offers the promise, as yet unproven, that prophylactic therapy in the first few days of life might prevent the reperfusion brain injury where recovery from brain injury and appearance of hypertension increases cerebral blood flow and causes brain disruption through extravasation or infiltration of blood into tissues devitalized by earlier hypoxic ischemic injury.

In a series of newborn admissions to the ICU, ranging from 27 to 35 weeks of gestational age, blood was obtained before 6 hours of life and assayed for adrenomedullin by radioimmunoassay. Multiple pregnancies and products of hypertensives, diabetics, and infected pregnancies as well as anomalous fetuses were excluded. Twenty-four infants subsequently proved to have IVH on 72-hour cranial US, and these were compared with 48 newborn neonatal ICU admissions matched for age without IVH with respect to plasma adrenomedullin concentration. Clinical and Doppler data were compared retrospectively.

As Figure 1 discloses, there was a striking increase in plasma adrenomedullin concentration in infants with the subsequent diagnosis of IVH. Retrospective analysis demonstrated these infants to have elevated internal cerebral artery pulsativity indexes which varied directly with the concentration of adrenomedullin and the severity of brain injury. Though more case experience is very desirable, this test may prove to be a reliable early indicator of subsequently diagnosable IVH in preterm newborns and open the door to their prophylactic management.

T. H. Kirschbaum, MD

Association Between Genetic Variation in the Gene for Insulin-Like Growth Factor-I and Low Birthweight
Vaessen N, Janssen JA, Heutink P, et al (Erasmus Med Centre, Rotterdam, The Netherlands)
Lancet 359:1036-1037, 2002   10–11

Introduction.—Low birth weight is strongly predictive of diabetes and cardiovascular disease in later life. The relationship between a polymorphism in the gene for insulin-like growth factor-I (IGF-I), which has been shown to increase the risk of type 2 diabetes and myocardial infarction, and low birth weight was examined.

Methods.—Birth weight data and DNA samples were obtained in 463 adults, 93 of whom had type 2 diabetes. Clinical data were collected without knowledge of genotype. A questionnaire was used to obtain data concerning health status, birth weight, and family history of diabetes mellitus. Height and weight were measured, and body mass index was ascertained.

Results.—Absence of the 192 bp allele was correlated with a 215 g decrease in birth weight, compared with persons homozygous for this allele (95% CI, −411 to −10). Heterozygous persons and those who were homozygous for the wild-type allele did not differ significantly. The difference in birth weight between genotypes was most notable for persons with a history of diabetes in the mother ($P = .001$). The mean birth weight was higher for persons with a history of maternal diabetes versus those with no maternal history of diabetes ($P = .03$) (Table 1). In the group with a history of maternal diabetes, the absence of the 192 bp allele was correlated with a 600 g lower birth weight versus those who were homozygous for this allele ($P = .03$). There was no correlation between genotype and weight or obesity in adulthood. The IGF-I genotype was strongly correlated with postnatal weight gain, defined as a shift within the weight distribution to a higher quartile. In persons homozygous for the 192 bp allele, just under one tenth had a shift toward the mean weight of the general population during life. In persons without the 192 bp allele, this weight gain was observed for more than one quarter of persons ($P = .001$).

Conclusion.—Genetic variation affecting fetal growth could be responsible for the relationship between low birth weight and susceptibility to diabetes and cardiovascular disease in later life.

► Although this work provides only supportive evidence for a hypothesis concerning the purported genetic basis for a relationship among fetal growth retardation, insulin resistance, and the increased risk of hypertension and arte-

TABLE 1.—Association Between a Polymorphism in IGF-I and Birthweight

| | | All | | Participants With a History of Maternal Diabetes | |
IGF-I genotype	n	Mean Difference (95% CI)	p*	n	Mean Difference (95% CI)	p†
Homozygous 192 bp allele	195	3299 (3196-3402)	—	37	3442 (3173-3657)	—
Heterozygous 192 bp allele	204	3296 (3196-3396)	0·74	42	3488 (3229-3714)	0·83
No 192 bp allele	64	3084 (2934-3234)	0·04	10	2842 (2354-3330)	0·03

Genotypes based on presence of wild-type (192 bp) allele
*Based on *t* test.
†Based on Mann-Whitney *U* test.
(Courtesy of Vaessen N, Janssen JA, Heutink P, et al: Association between genetic variation in the gene for insulin-like growth factor-I and low birthweight. *Lancet* 359:1036-1037, 2002. Reprinted with permission from Elsevier Science.)

riosclerotic heart disease in later life, it affords an opportunity to review some important research prospects. IGF-1 is a somatomedin (somatomedin C), one of several substances representing the intermediate response between human growth hormone and tissue growth.[1-3] Produced largely by the liver, its production is stimulated by fetal insulin and has a direct effect on newborn birth weight, pancreatic islet cell development, and newborn growth. Decreased IGF-1 concentrations have been implicated in type 2 diabetes mellitus and adult cardiovascular disease. The gene for its expression, located on chromosome 6, contains a promoter sequence for which a homozygous 192–base pair deletion results in decreased IGF-1 activity, decreased height at birth, decreased insulin production, and an increased risk of development of type 2 diabetes mellitus and myocardial infarction.[4] This study is based on demographic and clinical data coupled with birth weight, height, and body mass index, and DNA analyses in 463 women, 93 of whom have type 2 diabetes. Those homozygous for the deletional mutation showed a significant decrease in mean birth weight compared with those who lacked the mutation or were heterozygous for it. The reduced mean birth weight was maximal in maternal diabetics; presumably they also share the low capacity for insulin production imposed by the homozygous mutation. The smaller infants shared accelerated newborn weight increase, a common finding in infants with impaired glucose sensing, impaired insulin secretion, or both.

Some alternative explanations can't be excluded and need to be explored. Changes in the pattern of concentrations of 7 IGF-binding proteins may be important as are changes in IGF-2 which, acting directly or by binding to newborn IGF-1 receptors, may alter results. Genetic mechanisms for the impact of low birth weight on later life are currently actively being explored as an additional alternative to the Barker hypothesis, which posits fetal metabolic adjustments to placental nutrient deficiencies, and increasingly suffers from the lack of objective supportive data.[5,6] Defective expression of IGF-1 may explain the linkage of fetal growth retardation, insulin resistance, and later life cardiovascular events.

T. H. Kirschbaum, MD

References

1. 1992 YEAR BOOK OF OBSTETRICS, GYNECOLOGY, AND WOMEN'S HEALTH, pp 122-124.
2. 1995 YEAR BOOK OF OBSTETRICS, GYNECOLOGY, AND WOMEN'S HEALTH, pp 123-124.
3. 1996 YEAR BOOK OF OBSTETRICS, GYNECOLOGY, AND WOMEN'S HEALTH, pp 17-21.
4. Vaessen N, Heutink P, Janssen JA, et al: A polymorphism in the gene for IGF-I: Functional properties and risk for type 2 diabetes and myocardial infarction. *Diabetes* 50:637-642, 2001.
5. 2002 YEAR BOOK OF OBSTETRICS, GYNECOLOGY, AND WOMEN'S HEALTH, pp 73-77.
6. 2002 YEAR BOOK OF OBSTETRICS, GYNECOLOGY, AND WOMEN'S HEALTH, pp 254-256.

Maternal Folate Supplementation in Pregnancy and Protection Against Acute Lymphoblastic Leukaemia in Childhood: A Case-Control Study

Thompson JR, Fitz Gerald P, Willoughby MLN, et al (Cancer Found of Western Australia, West Perth; Univ of Newcastle, New South Wales, Australia; Princess Margaret Hosp, Perth, Australia; et al)
Lancet 358:1935-1940, 2001   10–12

Background.—The most common childhood cancer in developed countries is acute lymphoblastic leukemia. This disease has few recognized risk factors or preventive measures, but it has been associated with prenatal exposure to ionizing radiation, some chromosomal abnormalities, an infective agent, the child's immune response, socioeconomic status, maternal and perinatal factors, a variety of environmental exposures, and parental occupational history. Risk factors associated with common acute lymphoblastic leukemia were assessed.

Methods.—Known and suspected risk factors for common acute lymphoblastic leukemia were investigated from 1984 to 1992 in a population-based case-control study of children in Western Australia from ages 0 to 14 years. Eighty-three of the children were drawn from the state's sole referral center for pediatric cancer and matched with 166 control subjects for age and sex. The controls were recruited by a mail survey of people randomly selected from among the states' registered voters. The mothers of the children were interviewed, and the fathers completed a self-administered questionnaire.

Results.—A protective association was observed between iron or folate supplementation in pregnancy and the risk of common acute lymphoblastic leukemia in the children. The odds ratio for iron alone was 0.75. Only 1 mother reported taking folate without iron. On further analyses of the use of folate with or without iron, it was discovered that there is little variation in the protective effect by time of first use of supplements or for the duration of consumption. This association was not weakened by adjustment for potentially confounding variables.

Conclusions.—This investigation of the risk factors associated with acute lymphoblastic leukemia yielded unexpected findings, suggesting that the risk of common acute lymphoblastic leukemia in children can be reduced by folate supplementation during pregnancy.

▶ This unexpected, and as yet unexplained finding, came from a population-based cohort study of 83 children up to 14 years of age in western Australia in whom the diagnosis of acute lymphoblastic leukemia (ALL) was made. This is the most prevalent of childhood leukemias; other T- and B-cell-derived diseases were excluded from entry to avoid complexity. Univariate analysis was used to compare these 83 with 166 controls with respect to several demographic and environmental variables. Although relation to pesticides, paints, and solvents were noted, by far the strongest covariant appeared to be maternal use of iron or folate during pregnancy, inversely related to ALL occurrence. More specifically, the risk ratio associated with iron use alone was not significantly different from unity, but for folate with or without iron, independent of the time and duration of use of either during pregnancy, consistently strong *P* values ranging from .0009 to .0042 resulted. By using multivariate statistics to test for confounding relations with other variables, the relation between apparent folate protection against ALL remained strong. The authors' original intent was to search for new hypotheses regarding the origin of ALL. Because folate deficiencies result in decreased availability of tissue methionine, which in turn diminishes DNA methylation and impairs DNA production and repair, they have unearthed a relation and we're certain to learn more about as other investigators pursue it.

T. H. Kirschbaum, MD

Postnatal Adaptation of Brain Circulation in Preterm Infants
Pellicer A, Valverde E, Gayá F, et al (La Paz Univ, Madrid)
Pediatr Neurol 24:103-109, 2001   10–13

Background.—Coupling between cerebral blood flow (CBF) and metabolic and anatomical development has been well described in neonates. However, there is little information available regarding the regulation of the cerebral circulation in the newborn infant. In the human neonate, changes in brain hemodynamics have been assessed primarily by Doppler studies, which have yielded qualitative information on postnatal cerebral circulatory adaptation. Early serial quantitative data on brain hemodynamics, particularly in preterm infants, are few. This study was conducted to analyze adaptive changes in different parameters of brain perfusion in stable preterm infants in the early postnatal period. This period was selected for study because it is the time during which most brain lesions occur. Two noninvasive methods were used: color Doppler flow imaging and near-infrared spectroscopy. Of special interest were differences in behavior between large and small vessels. Also investigated was the association between brain damage documented by sonographic criteria and persistent distinctive patterns of brain perfusion.

Methods.—The studies were conducted on 35 preterm infants on the first and second days after delivery. Near-infrared spectroscopy was used to measure CBF and cerebral blood volume (CBV). Color Doppler flow imaging was used to determine the CBF velocity and resistance index in the internal carotid, anterior cerebral, and striate arteries. Serial cerebral US studies were also performed to detect changes in brain parenchymal echogenicity or intraventricular hemorrhage (IVH).

Results.—There was a significant increase in CBF and CBF velocity with time, independent of the mean blood pressure, partial pressure of oxygen, partial pressure of carbon dioxide, hematocrit, or glycemia. However, the CBV and resistance index were unchanged. Sonography demonstrated no differences in postnatal CBF or CBF velocity changes, regardless of whether patients had or did not have parenchymal lesions or IVH. Higher CBV values were noted on the second day in infants with IVH compared with those without IVH (Table 2).

TABLE 2.—Cerebral Hemodynamic Studies

		First Day	Second Day	P Value
CBF		25.1 ± 2	34 ± 3	P < 0.01
CBV		2.7 ± 0.3	2.9 ± 0.2	NS
TMFV	ACA	13.6 ± 1.1	15.9 ± 1.1	P < 0.05
RI	ACA	0.77 ± 0.01	0.74 ± 0.02	NS
TMFV	ICA	14.5 ± 1.0	20.3 ± 1.6	P < 0.01
RI	ICA	0.8 ± 0.01	0.77 ± 0.02	NS
TMFV	SA	5 ± 0.3	6 ± 0.3	P < 0.05
RI	SA	0.57 ± 0.01	0.58 ± 0.01	NS

Values expressed as mean ± S.E.M.

Note: Values are expressed as mean ± SEM.

Abbreviations: ACA, Anterior cerebral artery; *CBF,* cerebral blood flow (mL/hg/min); *CBV,* cerebral blood volume (mL/hg); *ICA,* internal carotid artery; *NS,* not significant; *RI,* resistance index; *SA,* striate artery; *TMFV,* temporal mean flow velocity (cm/s)

(Reprinted by permission of the publisher from Pellicer A, Valverde E, Gayá F, et al: Postnatal adaptation of brain circulation in preterm infants. *Pediatr Neurol* 24:103-109, 2001. Copyright 2001 with permission from Elsevier Science.)

Conclusion.—It appears that early coupling of CBF and metabolic demands is independent of blood pressure and that improved venous return, rather than vasodilation, could be important in this condition.

▶ This study aimed at evaluating preterm newborn normal circulatory adjustments, and the implications for IVH are important for giving us a chance to compare CBF rates obtained by classical means with Doppler velocimetry. Near-infrared spectroscopy allows both CBF measurements using the Fick principal and CBV measurements using indicator dilution techniques, all based on 6 to 8 seconds of transient increase in infant blood partial pressure of oxygen and oxygen saturation and subsequent changes in their concentrations in blood.

Thirty-five stable preterm infants weighing less than 1.5 kg at birth and free of anomalies were studied. CBF is measured by transiently increasing oxyhemoglobin, through increasing newborn ambient air oxygen concentration for 6 to 8 seconds, as an internal tracer, and measuring CBF as a quotient of tracer accumulation with time and tracer supplied and by using transmission light spectral differences between reduced and oxidized hemoglobin to measure oxyhemoglobin. Total cerebral hemoglobin, measurable to a depth of up to 8 cm across paired infrared sources, and sensors on the newborn skull, using the Beer-Lambert law and some algebraic manipulations and known physical constants, were involved in the calculations. Readers may wish to refer to the references below for the techniques.[1,2] At least 2 sets of measurements were done at mean ages of 16 and 38 hours. On both occasions, major infant cardiovascular and respiratory variables were normal.

During the roughly 24 hours between the first and second days of life, mean CBF increased by 35% without changes in CBV. During the same time, Doppler studies showed significant increase in temporal lone mean flow velocity, but at the same time no changes in color Doppler–derived resistance indexes from internal carotid, anterior cerebral, and striate arteries were noted. Evidence of hemorrhagic or ischemic brain lesions in the interim resulted in no changes in Doppler findings, CBF velocity, or CBF measurements using the Fick principle. In contrast, CBV measurements increased significantly in infants with hemorrhagic brain lesions. The findings indicate that increased CBF in the early neonatal period is driven neither by blood pressure nor brain blood volume changes. What is most interesting is the failure of Doppler velocimetry to reflect these changes, interpreted as resistance indexes, which were apparent from classic Fick-derived CBF measurements. The lesson is that one should beware of inferring CBF rate information from Doppler velocimetry studies in the newborn brain, at least in this weight range.

T. H. Kirschbaum, MD

References

1. Edwards AD, Wyatt JS, Richardson D, et al: Cotside measurement of cerebral blood flow in ill preterm infants by near infrared spectroscopy. *Lancet* 2:770-771,1988.
2. Wyatt JS, Cope M, Delpy DT, et al:. Quantitation of cerebral blood volume in human infants by near infrared spectroscopy: *J Apply Physiol* 68:1086-1091,1990.

Active Transport of Nitrofurantoin Into Human Milk
Gerk PM, Kuhn RJ, Desai NS, et al (Univ of Kentucky, Lexington)
Pharmacotherapy 21:669-675, 2001   10–14

Background.—Nitrofurantoin is a weakly acidic agent with a pKa of 7.2. Because it is actively excreted in the renal tubule, nitrofurantoin is bacteriostatic or bactericidal in the urine, depending on the concentration. It is prescribed to lactating women for the treatment of urinary tract infections and remains one of the top 200 prescription drugs in the United States. There are differing reports regarding the extent of transfer of nitrofurantoin into human milk. The American Academy of Pediatrics has classified the agent as usually compatible with breast-feeding. However, some patients who receive nitrofurantoin may have rare but serious side effects, such as chronic liver disease, cholestatic hepatitis, or hemolytic anemia in patients who are glucose-6-phosphate dehydrogenase deficient. Thus, there is a clinical concern regarding the transfer of nitrofurantoin into breast milk. The extent to which nitrofurantoin is transferred into human milk was investigated in a prospective, single-dose pharmacokinetic study.

Methods.—In a university-affiliated clinical research center, 4 healthy lactating women from 8 to 26 weeks post partum received a single, oral, 100-mg dose of nitrofurantoin macrocrystals with food. Serial serum and milk samples were obtained and analyzed by high-performance liquid chromatography. The milk pH, milk fat partitioning, and protein-binding in serum and milk were determined. The predicted milk-serum ratio (M:S) was compared with the observed M:S.

Results.—The predicted nitrofurantoin M:S was 0.28 ± 0.05, while the observed M:S was 6.21 ± 2.71. The average milk concentration was 1.3 mg/

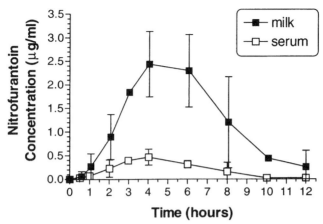

FIGURE 1.—Mean (±SD) milk and serum concentrations in 4 lactating women after a 100-mg dose of nitrofurantoin macrocrystals. Samples at 3 and 10 hours were not obtained for subjects 1 and 2; only the corresponding means are presented. (Courtesy of Gerk PM, Kuhn RJ, Desai NS, et al: Active transport of nitrofurantoin into human milk. *Pharmacotherapy* 21:669-675, 2001.)

L, and the estimated suckling infant dosage was 0.2 mg/kg/d, or 6% of the maternal dose (milligrams per kilogram) (Fig 1).

Conclusion.—Nitrofurantoin is actively transported into human milk at concentrations that are significantly in excess of the concentrations found in serum. These findings should raise concern for suckling breast-feeding infants under the age of 1 month and for infants with a high frequency of glucose-6-phosphate dehydrogenase deficiency or sensitivity to nitrofurantoin.

▶ Nitrofurantoin, often given as Macrodantin, is a common standard therapeutic for treating acute and preventing recurrent urinary tract infection in pregnancy. Its popularity is based on its bacteriostatic and bactericidal properties in urine (depending upon its concentration there) and the low incidence of side effects in newborns, likely related to its low maternal blood concentration. Basing their work on a simple diffusional model, the authors predicted the concentration of the drug in human milk and confirmed it by measuring milk concentrations generally 5 times higher than maternal blood concentrations 4 to 6 hours after the administration of 100 mg of nitrofurantoin. The estimated fetal transfer of approximately 10% of the maternal dose is likely to be of consequence only for very small infants less than 1 month of age; those receiving neonatal nitrofurantoin as well; and those with G6-P dehydrogenase deficiency, which complicates its metabolism.

T. H. Kirschbaum, MD

GYNECOLOGY

11 Gynecologic Urology

Tension-Free Vaginal Tape Operation: Results of the Austrian Registry
Tamussino KF, for the Austrian Urogynecology Working Group (Univ of Graz, Austria; et al)
Obstet Gynecol 98:732-736, 2001   11–1

Background.—The tension-free vaginal tape (TVT) system has rapidly become popular in Europe and elsewhere for the correction of stress urinary incontinence despite the absence of completed randomized trials comparing TVT with standard anti-incontinence operations. More than 150,000 TVT sets have been sold throughout the world, with more than 6700 in Austria by May 2001. The use of and perioperative complications associated with the TVT procedure for the correction of stress urinary incontinence were assessed.

Methods.—All 95 departments of gynecology in Austria were contacted by mail about participating in a central registry. A total of 55 units agreed to participate. These centers completed questionnaires regarding patients undergoing the TVT operation and collected information on patient, surgical, and postoperative data.

Results.—A total of 2795 patients in 55 centers were enrolled. Overall, 773 patients (28%) had undergone previous surgery for incontinence or prolapse. A total of 1540 TVT procedures (59%) were performed as isolated operations, and 1155 (41%) were performed in conjunction with other procedures. The median operating time for the TVT procedures alone was 30 minutes. In patients undergoing TVT only, 44% of the procedures were performed with local anesthesia, 43% with regional anesthesia, and 12% with general anesthesia. Postoperative bladder drainage in these patients was obtained by intermittent catheterization in 24% of the patients, an indwelling urethral catheter in 63% of the patients, and a suprapubic catheter in 9% of the patients. The overall rate of bladder perforation was 2.7%, with a higher rate (4.4%) among patients who had previously undergone surgery than among those without previous surgery. Most of the patients who underwent the isolate procedure were able to void the next day. A total of 68 patients (2.4%) required reoperation for reasons related to the tape.

Conclusions.—The tension-free vaginal tape procedure is frequently performed in Austria, with considerable variations in clinical practice. Severe complications were rare in this series, but the risk of bladder perforation was increased in patients with previous surgery.

▶ When a new surgical procedure is introduced, there is a tendency to report small series of patients from individual surgeons or centers, most of which extol the virtues of the procedure. Generally, there is a comparison with the results of other procedures that have been designed to correct the specific problem under consideration, and rarely is a randomized controlled trial attempted. Therefore, it takes the cumulative experience of several operators and centers to identify the actual benefits of the procedure, as well as to determine potential complications and long-range success rates. Recently, the TVT operation has enjoyed wide attention because of its ease of performance and, as expected, reports on the results of relatively small numbers of patients have begun to filter into the literature. The study reported here assessed the use and perioperative complications of the operations in 55 gynecology units in Austria representing 2795 patients, 773 of whom had undergone previous surgery for incontinence or prolapse. In this series, 59% of the patients underwent the TVT operation alone and 1155 in combination with other procedures. The authors were able to show that the operation could be performed quickly (average, 30 minutes) and could be performed with regional or local anesthesia. As with other sling-type procedures, one quarter of the patients required intermittent catheterization until voiding was re-established. The complication rate included 2.7% bladder perforation (which was noted to be 2-fold higher in patients with previous surgery) and an additional 2.4% of the patients required removal or cutting of the tape because of inability to void. Fortunately, there were only 19 hematomas and 1 bowel injury in the group.

The TVT operation appears to be a useful addition to the treatment tools for stress urinary incontinence. This study provided some good information about its performance and the complications that may occur with its use. The next step in assessing the efficacy of this procedure is to evaluate long-term follow-up, and hopefully this group will be able to provide us with that information.

M. A. Stenchever, MD

The Tension-Free Vaginal Tape Procedure in Women With Previous Failed Stress Incontinence Surgery
Azam U, Frazer MI, Kozman EL, et al (Warrington Gen Hosp, Cheshire, England; Royal Victoria Infirmary, Newcastle upon Tyne, England; Kirwan Hosp for Women, Townsville, Australia)
J Urol 166:554-556, 2001   11–2

Background.—An increased number of physicians now choose to use tension-free vaginal tape (TVT) procedures in women with urinary stress incontinence. However, most research in this area has focused on women who underwent TVT procedures as the primary treatment for urinary stress incontinence rather than women who had undergone previous failed surgeries. Researchers present 1-year follow-up results from TVT surgeries in women with histories of unsuccessful stress incontinence surgery.

Methods.—The TVT procedure was used in 67 women with previous histories of failed urinary stress incontinence surgery. Outcomes were measured at 3 months by cystometry, urinary pad loss, and subjective questioning, and outcome categories included whether there was a cure, significant improvement, or failure. At 1 year, further subjective questioning was done.

Results.—The procedure did not result in any serious morbidity. Eighty-one percent of the women (n = 54) were considered cured at 12 months; 6% (n = 4) were considered significantly improved; and 13% (n = 9) were considered no better. The median pad test values for patients considered significantly improved (n = 4) was 76 to 11.3 g. In patients with surgery that was considered to have failed (n = 9), the median pad test value ranged from 103 to 59 g.

Conclusions.—A success rate similar to that of conventional sling surgery was seen with use of the TVT procedure in candidates who had previous surgery for urinary stress incontinence that failed. Postoperative morbidity and operative complications occurred with low frequency. However, the authors believe that surgeons should not use TVT surgery as a procedure in this patient population until they gain considerable experience with the procedure in virgin cases.

▶ The results of this study of 67 women who had previously failed surgery for stress urinary incontinence and were now treated with a tension-free vaginal tape procedure offered 1-year follow-up information with respect to the success of the procedure. The authors evaluated success using cystometry and the findings of urine loss on pelvic pads at 3 months of follow-up and on subjective questioning at 3 months and 1 year of follow-up. By their definition, at 12 months, 54 women (81%) were cured, four (6%) were significantly improved, and 13% were considered no better than prior to surgery. Although the authors reported 13 cases (19%) of bladder perforation, most of these occurred in the early stages of the study, when, as they point out, they were in the learning curve for the procedure. They reported no hematomas. Interestingly, a few patients who did not have preoperative bladder instability suffered from it after the procedure.

The value of this study is that it demonstrated that the success rate of this procedure is similar to the success rate of other procedures utilized for the treatment of stress urinary incontinence, such as the Burch procedure. It also demonstrated that perforation of the bladder is possible, particularly after previous procedures have been utilized, and that cystoscopy should be part of the operative procedure to ensure that long-term damage does not occur.

M. A. Stenchever, MD

Combined Genitourinary Prolapse Repair and Prophylactic Tension-Free Vaginal Tape in Women With Severe Prolapse and Occult Stress Urinary Incontinence: Preliminary Results

Gordon D, Gold RS, Pauzner D, et al (Tel Aviv Univ, Israel)
Urology 58:547-550, 2001   11–3

Background.—Continent patients with positive stress test results on repositioning of severe genitourinary prolapse are thought to be at high risk for the development of symptomatic stress urinary incontinence (SUI) postoperatively. An assessment was made of whether a prophylactic, tension-free vaginal tape (TVT) procedure done during prolapse repair would prevent the development of postoperative SUI in such women.

Methods.—Thirty women with a mean age of 64.5 years, who were clinically continent but who had severe genitourinary prolapse and occult SUI, were enrolled in the study. All women had urethral hypermobility. None had intrinsic sphincter deficiency. The patients underwent genitourinary prolapse repair and concomitant TVT to prevent postoperative SUI. Follow-up lasted for at least 1 year, with urodynamic studies done at 3 to 6 months after surgery.

Findings.—Postoperative symptomatic SUI did not develop in any of the patients. However, 10% of the patients had a positive stress test response during their postoperative urodynamic assessment. Thirty percent had detrusor instability preoperatively, which persisted in 66% postoperatively. In another 13.3% of the patients, postoperative de novo detrusor instability was diagnosed. There were no cases of recurrent urogenital prolapse or evidence of bladder outlet obstruction.

Conclusions.—These preliminary findings are encouraging. In the current series, TVT was an effective prophylactic procedure in clinically continent women with severe prolapse and occult SUI. Longer-term follow-up is needed to verify the durability of these outcomes.

▶ This study suffered from the fact that it was a preliminary study in which no control group was used. All patients had also undergone anterior and posterior colporrhaphy, which may have contributed to the fact that at the relatively short follow-up time of 12 to 24 months, none demonstrated stress urinary incontinence symptomatically, although 3 demonstrated this on urodynamic study. Furthermore, the follow-up was too short to draw any conclusions about whether or not there was an improvement with use of tension-free vaginal tape (TVT). The authors suggested that further studies are necessary, and this is certainly true. A prospective study comparing patients so treated with those who are not treated with TVT, but are otherwise similar, would be extremely helpful.

M. A. Stenchever, MD

Effect of Tension-Free Vaginal Tape Procedure on Urodynamic Continence Indices

Mutone N, Mastropietro M, Brizendine E, et al (Indiana Univ, Indianapolis)
Obstet Gynecol 98:638-645, 2001   11–4

Background.—The tension-free vaginal tape (TVT) procedure has a reported cure rate of 86% at 3 years, which is comparable with other anti-incontinence operations. The TVT procedure is minimally invasive and can be performed with the patient under local anesthesia. This procedure also differs from other anti-incontinence procedures by being positioned at the midurethra rather than the urethrovesical junction and by not being anchored to a fixed anatomic structure. Although its effectiveness has been documented, the mechanism by which TVT induces urinary continence is not understood. The difference in measured urethral function before and after a TVT procedure was assessed.

Methods.—The study group included women undergoing a TVT procedure between January 1 and August 31, 2000. Inclusion criteria for the study included a diagnosis of urodynamically proved genuine stress incontinence with or without intrinsic sphincter deficiency. Multichannel urodynamic testing was performed preoperatively and at 6 weeks postoperatively, and maximum urethral closure pressure and pressure transmission ratio were recorded. Valsalva leak point pressures were determined at 150 mL and again when the bladder was at full capacity. The cotton swab technique was used to determine resting and straining urethral angles. In addition, all of the study subjects completed the Incontinence Impact Questionnaire and Urodynamic Distress Inventory preoperatively and postoperatively.

Results.—A total of 35 consecutive women were studied, and 23 women (65.7%) had a preoperative diagnosis of intrinsic sphincter deficiency. The subjective and objective success rates for TVT were 91% and 83%, respectively, and there was an 86.8% improvement in the Incontinence Impact Questionnaire score and a 72.9% improvement in the Urodynamic Distress Inventory score. The mean change in maximum urethral closure pressure was −1.3 cm water, whereas the pressure transmission ratio increased by a mean of 15.7%. The mean decrease in straining urethral angle was 16.3°. Patients who were cured and demonstrated hypermobility preoperatively also demonstrated hypermobility after the TVT procedure.

Conclusions.—The TVT procedure resulted in a significant increase in pressure transmission ratio but not maximum urethral closure pressure, changes that are similar to those reported after traditional sling procedures and retropubic urethropexy. It appears that the effectiveness of the TVT procedure is not dependent on a clinically significant change in the straining urethral angle.

▶ The TVT procedure for urinary stress incontinence is becoming quite popular internationally. It is therefore important, in addition to learning about its success and complication rates, that we also try to understand how it works. The authors of this study included both women with genuine stress incontinence and women who also had intrinsic sphincter deficiency. They studied patients urodynamically 6 weeks postoperatively and found an excellent subjective and objective improvement. They demonstrated that the increase in pressure transmission ratio seen following the procedure was consistent with studies of other retropubic urethropexy and sling procedures. This was in spite of the fact that they noted no change in resting urethral closure pressure. It is of interest that improvement occurred in the patients with intrinsic sphincter dysfunction, even though bladder neck hypermobility continued postoperatively. Unlike sling procedures, the tape in the TVT procedure is not anchored. The authors speculated that the improvement in support of the bladder neck with straining might have been due to the dense collagen that forms around the tape, thus giving support under stress. Hopefully, the authors will follow up these patients to determine to what degree the improvement persists.

M. A. Stenchever, MD

Vaginal Retropubic Urethropexy With Intraoperative Cystometry for Treating Urinary Stress Incontinence
Clark AD, Salloum MS (St Mary's Hosp, Portsmouth, Hampshire, UK)
BJU Internatl 88:49-52, 2001   11–5

Background.—Many surgical approaches for the treatment of urinary stress incontinence (USI) have been published. The urethropexy provides a new permanent artificial platform or hammock support to the deficient arcus tendineus fascia pelvis or pubocervical fascia, which stabilizes the urethra and the bladder neck. The efficacy of a vaginal retropubic urethropexy with intraoperative cystometry in women with USI was investigated.

Methods.—One hundred patients with genuine stress incontinence as seen on urodynamic evaluation were treated with vaginal retropubic urethropexy. Ninety-six patients were followed up for 1 year.

Findings.—Ninety-five percent of the patients were cured of USI at 1 year. In the remaining 5%, stress incontinence recurred. Complications consisted mainly of suture erosion, which occurred in 6% of the patients.

Conclusions.—This method of urethropexy has yielded excellent outcomes to date. Complication and morbidity rates have been low. A randomized, controlled study comparing this technique with standard established procedures is now needed.

▶ The authors demonstrate a procedure that can be carried out vaginally to position the bladder neck behind the pubic symphysis. They demonstrate a means of testing its efficacy utilizing intraoperative cystometry. Of the 95 patients in the series, 95% were considered cured at 1 year, and of this 91, 9 had previously had stress urinary incontinence surgery. The procedure was free of complications except for a few cases that had erosion of the suture, and thus the authors have demonstrated a good outcome with an acceptable complication rate. I have performed a variation of this procedure for a number of years with good results. It is often performed, as the authors point out, in conjunction with other procedures for pelvic relaxation, such as vaginal hysterectomy with anterior and posterior colporrhaphy. To obtain results that are comparable to a retropubic urethropexy using a vaginal approach is quite satisfying for both physician and patient.

M. A. Stenchever, MD

Early Results of Pubovaginal Sling Lysis by Midline Sling Incision
Nitti VW, Carlson KV, Blaivas JG, et al (New York Univ; Cornell Univ, New York; North Texas Ctr for Urinary Control, Fort Worth)
Urology 59:47-52, 2002   11–6

Background.—Sling procedures, shown to be effective in the long term, can be applied to all types of stress incontinence. These authors have been using sling incision as a primary procedure for obstruction after pubovaginal sling placement. The technique and its outcomes were reported.

Methods.—Nineteen women undergoing pubovaginal sling lysis for obstruction were included in the review. The mean age was 57 years. A midline incision of the sling was performed using a transvaginal approach without formal urethrolysis.

Findings.—Seventy-nine percent of the women had an autologous rectus fascial sling; 16%, an allographic fascia lata sling; and 5%, a polypropylene sling. Sixty-three percent of the women required catheterization initially for urinary retention. The mean time to sling lysis was 10.6 months from initial surgery. The patients were followed up for a mean of 12 months. Sling lysis was successful in 84% of the patients. In 17%, stress incontinence recurred. The procedure was associated with no significant perioperatuve complications.

Conclusion.—Pubovaginal sling lysis without formal urethrolysis appears to effectively alleviate obstruction. In the authors' experience, it is also safe. Rates of success and recurrent stress incontinence are similar to those associated with formal urethrolysis.

▶ Women who undergo operative procedures for urinary stress incontinence often suffer from urinary retention postoperatively and require intermittent catheterization. This problem is particularly common in women who have undergone urethral sling procedures. The authors reported a small series of 19 women who underwent a simple pubovaginal sling lysis, with an overall success rate (return to spontaneous voiding) of 84%. Stress incontinence recurred in 17% of patients, which is comparable to the recurrence rate of stress incontinence in other patients who have undergone procedures to relieve urinary retention following a sling procedure.

The success of this procedure in terms of restored continence in the majority of the patients is probably related to the fact that the bladder neck is supported by scarring following the operation, and that over time the sling itself is no longer necessary. However, the fact that 17% of the patients suffered a recurrence of their stress incontinence showed that this effect was by no means universal. How frustrating it must have been for these patients to undergo 2 procedures and still be incontinent.

M. A. Stenchever, MD

Laparoscopic Burch Colposuspension: A Randomized Controlled Trial Comparing Two Transperitoneal Surgical Techniques
Zullo F, Palomba S, Piccione F, et al (Univ of Catanzaro, Italy; Univ of Messina, Italy)
Obstet Gynecol 98:783-788, 2001   11–7

Background.—The transperitoneal and preperitoneal approaches to laparoscopic Burch procedures both allow fixation by different means, including mesh, clips, tacks, fibrin glue, and sutures. The efficacies of 2 transperitoneal laparoscopic Burch procedures were compared.

Methods.—Sixty women with genuine stress incontinence were assigned randomly to 1 of 2 groups. Treatment consisted of the transperitoneal laparoscopic Burch procedure using nonabsorbable sutures (group A) or prolene mesh fixed with tacks or staples (group B). Outcomes were assessed by subjective and objective measures.

Findings.—The subjective failure rate, defined by patients' rating of their urine loss on a visual analogue scale, did not differ significantly between groups at various follow-up evaluations. At 3 months after surgery, the failure rate was 0% in both groups. At 6 months, the rates were 3.7% and 3.8% in groups A and B, respectively, and at 12 months, they were 7.4% and 15.4%, respectively. The objective failure rate also did not differ between groups at 3 and 6 months. However, at 12 months, group A had a significantly lower failure rate, at 11.1%, than group B, at 26.9%.

Conclusion.—The use of sutures in transperitoneal laparoscopic Burch colposuspension was more effective than the use of mesh. In addition, the cost of suture is much lower than that of mesh fixed with tacks and staples.

▶ The Burch colposuspension procedure has been one of the standard procedures for the treatment of stress urinary incontinence for many years. In recent years, it has been demonstrated that it could be performed laparoscopically. This has led to various technical modifications including the number of sutures utilized and the utilization of materials affixed with tacks or staples.

In the current study, the authors demonstrated that in their hands, performing the transperitoneal laparoscopic Burch procedure with nonabsorbable sutures had a greater success rate than performing it with mesh and staples. Of interest was the fact that there was little difference in the subjective failure rate between the 2 groups of patients at 3 and 6 months postoperative. However, by 1 year, the failure rate was twice as great for the mesh and staple group than for the suture group. It is difficult to understand this, except that the placement with a needle may be more secure than the placement with a staple. Nevertheless, suturing has a further advantage because the cost is much less than the mesh and staple approach.

When a new procedure is introduced, there are bound to be variations performed by different surgeons. It is therefore important to carefully evaluate these variations to choose those that work best. The authors have done this with respect to these 2 techniques.

M. A. Stenchever, MD

High Failure Rate Using Allograft Fascia Lata in Pubovaginal Sling Surgery for Female Stress Urinary Incontinence
Huang Y-H, Lin ATL, Chen K-K, et al (Natl Yang-Ming Univ, Taipei, Taiwan, Republic of China)
Urology 58:943-946, 2001   11–8

Background.—The use of pubovaginal sling surgery has become a popular approach to the treatment of female stress urinary incontinence (SUI). There are several options available for use as the sling, including autologous fascia, synthetic materials, and allograft fascia. The harvest of autologous rectus fascia or fascia lata for use as a sling material has become commonplace. However, the harvest of fascia requires additional operating time and increases the morbidity and risk of other negative effects, including hematoma formation, wound infection, herniation, postoperative pain, and longer hospital stay. Synthetic materials have also been used recently for the sling material, but there are several chronic complications associated with these materials, including fistula formation, nonhealing of the vaginal wound, sinus tract formation, and chronic wound infection. Allograft fascia lata is tissue harvested from humans, usually from cadavers, and it has recently been proposed as an attractive option for sling material in pubovaginal sling surgery. The viability of allograft fascia lata as a sling material was explored.

Methods.—Sling surgery for SUI was performed in a total of 18 women with a mean age of 51.7 years from March 1999 to July 1999. Solvent-dehydrated gamma-irradiated human fascia lata measuring 7×2 cm was used to form the sling. A questionnaire was used to collect the results.

Results.—The patients were followed up for a mean of 9.2 months. Thirteen patients reported that they considered the surgery to be successful or to have improved their condition by a mean of 82.5% subjective improvement. Significant failure occurred in 5 patients (27.8%), with full recurrence of incontinence within 3 to 6 months.

Conclusions.—The use of solvent dehydrated gamma-irradiated allograft fascia resulted in a high failure rate within a short period. These findings prohibit the use of allograft fascia for the treatment of stress urinary incontinence.

▶ This is a small series; however, the outcome for the patients treated was clearly poor when a pubovaginal sling was performed using solvent-dehydrated gamma-irradiated human fascia lata. This is in keeping with reports from other surgeons. The results, therefore, are not surprising. First, the treatment of the fascia lata probably weakened the tissues. Second, it is likely that the host would reject autologous tissue in a relatively short period of time. This was certainly the case. Although autologous tissue is currently used by other specialties, such as ophthalmology and orthopedics, its value in treating stress urinary incontinence appears to be less than favorable and suggests that alternate materials should be used in this operation. Although this series is small, its results and the results of others imply that this is not a technique to be pursued.

M. A. Stenchever, MD

A New Injectable Bulking Agent for Treatment of Stress Urinary Incontinence: Results of a Multicenter, Randomized, Controlled, Double-Blind Study of Durasphere

Lightner D, Calvosa C, Andersen R, et al (Mayo Clinic, Rochester, Minn; Instituto Costaricense de Investigaciones Clinicas, San Jose, Costa Rica; Clinical Research of Washington, Seattle; et al)
Urology 58:12-15, 2001   11–9

Introduction.—Bovine collagen injection therapy is safe and effective in the treatment of intrinsic sphincter deficiency (ISD). The material completely degrades within 9 to 19 months, necessitating repeated injections to sustain a successful result. Durasphere is a new injectable bulking agent that is designed for permanent use. It is biocompatible and is made up of nonmigratory and nonabsorbable pyrolytic carbon-coated zirconium oxide beads suspended in a carrier gel. The safety and effectiveness of Durasphere, compared with bovine collagen, were examined in the treatment of stress urinary incontinence (SUI) caused by ISD in a multicenter, randomized, controlled, double-blind investigation.

Methods.—Three hundred fifty-five women with a diagnosis of SUI caused by ISD were evaluated using a standardized pad test and the Stamey continence grade as the primary end points. The patient age range was 26 to 84 years. All participants had an abdominal leak point pressure of below 90 cm H_2O (average, 51 cm H_2O).

Results.—The 2 materials were equivalent at 12 months after initial injection in terms of improvement in continence grade and pad weight testing. Less Durasphere was injected to achieve clinical results comparable to bovine collagen injections (4.83 mL vs 6.23 mL; $P < .001$). At 1 year after the final treatment, 49 (80.3%) of the 61 women treated with Durasphere had improvement of 1 continence grade or higher, compared with 47 (69.1%) of 68 women treated with bovine collagen (P value for difference = .162). The 2 groups were similar in reports of adverse effects. Participants in the Durasphere group had an increased short-term risk for urgency and urinary retention.

Conclusion.—Durasphere in the treatment of SUI caused by ISD was equally effective compared with bovine collagen and required less injectible material per case. The initial clinical data indicate the potential for greater durability of the clinical effect, with a potential for a permanent solution for SUI caused by ISD in some women.

▶ Durasphere and bovine collagen have equal efficacy and both appear to be safe and effective forms of treatment. Durasphere, however, was designed to be permanent, and may, in the long run, be capable of maintaining continence without repeat injection. Whereas the results of the study are encouraging, further follow-up studies will be necessary to prove its lasting value. The Food and Drug Administration has approved the substance for use as a bulking agent in the treatment of incontinence, so information on its further use for this purpose is probably forthcoming.

M. A. Stenchever, MD

The Routine Use of Cystoscopy With the Burch Procedure
Gill EJ, Elser DM, Bonidie MJ, et al (Virginia Commonwealth Univ, Richmond; Christ Hosp and Med Ctr, Chicago; Western Pennsylvania Hosp, Pittsburgh)
Am J Obstet Gynecol 185:345-348, 2001   11–10

Background.—Pelvic surgery can be complicated by injury to the lower urinary tract. The rate of injury to the lower urinary tract, as detected by routine intraoperative cystoscopy, attributable to the Burch procedure during pelvic surgery was established.

Methods.—One hundred eighty-one women undergoing pelvic surgery for genuine stress urinary incontinence in 1998 and 1999 were included in the retrospective analysis. In all procedures, Burch retropubic urethropexy was used. Intraoperative cystoscopy was done at completion of the procedure, after IV indigo carmine dye was administered.

Findings.—Injuries to the lower urinary tract occurred in 3.3% of the patients. Five of the 6 injuries were cystotomies recognized during surgery. The remaining injury was obstruction to a left ureter, detected by cystoscopy and alleviated by releasing the left paravaginal repair sutures. No unsuspected injuries detected by cystoscopy could be attributed to the Burch procedure.

Conclusions.—In this series, the lower urinary tract injury rate was 3.3%. Only 1 of the 6 injuries went unrecognized until cystoscopy. This injury was attributed to concomitant paravaginal repair rather than to the Burch procedure.

▶ A major current controversy among urogynecologists is whether or not cystoscopy should be performed routinely with all urogynecologic procedures. In fact, some have suggested that it should be performed with all pelvic procedures. Most studies have estimated that the risk of bladder or ureter compromise is somewhere between 1% and 3%. In the current study, it is 3.3%; however, all but 1 of the injuries were recognized at the time of the procedure and repaired. The injury that was not recognized was an obstructed ureter, and this was detected by cystoscopy. The authors are reporting only the problems associated with the Burch procedure, not pelvic operations in general. There is undeniably some risk of injury to the ureter and bladder, but the risk is probably small. However, is performing cystoscopy on all patients undergoing pelvic surgery cost-effective and will cystoscopy pick up all potential injuries? We know, for instance, that damage to the blood supply of the lower ureter may lead to ureteral complications such as ureterovaginal fistula. In addition, pelvic abscess may also cause erosion into the ureter and lead to fistula formation, but these complications would not be apparent on cystoscopy and dye injection. The authors have demonstrated the probable risk for the Burch procedure. It would be extremely useful to have some indication of what the risk might be for other pelvic procedures so that a cost-benefit ratio could be developed. At this point, in most centers, cystoscopy is performed based on clinical judgment dealing with the type and severity of the procedure, and the final answer to this problem remains unknown.

M. A. Stenchever, MD

The Role of Intraoperative Cystoscopy in Prolapse and Incontinence Surgery

Jabs CFI, Drutz HP (Regina Gen Hosp, Sask, Canada; Univ of Toronto)
Am J Obstet Gynecol 185:1368-1373, 2001   11–11

Background.—Unrecognized ureteral and bladder injury during gynecologic surgery is an important source of morbidity and mortality. The frequency with which intraoperative cystoscopy during prolapse and incontinence procedures resulted in a change in intraoperative management to prevent ureter and bladder injury was determined.

Methods.—The charts and operative reports of 235 routine intraoperative cystoscopies during prolapse and incontinence surgery over a 2-year period at 1 center were reviewed. Eleven cases were excluded from the final analysis.

Findings.—Cystoscopic findings prompted changes in intraoperative management during 5.3% of the procedures. Of the 12 patients with such changes, 8 had ureter blockage. Patients with abnormal cystoscopy results and those with normal findings did not differ significantly in age, weight, parity, maximum prolapse grade, estimated blood loss, or previous surgery. In 58% of patients with abnormal cystoscopy results, there had been no suspicion of technical difficulty based on surgical history. Preoperative renal imaging findings did not predict which patients would have abnormal cystoscopy results. No complications resulted from the intraoperative cystoscopy.

Conclusion.—Intraoperative cystoscopy can identify otherwise undetected intraoperative compromise of the urinary tract during prolapse and incontinence surgery. Cystoscopy should be used liberally to decrease the frequency of serious consequences from urinary tract injury.

▶ Unrecognized ureteral and bladder injuries occur in a small percentage of gynecologic procedures and may be more common in patients who undergo procedures for prolapse and incontinence. Many authors have advocated routine intraoperative cystoscopy and IV dye injection in order to detect these injuries. It is not known whether universal application of this recommendation would be totally safe and cost effective. In this particular study of 235 patients who underwent operations for prolapse or urinary incontinence, the intraoperative management was changed for 12 (5.3%) patients because of the cystoscopy findings. Eight of these patients had blockage of the ureter and in more than half of patients with abnormal cystoscopy results, there had been no indication that the ureter had been compromised during the operation. The authors advocated the use of intraoperative cystoscopy, and at least in this high-risk group of patients—ie, those with prolapse and urinary incontinence—this may be an appropriate recommendation.

M. A. Stenchever, MD

Annual Direct Cost of Urinary Incontinence
Wilson L, Brown JS, Shin GP, et al (Univ of California, San Francisco; Univ of Illinois, Chicago)
Obstet Gynecol 98:398-406, 2001   11–12

Background.—Incontinence is one of the most prevalent chronic disorders. Recently reported increases in cost associated with incontinence is greater than can be explained by medical inflation. The annual direct costs of urinary incontinence for all age groups in the United States were determined.

Methods.—The direct costs of urinary incontinence were estimated using epidemiologically based models involving diagnostic and treatment algorithms from published clinical practice guidelines and current disease prevalence data. Prevalence and event probability estimates were based on published studies, national data sets, small surveys, and expert opinion. The mean national Medicare reimbursement was used to estimate costs in different patient subgroups.

Findings.—The estimated annual direct cost of urinary incontinence in 1995 US dollars was $16.3 billion. Seventy-six percent of this cost was for women. Community-dwelling women accounted for 69% of the cost and institutionalized women, 31%. Costs for women older than 65 years were more than double those for younger women. Routine care was the largest cost category, at 70%, followed by nursing home admissions (14%), treatment (9%), complications (6%), and diagnosis and evaluations (1%). Changes in the prevalence of incontinence, routine care, and institutionalization rates and charges had the greatest effects on costs.

Conclusion.—The cost of urinary incontinence appears to be very high. Annual expenditures are comparable to those for other chronic diseases in women.

▶ Urinary incontinence is a common problem in the United States, particularly in women. It increases with age and with degree of disability. The authors have utilized epidemiologically based models to estimate the annual cost of managing these patients in the United States. They estimated that this cost is $16.3

billion (in 1995 dollars), with 76% of this cost toward the care of women. These costs are comparable with those of previous studies and when the cost is reduced to 1995 dollars, have been relatively constant for a few years.

However, during the next 10 years, 40% of American women will be past the age of 60. As the authors have shown that costs for women 65 years and older are more than twice that of women under 65 years, we can anticipate a rise in these expenditures. Therefore, developing strategies to identify and treat women with incontinence is not only important from the standpoint of the comfort and well being of the patient, but also in terms of the cost to society.

A large majority of women who are community dwelling and incontinent do not bring this to the attention of their physician. Instead they utilize sanitary products that are costly and discomforting and settle for a less than optimal quality of life. Many do so out of embarrassment; others do so because they believe that nothing can be done about their problem and that incontinence is simply an aspect of aging. Thus, gynecologists have an important responsibility in detecting cases of incontinence, evaluating them, and offering patients options to incontinence.

M. A. Stenchever, MD

Urinary Incontinence in Older People in the Community: A Neglected Problem?
Stoddart H, Donovan J, Whitley E, et al (Univ of Bristol, England; Univ of East Anglia, Norwich, England)
Br J Gen Pract 51:548-554, 2001   11–13

Background.—The prevalence and impact of urinary incontinence have been investigated more in older women than in older men. Many elderly persons do not seek medical help, even when they may be severely affected. The prevalence and impact on daily life of urinary incontinence in elderly men and women were further investigated.

Methods.—The cross-sectional survey included a stratified random sample of 2000 community-living elderly persons in 11 general practices in a city in the United Kingdom. The sample consisted of equal numbers of men and women, aged 65 years and older. Seventy-nine percent of the subjects responded to the survey.

Findings.—Overall, the prevalences of incontinence in the preceding month for men and women were 23% and 31%, respectively. The frequency of incontinence was generally more severe and the degree of wetness was greater in women than in men. Only 45% of women and 40% of men had sought medical help for their incontinence. Factors that significantly predicted the use of health services were reporting incontinence as a problem, increased frequency of incontinence, and a greater degree of wetness. However, about one third of those reporting leaks with severe frequency or reporting that this was a problem had not accessed health services.

Conclusion.—Urinary incontinence is common among community-living elderly women and men. A combination of increased public and professional awareness may lead to earlier patient presentation and treatment, resulting in improved quality of life for the elderly.

▶ The authors of this British study sent a postal questionnaire about incontinence to 2000 older individuals who were stratified to 65-74 years and 75 years and older. Although the study was cross-sectional in nature, it did demonstrate that 31% of the women and 23% of the men in the study had been incontinent in the previous month. Women had a more severe frequency of incontinence and a greater degree of wetness than the men. Only 45% of the women had sought medical help for this problem, and of those with severe wetness that caused a social problem, only one third had sought medical help. It is likely that the results of this study would be similar if the study were performed in the United States. The huge market for wetness protection products in the United States indicates that the problem is a large one. During this decade, 40% of the female population in the United States will be past the age of 60; therefore, it behooves practitioners to ask questions specifically aimed at detecting incontinence so that medical intervention can be offered.

M. A. Stenchever, MD

The Cause and Natural History of Isolated Urinary Retention in Young Women

Swinn MJ, Wiseman OJ, Lowe E, et al (Natl Hosp for Neurology and Neurosurgery, London)
J Urol 167:151-156, 2002   11–14

Background.—Urinary retention in women is attributed to abnormal results of electromyography of the striated urethral sphincter. In young women, urinary retention had often been thought to be caused by multiple sclerosis or a psychogenic disorder. The course and natural history of urinary retention in women was investigated.

Methods.—Two hundred sixteen women with abnormal sphincter electromyography results and urinary retention were mailed a questionnaire. One hundred twelve responses were received. Ninety-one from women who had been in complete urinary retention were analyzed.

Findings.—Patient age at the onset of complete retention ranged from 10 to 50 years, with a mean of 27.7 years. None of the patients had neurologic features suggesting cauda equina lesions or central demyelination. None had progressed to features of general neurologic disorder. At the initial episode of complete retention, the mean maximum bladder capacity was 1208 ml. Sixty-five percent of the patients reported an event that appeared to precipitate urinary retention, most commonly a gynecologic surgical procedure with general anesthesia. The only intervention that restored voiding was sacral neuromodulation.

Conclusion.—In this series of otherwise healthy young women with urinary retention, no underlying neurologic disorders were identified. This disorder appears to be a primary failure of relaxation of the striated urethral sphincter.

▶ The authors described a relatively rare and very interesting condition of urinary retention in otherwise healthy women. As they pointed out, urinary retention is usually thought to be related to a neurologic problem, such as multiple sclerosis or another spinal cord condition, and in patients found not to have a neurologic condition, the cause is often thought to be psychogenic. The authors noted that in as many as two thirds of patients in their series, there was an association with an operative procedure or an anesthetic, and the majority of these were gynecologic procedures or childbirth. As 44% of patients in their series experienced polycystic ovary syndrome, the authors speculated on a possible hormonal cause of the condition. On electromyography, there was impaired stability of the muscle membrane of the striated urethral sphincter with a direct muscle fiber end to end muscle fiber spread of excitation, leading to a state of hyperexcitability of the muscle fibers and spasm of the sphincter.

Other investigators have shown that when women undergo sphincter electromyography for various reasons, 8% to 10% will express this hyperexcitability, but urinary retention is rarely present. The authors therefore postulated that urinary retention is due to abnormal activity of the striated urethral sphincter muscles impairing relaxation. Recently, sacral nerve stimulation has been effective in patients with this condition, whereas previous therapies have not been uniformly successful.

The authors observed that since there is frequently a relationship to operative procedures or anesthesia, there might be a medicolegal implication, making the understanding of the problem rather imperative. In any event, though this condition is not common, it is important that gynecologists are aware of it, especially if the patient has polycystic ovary syndrome.

M. A. Stenchever, MD

Maximum Urethral Closure Pressure and Sphincter Volume in Women With Urinary Retention
Wiseman OJ, Swinn MJ, Brady CM, et al (Natl Hosp for Neurology and Neurosurgery, London)
J Urol 167:1348-1352, 2002   11–15

Background.—In 1988, a syndrome of isolated urinary retention in young women associated with electromyographically revealed abnormality of the striated urethral sphincter was reported, leading to the hypothesis that urinary retention is caused by failure of sphincter relaxation. If the electromyographically shown abnormality is caused by urinary retention, the urethral sphincter would be expected to be enlarged and the urethral pressure profile increased in affected women. The role of static urethral pressure profilometry and transvaginal US was assessed in women with urinary retention.

Methods.—Sixty-six women in complete or partial urinary retention underwent electromyography of the striated urethral sphincter. A concentric needle electrode was used. The patients then underwent urethral pressure profile and/or urethral sphincter volume measurements by transvaginal US.

Findings.—Patients with abnormal results electromyographically had significantly higher maximum urethral closure pressure than those without such abnormality; the mean values were 103 and 76.7 cm water, respectively. In addition, women with the abnormality had an increased maximum urethral sphincter volume compared with women without the abnormality, at 2.29 and 1.62 cm^3, respectively.

Conclusion.—These data support the hypothesis that, in a subgroup of women, a local sphincter abnormality is the cause of urinary retention. For such patients, urethral pressure profilometry and sphincter volume measurements are useful, especially when sphincter electromyography is unavailable.

▶ The authors have an interest in studying young women with isolated urinary retention using electromyography. In this study, they demonstrated that when an electromyographic abnormality consistent with striated urethral sphincter spasm was found, the maximum urethral closure pressure was significantly increased compared with women without the electromyographic abnormality. These patients also had an increased urethral sphincter volume compared with women without the abnormality. Thus, they demonstrated that urethral pressure profilometry and sphincter volume measurements are helpful in assessing women with urinary retention and that the findings are comparable with those found with electromyographic techniques. The syndrome of isolated urinary retention was first described as an abnormality of striated urethral sphincter in 1988. The results of the current study support our understanding of the underlying pathophysiology.

M. A. Stenchever, MD

Urethral Sphincter Morphology in Women With Detrusor Instability
Major H, Culligan P, Heit M (Univ of Louisville, Ky)
Obstet Gynecol 99:63-68, 2002   11–16

Background.—In 20% to 30% of women with urinary incontinence, the cause is detrusor instability. Whether sonographic urethral sphincter morphology differs between patients with detrusor instability and those with normal urodynamic testing was determined.

Methods.—Seventeen patients with detrusor instability and 16 with normal urodynamic testing results were studied. All had been seen for assessment of urinary incontinence or pelvic organ prolapse and had undergone intraurethral US before multichannel urodynamic testing.

Findings.—The 2 groups did not differ in age, vaginal parity, race, weight, body mass index, previous continence surgery, or maximal total urethral closure pressure. However, compared with patients with normal test results, patients with detrusor instability had reduced urethral longitudinal smooth muscle thickness, total urethral diameter, and total urethral circumference.

Rhabdosphincter thickness was associated linearly with strength of involuntary detrusor contraction.

Conclusion.—Patients with detrusor instability have a different urethral sphincter morphology than patients with normal urodynamic test results. These data provide an anatomical basis for the physiologic findings seen in "urethrogenic" detrusor instability.

▶ The authors used intraurethral US to compare urethral sphincter morphology in 17 women with detrusor instability and 16 women with normal urodynamic testing results. The 2 groups were similar with respect to age, parity, race, weight, body mass index, prior continence surgery, and maximal total urethral closure pressure. The authors demonstrated by intraurethral US that the group with detrusor instability had decreased urethral longitudinal smooth muscle thickness, total urethral diameter, and total urethral circumference compared with the normal patients. This demonstrated that there might be anatomical differences between patients with and without detrusor instability.

The authors speculated that the changes that led to a decrease in urethral resistance might allow urine to enter the bladder neck, thereby stimulating a detrusor contraction. The theory is appealing but may be difficult to prove. Nevertheless, it is encouraging that there may be an anatomical reason in at least some of the patients who suffer from detrusor instability. The authors speculated that this group of patients may be those who do not respond to anticholinergic therapy. Clearly, bladder instability is a multifactorial problem. The authors may have uncovered 1 facet of it.

M. A. Stenchever, MD

Urinary Tract Infections in Postmenopausal Women: Effect of Hormone Therapy and Risk Factors
Brown JS, for the Heart and Estrogen/Progestin Replacement Study Research Group (Univ of California, San Francisco; et al)
Obstet Gynecol 98:1045-1052, 2001   11–17

Background.—Urinary tract infection (UTI) is common among women of all age groups. The incidence peaks at 17.5% in 18- to 24-year-olds but is still high at 9% in women aged 50 years and older. The effects of hormone therapy on UTI frequency was investigated.

Methods.—Data were obtained from the Heart and Estrogen/Progestin Replacement Study, a randomized study of the effects of hormone treatment on coronary heart disease in 2763 postmenopausal women with established coronary heart disease. Participants' ages ranged from 44 to 79 years. By random assignment, the women received 0.625 mg of conjugated estrogens plus 2.5 mg of medroxyprogesterone acetate or placebo. The mean follow-up was 4.1 years.

Findings.—The frequency of UTI was higher in the hormone recipients, although nonsignificantly. In a multivariate analysis, significant risk factors for UTI were the presence of treated diabetes, with an odds ratio of 1.81;

taking oral medications, at 1.44; having poor health, at 1.34; having had children, at 1.38; and having vaginal itching, vaginal dryness, and urge incontinence, at 1.63, 1.30, and 1.51, respectively.

Conclusion.—Oral hormone therapy does not appear to reduce the frequency of UTI in postmenopausal women. Potentially modifiable risk factors in this age group differ from those in younger women. These include diabetes, vaginal symptoms, and urge incontinence.

▶ UTIs are common in women, and more so during the reproductive years. As estrogen therapy produces many important beneficial changes in the genitourinary tract, it was reasonable to assume that it might have a preventive effect with respect to UTIs. In fact, many physicians believe this to be true, but in the authors' study, this did not seem to be the case. Rather, they demonstrated that older women differ from younger women with respect to UTI and that the risk factors in older women include the presence of diabetes, vaginal dryness and itching, and urge incontinence.

Estrogen should have a positive effect on the treatment of vaginal dryness and irritation, and though it is not known whether the study had the power to determine that there was a relationship between estrogen and the prevention of these symptoms, it probably did not. The authors also noted that poor health, as determined by the patient's personal assessment, also seemed related to UTIs in this age group. The effect of estrogen might or might not have an effect on improving general health quality. Clearly, UTI in all age groups, and particularly in the elderly, is a mixed problem with respect to etiology. Although the authors did not demonstrate a direct relationship between estrogen therapy and the reduction of UTIs in postmenopausal women, the benefits of estrogen are so numerous in this age group that these data should not preclude its use.

M. A. Stenchever, MD

Prevalence of Urinary Incontinence in Women With Cystic Fibrosis
Cornacchia M, Zenorini A, Perobelli S, et al (Ospedale Civile Maggiore, Verona, Italy)
BJU Internatl 88:44-48, 2001   11–18

Background.—To date, no one has reported on urinary incontinence (UI) in women with cystic fibrosis (CF). The prevalence of UI in female patients, aged 15 years and older, attending a CF center was determined.

Patients and Findings.—One hundred seventy-six patients with CF completed an anonymous questionnaire during routine outpatient evaluations. Forty-one percent were classified as never incontinent and 35% as occasionally incontinent. Twenty-four percent reported UI occurring 2 or more times a month for at least 2 consecutive months in the previous year. Such regular UI correlated with increasing age and a lower mean forced expiratory volume per second than that predicted for women with no urinary symptoms.

All patients with UI reported stress UI. Coughing was associated with UI in 92%, laughing in 33%, and physical activity in 21%.

Conclusion.—Stress UI is common in women with CF. Such patients should be asked about incontinence as part of routine follow-up. Pelvic floor muscle exercises may be recommended as treatment.

▶ Patients with CF are living longer due to modern medical management. As CF patients suffer with chronic cough associated with progressive lung disease and frequent pulmonary infections, the authors suspected that they might be at greater risk for stress UI than women of comparable age. Indeed, 24% of their patients reported moderate UI, and only 41% reported that they were never incontinent. Considering the fact that these women had a mean age of 24.6% years (range, 15-41.5 years), this was a fairly significant finding. The authors did not have a control group, and we do not know what comparable UI rates would be in women without CF in a population of comparable age. However, the rate of moderate-to-severe incontinence seems high for this age group, and it seems reasonable to discuss UI problems with CF patients. Given the knowledge that many women who are incontinent do not discuss their condition with their physician, awareness on the part of physicians is important when caring for this patient group.

M. A. Stenchever, MD

Is the Irritable Bladder Associated With Anterior Compartment Relaxation? A Critical Look at the 'Integral Theory of Pelvic Floor Dysfunction'
Dietz HP, Clarke B (Royal Hosp for Women, Sydney, New South Wales, Australia; Royal Women's Hosp, Brisbane, Queensland, Australia)
Aust N Z J Obstet Gynaecol 41:317-319, 2001   11–19

Background.—First proposed in 1990, the integral theory of pelvic floor dysfunction states that anterior vaginal wall relaxation is associated with symptoms of urgency, frequency, nocturia, and urge incontinence. This hypothesis was tested in a retrospective study.

Methods.—Two hundred seventy-two women with symptoms of lower urinary tract dysfunction were included in the study. Imaging data and urodynamic reports were reviewed. Anterior vaginal wall laxity was quantified by opening of the retrovesical angle, bladder neck descent, urethral rotation, and descent of a cystocele during Valsalva.

Findings.—None of the parameters tested correlated with symptoms or signs of detrusor overactivity. In fact, patients with higher grades of urethral and bladder descent were less likely to have nocturia and urge incontinence. These patients were also less likely to have sensory urgency and detrusor instability diagnosed on urodynamic testing.

Conclusions.—These data do not support the integral theory of pelvic floor dysfunction. Anterior vaginal wall relaxation is unlikely to be positively associated with or related to symptoms and signs of bladder irritability.

▶ In most studies of urinary stress incontinence approximately one third of the patients also have some form of unstable bladder, a so-called "mixed incontinence." It has always seemed important to attempt to clear up the unstable bladder problem before subjecting the patient to reparative surgery. Since it has been supposed that patients treated surgically would still have their unstable bladder problem, the surgery has not been considered successful. During the last decade some authors have suggested that the irritable bladder component may be related to the anterior vaginal wall defect that is associated with stress urinary incontinence and that simply repairing the anatomical defect might also treat the unstable bladder. The authors of the current article were able to investigate all of the potential signs of anterior vaginal wall relaxation, including the opening of the retrovesical angle, bladder neck descent, urethral rotation, and descent of a cystocele during the Valsalva maneuver, and compared these with the symptoms of bladder irritability and with the results of urodynamic assessment. Neither the subjective or urodynamic parameters of bladder dysfunction correlated with the measures of anterior compartment relaxation that were seen on ultrasonography. In fact, these correlations were consistently negative. Thus, the presence of a cystocele usually decreased the likelihood of symptoms and signs of bladder irritability. Therefore, it seems important to continue to investigate patients with mixed incontinence in order to understand the contribution of both anatomical defect and bladder irritability. The authors have shown reasonably well that these are separate issues.

M. A. Stenchever, MD

Role of Urethrocystoscopy in the Evaluation of Refractory Idiopathic Detrusor Instability

Groutz A, Samandarov A, Gold R, et al (Tel Aviv Univ, Israel)
Urology 58:544-546, 2001   11–20

Background.—A common cause of lower urinary tract symptoms in women is detrusor instability (DI). The role of diagnostic urethrocystoscopy in the assessment of women with idiopathic DI refractory to conventional drug therapy was investigated.

Methods.—One hundred consecutive women, with a mean age of 62.1 years, who had idiopathic DI refractory to conventional pharmacotherapy were enrolled in the prospective study. All women underwent a meticulous examination, including diagnostic urethrocystoscopy.

Findings.—Urinalysis was normal in all patients. In addition, all cytologic findings were negative. However, diagnostic urethrocystoscopy demonstrated isolated bladder tuberculosis in 1 patient and transitional cell carcinoma in another patient. Another 7 patients were found to have bladder diverticula; in only 1 of these was the condition also diagnosed by sonographic evaluation. Twenty-two patients had mild to moderate bladder trabeculations.

Conclusions.—In patients with refractory DI, the absence of other serious signs, such as recurrent urinary tract infection, hematuria, and significant residual urinary volume, does not confirm the lack of significant lower urinary tract abnormalities. Diagnostic urethrocystoscopy is a safe, simple procedure that facilitates timely diagnosis and proper treatment for such patients.

▶ The authors defined DI that was treated for at least 6 months without response to single or multiple medications as refractory DI. Their further testing included sonographic imaging of the urinary tract and diagnostic urethroscopy. All patients had normal urinalysis and negative cytologic findings. In the study group, 84% were postmenopausal; of these, 20% were using hormone replacement therapy. The control group comprised randomly selected patients who had idiopathic DI that responded to medical therapy. Various bladder and urethra problems were noted in 38% of patients in the refractory group and in only 1 patient in the nonrefractory group. The value of this article is that it points out that further evaluation is necessary in patients who are refractory to the usual therapy. The problem with the article is that the control group was not studied in a similar fashion and therefore we do not know what pathologic problems might be present in these women, even though they are asymptomatic. The control group was merely used to compare demographic and clinical characteristics with those of the study group.

Nonetheless, the take-home message of this study is that if patients do not respond appropriately to treatment, they should be evaluated further, as many will still have pathologic conditions that can be treated.

M. A. Stenchever, MD

Assessment and Grading of Pelvic Organ Prolapse by Use of Dynamic Magnetic Resonance Imaging
Singh K, Reid WMN, Berger LA (Univ College, London)
Am J Obstet Gynecol 185:71-77, 2001   11–21

Background.—Pelvic organ prolapse is commonly assessed by clinical examination, but there are limitations to this approach. One third of the patients who undergo prolapse surgery will require a second operation. Therefore, the preoperative assessment must be as accurate and definitive as possible in characterizing the defects in the fascial supports that led to prolapse. The grading system proposed by the International Continence Society is reproducible and site specific, but it can be difficult to correctly identify the prolapsing organ by vaginal examination and to demonstrate objectively the anatomic changes that result from surgical correction. The introduction of MRI has revolutionized assessment of the pelvic floor. It not only demonstrates pelvic floor anatomy in detail but also objectively demonstrates pelvic organ prolapse. MRI can assess all 3 pelvic floor compartments simultaneously and can also dynamically assess pelvic floor descent and objectively grade prolapse. This study assessed the utility of dynamic MRI with the clinical staging proposed by the International Continence Society.

Methods.—Twenty patients participated in this cross-sectional study and underwent dynamic MRI. Clinical staging according to the International Continence Society was compared with staging by MRI. The midpubic line was used as a new reference line and was drawn on the MR image to correspond to the hymenal ring marker used in the clinical staging. Vaginal supports were indicated by the levator-vaginal angle and the area of the genital hiatus. A control group comprising 10 nulliparous symptom-free women was also studied.

Results.—There was good correlation between the proposed staging by MRI and clinical staging. MRI improved clinical assessment by measuring the actual pelvic organ descent and accurately delineating prolapse of the pouch of Douglas. The midpubic line was found to be a useful reference for grading prolapse on MRI, and the levator-vaginal angle and the area of the genital hiatus were found to be useful in assessing vaginal support at different anatomic levels.

Conclusions.—The use of MRI to grade pelvic organ prolapse relies on the same landmarks used in clinical grading and provides a uniform approach to and objective assessment of the results of surgical correction of pelvic organ prolapse.

▶ The International Continence Society recently developed a clinical staging system that numerically quantifies pelvic organ prolapse. The system is reproducible and has demonstrated minimal intraobserver and interobserver variation. It is site-specific and can be used to evaluate the effect of surgical repair as well as communicate findings among physicians. MRI has the advantage of assessing pelvic floor anatomy in detail and allows for the assessment of all 3 pelvic floor compartments simultaneously. It also allows for the objective grading of the prolapse. It is often more accurate in evaluating an enterocele and is a clinical vaginal examination and can provide a more accurate assessment of vaginal support at the different anatomical levels. The authors have devised a method of grading by MRI that uses the same landmarks as the clinical grading and therefore should allow uniformity of reporting. The major problem with this procedure, which is so often seen in other imaging procedures, is that of cost. Still, for complex cases, particularly those that have involved multiple operative procedures, this approach should be extremely useful.

M. A. Stenchever, MD

Outcome of Sphincteroplasty Combined With Surgery for Urinary Incontinence and Pelvic Organ Prolapse

Halverson AL, Hull TL, Paraiso MF, et al (Cleveland Clinic Found, Ohio)
Dis Colon Rectum 44:1421-1426, 2001   11–22

Background.—A combined approach may be used to treat patients with fecal incontinence and urinary incontinence or pelvic organ prolapse. However, whether performing a combined procedure would adversely affect patient outcomes is of concern. The current prospective study is the first to compare outcomes and cost associated with sphincteroplasty for anal incontinence and sphincteroplasty combined with 1 or more procedures for urinary incontinence, pelvic organ prolapse, or both.

Methods.—Forty-four patients with fecal incontinence were included. Twenty underwent sphincter repair alone, and 24 underwent sphincter repair combined with procedures for urinary incontinence or pelvic organ prolapse. A cohort of case-matched patients undergoing only urogynecologic procedures was also analyzed retrospectively for comparison.

Findings.—No major complications occurred. All 3 groups had similar functional outcomes and physical, social, and sexual activity. Twenty-two of the patients undergoing combined procedures reported that they were pleased to have had the concomitant procedures.

Conclusions.—Combination pelvic floor surgery yielded good outcomes in this series. This approach is also cost-effective. Clinicians should offer combined surgery to women with the concurrent problems of fecal and urinary incontinence or pelvic organ prolapse.

▶ The authors demonstrated that it is safe and reasonable to combine anal sphincter damage repair with a procedure for urinary incontinence or pelvic organ prolapse. They utilized preoperative mechanical bowel preparation and parenteral antibiotics. There was an appropriate control group of patients who were undergoing sphincter repair alone. There were no significant differences between the groups with respect to fecal incontinence for either gas or stool, and there were no limitations to physical, social, or sexual activity. There were no major complications in either the sphincter repair only group or the combined procedure group, and no infection problems occurred as a result of the combined procedure.

It is reassuring that women who are incontinent of both urine and stool can be treated at the same time operatively without the need for a separate procedure and its associated discomfort, cost, and inconvenience.

M. A. Stenchever, MD

12 Infection

Oral Versus Intra-vaginal Imidazole and Triazole Anti-fungal Agents for the Treatment of Uncomplicated Vulvovaginal Candidiasis (Thrush): A Systematic Review

Watson MC, Grimshaw JM, Bond CM, et al (University of Aberdeen, Scotland)
Br J Obstet Gynaecol 109:85-95, 2002   12–1

Background.—Vulvovaginal candidiasis (thrush) is very common, affecting 75% of women before menopause. The relative efficacy, cost-effectiveness, and safety of oral and intravaginal imidazole and triazole antifungal agents in the treatment of uncomplicated vaginal candidiasis were compared.

Comparison: 06 Fluconazole vs Clotrimazole
Outcome: 02 Long term mycological cure

Study	Intravaginal n/N	Oral n/N	OR (95%CI Random)	OR (95%CI Random)
Stein 1991	57/74	64/74		0.52[0.22,1.24]
0-Prasertsawat 1995	32/53	33/50		0.78[0.35,1.75]
Sobel 1995	90/131	80/125		1.23[0.73,2.08]
Mikamo (1) 1995	35/50	30/50		1.56[0.68,3.56]
Anonymous 1989	115/160	90/145		1.56[0.97,2.53]
Mikamo (2) 1995	40/50	30/50		2.67[1.09,6.52]
Adetoro 1990	20/23	12/20		4.44[0.98,20.07]
Goode 1992	3/3	4/7		5.44[0.21,144.11]
Total (95%CI)	392/544	343/521		1.36[0.92,2.00]

Test for heterogeneity chi-square=12.31 df=7 p=0.091
Test for overall effect z=1.54 p=0.12

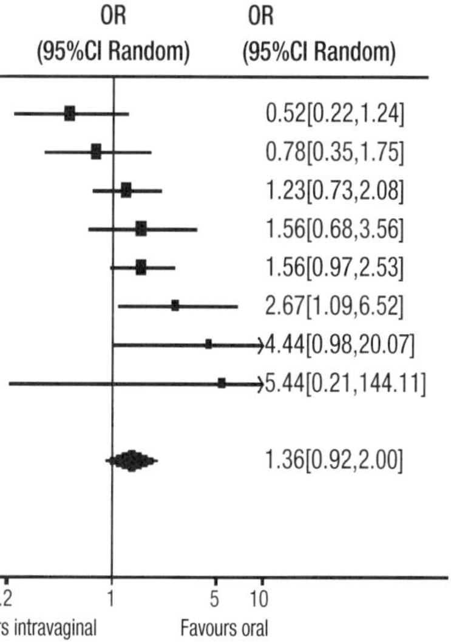

.1   .2   1   5   10
Favours intravaginal   Favours oral

Test for heterogeneity: if χ^2 <0.1 this indicates that there is heterogeneity amongst the trials (i.e. there is significant variation between the trials), therefore the results of the meta-analysis should be interpreted with caution.

FIGURE 3.—Long-term myocologic cure. (Reprinted from Watson MC, Grimshaw JM, Bond CM, et al: Oral versus intra-vaginal imidazole and triazole anti-fungal agents for the treatment of uncomplicated vulvovaginal candidiasis (thrush): A systematic review. *Br J Obstet Gynaecol* 109:85-95, 2002. With permission from Elsevier Science.)

Methods.—Studies comparing oral and intravaginal antifungal treatments for uncomplicated vulvovaginal candidiasis were reviewed systematically. Seventeen randomized controlled studies conducted worldwide were included. A total of 19 oral versus intravaginal antifungal treatment comparisons were reported. The primary outcome measure was clinical cure, and secondary measures were mycologic cure, patient preference, and safety.

Findings.—Oral and intravaginal antifungal treatments did not differ significantly in clinical or mycologic cure (Fig 3). All 10 studies that reported preferences indicated that patients favored oral treatment over intravaginal treatment. No cost data were reported.

Conclusions.—Oral and intravaginal antifungal treatments for thrush are equally effective. Patients appear to favor oral treatment.

▶ This review of randomized trials reported that both oral and vaginal administration of antifungal agents provided a similar and high rate of cure of vulvovaginal candidiasis. In the majority of trials the oral agent was a single 150-mg dose of fluconazole. The vaginal therapy in most of the trials was 1 or more doses of different amounts of clotrimazole. When the data from all the trials were analyzed, no significant differences were found between the effectiveness or side effects of these 2 agents. Patient preference and cost of drug will influence the clinician's decision about which agent to use.

D. R. Mishell, Jr, MD

Two-Day Regimen of Acyclovir for Treatment of Recurrent Genital Herpes Simplex Virus Type 2 Infection

Wald A, Carrell D, Remington M, et al (Univ of Washington, Seattle; Fred Hutchinson Cancer Research Ctr, Seattle)
Clin Infect Dis 34:944-948, 2002   12–2

Background.—In patients with recurrent genital herpes, the standard course of antiviral treatment requires that multiple doses of medication be administered for 5 days. Whether a shorter regimen of antiviral medication would reduce the duration of an episode of recurrent genital herpes was determined.

Methods.—One hundred thirty-one otherwise healthy adults with recurrent genital herpes simplex virus type 2 infection were enrolled in the randomized, double-blind trial. Patients were assigned to acyclovir, 800 mg, given orally 3 times a day for 2 days. Eighty-four patients were observed for 1 or more recurrences, and 65 were observed for 2 recurrences (for which patients received the same study drug, acyclovir or placebo).

Findings.—Acyclovir treatment significantly decreased the duration of lesions. The median duration of lesions in acyclovir and placebo recipients was 4 days and 6 days, respectively. Duration of the episode was also 4 and 6 days, respectively, and of viral shedding, 25 hours and 58.5 hours, respectively (Fig 1). Acyclovir treatment increased the proportion of aborted episodes.

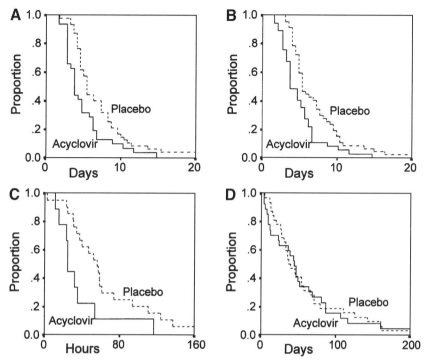

FIGURE 1.—Time to resolution of lesions (**A**), episode (**B**), viral shedding (**C**), and time to next recurrence (**D**), by study arm. (Courtesy of Wald A, Carrell D, Remington M, et al: Two-day regimen of acyclovir for treatment of recurrent genital herpes simplex virus type 2 infection. *Clin Infect Dis* 34:944-948, 2002, copyright by the Infectious Diseases Society of America; publisher, University of Chicago.)

Conclusions.—A 2-day course of oral acyclovir, 800 mg 3 times per day, shortened the duration of genital herpes episodes, lesions, and viral shedding in these patients. The low cost of generic acyclovir and ease of the 2-day, 6-pill treatment should encourage clinicians to consider this treatment regimen.

Valacyclovir for Episodic Treatment of Genital Herpes: A Shorter 3-Day Treatment Course Compared With 5-Day Treatment

Leone PA, Trottier S, Miller JM (Univ of North Carolina, Chapel Hill; Glaxo-SmithKline, Research Triangle Park, NC; Centre de Recherche Infectiologie Universite Laval, Sainte Foy, Quebec, Canada)
Clin Infect Dis 34:958-962, 2002   12–3

Background.—A 5-day regimen of 500 mg valacyclovir twice a day is an effective short-term treatment for recurrent genital herpes. The efficacy of a shorter, 3-day course was compared in a double-blind, controlled study with that of the 5-day treatment.

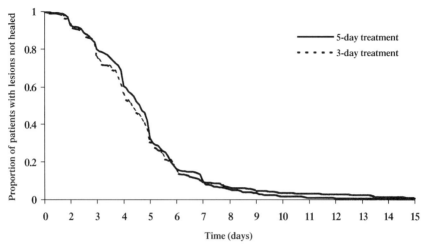

FIGURE 2.—Time to lesion healing in a comparative study of 3- and 5-day regimens of valacyclovir for episodic treatment of genital herpes. Hazard ratio, 0.95; 95% CI, 0.81-1.13; *P* = .59. (Courtesy of Leone PA, Trottier S, Miller JM: Valacyclovir for episodic treatment of genital herpes: A shorter 3-day treatment course compared with 5-day treatment. *Clin Infect Dis* 34:958-962, 2002, copyright by the Infectious Diseases Society of America; publisher, University of Chicago.)

Methods.—Four hundred two patients were assigned to 3 days of valacyclovir, 500 mg twice daily, and 398 were assigned to 5 days of valacyclovir, 500 mg twice daily. All patients were aged 18 or older, were otherwise healthy, and had a history of at least 4 episodes of genital or perianal herpes virus type 2 outbreaks in the preceding year or 2 episodes in the preceding 6 months.

Findings.—None of the treatment end points differed significantly between groups. Median time to lesion healing was 4.7 days in the patients receiving the 5-day regimen and 4.4 days in those receiving the 3-day regimen (Fig 2). Median length of pain duration was 2.5 and 1.9 days, respectively, and median episode length was 4.4 and 4.3 days. Lesions were aborted in 26.6% of the patients on the 5-day regimen and 25.4% of those on the 3-day regimen.

Conclusions.—A 3-day regimen of valacyclovir is as effective as a 5-day course for the episodic treatment of recurrent genital herpes. The shorter treatment course is more convenient and reduces cost.

▶ The standard course of antiviral therapy to treat recurrent lesions of genital herpes is 5 days of multiple doses of medication. The results of these 2 studies (Abstracts 12–2 and 12–3) indicate that a shorter duration of therapy provides equivalent reduction in the duration of lesions and percentage of individuals with aborted lesions. Thus, clinicians can administer 800 mg of acyclovir 3 times a day for 2 days or 500 mg of valacyclovir twice daily for 3 days instead of the standard 5-day treatment course of each of these agents to alleviate the acute symptoms of recurrent herpes.

D. R. Mishell, Jr, MD

CO_2 Laser Vaporization as Primary Therapy for Human Papillomavirus Lesions: A Prospective Observational Study

Savoca S, Nardo LG, Rosano TF, et al (Univ of Catania, Italy)
Acta Obstet Gynecol Scand 80:1121-1124, 2001   12–4

Background.—Human papillomavirus (HPV) is more frequent and severe in sexually active persons. Several treatment options are available. A study was undertaken to determine the efficacy of CO_2 laser vaporization for HPV warts.

Methods.—Eighty healthy, sexually active women were enrolled in the prospective trial. All had cytologically, colposcopically, histologically diagnosed HPV urogenital and perinatal warts. Treatment with CO_2 laser, 16 to 18 W, was administered. Patients' partners were also investigated. Subsequently, interferon-β was given. Patients were followed up for 12 months.

Findings.—At the most recent follow-up, 87.5% of the women were clear of warts. Recurrence, noted in 12.5% of the women with multiple partners, was affected by flat or endophytic condyloma of the cervix. None of the patients reported pain, scar tissue, deformity, or other adverse effects.

Conclusions.—Treatment with CO_2 laser vaporization is effective and safe for the treatment of HPV warts. This approach is recommended for condyloma acuminata unassociated with malignancy and during pregnancy.

▶ There are many therapies used to treat the genital lesions produced by human HPV. The results of this prospective observational study found that use of CO_2 laser was an effective way to remove the genital or perinatal lesions. Local anesthesia was used, and side effects of therapy were minimal.

D. R. Mishell, Jr, MD

Endometritis: The Clinical-Pathologic Syndrome

Eckert LO, Hawes SE, Wölner-Hanssen PK, et al (Univ of Washington, Seattle; Univ of Lund, Sweden; Fred Hutchinson Research Ctr, Atlanta, Ga; et al)
Am J Obstet Gynecol 186:690-695, 2002   12–5

Background.—Recent studies of women with suspected pelvic inflammatory disease (PID) have reported histologic evidence of endometritis in some patients without laparoscopic evidence of salpingitis. Risk factors, clinical manifestations, and microbial causes among consecutive, prospectively studied women with suspected PID undergoing laparoscopy and endometrial biopsy were reported.

Methods.—One hundred fifty-two women were included in the cross-sectional study. Standard medical histories were obtained, and physical examinations, endometrial biopsies, and laparoscopies were performed. Endometritis was defined as the presence of plasma cells in endometrial stroma and neutrophils in the endometrial epithelium.

Findings.—Forty-three women were found to have neither endometritis nor salpingitis. Twenty-six had endometritis without salpingitis, and 83 had salpingitis. Compared with women with no endometritis or salpingitis and those with acute salpingitis, women with endometritis alone more often reported douching recently, had a current intrauterine device, and were in menstrual cycle day 1 to 7. In addition, *Neisseria gonorrhoeae* and/or *Chlamydia trachomatis* infection was more common in women with endometritis alone than in those with no endometritis or salpingitis and less common in women with salpingitis. Compared with women with salpingitis, women with endometritis alone had significantly less common lower quadrant, adnexal, cervical motion, rebound tenderness, peritonitis, tenderness score, fever, and laboratory findings indicating inflammation as well as detection of gonorrheal or chlamydial infection. However, these findings were somewhat more common in women with endometritis alone than in women with no salpingitis or endometritis.

Conclusions.—Twenty-six of the 152 women with clinically suspected PID enrolled in this study were found to have histologic manifestations of endometritis without laparoscopic evidence of acute salpingitis. The risk factors for endometritis in this series included gonococcal and chlamydial infection as well as current IUD use, recent douching, and being between days 1 and 7 of the menstrual cycle.

▶ The signs and symptoms as well as the natural history of acute and chronic endometritis are not well defined. It is of interest that 17% of women with clinical manifestations of upper genital tract pelvic infection had evidence of endometritis without laparoscopic findings of salpingitis. It is also of interest that 85% of women with laparoscopic findings of salpingitis had histologic findings of endometritis. Studies should be performed to determine the effect of antimicrobial therapy on acute and chronic endometritis in symptomatic and asymptomatic women and to compare this effect to withholding treatment.

D. R. Mishell, Jr, MD

Effectiveness of Inpatient and Outpatient Treatment Strategies for Women With Pelvic Inflammatory Disease: Results From the Pelvic Inflammatory Disease Evaluation and Clinical Health (PEACH) Randomized Trial
Ness RB, for the PID Evaluation and Clinical Health (PEACH) Study Investigators (Univ of Pittsburgh, Pa; et al)
Am J Obstet Gynecol 186:929-937, 2002   12–6

Background.—Pelvic inflammatory disease (PID), a common intraperitoneal infection, is usually treated on an outpatient basis. However, the efficacy of this treatment approach has not been proved.

Methods.—Eight hundred thirty-one women with clinical signs and symptoms of mild to moderate PID were enrolled in a multicenter, randomized clinical trial. Inpatient treatment initiated by IV cefoxitin and doxycycline was compared with outpatient treatment consisting of a single IM injection of cefoxitin and oral doxycycline.

Findings.—The inpatient and outpatients groups were similar in short-term clinical and microbiologic improvement. At a mean follow-up of 35 months, pregnancy rates were 42% in the outpatient group and 41.7% in the inpatient group. The 2 groups also did not differ in length of time to pregnancy or in proportion of women with PID recurrence, chronic pelvic pain, or ectopic pregnancy.

Conclusions.—In these women with mild to moderate PID, outpatient and inpatient treatment yielded similar reproductive outcomes. Because outpatient treatment is the less costly approach, it appears to be preferable.

▶ Women with severe upper genital tract pelvic infection as well as those with evidence of a tubo-ovarian abscess are best treated as inpatients with IV antimicrobial therapy. It was previously believed that treating women with mild or moderate salpingitis as inpatients would result in less permanent tubal damage and infertility than when they are treated as outpatients. The results of this randomized trial indicate that there is no difference in symptomatic improvement, persistence of pathogens, recurrence of salpingitis, chronic pelvic pain, or ectopic pregnancy between inpatient and outpatient therapy of mild or moderate salpingitis. Furthermore, the pregnancy rates and mean time to pregnancy were similar after inpatient and outpatient therapy. The results of this study indicate that clinicians should treat women with mild to moderate acute salpingitis as outpatients because it is less costly and as effective as inpatient therapy.

D. R. Mishell, Jr, MD

13 Endocrinology

Menstrual Cycle Irregularity and Risk for Future Cardiovascular Disease
Solomon CG, Hu FB, Dunaif A, et al (Brigham and Women's Hosp, Boston; Harvard School of Public Health, Boston; Harvard Med School, Boston)
J Clin Endocrinol Metab 87:2013-2017, 2002   13–1

Background.—Menstrual irregularity may be caused by polycystic ovary syndrome (PCOS), which is also characterized by anovulation, androgen excess, and insulin resistance. It has been suggested that PCOS is associated with an increased risk of coronary heart disease (CHD). The association between irregular menstrual cycles and CHD was investigated, using The Nurses' Health Study database.

Study Design.—The Nurses' Health Study is a prospective, multicenter cohort study of 121,700 American female nurses, aged 30 to 55 years at the study inception in 1976. The present study included 82,439 women who responded to a 1982 question about prior menstrual cycle regularity at ages 20 to 35 years and who did not have a history of CHD. Biennial questionnaires were analyzed for data concerning MI and stroke and confirmed with medical records. Pooled logistic regression with 2-year increments was used to model CHD and stroke risk relative to cycle regularity, and was adjusted for age, body mass index (BMI), smoking, menopausal status, parental history of early CHD, parity, alcohol intake, aspirin use, physical activity, and history of oral contraceptive use.

Findings.—Women reporting irregular cycles tended to have a higher BMI, a history of diabetes, hypertension, and hypercholesterolemia than women with regular menstrual cycles. During 14 years or 1,155,915 person years of follow-up, 2255 cardiovascular events occurred in this population. Women with irregular cycles were at a significantly increased risk for CHD, even after adjusting for potential confounding factors. The association between menstrual cycle irregularity and CHD was even stronger for overweight women. The risk for stroke was also slightly elevated for these women, but not significantly.

Conclusions.—These findings, from a large prospective data set, indicate that a history of irregular menstrual cycles may be a marker for increased risk of coronary heart disease. This finding may be explained by the association of irregular menstrual cycles and polycystic ovary syndrome. Appropriate screening and counseling to reduce coronary risk factors may be appropriate for women with a history of irregular menstrual cycles.

▶ The results of this large prospective cohort study found that women with irregular menses during the reproductive years have a greater risk of developing CHD than women with regular cycles. The increased risk of developing CHD in women with irregular menses is greater for obese than for nonobese women. The most likely reason for the increased risk of CHD among women with irregular menses is the presence of PCOS, which has been shown in some, but not all studies, to be associated with a greater risk of CHD. Clinicians should measure glucose, insulin, and lipid levels in women with PCOS, and if they are abnormal, should institute appropriate therapy. In addition, dietary alterations, exercise, and weight loss should be advised for women with PCOS to improve their cardiovascular status.

D. R. Mishell, Jr, MD

Polycystic Ovaries in Hirsute Women With Normal Menses
Carmina E, Lobo RA (Columbia Univ, New York)
Am J Med 111:602-606, 2001   13–2

Background.—Hirsute women with normal ovulation commonly are diagnosed as having idiopathic hirsutism. A group of hirsute ovulatory women was studied to determine whether the subjects had a subtle form of polycystic ovary syndrome (PCOS) and any of the metabolic abnormalities associated with classic PCOS.

Methods.—Sixty-two women were assessed prospectively. Baseline hormonal profiles, ovarian responses to gonadotropin-releasing hormone agonist, and ovarian morphology on US were compared with those in 2 nonhirsute ovulatory control groups. One control group comprised 10 women matched for body mass index (overweight), and the other control group comprised 30 women with normal weight.

Findings.—Only 13% of the 62 hirsute ovulatory women had normal androgen levels and were judged to have idiopathic hirsutism. Thirty-nine percent had characteristic polycystic ovaries and/or an exaggerated 17-hydroxyprogesterone response to leuprolide, suggesting ovarian hyperandrogenism and the diagnosis of mild PCOS. The remaining 48% of the women were considered to have unspecified hyperandrogenism. The hyperandrogenic subgroups had similar age, body weight, and androgen levels. Compared with normal and overweight control subjects and with patients with idiopathic hirsutism, the women with mild PCOS had greater fasting insulin levels, lower glucose-insulin ratios, higher low-density lipoprotein cholesterol levels, and lower high-density lipoprotein (HDL) cholesterol levels. Compared with patients with unspecified hyperandrogenism, these women had higher fasting insulin concentrations, lower glucose-insulin ratios, and decreased high-density lipoprotein cholesterol levels.

Conclusions.—Mild PCOS appears to be more common than idiopathic hirsutism. Subtle metabolic abnormalities were associated with mild PCOS.

▶ The data in this study indicate that about 40% of women with hirsutism and regular ovulatory menstrual cycles have a mild form of PCOS. Of the 54 women with hyperandrogenism and ovulatory cycles, 22 had sonographic findings of polycystic ovaries. These women also had insulin resistance and lipid abnormalities. Thus, a high proportion of women who have hyperandrogenism with normal ovulatory cycles and normal body weight have a mild form of PCOS with some degree of metabolic abnormalities. It is probably worthwhile to measure serum androgens and perform pelvic sonography in all hirsute women with irregular or regular ovulatory cycles to determine whether they have PCOS.

D. R. Mishell, Jr, MD

Ultrasound and Menstrual History in Predicting Endometrial Hyperplasia in Polycystic Ovary Syndrome
Cheung AP (Univ of Alberta, Edmonton, Canada)
Obstet Gynecol 98:325-331, 2001   13–3

Background.—The clinical hallmarks of women with polycystic ovary syndrome (PCOS) are chronic anovulation and hyperandrogenism. Anovulation and PCOS are recognized risk factors for endometrial hyperplasia, with or without cytologic atypia. However, it is not clear whether anovulation and PCOS translate into risk factors for endometrial adenocarcinoma. This study assessed the role of endometrial thickness on vaginal US and menstrual history in the prediction of endometrial hyperplasia in women with PCOS seen with infertility caused by anovulation.

Methods.—A total of 56 women with PCOS were enrolled in a prospective study in a university referral-based fertility and endocrine clinic. All of the patients were seen with infertility caused by anovulation. They underwent both vaginal US assessment and endometrial biopsies. The main outcome measures were the predictive value of sonographic endometrial thickness and the menstrual history with other clinical characteristics for proliferative endometrium and endometrial hyperplasia on logistic regression analysis. Receiver operating characteristic curve analysis was also performed.

Results.—Proliferative endometrium was present in 36 (64.3%) patients with PCOS, while 20 (35.7%) had cytologic atypia. Endometrial thickness of less than 7 mm or an intermenstrual interval of less than 3 months was associated with proliferative endometrial hyperplasia. These factors, along with the average intermenstrual interval, were found to be significant predictors of endometrial hyperplasia (Fig 1).

Conclusion.—These findings underscore the utility of a detailed menstrual history in women with PCOS for the identification of those who are at increased risk for endometrial hyperplasia and thus in need of an endometrial

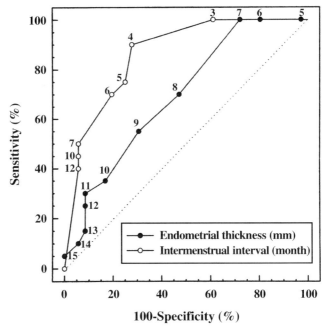

FIGURE 1.—Receiver operating characteristic curves (ROCs) for endometrial thickness and intermenstrual interval. The closer the ROC plot is to the upper left corner, the higher the overall accuracy of the test. When the variable under study cannot distinguish between the 2 groups, the area under the ROC curve is equal to 0.5 (*diagonal straight line*). (Reprinted with permission from The American College of Obstetricians and Gynecologists from Cheung AP: Ultrasound and menstrual history in predicting endometrial hyperplasia in polycystic ovary syndrome. *Obstet Gynecol* 98:325-331, 2001.)

biopsy. This clinical impression is corroborated by the endometrial thickness, which is particularly helpful when the patient's menstrual history is uncertain. In these women, endometrial hyperplasia is excluded when the endometrial thickness is less than 7 mm.

▶ Women with anovulation and PCOS have a high risk of endometrial hyperplasia with or without cytologic atypia. In this study, 36% of the women with infertility and PCOS had endometrial hyperplasia and one fourth of these had cytologic atypia. Sonographic measurement of endometrial thickness of more than 7 mm and intermenstrual intervals of more than 3 months were risk markers for endometrial hyperplasia and indicators for endometrial biopsy before initiating therapy for anovulation. In this study, women with menstrual intervals less than 3 months or endometrial thickness less than 7 mm did not have endometrial hyperplasia. Therefore, with these characteristics, it is not always necessary to perform an endometrial biopsy before initiating therapy for anovulation in women with PCOS.

D. R. Mishell, Jr, MD

Metformin Therapy Throughout Pregnancy Reduces the Development of Gestational Diabetes in Women With Polycystic Ovary Syndrome

Glueck CJ, Wang P, Kobayashi S, et al (Jewish Hosp, Cincinnati, Ohio)

Fertil Steril 77:520-525, 2002   13–4

Purpose.—Polycystic ovary syndrome (POS) is associated with gestational diabetes. The insulin-sensitizing drug metformin has proven useful in treating the metabolic and endocrine abnormalities observed in women with POS. Metformin's effects on the development of gestational diabetes in pregnant women with POS were examined in an observational study.

Methods.—The study included a prospective cohort of 33 women with POS who were taking metformin when they became pregnant and subsequently gave birth to a live infant. Mean metformin dose at the time of conception was 2.55 g/d. Twenty-eight women continued to take metformin during their pregnancy. Their rate of gestational diabetes was compared with that in a retrospective cohort of 39 women with POS who had pregnancies with live births in the absence of metformin therapy.

Results.—For the women who conceived while taking metformin, the gestational diabetes rate in 12 previous pregnancies without metformin was 67%. In the current study, the 2 comparison groups were similar in most characteristics, including height, weight, body mass index, fasting serum insulin, insulin resistance, and insulin secretion. The gestational diabetes rate was 3% in women taking metformin versus 27% in those not taking metformin. On a per-pregnancy basis, the rates were 3% and 23%, respectively. On analysis including all live births without metformin in both cohorts, the gestational diabetes rate increased to 31%. On logistic regression adjusting for age at delivery, the odds ratio for gestational diabetes with and without metformin was 0.093 (95% CI, 0.011 to 0.795). On a per-pregnancy basis, the odds ratio was 0.115 (95% CI, 0.014 to 0.938). Metformin was also associated with significant reductions in weight, body mass index, insulin, and insulin resistance. There were no major fetal complications associated with metformin.

Conclusions.—For women with POS, taking metformin may reduce the prevalence of gestational diabetes by 10-fold. By reducing insulin resistance and insulin secretion, metformin therapy also reduces the demands on the pancreatic β-cells. A randomized, placebo-controlled trial of metformin to prevent gestational diabetes in women with POS is needed.

▶ The data from this observational study suggest that if obese women with POS conceive while taking metformin, the likelihood of developing gestational diabetes during the subsequent pregnancy is markedly reduced if metformin use is continued throughout gestation. These findings need to be confirmed by a randomized, placebo-controlled trial. Until such a trial is performed, if non-pregnant women with POS who are receiving metformin become pregnant it appears advisable to continue metformin throughout their pregnancy. In addition to decreasing the risk of developing gestational diabetes, metformin also may reduce the rate of early miscarriage.

D. R. Mishell, Jr, MD

▶ Metformin is effective in increasing insulin sensitivity in the face of insulin resistance. It is of special interest in pregnant women with gestational diabetes and nonpregnant women who carry the diagnosis of polycystic ovarian disease (PCOS). Both groups share the likelihood of obesity, insulin resistance, increased insulin secretion rates, impaired reproductive capacity, and in the case of PCOS, hyperandrogenicity and menstrual abnormalities. On the basis of those similarities, this pilot study of the use of metformin in pregnancy compares its performance in 2 populations, both of them of clinical interest. The first is a prospective study of 33 gravidas with PCOS who conceived and delivered 34 newborns while receiving metformin. They were compared with a retrospective study of 39 women with PCOS who conceived without use of metformin and had 60 births. Women in the prospective group had diet prescriptions and weight reduction programs not necessarily shared by members of the retrospective group. Experience of the latter group clearly extended during a longer time than did the prospective group for which the average duration of care was approximately 15.5 months. PCOS was defined by oligo/amenorrhea evidence of hyperandrogenism or typical ovarian morphology and by exclusion of other endrocrinopathies.

Of the prospective group, prior to the index pregnancy and the use of metformin, there were 46 conceptions with 12 live births (26%), and 97% had menstrual abnormalities. Gestational diabetes developed in 67% of their pregnancies; 15 were sterile without metformin. Sixty-six percent had body mass indices greater than the 90th percentile. All infants born to women receiving metformin were live born, 15% prior to 37 weeks, with normal distributions of height and body weight at birth. Most important, all 34 newborns showed normal growth and development, and none showed evidence of hypoglycemia as newborns, as one might expect from fetal metformin exposure. The incidence of gestational diabetes mellitus in this group was 3%, and 21 women on metformin, studied at depth, showed decreased body weight, decreased serum insulin concentration and secretion rates, and reduced insulin resistance. In comparison, the retrospective group without metformin, also generally obese, had a 31% rate of development of gestational diabetes and a 28% spontaneous abortion rate. Although using internal control subjects would certainly have been preferred, the authors claim that use of metformin during pregnancy decreases the likelihood of gestational diabetes mellitus seems appropriate. The advantage to women with PCOS studied prospectively rested with their prepregnancy evaluation, dietary management, and antepartum care—all of them possibly serving to improve patient outcome. Whether fetal exposure to transplacental metformin from maternal blood is safe remains an important and viable question, but this experience is certainly reassuring in that regard.

T. H. Kirschbaum, MD

The Effect of the Menopause on Prolactin Levels in Patients With Hyperprolactinaemia

Karunakaran S, Page RCL, Wass JAH (Radcliffe Infirmary, Oxford, England)
Clin Endocrinol (Oxf) 54:295-300, 2001   13–5

Introduction.—Microprolactinomas can resolve spontaneously after pregnancy. It may be that estrogen therapy increases the size of microprolactinomas. Little is understood about the effect of menopause in women previously known to be hyperprolactinemic. The effects of pregnancy or menopause on prolactin levels were examined in a retrospective investigation of 148 patients with hyperprolactinemia and microprolactinemias treated between 1976 and 1996.

Methods.—Sixty-nine women who had not had pituitary surgery for treatment of microprolactinemia served as controls. None of these patients became pregnant or reached menopause. They were compared with 25 women who became pregnant, 11 who reached menopause, and 11 who were male. Participants were excluded from analysis if there were no follow-up data on dopamine agonist treatment of if they were surgically cured. Data were gathered concerning demographic parameters, treatment, scan abnormalities, prolactin levels at diagnosis and last follow-up, prolactin levels before and after pregnancy and before and after menopause. The pregnancy, postmenopausal, and male patient groups were compared with controls and with each other to ascertain whether they had a higher frequency of normalization of their prolactin levels during follow-up. Various factors were examined as possible variables for the normalization of prolactin, including the detection of scan abnormalities at diagnosis, prolactin levels at diagnosis, treatment with dopamine agonists, and duration of follow-up.

Results.—Prolactin levels normalized during the evaluation period in 45%, 24%, 18%, and 7% of the menopausal, pregnancy, male, and control groups. The menopausal group had a significantly higher possibility for normalization, compared with controls ($P < .005$); the pregnant group had a nonsignificant trend toward normalization ($P = .06$). Scan abnormalities, treatment with dopamine agonist, and duration of follow-up were not correlated with normalization of prolactin levels.

Conclusion.—Women with hyperprolactinemia who go through menopause have a significant chance of normalizing their prolactin levels. Those who go through pregnancy may have a nonsignificant higher chance of normalization. Menopause and pregnancy are indications for re-evaluation of treatment.

▶ There are few published data regarding the effects of menopause on functional hyperprolactinemia or hyperprolactinemia due to prolactin-secreting microadenomas of the pituitary gland. The results of this long-term follow-up study indicate that about half the women with hyperprolactinemia due to these causes normalize their prolactin levels after menopause. Clinicians should counsel their patients with hyperprolactinemia that prolactin levels will probably decrease after menopause. If a woman is receiving medical therapy for hyperprolactinemia, such therapy should be stopped for a few months after menopause or pregnancy to determine whether prolactin levels have returned to normal.

D. R. Mishell, Jr, MD

Treatment of Menorrhagia With the Levonorgestrel Intrauterine System Versus Endometrial Resection
Istre O, Trolle B (Central Hosp of Hedmark County, Hamar, Norway)
Fertil Steril 76:304–309, 2001   13–6

Background.—Two methods of treatment for uterine bleeding disorders (menorrhagia) are the levonorgestrel intrauterine system (LNG IUS) and transcervical endometrial resection (TCRE). Advantages of the LNG IUS include significant reduction in bleeding, avoidance of surgery, and contraceptive efficacy. Those for TCRE include few complications and promising clinical results. Disadvantages of LNG IUS are the incidence of side effects leading to discontinuation of therapy (irregular bleeding, breast tension, mood changes, and acne). Those for TCRE are the need for hospitalization and its contraindication for women who wish to preserve their fertility. These 2 methods were compared in a randomized open therapeutic setting.

Methods.—Two randomly determined groups were formed consisting of 30 premenopausal women each. Uterine bleeding was measured using a semiquantitative pictorial blood loss assessment score, which all women completed in the 2 months before enrollment. Excessive bleeding was defined as a monthly score of 75 or greater on this instrument, which corresponded to blood loss of 60 mL or greater. The endometrial resection was performed without simultaneous laparoscopy. A mixed diathermal current of 120 W from a diathermia unit was routinely used for resection of fibroids and endometrium. Follow-up examinations were conducted 6 weeks, 6 months, and 12 months after the resection or LNG IUS placement. None of the women underwent any additional treatment for menorrhagia. The outcome sought was a pictorial blood loss assessment score of 75 or less at 12 months. Menstrual blood loss and adverse events accompanying the 2 methods were documented.

Results.—A significant reduction in monthly blood loss was achieved in 20 patients (83%) with the LNG IUS after 12 months; success was achieved in 67% of patients. Six patients discontinued LNG IUS and had successful endometrial resection. Of the 29 patients who had TCRE, the procedures were uneventful, and 25 of 27 patients (90%) with primary TCRE had significantly reduced monthly blood losses at 12 months; the average blood loss per month fell from 378 to 7 mL. No difference in the number of pain days at each period was noted between the groups.

Conclusion.—Primary treatment with LNG IUS is possible for 60% to 70% of patients who currently undergo operative procedures. Menstrual blood loss is significantly reduced with both LNG IUS and TCRE. LNG IUS is reversible, may be useful as first-line treatment for younger women, and is accompanied by few mild adverse side effects. TCRE is perhaps more effective in reducing blood loss but requires operation facilities, is irreversible, and, if it fails, a new operation is needed. These factors must all be weighed in making the decision as to which technique to use for menorrhagia.

▶ Several groups have reported that insertion of the LNG IUS is an effective treatment for idiopathic menorrhagia. In this study, the mean monthly menstrual blood loss decreased from 410 to 42 mL 1 year after insertion of the LNG IUS. TCRE yielded slightly greater effectiveness than insertion of a LNG IUS. However, insertion of a LNG IUS requires less training, is less expensive, and is easier and more rapid to perform than endometrial resection. Furthermore, the use of the LNG IUS, unlike TCRE, is completely reversible. Clinicians should consider insertion of the LNG IUS as the initial treatment for idiopathic menorrhagia.

D. R. Mishell, Jr, MD

Recurrence of Endometriosis in Women With Bilateral Adnexectomy (With or Without Total Hysterectomy) Who Received Hormone Replacement Therapy

Matorras R, Elorriaga MA, Pijoan JI, et al (País Vasco Univ, Baracaldo, Spain)
Fertil Steril 77:303-307, 2002   13–7

Background.—Recurrence of endometriosis is common, even after surgical treatment. Given that endometriosis is a hormone-dependent condition, many clinicians advise that hormone replacement therapy (HRT) not be used in women with endometriosis who have undergone bilateral salpingo-oophorectomy (BSO). However, empirical data for supporting this recommendation are lacking. Whether HRT after BSO for endometriosis increases the risk of recurrence was evaluated prospectively.

Methods.—The patients were 172 women (mean age, 47.7 years) with endometriosis who underwent BSO during a 5-year period. Most of the patients (158 or 91.8%) had a total hysterectomy. None of the patients had received medical treatment for endometriosis, and none had taken hormone treatment for 6 months or longer before surgery. Four weeks after BSO, patients were randomly assigned either placebo (57 patients) or HRT (115 patients). HRT consisted of the sequential administration of estrogens (two 1.5-mg estradiol patches each week, which released 50 µg/d) and micronized progesterone (200 mg orally per day for 14 days, then no treatment for 16 days). Patients were followed up every 6 months for a mean of 45 months.

Results.—During follow-up, 4 patients in the HRT group (3.5%) had a recurrence, for a rate of 0.91 per 100 person-years. In contrast, none of the patients in the control group had a recurrence. However, the between-group difference in the risk of recurrence was not significant. The recurrence rate was higher in patients who did not undergo hysterectomy (5.9% per year) than in patients whose uterus was completely extirpated (0.5% per year) ($P = .02$; relative risk, 11.8). The recurrence rate was also higher in patients with peritoneal involvement of 3 cm diameter or greater (2.4% per year) than in those without such involvement (0.3% per year) (P = NS; relative risk, 8.1). None of the patients with stage I or II cancer had a recurrence. Two of the 58 patients with stage III cancer (3.4%) had recurrence, as did 2 of the 36 patients with stage IV disease (5.6%) (P = NS).

Conclusion.—Women with endometriosis who undergo total hysterectomy plus BSO have a low risk of recurrence (0.5% per year) when taking HRT after surgery. Given the benefits of HRT, it would seem to be a reasonable option. However, HRT appears to increase the risk of recurrence in patients whose uterus remains intact. Severe peritoneal involvement may also increase the risk of recurrence; while HRT is not completely contraindicated in this group, these patients should be monitored closely, and HRT should be discontinued if there is any suspicion of recurrence.

▶ The decision whether or not to administer estrogen with or without progestins after performing a BSO to treat endometriosis remains controversial. In this study, no recurrence occurred in the 57 women who did not receive exogenous hormones after BSO with or without hysterectomy for treatment of endometriosis. Among the women receiving exogenous hormones, 4 out of 115 women (3.5%) had recurrence of endometriosis for a rate of 1% per year. After BSO is performed for the treatment of endometriosis surgically, the benefit of administering exogenous hormones needs to be compared with the risk of recurrence in each individual woman. The low risk of recurrence may be further reduced by administering the estrogen and progestin continuously instead of sequentially as was done in this study.

D. R. Mishell, Jr, MD

14 Menopause

Hormones, Weight Change and Menopause
Davis KM, Heaney RP, Recker RR, et al (Creighton Univ, Omaha, Neb)
Int J Obes 25:874-879, 2001   14–1

Introduction.—Estrogen or hormone replacement therapy (ERT/HRT) after menopause is widely recommended; yet more than half of the women in North America who might benefit from long-term therapy adherence abandon treatment after a brief period. Total body mass was observed in 2 cohorts of women followed up longitudinally during extended observations both before and after menopause to determine total body weight change, specifically with respect to occurrence of menopause and the use of estrogen.

Methods.—Cohort 1 consisted of 191 healthy nuns aged 35 to 45 years at enrollment in 1967. They were participating in a prospective evaluation of calcium metabolism and bone health at 5-year intervals. Cohort 2 was participating in a trial of bone remodelling dynamics and biochemical markers. These 75 healthy perimenopausal women were observed at 6-month intervals over a 9-year evaluation period. At enrollment in 1988, the women in this cohort were aged 46 years or older and were still menstruating. About one third of each group received HRT after menopause. Patients were followed up for body weight and height, age, menstrual status, and use of estrogen replacement. For cohort 1, 608 measurements were obtained at 5-year intervals spanning a period from 17 years before to 22 years after menopause. For cohort 2, 1180 measurements were obtained at 6-month intervals spanning a period from 5 years before to 5 years after menopause.

Results.—The time course of relative body mass in cohort 1 was separated into 3 trajectories: 2 for women who ultimately received ERT/HRT and 1 for those who did not use these therapies. For this cohort, weight rose as a linear function of age (both chronologic and menopausal), both before and after cessation of ovarian function, at a rate of $\sim 0.43\%$ per year^{-1}. Neither menopausal transition nor use of estrogen had an appreciable influence on this rate of gain. For cohort 2, the rate of gain seemed to drop slightly at menopause. As for cohort 1, HRT (or its absence) had no appreciable influence on weight.

Conclusion.—The long-term, total body weight trajectory from at least age 35 to at least age 65 is not appreciably affected by either cessation of ovarian function or HRT.

▶ The results of this study of 2 different cohorts of women with similar changes in body weight over time indicate that women steadily gain weight as they age. This increase in weight is unaffected by the onset of menopause or by whether or not they take estrogen or estrogen-progestin hormonal replacement. One of the main reasons women discontinue HRT is the belief that the hormones make them gain weight. These data, as well as data from the randomized prospective estrogen-progestin intervention (PEPI) study, provide good information that postmenopausal estrogen or estrogen-progestin replacement does not cause an additional increase in body weight. Clinicians should counsel postmenopausal women about this information, especially if they wish to discontinue HRT because of fear of weight gain.

D. R. Mishell, Jr, MD

***

Discontinuation of Postmenopausal Hormone Therapy in a Massachusetts HMO

Reynolds RF, Walker AM, Obermeyer CM, et al (Pfizer Inc, New York; Harvard School of Public Health, Boston; Fallon Clinic Inc, Worcester, Mass)
J Clin Epidemiol 54:1056-1064, 2001   14–2

Background.—Most studies indicate that postmenopausal hormone therapy has significant benefits, but risks have also been identified. It is usually recommended that women use hormone therapy for a minimum of 3 to 5 years to obtain preventive effects on osteoporosis and cardiovascular disease, yet women rarely use this therapy for more than 2 years, with almost half of all women in the United States who initiate therapy discontinuing it within the first year. Generally the reasons given are adverse or bothersome side effects and fear of cancer. The rate and significant predictors of discontinuing hormone therapy were assessed in women cared for through an HMO in central Massachusetts. In addition, the role of medical, health service, and other prescription drug use in hormone therapy discontinuance was assessed, as was how these determinants vary over time.

Methods.—The 992 women assessed ranged in age from 45 to 59 years. They began taking hormone therapy between 1993 and 1995. Follow-up extended for 2 years after the first filling of their prescription for estrogen. Medical diagnoses, treatment characteristics at initiation, and health service and medication use were determined from pharmacy, ambulatory, hospital, and laboratory data covering 1 year before and 2 years after beginning the study.

Results.—The women's median age at initiation of estrogen therapy was 51 years. Therapy was discontinued by 53% of the women by the first year of follow-up, with 20% discontinuing treatment after the first month, 33% by the fourth month, and 65% by the end of the study. Among the factors linked to discontinuing therapy were the prescribing physician's specialty; previous breast cancer diagnostic test, mammogram, Pap smear or hospitalization; use of monoamine oxidase (MAOI)/selective serotonin reuptake inhibitors (SSRIs), antidepressants, or antilipidemics 3 months before initiating hormone therapy; number of years enrolled at the HMO; and year of entry into the study.

Adjustments were made, and it was shown that a prescription from a gynecologist and a mammogram 1 year before beginning hormone treatment were linked to a lower rate of discontinuation. Higher rates were associated with use of an MAOI/SSRI antidepressant and number of years enrolled in the health maintenance organization. Women who enrolled in the study in 1994 and 1995 had a higher annual likelihood of discontinuing treatment than those enrolled in 1993. The rate of discontinuing therapy during the first 2 months of use was the highest.

Conclusion.—The factors found to be most closely linked to continuing or discontinuing hormone therapy in these women were as follows: receiving the initial prescription from a gynecologist, having had a previous mammogram, and number of years enrolled in the HMO. Factors that were not significant included the woman's age, the mode of estrogen administration, the use of progestin, and the type of progestin regimen used. However, long-term hormone therapy use was noted to be uncommon in clinical practice.

▶ Despite the many reported benefits of postmenopausal estrogen replacement therapy (ERT), about half the women who initiated ERT in this HMO stopped taking it within 1 year. The incidence of discontinuation of ERT steadily increased among women initiating therapy between 1993 and 1995. Clinicians prescribing ERT need to thoroughly counsel women about the long-term benefits and risks of taking ERT. Therefore, if they decide to initiate this therapy, they will be more likely to continue its use in order to maximize the beneficial effect of ERT.

D. R. Mishell, Jr, MD

Benefits of Soy Isoflavone Therapeutic Regimen on Menopausal Symptoms

Han KK, Soares JM Jr, Haidar MA, et al (Federal Univ of Sao Paulo, Brazil)
Obstet Gynecol 99:389-394, 2002   14–3

Background.—Prolonged exposure to unopposed estrogens stimulates endometrial growth, which increases the risk of endometrial hyperplasia and neoplasia. Isoflavones, a group of biologically active compounds, have estrogenic and anti-estrogenic effects, depending on the target tissue. The change in menopausal symptoms and cardiovascular risk factors in postmenopausal women in response to 4 months of daily 100-mg soy isoflavone was studied.

Methods.—Eighty women were enrolled in the double-blind, placebo-controlled study. By random assignment, 40 received isoflavone and 40 received placebo. The menopausal Kupperman index was used to determine changes in menopausal symptoms. Plasma lipid levels, body mass index, blood pressure, and glucose concentrations were measured to determine cardiovascular risk factors. In addition, the effects of the regimen on endogenous hormone levels were assessed. Transvaginal sonography was performed to determine endometrial thickness.

Findings.—The isoflavone recipients had a significant decrease in menopausal symptoms compared with baseline and placebo group measurements. Total cholesterol and low-density lipoprotein declined significantly in the isoflavone group. Isoflavone treatment did not appear to affect blood pressure or plasma glucose, high-density lipoprotein, or triglyceride levels.

Conclusion.—This regimen of isoflavone appears to be a safe, effective alternative for the treatment of menopausal symptoms. It may also benefit the cardiovascular system.

▶ Soy isoflavone has a modest beneficial effect on vasomotor symptoms as well as other subjective symptoms found in women who are recently postmenopausal. Some other studies have confirmed that soy isoflavone has a beneficial effect upon vasomotor symptoms, while other studies have not shown significant benefit. There is no evidence that soy isoflavones or other alternative medicines have a beneficial effect on the risk of myocardial infarction, hip fractures, or Alzheimer's disease as has been shown for estrogen. Estrogen has also been shown to effectively reduce the incidence of vasomotor symptoms in comparison with placebo. Thus, because of the many benefits and few risks of estrogen, it would be preferable for most women to take estrogen for relief of vasomotor symptoms instead of soy isoflavone.

D. R. Mishell, Jr, MD

Hormone Replacement Therapy and Lens Opacities: The Salisbury Eye Evaluation Project
Freeman EE, Munoz B, Schein OD, et al (Wilmer Eye Inst, Baltimore, Md)
Arch Ophthalmol 119:1687-1692, 2001   14–4

Background.—Cataract is the leading cause of visual impairment in adults worldwide. It is estimated that by 2020, 52 million Americans will be over age 65 years. More than 1 million cataract operations are performed annually in the United States at a cost of $3.4 billion. Cataract surgery consumes 12% of the Medicare budget at present, and a steady increase is projected. Identification of a factor to slow the progression of lens opacification would lead to a significant reduction in cataract operations and greatly improve the quality of life for older adults.

It has been noted that after menopause, women begin to have higher rates of cataract than men. Data have suggested a possible protective effect against lens opacity with the use of hormone replacement therapy (HRT). However, there is no agreement as to the type of opacity that is affected. This study was conducted to determine whether there is an association between

HRT and the prevalence of different lens opacity types after controlling for endogenous estrogen exposure.

Methods.—The Salisbury Eye Evaluation is a population-based prevalence survey conducted among residents of Salisbury, Md, in 1993. Participants were aged 65 through 84 years. For this particular study, only women participants were included. A total of 1239 women underwent clinical examination, including a 4-hour eye examination. Pupils were dilated, and 2 nuclear photographs of each eye were obtained. Cortical photographs were also obtained. The main outcome measures were nuclear, cortical, and posterior subcapsular opacity.

Results.—A protective association was noted between nuclear opacity and current and recent use of HRT. An increasing number of births for younger women was also found to be associated with a protective effect. Only women who had never been pregnant benefited from past HRT use in this regard. Past and current use of HRT was associated with a lower prevalence of posterior subcapsular opacity.

Conclusion.—This study identified a protective benefit for HRT against nuclear and posterior subcapsular opacities. These findings should be confirmed in prospective studies.

▶ The results of this study, if confirmed in other studies, demonstrate an additional health benefit of postmenopausal HRT. Cataract formation is the leading cause of visual impairment in older adults and cataracts are more common in women than men. Therefore, women should be informed about the results of this observational study as it may influence their decision whether or not to use HRT.

D. R. Mishell, Jr, MD

Identification and Fracture Outcomes of Undiagnosed Low Bone Mineral Density in Postmenopausal Women: Results From the National Osteoporosis Risk Assessment

Siris ES, Miller PD, Barrett-Connor E, et al (Columbia Univ, New York; Colorado Ctr for Bone Research, Lakewood; Univ of California, San Diego, La Jolla; et al)
JAMA 286:2815-2822, 2001   14–5

Background.—Osteoporotic fractures are an important cause of disability. Low bone mineral density (BMD) is the single best predictor of fracture risk in aysmptomatic postmenopausal women. Currently, the gold standard for the measurement of BMD is dual-energy x-ray absorptiometry of the hip and spine. However, central dual-energy x-ray equipment is large, expensive, and not universally available, and testing costs are not covered by all insurance companies, particularly for women under age 65 years. As a result, many women potentially at risk for osteoporosis and fracture have not been evaluated.

Access to testing has been improved recently with the availability of lower-cost, small, portable technologies that test peripheral skeletal sites.

However, the usefulness of peripheral measurements for short-term prediction of fracture risk is uncertain. The National Osteoporosis Risk Assessment is a longitudinal observational study of osteoporosis among postmenopausal women in primary care practices in the United States. It has measured BMD and is now collecting longitudinal data from over 200,000 postmenopausal women. The prevalence of low appendicular BMD within the National Osteoporosis Risk Assessment cohort was reported, as well as its association with risk factors for osteoporosis and its relationship to fracture incidence.

Methods.—A total of 200,160 ambulatory, postmenopausal women aged 50 years and older were enrolled from over 4200 primary care practices in 34 states. The main outcome measures were baseline BMD T scores, risk factors for low BMD, obtained from questionnaire responses, and clinical fracture rates at 12-month follow-up.

Results.—On the basis of World Health Organization criteria, 39.6% of the women had osteopenia and 7.2% had osteoporosis. Age, personal or family history of fracture, Asian or Hispanic descent, smoking, and use of cortisone were factors associated with a significantly increased likelihood of osteoporosis. Exercise, higher body mass index, African American heritage, diuretic or estrogen use, and alcohol consumption significantly decreased the likelihood of osteoporosis. Follow-up information was available for 163,979 participants. Osteoporosis was associated with a fracture rate about 4 times hither than that with normal BMD.

Conclusion.—Nearly half the population in this study had low BMD that was previously undetected, and 7% had osteoporosis. Peripheral BMD results were found to be highly predictive of fracture risk.

▶ Peripheral BMD measurements are a good predictor of subsequent fracture due to osteoporosis. Clinicians may find it useful to perform screening of BMD in all postmenopausal women to determine those women at increased risk of fracture from this asymptomatic disorder so that appropriate therapy to prevent further bone loss can be initiated in these women.

D. R. Mishell, Jr, MD

A Prospective, Controlled Study of the Effects of Hormonal Contraception On Bone Mineral Density

Berenson AB, Radecki CM, Grady JJ, et al (Univ of Texas, Galveston; Wilford Hall Med Ctr, San Antonio, Tex)
Obstet Gynecol 98:576-582, 2001   14–6

Background.—Recent studies have suggested that bone loss may be caused or accelerated by the use of depot medroxyprogesterone acetate (DMPA). It is also unclear as to whether the use of oral contraceptives during the reproductive years affects bone mineral density (BMD). This study compared the effects of (DMPA) and 2 types of oral contraceptives on BMD among women between the ages of 18 and 33 years with similar women who did not use hormonal contraception.

Methods.—The study used data from 155 women. DMPA was administered to 33 women, while 63 women who chose to use oral contraception were randomly assigned to either a pill containing norethindrone (28 women) or one containing desogestrel (35 women). A control group comprised 59 women who did not use hormonal contraception. Lumbar spine BMD was determined by dual-energy x-ray absorptiometry at baseline and after 12 months of contraceptive use. The method-related percentage change in BMD was analyzed, with control for body mass index, calcium intake, exercise, and smoking. The study had approximately 90% power to detect a 2.5% difference between any 2 groups.

Results.—Women who used DMPA experienced a mean loss of BMD of 2.74% over 12 months compared with a 0.37% loss among the control group. Women who used oral contraceptives demonstrated a gain of 2.33% for norethindrone-containing pills and 0.33% for desogestrel-containing pills. These results differed from controls among the users of norethindrone-containing pills but not among users of desogestrel-containing pills. The changes in BMD among users of DMPA differed from changes in BMD among women who used either type of oral contraceptive.

Conclusion.—DMPA adversely affects BMD in comparison with oral contraceptives or nonhormonal methods when used for 12 months. However, caution is advised in the interpretation of these findings until it can be determined whether these effects are transient and reversible or long lasting.

▶ This prospective study provides additional evidence that the use of DMPA injections is associated with a reduction in BMD of the spine while the use of combination oral contraceptives increases spinal BMD. To date, no studies have reported an increased rate of fracture in former or current DMPA users. Therefore, studies need to be undertaken to clarify the long-term effect of decreased BMD in short- and long-term users of DMPA.

D. R. Mishell, Jr, MD

Effect of Lower Doses of Conjugated Equine Estrogens With and Without Medroxyprogesterone Acetate on Bone in Early Postmenopausal Women

Lindsay R, Gallagher JC, Kleerekoper M, et al (Helen Hayes Hosp, West Haverstraw, NY; Creighton Univ, Omaha, Neb; Wayne State Univ, Detroit; et al)
JAMA 287:2668-2676, 2002   14–7

Background.—Treatment with conjugated equine estrogens (CEEs) at doses lower than commonly prescribed plus medroxyprogesterone acetate (MPA) has been found to improve vasomotor symptoms and vaginal atrophy. In addition, the associated bleeding and lipid profiles are acceptable, and endometrial protection is provided. Protection against the loss of bone mineral density (BMD) associated with menopause, however, has not been studied thoroughly.

Methods.—In this double-blind, placebo-controlled substudy of the Women's Health, Osteoporosis, Progestin, Estrogen trial, the effects of lower doses of CEEs only and of CEEs-MPA on spine and hip BMD, total body bone mineral content (BMC), and biochemical markers of bone turnover were documented. The 19 participating centers enrolled 822 healthy postmenopausal women between 1995 and 2000. The women were aged 40 to 65 years and were within 4 years of their last menstrual period. Participants were assigned randomly to varying dosages and combinations of treatment.

Findings.—At 24 months, women in all the active treatment groups showed significant increases in spine and hip BMD as well as total body BMC compared with baseline. The one exception was no gain in total body BMC in women receiving CEEs, 0.3 mg/d. The changes observed differed significantly from those in the placebo group. Losses of bone mass in the spine and total body were evident in the placebo recipients. In the placebo group, hip BMD loss from baseline was significant at 18 but not 24 months. In all active treatment groups at all time points, levels of serum osteocalcin and urinary cross-linked N-telopeptides of type I collagen were decreased significantly from baseline. No such changes occurred in the placebo recipients. Among women treated with CEEs alone, the increase in spine BMD for those taking 0.625 mg/d was significantly greater than for those taking 0.3 mg/d, but not those taking 0.45 mg/d.

Conclusions.—In early postmenopausal women, CEE and CEE-MPA doses lower than 0.625 mg/d increase BMD and BMC. Lower estrogen and progestin doses may improve compliance with therapy by enhancing the risk-benefit ratio.

▶ Earlier studies found that doses of CEE less than 0.625 mg per day did not prevent a decrease in BMD in postmenopausal women. For this reason, 0.625 mg of CEE has been considered to be the physiologic replacement dose of estrogen in postmenopausal women. The results of this 2-year trial found that doses of CEE of 0.3 and 0.45 mg daily with calcium supplements, with and without the addition of the progestin MPA, cause a mean increase in BMD of the spine and hip compared with a decrease in mean BMD in the women receiving placebo. The results of this study suggest that doses of CEE less than 0.625 mg with daily calcium supplementation may be used by asymptomatic postmenopausal women to prevent osteoporosis.

D. R. Mishell, Jr, MD

Noninvasive Assessment of Coronary Microcirculatory Function in Postmenopausal Women and Effects of Short-term and Long-term Estrogen Administration

Campisi R, Nathan L, Pampaloni MH, et al (Univ of California, Los Angeles)
Circulation 105:425-430, 2002   14–8

Background.—Estrogen is known to improve endothelial function in the coronary conduit vessels of animals. Its effect on the coronary microcirculation in humans was further investigated.

Methods.—Fifty-four postmenopausal women with no coronary artery disease were included in the study. Thirty-one women were long-term hormone replacement therapy (HRT) users, who took estrogen alone or with a progestogen, and 23 were not. Myocardial blood flow (MBF) was studied with a positron emission tomography scan at rest, during cold pressor testing (CPT), and during dipyridamole hyperemia. Twelve healthy young women composed a control group. In nonusers, MBF measurements were repeated after 25 mg of conjugated equine estrogens were delivered IV.

Findings.—In women with and without coronary risk factors, neither short-term nor long-term HRT affected MBF at rest. Only women with risk factors who did not take HRT had attenuated dipyridamole MBF. Neither short-term estrogen nor long-term HRT reversed the abnormal response. In HRT nonusers, MBF responses to CPT were abnormal, irrespective of risk factors. These responses remained unchanged after short-term estrogen administration. Long-term HRT normalized CPT response only in women with no coronary risk factors. Women taking estrogen alone or with a progestogen had similar MBF, whether or not they had coronary risk factors.

Conclusion.—Menopause is associated with abnormal CPT, which can be reversed by long-term HRT only in women without coronary risk factors. Progestogens do not appear to antagonize this effect. Thus, long-term HRT may be beneficial in the primary prevention of coronary artery disease in women with no coronary risk factors.

▶ CPT provides an indirect measurement of endothelial function. The results of this carefully done study indicate that when estrogen or estrogen plus progestin is given to healthy postmenopausal women without coronary risk factors, there is a normal response of MBF to CPT. Postmenopausal women not taking estrogen or those taking estrogen with coronary risk factors had an abnormal MBF following CPT. These findings are in agreement with epidemiologic data that show when estrogen is given to healthy postmenopausal women, there is a reduction in the risk of myocardial infarction compared with women of similar age not taking estrogen. However, estrogen does not have this beneficial effect in women with established coronary artery disease, as shown in the Heart and Estrogen/Progestin Replacement Study (HERS).

D. R. Mishell, Jr, MD

Endogenous Estrogen Exposure and Cardiovascular Mortality Risk in Postmenopausal Women

de Kleijn MJJ, van der Schouw YT, Verbeek ALM, et al (Univ Med Ctr Utrecht, The Netherlands; Univ of Nijmegen, The Netherlands)
Am J Epidemiol 155:339-345, 2002   14–9

Background.—Several studies have shown that age at menopause correlates with the risk of cardiovascular disease. However, age at menopause is not the only factor associated with endogenous estrogen exposure. Whether combined information on reproductive factors has additive value to the single reproductive factor of age at menopause for determining endogenous estrogen exposure and cardiovascular mortality risk in postmenopausal women was studied.

Methods.—The population-based cohort study included 9450 postmenopausal women from Nijmegen, The Netherlands, aged 35 to 65 years at enrollment in 1975. The median follow-up was 20.5 years.

Findings.—Women aged 52 years or older at menopause had an 18% decrease in cardiovascular mortality rate compared with those aged 44 or younger. Women exposed to endogenous estrogen for more than 18 years had a significant 20% decrease in cardiovascular mortality rate compared with women with 13 years of exposure or less.

Conclusions.—Age at menopause correlated with cardiovascular disease mortality. The newly developed composite measure of endogenous estrogen exposure did not improve the predictive value of age at menopause for cardiovascular mortality.

▶ The results of this interesting epidemiologic study found that having a late menopause, 52 years of age or older, as well as more than 18 years of premenopausal exposure to endogenous estrogen without progesterone were each associated with a 20% reduction in overall cardiovascular mortality rate compared with women at a younger age of menopause or 13 years or less of exposure to endogenous estrogen. These findings lend support to the belief that estrogen exposure reduces the risk of coronary artery atherosclerosis.

D. R. Mishell, Jr, MD

Postmenopausal Hormone Use and Secondary Prevention of Coronary Events in the Nurses' Health Study: A Prospective, Observational Study

Grodstein F, Manson JE, Stampfer MJ (Harvard Med School, Boston; Harvard School of Public Health, Boston)
Ann Intern Med 135:1-8, 2001   14–10

Introduction.—The Heart and Estrogen/progestin Replacement Study (HERS) found no significant reduction in the overall rate of recurrent coronary heart disease among women receiving combined hormone therapy. However, further analyses showed an unexpected increase in the risk of major coronary events during the first year of hormone replacement therapy,

TABLE 2.—Risk for Major Coronary Heart Disease Among Users and Nonusers of Postmenopausal Hormone Therapy in Women With Previous Myocardial Infarction or Coronary Atherosclerosis in the Nurses' Health Study (1976-1996)

Homone Use	Follow-Up	Cases	Relative Risk (95% CI)	
			Age-Adjusted	Multivariable-Adjusted*
	person-years	*n*		
Never	6652	99	1.0 (referent)	1.0 (referent)
Current†	4997	42	0.56 (0.39-0.80)	0.65 (0.45-0.95)
<1 y	1549	24	1.06 (0.67-1.66)	1.25 (0.78-2.00)
1-1.9 y	1522	6	0.26 (0.11-0.60)	0.55 (0.13-2.27)
≥2 y	1926	12	0.38 (0.20-0.71)	0.38 (0.22-0.66)‡

*Adjusted for age, cigarette smoking, diabetes, high blood pressure, high cholesterol level, body mass index, age at menopause, and parental history of premature myocardial infarction.

†Duration of use is underestimated by an average of 1 year because duration during each 2-year follow-up period is established at the start of each period.

‡P for trend = .002. Test of trend was calculated by using categories of less than 1 year, 1-1.9 years, or 2 years or more of current hormone use.

(Courtesy of Grodstein F, Manson JE, Stampfer MJ: Postmenopausal hormone use and secondary prevention of coronary events in the Nurses' Health Study: A prospective, observational study. *Ann Intern Med* 135:1-8, 2001.)

followed by a significant decrease during the fourth and fifth years. Data from the Nurses' Health Study were used to further evaluate time trends in the effects of postmenopausal hormone replacement therapy on secondary prevention of coronary heart disease.

Methods.—From the Nurses' Health Study database, the investigators identified 2489 postmenopausal women with histories of myocardial infarction or confirmed atherosclerosis. Overall follow-up through 20 years totaled 17,239 person-years. From this group, 213 patients with recurrent, nonfatal myocardial infarction or coronary death were identified. Study participants provided data on hormone status and recurrent disease in regular follow-up questionnaires. The relationship between hormone use over time and coronary events was assessed with adjustment for potential confounders.

Results.—As the duration of hormone replacement therapy increased, the risk of recurrent coronary events decreased significantly. The adjusted relative risk of major coronary heart disease among women who were current, short-term hormone users was 1.25 (95% CI, 0.78-2.00) compared with that of women who had never used hormones. However, the relative risk decreased to 0.38 (95% CI, 0.22-0.66) for women who were long-term hormone users compared with women who had never used hormones. No consistent patterns were noted for women who used estrogen alone versus those who used estrogen combined with progestin. At last follow-up, the overall relative risk for women who were currently using hormones was 0.65 (95% CI, 0.45-0.95) compared with that of women who had never used hormones (Table 2).

Conclusion.—The analysis suggest that short-term use of hormone replacement therapy may increase the risk of recurrent coronary events among postmenopausal women. However, the ultimate risk of recurrent events seems to decrease with long-term hormone use. Additional data are needed, but the results indicate that hormone replacement therapy should not be given for the sole indication of preventing recurrent heart disease.

▶ The results of this large, prospective observational study are in agreement with those of the randomized clinical trial called the Heart and Estrogen/progestin Replacement Study (HERS). Both of these studies indicated that when postmenopausal estrogen replacement is given to women with a prior myocardial infarction or evidence of serious coronary artery atherosclerosis, the risk of a subsequent coronary artery event is increased in the first year after the initial event but decreased 4 or more years after the first coronary artery problem. Thus, postmenopausal women who have a myocardial infarction should not initiate estrogen replacement in order to decrease the risk of a subsequent event. However, women who have been taking estrogen for more than 1 year when they have a coronary artery event should be advised to continue taking estrogen as its use is associated with a decreased risk of a subsequent event.

D. R. Mishell, Jr, MD

Estrogen in the Prevention of Atherosclerosis: A Randomized, Double-blind, Placebo-controlled Trial

Hodis HN, for the Estrogen in the Prevention of Atherosclerosis Trial Research Group (Univ of Southern California, Los Angeles; et al)
Ann Intern Med 135:939-953, 2001   14–11

Background.—Mortality from coronary heart disease among women rises steadily after menopause, but estrogen reduces disease incidence. Endogenous estrogens have a cardioprotective effect on women before menopause. In postmenopausal women, hormone replacement therapy reduces cardiovascular morbidity and mortality. Unopposed estrogen replacement therapy is rarely studied in healthy postmenopausal women who have no cardiovascular disease. The Estrogen in the Prevention of Atherosclerosis Trial is a randomized, double-blind, placebo-controlled trial testing whether unopposed 17β-estradiol can influence subclinical atherosclerosis in healthy

---

FIGURE 2.—Time course of progression of common carotid artery intima-media thickness in the estradiol (*solid lines*) and placebo (*dotted lines*) groups. **Top,** Stratified by treatment group. The mean (± standard deviation [SD]) baseline intima-media thickness in all 199 evaluable participants (102 placebo recipients and 97 estradiol recipients) was 0.776 ± 0.149 mm compared with 0.752 ± 0.111 mm ($P < .2$). The mean rate of change in intima-media thickness in the placebo and estradiol groups was 0.0036 mm/y versus −0.0017 mm/y ($P = .046$). **Center,** Participants not taking lipid-lowering medications. The mean (± SD) baseline intima-media thickness in 77 evaluable participants (35 placebo recipients and 42 estradiol recipients) not taking lipid-lowering medications was 0.799 ± 0.182 mm compared with 0.734 ± 0.111 mm ($P = .07$). The mean rate of change in intima-media thickness in the placebo and estradiol groups was 0.0134 mm/y versus −0.0013 mm/y ($P = .002$). **Bottom,** Participants taking lipid-lowering medications. The mean (± SD) baseline intima-media thickness in 122 evaluable participants (67 placebo recipients and 55 estradiol recipients) taking lipid-lowering medications was 0.764 ± 0.128 mm compared with 0.766 ± 0.110 mm ($P > .2$). The mean rate of change in intima-media thickness in the placebo and estradiol groups was −0.0016 mm/y versus −0.0019 mm/y ($P > .2$). (Courtesy of Hodis HN, for the Estrogen in the Prevention of Atherosclerosis Trial Research Group: Estrogen in the prevention of atherosclerosis: A randomized, double-blind, placebo-controlled trial. *Ann Intern Med* 135:939-953, 2001.)

FIGURE 2

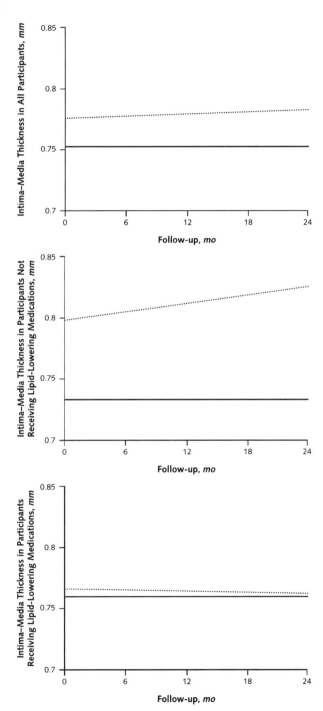

postmenopausal women with no previous cardiovascular disease. Results of the trial were reported.

Methods.—Characteristics of participants were serum estradiol levels less than 73.4 pmol/L, age at least 45 years, and a low-density lipoprotein (LDL) cholesterol level at least 3.37 mmol/L. No women had had breast or gyneco-logic cancer within 5 years or used hormone replacement therapy for more than 10 years or within 1 month of the first screening visit. Participants were randomly assigned to receive unopposed estradiol or placebo. All were counseled about dietary choices. At baseline and every 6 months thereafter, patients had carotid artery US. The outcome criterion was rate of change in intima-media thickness of the right distal common carotid artery far wall as detected by US.

Results.—Of 222 participants, 111 were in each treatment group. Ages ranged from 46 to 80 years (mean age, 62.2 years). Only 166 completed the 2-year study. The only significant differences noted at baseline were in rates of oophorectomy. The mean adherence to the protocol was 95% for women receiving estradiol and 92% for women taking placebo. The women taking estradiol had their mean serum estradiol level increase from 49.5 to 218.7 pmol/L. Sixty-one percent of the participants were taking lipid-lowering medications. Baseline carotid intima-media thicknesses were similar regard-less of group in those taking lipid-lowering drugs and those not doing so. The subclinical atherosclerosis progressed 0.0036 mm/y in the placebo group, but it regressed 0.0017 in women taking estradiol.

Women not taking lipid-lowering drugs had a change in intima-media thickness of 0.0134 mm/y in the placebo group and −0.0013 mm/y in the estradiol group. Regardless of group, these women had similar rates of pro-gression of atherosclerosis (Fig 2). Women taking placebo who received lipid-lowering drugs had less atherosclerotic progression than those not tak-ing those drugs, with a difference of 0.015 mm/y. No statistically significant difference (0.0008 mm/y) in atherosclerotic progression occurred between those women in the estradiol group taking and not taking lipid-lowering drugs. A comparison of women in the placebo group who took lipid-lowering drugs and women in the estradiol group who did not showed no difference in atherosclerotic progression.

In the estradiol group, the percentage increase in high-density lipoprotein (HDL) cholesterol and triglyceride levels was higher than in women taking placebo; their decrease in LDL cholesterol level had a greater percentage de-crease. The increased HDL cholesterol and decreased LDL cholesterol levels were always greater in the estradiol than in the placebo group, regardless of whether lipid-lowering medications were involved. Compared with place-bo, carbohydrate metabolism was positively affected by estradiol.

Conclusion.—Healthy postmenopausal women with no past cardiovas-cular disease who received unopposed estrogen replacement therapy had slower atherosclerotic progression than those receiving placebo. Women not taking lipid-lowering drugs had the greatest disparity in progression; no dif-ference was seen in women who took lipid-lowering drugs.

▶ More than 40 observational studies have consistently found that use of postmenopausal estrogen replacement therapy given to healthy women reduces the risk of cardiovascular disease, particularly myocardial infarction. Nevertheless, there is currently a great amount of controversy about whether estrogen causes the reduction in cardiovascular disease or whether the observed reduction is due to confounding factors.

The main basis for this controversy is the results of a randomized trial comparing the use of estrogen plus progestin (hormone replacement therapy) with placebo in older women with established coronary artery disease. After 4 to 5 years of the trial, no significant difference in the incidence of subsequent cardiac events was found between women using hormone replacement therapy or placebo. The results of this randomized trial reported by Hodis and colleagues convincingly demonstrated that estrogen prevented the progression of atherosclerosis in the carotid arteries during the 2 years of the study.

In addition to the beneficial effects estrogen has on the lipid profile, there are other direct beneficial local effects of estrogen upon the coronary arteries to retard atherosclerosis. Nearly all women who initiate estrogen replacement therapy do not have established coronary artery disease. The results of this study, as well as numerous epidemiologic studies, indicate that when estrogen is given to healthy women it retards the rate of subclinical progression of atherosclerosis and reduces the risk of myocardial infarction.

D. R. Mishell, Jr, MD

Intrauterine 10 µg and 20 µg Levonorgestrel Systems in Postmenopausal Women Receiving Oral Oestrogen Replacement Therapy: Clinical, Endometrial and Metabolic Response
Raudaskoski T, Tapanainen J, Tomś E, et al (Oulu Univ, Finland; Tampere Univ, Finland; Med Centre Gyne-Praxis, Jyväskylä, Finland; et al)
Br J Obstet Gynaecol 109:136-144, 2002   14–12

Background.—During the menopausal years, the size of the uterus declines. Thus, a smaller intrauterine hormone-releasing system has been developed. The menopausal levonorgestrel system has a daily release rate of 10 µg levonorgestrel. The endometrial response and bleeding patterns in postmenopausal women using the menopausal levonorgestrel system combined with continuous oral estrogen were investigated. In addition, the effects with the established levonorgestrel intrauterine system with a daily release rate of 20 µg or with cyclic oral medroxyprogesterone acetate combined with continuous oral estrogen were compared.

Methods.—One hundred sixty-three healthy postmenopausal women with climacteric symptoms or already using hormone replacement therapy (HRT) volunteered for the prospective, randomized, 1-year study. Women received a new intrauterine system releasing 10 µg levonorgestrel daily, an established intrauterine system releasing 20 µg levonorgestrel daily, or sequential oral medroxyprogesterone acetate, 5 mg/day, on 14 out of 30 days. These 3 regimens were combined with an oral daily dose of 2 mg E_2-valerate.

Findings.—Inserting the smaller, 10-µg levonorgestrel system was easy in 70% of the participants and difficult in 4%. Inserting the established intrauterine system was easy in 46% and difficult in 21%. After 6 months of treatment, 95.6% of the participants receiving 10 µg levonorgestrel and 98.2% of those receiving 20 µg levonorgestrel had no bleeding. The sequential medroxyprogesterone acetate treatment produced typical cyclic withdrawal bleeding. No endometrial hyperplasia occurred. After 12 months, strong endometrial suppression was documented in virtually all participants receiving 10 and 20 µg of levonorgestrel. However, the endometrium was proliferative in 18 of 47 participants in the medroxyprogesterone acetate group. The serum total cholesterol value was reduced in all groups. In women receiving medroxyprogesterone acetate or the smaller intrauterine dose of levonorgestrel, HDL cholesterol levels increased.

Conclusions.—Both levonorgestrel doses provided good endometrial protection in these women. The advantage of the 10 µg system with a smaller size is ease of insertion as well as minimal attenuation of the positive effects of oral estrogen on the serum lipid profile.

▶ Many women who take estrogen replacement therapy postmenopausally have adverse symptoms when they also take a progestin orally to prevent the increased risk of endometrial hyperplasia and adenocarcinoma that occurs with the use of estrogen alone. The intrauterine system described in this report releases levonorgestrel locally and thus prevents endometrial hyperplasia in women receiving estrogen. The intrauterine system also provided an acceptable bleeding pattern. The smaller levonorgestrel intrauterine system was easier to insert into postmenopausal women than the larger levonorgestrel-releasing contraceptive system now being marketed. Both systems provide adequate endometrial suppression. Development of the smaller system that releases 10 mg of levonorgestrel per day will provide an alternative for clinicians to administer progestins to postmenopausal women receiving estrogen.

D. R. Mishell, Jr, MD

A 5-Year Follow-up Study on the Use of a Levonorgestrel Intrauterine System in Women Receiving Hormone Replacement Therapy
Varila E, Wahlström T, Rauramo I (Univ of Tampere, Finland; Univ of Helsinki; Helsinki)
Fertil Steril 76:969-973, 2001   14–13

Background.—In addition to relief of climacteric symptoms, hormone replacement therapy (HRT) has been used to minimize the risks of osteoporosis and cardiovascular disease. HRT has also been suggested as having a role in the reduction of risk of Alzheimer disease. Thus, HRT could be extended for several years or even for the rest of a woman's life. The avoidance of withdrawal bleeding may be the primary motivating factor for long-term HRT, and the continuous use of estrogen and progestin therapy is effective for this purpose. However, oral progestin is accompanied by some undesirable side effects, such as irritability and fluid retention, which discourage compliance with long-term HRT. A novel method for continuous combined HRT is the administration of progestin directly into the uterine cavity via a levonorgestrel intrauterine system (LNG IUS). This study investigated endometrial histology, bleeding, and the effects of this system after 5 years of combined use with estrogen.

Methods.—A prospective cohort study enrolled 40 postmenopausal women who started HRT with LNG IUS and either a patch (50 µg/24 h) or oral (2 mg) estradiol valerate. Thirty-nine patients completed 12 months of treatment. Of these, 29 had used LNG IUS with continuous estradiol replacement therapy for 5 years. Seven patients volunteered to undergo a 3-month treatment-free period before reinsertion; 22 patients chose immediate reinsertion. The women completed bleeding diaries from 3 months before to 3 months after reinsertion. Endometrial histology was evaluated, the effects of estrogen and progestin were investigated, and endometrial thickness was measured.

Results.—Endometrial histology was nonproliferative at 6 and 12 months. At removal, all endometria were suppressed, and a strong progestin effect was observed. The thickest endometrium was 3.6 mm. In all 7 women were atrophic after washout. Twenty-six women were amenorrheic before the IUS was replaced, while 3 women had minor spotting. After replacement, 5 women had no bleeding, and 10 women experienced only spotting, which ended within 18 days. Investigators found the insertion of the LNG IUS was easy, and the women reported that it was well tolerated. In 10 insertions, cervical dilation or paracervical blockade was used.

Conclusions.—LNG IUS provides effective protection against endometrial hyperplasia. In most women, intrauterine levonorgestrel induced amenorrhea, with transient or short-term spotting or bleeding after reinsertion.

▶ To prevent development of endometrial hyperplasia and adenocarcinoma in women receiving estrogen replacement therapy (ERT), progestins are usually given orally. With the use of oral progestins, many women have uterine bleeding and spotting as well as such undesirable side effects as mood changes. The results of this observational study confirm results of other studies that have shown that insertion of an LNG IUS into the endometrial cavity prevents endometrial hyperplasia for at least 5 years in women receiving ERT and is accompanied by amenorrhea in two thirds of the women. Some women taking ERT may wish to have a levonorgestrel-releasing intrauterine system inserted into their endometrial cavity instead of taking oral progestins each day.

D. R. Mishell, Jr, MD

Postmenopausal Estrogen Replacement and Risk for Venous Thromboembolism: A Systematic Review and Meta-analysis for the US Preventive Services Task Force
Miller J, Chan BKS, Nelson HD (Veterans Affairs Med Ctr, Portland, Ore; Oregon Health & Science Univ, Portland)
Ann Intern Med 136:680-690, 2002   14–14

Background.—The risk of venous thromboembolism (VTE) with the use of estrogen replacement therapy (ERT) in postmenopausal women was evaluated.

Methods.—MEDLINE (1966 to December 2000), HealthSTAR (1975 to December 2000), the Cochrane Controlled Trials Register, and relevant reference lists were searched to identify English-language studies of postmenopausal ERT that reported VTE as an outcome or an adverse event. Data were abstracted from each study regarding the number of patients, intervention, event rates, confounders for which data were adjusted, method of outcome measurement, and duration of study. Each study's quality was independently rated by 2 reviewers using criteria developed by the US Preventive Services Task Force.

Results.—Twelve studies met the inclusion criteria; they included 159,684 women who were exposed to ERT and 342,380 women who were not exposed. None of the 3 randomized controlled trials (RCTs) included VTE as a primary outcome, and all 3 used conjugated estrogen at a dosage of 0.625 mg/day. Two of these trials were rated as being of fair quality, and 1 was rated as good. Venous thromboembolic events occurred in 51 of 2266 patients (2.3%) exposed to estrogen and in 13 of 1653 patients (0.8%) in the placebo groups. One RCT indicated that the risk of VTE was higher during the first 2 years of ERT. Relative risk of VTE among ERT users ranged from 2.89 to 5.10. Of the 8 case-control studies, quality was poor in 3, fair in 2, and good in 3. Six studies reported an increased risk of VTE with ERT use. Five studies indicated that the risk of VTE was higher in the first year of ERT use, and 3 studies reported that a conjugated estrogen dosage greater than 0.625 mg/day was associated with higher VTE risk than lower dosages. In 3 studies the risk of VTE was higher among users of estrogen combined with a progestin than with the use of estrogen alone. One study reported a higher risk with oral estrogen than with transdermal estrogen. Overall, relative risks (RRs) of VTE among ERT users ranged from 0.79 to 3.6. The only cohort study (of good quality) included 16 years of follow-up and reported an RR of VTE of 2.1 for ERT users. In meta-analysis, ERT use was associated with an increased risk of VTE (Fig 2). Pooled RR estimates were 3.75 for the RCTs and 2.05 for the case-control studies. The overall RR of VTE in postmenopausal ERT users was 2.14. All 6 studies that reported results by year of use (1 RCT, 5 case-control studies) indicated that the risks of VTE were higher in the first 2 years of ERT use (RR of VTE during first year, 3.49; RR of VTE during second year, 1.91). The RR of VTE with ERT use was 2.25 in the 9 studies with good or fair quality and 2.44 when only the good-quality studies were included. The RR of VTE with ERT use was 2.73 among the 6

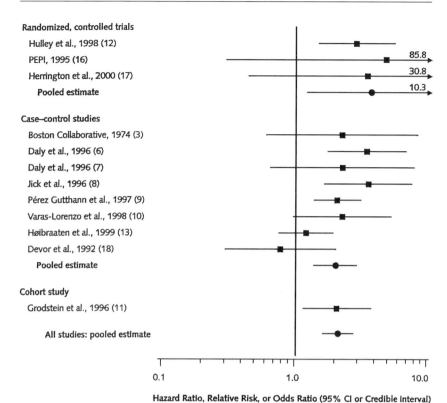

Randomized, controlled trials
Hulley et al., 1998 (12)
PEPI, 1995 (16) 85.8
Herrington et al., 2000 (17) 30.8
    Pooled estimate 10.3

Case–control studies
Boston Collaborative, 1974 (3)
Daly et al., 1996 (6)
Daly et al., 1996 (7)
Jick et al., 1996 (8)
Pérez Gutthann et al., 1997 (9)
Varas-Lorenzo et al., 1998 (10)
Høibraaten et al., 1999 (13)
Devor et al., 1992 (18)
    Pooled estimate

Cohort study
Grodstein et al., 1996 (11)

    All studies: pooled estimate

0.1   1.0   10.0

Hazard Ratio, Relative Risk, or Odds Ratio (95% CI or Credible Interval)

FIGURE 2.—Meta-analysis of estrogen studies. The pooled estimate of venous thromboembolism risk for all 12 studies meeting eligibility criteria was 2.14 (95% credible interval, 1.64-2.81). Numbers above the lines ending in *arrows* indicate the outer limits of the confidence intervals. *Abbreviation:* PEPI, Postmenopausal Estrogen/Progestin Interventions Trial. *Note:* Numbers appearing in parentheses are references available in original journal article. (Courtesy of Miller J, Chan BKS, Nelson HD: Postmenopausal estrogen replacement and risk for venous thromboembolism: A systematic review and meta-analysis for the US Preventive Services Task Force. *Ann Intern Med* 136: 680-690, 2002.)

studies that excluded patients with known coronary artery disease and 3.25 among the 2 studies that included these patients.

Conclusion.—Postmenopausal women who are currently using ERT have an approximately doubled risk of VTE. ERT increased the baseline risk of VTE from 1.3 events/10,000 woman-years by an additional 1.5 events/ 10,000 woman-years. This additional risk reflects an absolute incremental risk of 3.2 events/10,000 woman-years during the first 12 months of use and 1.2 events/10,000 woman-years thereafter.

▶ This comprehensive review and meta-analysis of 3 randomized controlled trials, 8 case-control studies, and 1 cohort study found that use of postmenopausal ERT increases the risk of developing VTE by about 2-fold. The absolute rate increase of VTE with ERT is about 1.5 events per 10,000 women in 1 year. The risk is greatest in the first year of ERT use and declines substantially or disappears after 2 years of use of ERT. The data in all but 1 of the studies are derived exclusively from oral estrogen use and may be less with transdermal estrogen. Women considering the use of ERT should be counseled about its associated increase in the risk of developing VTE, especially if they have a past history of VTE or an inherited thrombophilia. If women with these conditions wish to use ERT, it may be better to treat them with transdermal instead of oral estrogen. This suggestion is theoretical because to date there are no data showing a lower risk of VTE with transdermal ERT than with oral ERT.

D. R. Mishell, Jr, MD

Hormone Replacement Therapy in Relation to Breast Cancer

Chen C-L, Weiss NS, Newcomb P, et al (Univ of Washington, Seattle)
JAMA 287:734-741, 2002   14–15

Background.—Women receiving long-term hormone replacement therapy (HRT) appear to have an elevated risk of breast cancer. Few data exist on the effects of HRT use on the risk of cancer of different histologic types. This issue was addressed in a case-control study, including the impact of different HRT formulations and different breast cancer histologic diagnoses.

Methods.—The study included 705 women, aged 50 to 74 years, with a new diagnosis of first primary invasive breast cancer. The diagnoses were made from 1990 to 1995, when the women were enrolled in a large HMO. The women with breast cancer were matched for year of diagnosis, age, and years of HMO enrollment to 692 random controls. Use of HRT was assessed from pharmacy data; additional data on lifetime exposure were gathered from a breast cancer screening questionnaire. Incidence and histologic type of breast cancer were analyzed by duration of HRT.

Results.—Women who were current users of combination estrogen-progestin HRT had an elevated risk of breast cancer, although past users of any type of HRT were not at increased risk. For the 5-year period ending 1 year before diagnosis, women with a longer duration of oral HRT were at higher risk of breast cancer compared with those using no HRT during this period (odds ratio, 1.70). This increase in risk was similar for women using oral estrogens alone versus combination HRT and for those using sequential versus continuous combination HRT.

The association with HRT use was somewhat stronger for women with estrogen or progestin receptor-positive cancer, for thinner women, and for those with surgical menopause. The relation between HRT use and cancer risk was stronger for lobular than for nonlobular breast cancer. Risk of lobular cancer was increased for current users of oral estrogen, alone or in combination with oral progestin. This risk was particularly high for users of current combination therapy (odds ratio, 3.91). The risk of lobular cancer was tripled for women with a recent history of long-term ($\geq$57 mo) HRT use compared with a 50% increase in the risk of nonlobular tumors. For both types of tumors, the extent of risk associated with estrogen alone and with combination therapy was similar to that associated with total oral HRT use.

Conclusions.—Postmenopausal women with a recent history of long-term oral estrogen use are at increased risk of invasive breast cancer. The risk is similar for estrogen alone versus combined estrogen-progestin; for combined HRT, this risk is similar for sequential versus continuous therapy. The extent of risk is significantly greater for lobular breast cancer, including a 3-fold increase with longer duration of HRT and a 4-fold increase for current use of combination therapy.

▶ The results of this observational study suggest that long-term current users of postmenopausal estrogen replacement therapy (ERT) or estrogen plus either combined or sequential use of progestins (HRT) increases the risk of breast cancer. Incidence of the less common, less lethal lobular type of breast cancer was higher than that for the more common, more lethal ductal form of breast cancer. The data from this study also revealed that there was no increase in risk of breast cancer in former users of either ERT or HRT, which agrees with the results of most other studies. Therefore, it is unlikely that administration of estrogen or progestin initiates breast cancer because there is no longer an increased risk of diagnosis in former users. However, the increased risk of diagnosis in current hormone users could be caused by detection bias, possibly by greater use of screening mammography in users of hormones than in nonusers. The increased risk of diagnosis could also be caused by a promotional effect of hormones on the growth of breast cancer, increasing the likelihood of diagnosis while women are taking hormones but not thereafter. Perhaps ERT and HRT stimulate the growth of the lobular type of breast cancer more than the more common ductal type. It would be helpful to study the lifetime risk of breast cancer occurrence in women who have and have not used ERT or HRT.

D. R. Mishell, Jr, MD

Menopausal Hormone Replacement Therapy and Risk of Ovarian Cancer
Lacey JV Jr, Mink PJ, Lubin JH, et al (Natl Cancer Inst, Rockville, Md)
JAMA 288:334-341, 2002   14–16

Introduction.—Most trials assessing hormone replacement therapy in postmenopausal women have done so without distinguishing between estrogen replacement therapy (ERT) and combined estrogen-progestin replacement therapy (EPRT). The relationship between menopausal hormone replacement therapy and ovarian cancer is not clear. The potential association between ERT and EPRT and ovarian cancer was examined by using data from the Breast Cancer Detection Demonstration Project follow-up investigation, a nationwide breast cancer screening program.

Methods.—A large prospective cohort of 44,241 postmenopausal women was evaluated in 29 clinical centers in the United States. The cohort was evaluated between 1979 and 1998. Excluded were 12,581 women who reported a bilateral oophorectomy, 4 who died, 30 diagnosed as having ovarian cancer, and 4086 diagnosed as having breast cancer before initiation of the trial. The primary outcome measure was incident ovarian cancer.

Results.—A total of 329 women developed ovarian cancer during follow-up. In time-dependent analyses adjusted for age, menopause type, and oral contraceptive use, ever use of ERT-only was significantly correlated with ovarian cancer (rate ratio [RR], 1.6; 95% CI, 1.2-2.0). Increasing duration of ERT-only use was significantly correlated with ovarian cancer: RRs for 10 to 19 years and 20 or more years were 1.8 (95% CI, 1.1-3.0) and 3.2 (95% CI, 1.7-5.7), respectively (*P* value for trend < .001). A 7% (95% CI, 2%-13%) increase in RR was observed per year of use. Significantly elevated RRs were seen with increasing duration of ERT-only use across all strata of other ovarian cancer risk factors, including women with hysterectomy. The RR for EPRT use after previous ERT-only use was 1.5 (95% CI, 0.91-2.4). The RR for EPRT use was 1.1 (95% CI, 0.64-1.7). The RRs for shorter than 2 years and 2 or more years of EPRT-only use were 1.6 (95% CI, 0.78-3.3) and 0.80 (95% CI, 0.35-1.8), respectively. There was no indication of a duration response (*P* value for trend = .30).

Conclusion.—Women who used ERT-only, especially for 10 years or more, were at significantly increased risk for ovarian cancer. Those who used short-term EPRT-only were not at increased risk. The risks of both short-term and longer-term EPRT use should be evaluated further.

▶ The results of this large prospective observational study suggest that long-term use of estrogen alone, but not estrogen plus progestin, significantly increases the risk of a woman developing epithelial ovarian cancer. There have been numerous other observational epidemiologic studies investigating the association between postmenopausal estrogen use and the risk of developing ovarian cancer. The results have been inconsistent with the majority of studies, and a recent meta-analysis reporting no increased risk of ovarian cancer with estrogen use. However, another meta-analysis indicated that estrogen was associated with a small—but significantly increased—risk of ovarian cancer. Thus, these epidemiologic data are conflicting, not consistent, regarding the relationship of estrogen and ovarian cancer. Clinicians should inform patients that a relationship may exist but most studies show no association.

D. R. Mishell, Jr, MD

Risks and Benefits of Estrogen Plus Progestin in Healthy Postmenopausal Women: Principal Results From the Women's Health Initiative Randomized Controlled Trial

Rossouw JE, for the Women's Health Initiative Investigators (Natl Heart Lung and Blood Inst, Bethesda, Md; et al)

JAMA 288:321-333, 2002   14–17

Introduction.—There are decades of accumulated observational evidence, but the balance of risks and benefits for hormone use in healthy postmenopausal women has yet to be determined. The Women's Health Initiative (WHI) examined the risks and benefits of strategies that could potentially diminish the incidence of heart disease, breast and colon cancer, and fractures in postmenopausal women.

Methods.—A total of 161,809 postmenopausal women aged 50 to 79 years were enrolled between 1993 and 1998. The estrogen plus progestin component of the WHI was a randomized, controlled primary prevention trial (planned duration, 8.5 years) in which 16,608 postmenopausal women aged 50 to 79 years with an intact uterus at baseline were evaluated at 40 clinical centers in the United States between 1993 and 1998. Participants were randomized to either conjugated equine estrogens, 0.625 mg/day plus medroxyprogesterone acetate, 2.5 mg/day in 1 tablet or placebo (8506 and 8102 participants, respectively). The primary outcome measure was coronary heart disease (CHD). The primary adverse outcome was invasive breast cancer. A global index summarizing the balance of risk and benefits included the 2 primary outcomes, along with stroke, pulmonary embolism, endometrial cancer, colorectal cancer, hip fracture, and death from other causes.

Results.—On May 31, 2002, after a mean of 5.2 years of follow-up, the data and safety monitoring board recommended ceasing the trial of estrogen plus progestin versus placebo because the test statistic for invasive breast cancer exceeded the stopping boundary for this adverse effect. The global index statistic supported risks exceeding benefits. Data are available on the major clinical outcomes through April 30, 2002. Estimated hazard ratios (nominal 95% CIs) were as follows: CHD, 1.29 (1.02-1.63) for 286 patients; breast cancer 1.26 (1.00-1.59) for 290 patients; stroke, 1.41 (1.07-1.85) for 212 patients; pulmonary embolism, 2.13 (1.39-3.25) for 101 patients; colorectal cancer, 0.63 (0.43-0.92) for 112 patients; endometrial cancer, 0.83 (0.47-1.47) for 47 patients; hip fracture, 0.66 (0.45-0.98) for 106 patients; and death attributable to other causes, 0.92 (0.74-1.14) for 331 patients. Corresponding hazard ratios for composite outcomes were 1.22 (1.09-1.36) for total cardiovascular disease (arterial and venous disease), 1.03 (0.90-1.17) for total cancer, 0.76 (0.69-0.85) for combined fractures, 0.98 (0.82-1.18) for total mortality, and 1.15 (1.03-1.28) for the global index. The absolute excess risks per 10,000 person-years attributable to estrogen plus progestin were 7 more CHD events, 8 more strokes, 8 more pulmonary embolisms, and 8 more invasive breast cancers. The absolute risk reductions per 10,000 person-years were 6 fewer colorectal cancers, and 5 fewer hip fractures. The absolute excess risk of events involved in the global index was 19,000 person-years.

Conclusion.—The overall health risks exceeded benefits from the use of combined estrogen plus progestin for an average 5.2-year follow-up among healthy postmenopausal women. All-cause mortality was not affected. The risk-benefit profile was not consistent with the requirements for a viable intervention for primary prevention of chronic diseases. This regimen should not be initiated or continued for the primary prevention of CHD.

▶ This large randomized, controlled trial provides a high level of evidence that t12b combination of 0.625 mg conjugated equine estrogen plus 2.5 mg medroxyprogesterone acetate significantly increases the risk of developing coronary heart disease, stroke, breast cancer, and venous thromboembolism and decreases the risk of developing hip fracture and colorectal cancer. The data about CHD and stroke differ from the results of prior observational studies, but the data regarding other events are consistent with the findings of observational studies. Another arm of this study in which women without a uterus received estrogen alone did not demonstrate an increased risk of breast cancer after the same duration of this study; that arm is scheduled to complete the planned duration of 8.5 years. This study did not address the effect of estrogen and progestin upon hot flushes, vaginal atrophy, and Alzheimer's disease. Observational studies have shown that estrogen reduces the risk of developing these events. It is possible that formulations other than the one studied, such as transdermal estrogen, may have greater benefits and less risks. Unfortunately, it is unlikely that randomized, controlled trials of other hormonal regimens will ever be undertaken and the results of the estrogen alone arm of this study will not be available for 3 years. Therefore, clinicians and women need to decide whether the benefits of taking estrogen with progestin outweigh the risks for the individual woman based upon the epidemiologic data now available.

D. R. Mishell, Jr, MD

15 Infertility

Chronological Aspects of Ultrasonic, Hormonal, and Other Indirect Indices of Ovulation

Ecochard R, Boehringer H, Rabilloud M, et al (Hospices Civils de Lyon, France; Quidel Corp, San Diego, Calif)

Br J Obstet Gynaecol 108:822-829, 2001   15–1

Background.—There are many techniques, most of them indirect methods, that are purported to be predictive of ovulation. Laparoscopy is the direct reference method for observing ovulation, but it is technically difficult and impractical to perform routinely. As a result, new techniques for prediction of ovulation are often evaluated with reference to the midcycle luteinizing hormone peak or US investigation. It is less accurate than laparoscopy, but US detection of the day of ovulation (US-DO) is a direct method. However, US-DO has the disadvantage of the risk of subjective interpretations of the ovaries' US morphology. This study was designed to assess discrepancies between the luteinizing hormone–expected date of ovulation and the US-DO and to describe the temporal relationships between these indexes and other indirect indexes of ovulation.

Methods.—One hundred seven normally fertile and cycling women (age, 18 to 45 years) were enrolled at 8 natural family planning clinics. All of the women were followed up for at least 3 cycles. The interventions included daily measurements of urinary luteinizing hormone, follicle-stimulating hormone, estrone-3-glucuronide, and pregnanediol-3α-glucuronide; basal body temperature recording and checking of cervical mucus; and transvaginal US examination of the ovaries. The main outcome measures were delays between the expected day of ovulation according to the luteinizing hormone peak or US evidence and the expected day of ovulation according to the other indexes of ovulation.

Results.—US demonstrated evidence of ovulation in 283 of 326 cycles (Fig 1). The average time lag between luteinizing hormone peak and US evidence was less than 1 day, but premature and late luteinizing hormone–expected date of ovulation were noted in almost 10% and 23% of patients, respectively. There was a rise in basal body temperature in 98% of cycles. Cervical mucus peak symptom, rapid drop in the ratio of urinary metabolites, and initial rise in luteinizing hormone were close to US evidence in more than 72% of cycles.

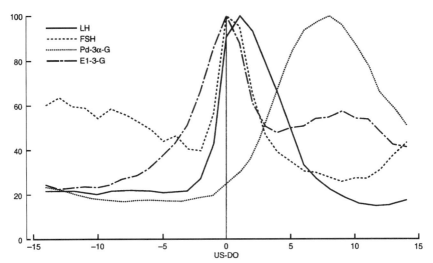

FIGURE 1.—Mean urine estrone-3-glucuronide (*E1-3-G*), pregnanediol-3α-glucuronide (*Pd-3α-G*), follicle stimulating hormone (*FSH*), and luteinising hormone (*LH*) concentrations with regard to ovulation day as determined by US (*US-DO*). Hormone concentrations were first expressed in convenient units (nanograms per milliliter, micrograms per milliliter, and milli-IU per milliliter, respectively), adjusted for creatinine, then transformed into percentage of the maximum mean value for each hormone. (Reprinted from Ecochard R, Boehringer H, Rabilloud M, et al: Chronological aspects of ultrasonic, hormonal, and other indirect indices of ovulation. *Br J Obstet Gynaecol* 108:822-829. Copyright 2001, with permission from Elsevier Science.)

Conclusion.—It would appear from the findings that, in terms of accuracy and feasibility, the cervical mucus peak symptom, the ratio of urinary metabolites, and luteinizing hormone initial rise may be better indexes of ovulation than the luteinizing hormone peak.

▶ The hormonal content of the first morning urine specimen usually reflects hormonal patterns occurring in the circulation during the previous day. Thus, the day of the luteinizing hormone (LH) peak concentration in first morning urine usually occurs on the day of or the day following US detection of ovulation. In order to predict ovulation, it is best to determine when urinary LH concentrations begin to rise and to detect LH concentrations in a urine specimen obtained sometime during the day after the first morning urine is voided.

D. R. Mishell, Jr, MD

Determinants of Pregnancy Rate and Obstetric Outcome After Laparoscopic Myomectomy for Infertility

Dessolle L, Soriano D, Poncelet C, et al (Hôpital Hôtel-Dieu de Paris; Hôpital Bichat-Claude Bernard, Paris)
Fertil Steril 76:370-374, 2001   15–2

Background.—The most common tumors of the female genital tract are uterine fibroids, which are estimated to occur in 20% to 50% of women. The occurrence of uterine fibroids increases in frequency during the later reproductive years. Infertile women with fibroids who undergo assisted reproductive therapy have lower pregnancy rates than those for age-matched women without fibroids. However, the characteristics of infertile patients suitable for myomectomy are unclear. The effects of myomectomy on infertility were evaluated, and the factors affecting reproductive outcome in this setting were assessed.

Methods.—The study enrolled 103 infertile women with uterine leiomyoma who had experienced infertility for more than 2 years. Follow-up was 12 months. The follow-up was completed by 88 patients, including 28 women (31.8%) with primary infertility and 44 (50%) with unexplained infertility. The patients had a mean age of 36.1 ± 2.1 years. All of the patients underwent laparoscopic myomectomy. The main outcome measure was the rate of pregnancy according to patient and fibroid characteristics.

Results.—A total of 42 patients (40.7%) became pregnant, and almost 80% of the women conceived spontaneously. The mean delay in conception was 7.5 ± 2.6 months. Of the 44 pregnancies in these 42 women, 36 live births resulted. There were no incidents of dehiscence or uterine scar. The pregnancy rate was significantly higher in women under age 35 years or with a history of infertility of less than 3 years. The pregnancy rate was higher for women with unexplained fertility than for women with multifactorial infertility. There were no differences in pregnancy rates according to fibroid characteristics.

Conclusion.—The most significant factors in fertility and pregnancy after laparoscopic myomectomy are patient age, duration of infertility before myomectomy, and existence of associated infertility factors.

▶ The results of this retrospective observational study are in agreement with the findings of other observational studies, which indicate that myomectomy improves fertility rates in women with no other explanation for their infertility and the presence of uterine leiomyomas. In this study of 88 women with infertility treated with myomectomy with adequate follow-up, 42 (47.7%) conceived. Among the 44 women with unexplained infertility 32 (72.7%) conceived after myomectomy. No woman over 40 years of age conceived after myomectomy. Although this was not a randomized trial, it appears that myomectomy enhances the chance of fertility in women younger than age 40 with unexplained infertility and intramural or subserous uterine leiomyomas.

D. R. Mishell, Jr, MD

Ovarian Function and Metabolic Factors in Women With Oligomenorrhea Treated With Metformin in a Randomized Double Blind Placebo-Controlled Trial

Fleming R, Hopkinson ZE, Wallace AM, et al (Royal Infirmary, Glasgow, Scotland)
J Clin Endocrinol Metab 87:569-574, 2002   15–3

Background.—Women with oligomenorrhea and polycystic ovaries have a high incidence of ovulation failure, possibly related to insulin resistance and associated metabolic features. The biguanide metformin may improve ovarian function. A detailed assessment of ovarian activity was used to test the value of this treatment.

Methods and Findings.—Ninety-two patients were randomly assigned to placebo or metformin, 850 mg twice daily. Fifteen patients in the treatment group, compared with only 5 in the placebo group, left the study prematurely. Ovulation frequency, expressed as the ratio of luteal phase weeks to observation weeks, was significantly greater in the treatment group than in the placebo group, at 23% and 13%, respectively. In addition, time to first ovulation was significantly shorter. A higher proportion of women in the placebo group did not ovulate during the study period. Most ovulations in both groups were characterized by normal progesterone levels. The effect of metformin on follicular maturation was rapid, the E2 circulating level increasing in the first week of metformin treatment. The metformin recipients had significant weight loss, whereas placebo recipients gained weight. Only the metformin recipients had a significant increase in circulating high-density lipoprotein. However, the metabolic risk factor benefits of metformin were not evident in the subgroup of morbidly obese participants. After 14 weeks, there was no change in fasting glucose levels, fasting insulin, or insulin response to glucose challenge. Body mass correlated inversely with treatment efficacy.

Conclusions.—Metformin treatment can improve ovulation frequency in women with abnormal ovarian function and polycystic ovaries. This improvement in the current series was significant, though modest. In addition, prolonged treatment appears to improve cardiovascular risk factors.

▶ A steadily increasing amount of information is being accumulated regarding the effect of metformin on endocrinologic, metabolic, and antithropometric parameters in women with polycystic ovarian syndrome (PCOS). In this study, the women with PCOS treated with metformin had a significant decrease in their body mass index, and one third had regular ovulatory cycles develop. Interestingly, metformin did not affect glucose metabolism but was associated with an increase in HDL cholesterol levels. The high dose of metformin used in this study was associated with a high incidence of gastrointestinal side effects. Additional studies are warranted to determine the appropriate dosage and duration of metformin therapy in women with PCOS. It also remains to be determined whether all women with PCOS should be treated with this agent or only women with certain abnormalities.

D. R. Mishell, Jr, MD

Strategies for the Use of Insulin-Sensitizing Drugs to Treat Infertility in Women With Polycystic Ovary Syndrome
Nestler JE, Stovall D, Akhter N, et al (Virginia Commonwealth Univ, Richmond; Hospital de Clinicas Caracas, Venezuela)
Fertil Steril 77:209-215, 2002   15–4

Introduction.—Treatment with insulin-sensitizing drugs has emerged as a new option for women with polycystic ovary syndrome (PCOS). A practical review of the use of insulin-sensitizing drugs to treat infertility associated with PCOS is presented.

Role of Hyperinsulinemic Insulin Resistance.—Most patients with PCOS have insulin resistance with compensatory hyperinsulinemia, a condition that likely interferes with spontaneous ovulation. In clinical practice, it is not necessary to measure the extent of insulin resistance; all women with PCOS may be regarded as being insulin resistant. Several research groups have examined the use of insulin-sensitizing drugs to improve peripheral insulin sensitivity and lower plasma insulin level for women with PCOS, with benefits in terms of menstrual cyclicity, ovulation, and fertility.

Insulin-Sensitizing Drugs and Their Uses.—Metformin—given at a dosage of 500 mg 3 times daily—is the best-studied insulin-sensitizing drug for the treatment of PCOS. The evidence to date suggests that insulin-sensitizing drugs might be the treatment of choice for initial induction of ovulation, although clomiphene citrate remains the standard of case. One trial found that 34% of women with PCOS ovulated while taking metformin alone compared with 8% taking clomiphene citrate plus placebo. A head-to-head randomized comparison of these 2 treatments for initial ovulation is needed.

It has also been suggested that giving metformin and clomiphene together might be more effective than either treatment. In the same trial mentioned, the ovulation rate with metformin plus clomiphene was 90%; metformin increased the spontaneous ovulation rate by more than 8-fold and the clomiphene-induced ovulation rate by more than 11-fold. Another study found metformin effective in promoting ovulation and conception among women in whom clomiphene treatment had failed. Metformin may also reduce the risk of ovarian hyperstimulation in response to follicle-stimulating hormone therapy, thus lowering the rate of multiple gestation. Given its safety record, metformin is currently the insulin-sensitizing agent of choice for treatment of PCOS-related infertility.

Treatment Algorithm.—Based on the available data, the authors present a recommended approach to insulin-sensitizing drug therapy for treatment of infertility in women with PCOS. For patients who do not ovulate in response to clomiphene 150 mg, it is reasonable to add metformin in an attempt to induce ovulation. Pending a randomized trial, the use of metformin as the initial approach to ovulation induction remains speculative.

Discussion.—A growing body of evidence suggests that treatment for insulin resistance can improve fertility outcomes in women with PCOS. The authors review current data supporting the use of metformin for this indication, including specific recommendations for clinical treatment.

▶ A high proportion of anovulatory infertile women with PCOS do not ovulate when treated with clomiphene citrate. It is difficult to treat these women who do not ovulate after use of clomiphene citrate with gonadotrophins because of the high incidence of multiple ovulations and multiple gestations as well as the frequent occurrence of the ovarian hyperstimulation syndrome. Several studies have reported that the use of the insulin-sensitizing agent metformin increases the likelihood that anovulatory women with PCOS will ovulate after use of clomiphene citrate. This review summarizes the data supporting the use of metformin in women with PCOS who do not ovulate with clomiphene citrate. Although induction of ovulation is not an approved use for metformin, there is sufficient published evidence for clinicians to use metformin in a dose of 500 mg 3 times a day to treat anovulatory women with PCOS who do not ovulate with clomiphene citrate.

D. R Mishell, Jr, MD

Pregnancies Following Use of Metformin for Ovulation Induction in Patients With Polycystic Ovary Syndrome
Heard MJ, Pierce A, Carson SA, et al (Baylor College of Medicine, Houston)
Fertil Steril 77:669-673, 2002   15–5

Introduction.—Polycystic ovary syndrome (PCOS) is considered a common cause of infertility. The condition is associated with chronic anovulation, and many patients have insulin resistance with elevated insulin levels. Metformin, when used for patients with PCOS, corrects hyperinsulinemia and induces resumption of regular menses and ovulation. A group of anovulatory infertile patients with a diagnosis of PCOS was studied for pregnancy outcome after treatment with metformin.

Methods.—The study included 48 patients (mean age, 29.9 years) who were treated with metformin, with or without clomiphene citrate (CC), from December 1, 1999, through February 15, 2001. Metformin was administered initially at 500 mg twice daily for 6 weeks, with dosage varied to accommodate side effects. Patients who did not respond to the initial dose with ovulation received increased doses, and CC was added (50 mg/d for 5 days) when no response occurred in 6 more weeks. Women who conceived while receiving metformin continued this medication through 12 weeks of gestation.

Results.—Of the 48 patients, 19 (40%) resumed spontaneous menses after treatment and showed presumptive evidence of ovulation with metformin alone. Of 15 women who required CC in conjunction with metformin therapy, 10 had evidence of ovulation. Overall, 20 (42%) members of the study group conceived with a median time to conception of 3 months; Of these women, however, 7 (35%) had spontaneous abortions. No multiple gestations occurred. Gastrointestinal side effects were common (40% of patients), and the dosage of metformin had to be decreased in 5 patients. Only 1 patient discontinued therapy because of side effects.

Conclusion.—This is the second and largest study to date in which metformin, in conjunction with CC, was used to increase ovulatory and pregnancy rates in women with PCOS. A substantial number of pregnancies were achieved, and 42% of women who ovulated achieved conception in less than 6 months of therapy.

▶ Anovulatory women with polycystic ovarian syndrome (PCOS) frequently fail to ovulate when treated with clomiphene citrate (CC). It has been shown that the ovulatory rate of women with PCOS who fail to ovulate when treated with CC alone can be increased if they are also given metformin. This study shows that when metformin is used initially in anovulatory women with PCOS, the ovulation rate was 40%. When clomiphene citrate was added to metformin in the women who failed to ovulate with metformin alone, the ovulation rate increased to 60%. The conception rate of these ovulatory women was high, reaching 68% within 6 months. Randomized trials of initiating therapy with either clomiphene citrate or metformin need to be performed in anovulatory women with PCOS to help enable clinicians to decide which agent should be used initially to induce ovulation. At present, initiating therapy with either metformin or CC and adding the other agent if ovulation does not occur provide good rates of ovulation.

D. R. Mishell, Jr, MD

Metformin Therapy Improves Ovulatory Rates, Cervical Scores, and Pregnancy Rates in Clomiphene Citrate–Resistant Women With Polycystic Ovary Syndrome
Kocak M, Caliskan E, Simsir C, et al (SSK Ankara Maternity and Women's Health Teaching Hosp, Turkey)
Fertil Steril 77:101-106, 2002   15–6

Background.—Polycystic ovary syndrome (PCOS) is characterized by oligomenorrhea and is often treated with clomiphene citrate (CC) for ovulation induction. As evidence has pointed to a link among hyperinsulinemia, insulin resistance, and increased androgen secretion in PCOS, insulin sensitizers such as metformin have been suggested to improve symptoms in women with PCOS. This prospective, randomized, double-blind, placebo-controlled study examined whether metformin administration improved response to CC in patients with CC-resistant PCOS.

Study Design.—The study group consisted of 56 primary infertile patients with PCOS who were resistant to CC. On the first day of their menstrual cycles, these patients' weight, height, waist-to-hip ratio, and body mass index were assessed. Baseline steroid, fasting insulin, and glucose levels were obtained. The women were then randomly assigned to receive CC with either metformin or placebo. Assessments were repeated on the second day of their second menstrual cycle. Endometrial thickness, cervical score, ovulation, and pregnancy rates were compared between the two groups by using the Student *t*-test or the Mann-Whitney rank sum test.

Findings.—Metformin therapy was associated with a significant decrease in total testosterone, luteinizing hormone, luteinizing hormone/follicle-stimulating hormone ratio, insulin resistance, and mean body mass index. No differences were noted between the 2 groups in waist-to-hip ratio, dehydroepiandrosterone sulfate level, or fasting insulin level. CC induction was more successful in the metformin group and resulted in higher ovulation rates and thicker endometrium. A higher pregnancy rate occurred in the metformin group, but the difference did not reach statistical significance.

Conclusions.—In CC-resistant women with PCOS, treatment with the insulin sensitizer metformin reduced serum androgens and luteinizing hormone and increased ovulation, endometrial thickening, and pregnancy rates. Metformin may be useful in the treatment of women with PCOS.

▶ The results of this randomized study provide additional evidence that administration of the insulin sensitizer metformin improves the likelihood of ovulation in women with PCOS treated with CC. If anovulatory women with PCOS wish to conceive, they should be treated with CC. If it fails to induce ovulation, administration of metformin in addition to CC should increase the incidence of ovulation.

D. R. Mishell, Jr, MD

Use of Fertility Drugs and Risk of Ovarian Cancer
Parazzini F, Pelucchi C, Negri E, et al (Istituto di Ricerche Farmacologiche 'Mario Negri', Milan, Italy; Università degli Studi di Milano, Milan, Italy; Internatl Agency for Research on Cancer, Lyon, France; et al)
Hum Reprod 16:1372-1375, 2001   15–7

Background.—Whether the use of fertility drugs increases the risk of ovarian epithelial cancer is still unresolved. This retrospective case-control study explored this possibility.

Methods.—The patients were 1031 women (median age, 56 years) with incident epithelial ovarian cancer who resided in 1 of 4 regions of Italy between January 1992 and September 1999. In all cases, cancer was confirmed by histologic examination. The control subjects were 2411 women (median age, 57 years) who resided in the same regions and who were admitted to the same hospitals for acute nonneoplastic conditions. All subjects were interviewed to determine demographic and pregnancy-related characteristics, including whether they had ever used fertility drugs.

Results.—Fifteen patients (1.5%) and 26 controls (1.1%) had used fertility drugs. Odds ratios (ORs) for ovarian epithelial cancer were not significant for the group as a whole (OR, 1.3), for nulliparous women (OR, 0.6), or for parous women (OR, 1.9). Similarly, ORs did not differ for women who last used a fertility drug more than 25 years previously (OR, 1.2) or for women whose use was more recent (OR, 1.3).

Conclusion.—There does not appear to be a strong relationship between the use of fertility drugs and ovarian epithelial cancer. Nonetheless, the data cannot exclude a moderate association, especially among parous women. Further large studies are needed to examine this possible association and to evaluate whether the specific fertility drug used affects the risk of ovarian epithelial cancer.

▶ The risk of developing epithelial ovarian cancer is directly related to the number of times a woman ovulates in her lifetime. Both pregnancy and the use of oral contraceptives decrease the risk of the development of epithelial ovarian cancer. Therefore, there is concern that the use of agents that induce multiple ovulations increase the risk of this type of cancer. The epidemiologic evidence is conflicting. The data obtained in this study are somewhat reassuring, but, because of the small sample size, the findings cannot exclude the possible association between use of agents that induce ovulation and an increased risk of epithelial ovarian cancer developing later in life. More data in larger groups of women need to be obtained to help determine if a relation exists between the use of specific ovulatory-inducing agents and the risk of epithelial ovarian cancer developing.

D. R. Mishell, Jr, MD

Assisted Reproductive Technology in the United States: 1998 Results Generated From the American Society for Reproductive Medicine/ Society for Assisted Reproductive Technology Registry
Society for Assisted Reproductive Technology and the American Society for Reproductive Medicine (Birmingham, Ala)
Fertil Steril 77:18-31, 2002   15–8

Background.—The Society for Assisted Reproductive Technology (SART) began publishing annual reports of assisted reproductive technology (ART) activities in 1988. These early reports were based on voluntarily submitted data and provided a forum for sharing information as the technology emerged. In 1992, the Fertility Clinic Success Rate and Certification Act mandated the Centers for Disease Control and Prevention to publish clinic-specific pregnancy success rates for ART procedures in the United States. SART has continued to augment the annual Centers for Disease Control and Prevention report with reviews and analyses of annual data to explore trends in ART activities in greater detail. The procedures and outcomes of ART undertaken in the United States in 1998 were summarized.

Methods.—Data on procedures performed in 1998 were submitted by 360 programs. The data were collated after November 1999 so that the outcomes of all pregnancies would be known. The data were gathered electron-

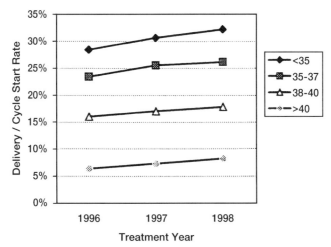

Treatment Year

FIGURE 1.—Delivery rates in 1996, 1997, and 1998. (Reprinted by permission from the American Society for Reproductive Medicine courtesy of Society for Assisted Reproductive Technology and the American Society for Reproductive Medicine: Assisted reproductive technology in the United States: 1998 results generated from the American Society for Reproductive Medicine/Society for Assisted Reproductive Technology Registry. *Fertil Steril* 77:18-31, 2002.)

ically with the use of the SART Clinical Outcome Reporting System. The main outcome measures were the incidence of clinical pregnancy, abortion, stillbirth, and delivery.

Results.—A total of 81,899 cycles of ART treatment were reported. Of these, 58,937 cycles involved in vitro fertilization (with and without micromanipulation), with a delivery rate per retrieval of 29.1%. Gamete intrafallopian transfer was involved in 1293 cycles, with a delivery rate per retrieval of 27.4%. Zygote intrafallopian transfer was involved in 1054 cycles, with a delivery rate per retrieval of 29.6%. Other ART procedures initiated were 5273 fresh donor oocyte cycles (a delivery rate per transfer of 41.2%); 11,228 frozen embryo transfer procedures (a delivery per transfer of 19.3%); 1913 frozen embryo transfers using donated oocytes or embryos (a delivery rate per transfer of 23.5%); and 809 cycles with the use of a host uterus (a delivery rate per transfer of 31.6%). There were also 969 cycles that were combinations of multiple treatment techniques, 25 cycles as research, and 398 as embryo banking. A total of 20,241 deliveries resulting in 29,128 neonates were reported.

Conclusion.—There were more programs reporting ART treatment in 1998 and a significant (12.1%) increase in reported cycles compared with 1997. Overall, there was an increase of 4.7% in the success rate compared with 1997 results (Fig 1).

▶ The data collected from this registry are of great importance for counseling infertile couples in the United States about their chance of having a successful pregnancy after undergoing various types of ART. The data confirm the profound influence of increasing female age decreasing the likelihood of having a successful outcome. It is encouraging to observe that the incidence of having a successful pregnancy has shown a modest but steady increase in each female age group between 1996 and 1998. It is also of interest that when intracytoplasmic sperm injection (ICSI) was utilized to achieve fertilization, pregnancy rates and delivery rates were similar to cycles in which fertilization was performed without ICSI.

D. R. Mishell, Jr, MD

What Is the Probability of Conception for Couples Entering an IVF Program?
Kovacs GT, MacLachlan V, Brehny S (Box Hill Hosp, Melbourne, Australia)
Aust N Z J Obstet Gynaecol 41:207-209, 2001   15–9

Introduction.—One of the challenges of evaluating the outcome of treatment by in vitro fertilization (IVF) is that there will always be some women who have not completed their treatment. This is best compensated for by using life table analysis, which considers what is likely to happen to these patients if they undergo further treatment. The outcomes of 4225 couples undergoing 8207 IVF cycles between January 1992 and December 1997 were analyzed with the use of life table analysis.

Methods.—Pregnancy for this analysis was defined as a "clinical pregnancy" if a fetus was present at US examination. Only 20 (0.5%) of the couples proceeded beyond 6 cycles, accounting for 34 of a total of 8207 cycles (0.5%) (Fig 1).

Results.—Only 1 in 200 patients continued beyond 6 cycles. Of 4225 patients who had their first stimulated cycle in 1993-1997, 777 conceived with fresh embryos/oocytes and 99 conceived with frozen embryos collected in their first stimulated cycle. Thus, 20.7% of the patients conceived after the initial oocyte collection. Nearly half of the patients were pregnant within 3 cycles and more than two thirds were pregnant within 6 cycles.

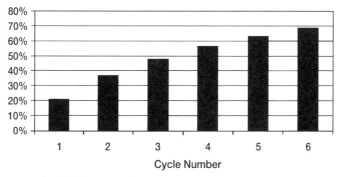

FIGURE 1.—Life table of compounded outcome. (Courtesy of Kovacs GT, MacLachlan V, Brehny S: What is the probability of conception for couples entering an IVF program? *Aust N Z J Obstet Gynaecol* 41:207-209, 2001.)

Conclusion.—These data may be useful in presenting the chance of pregnancy to prospective couples.

▶ This study was started in 1992, and the rates of pregnancy after IVF have been steadily increasing since that time. Thus, pregnancy rates after IVF are currently higher than those published in this report. However, the rate of fecundity reported in this study is similar to that of normal fertile couples—20% at 1 month, 50% at 3 months, and 70% at 6 months. Couples who do not conceive during their first cycle of IVF will have a steadily decreasing chance of conceiving in subsequent IVF cycles and should be counseled accordingly.

D. R. Mishell, Jr, MD

Cumulative Probability of Live Birth After Three in Vitro Fertilization/ Intracytoplasmic Sperm Injection Cycles
Olivius K, Friden B, Lundin K, et al (Göteborg Univ, Sweden)
Fertil Steril 77:505-510, 2002   15–10

Background.—In Sweden, infertile couples may receive up to 3 state-subsidized cycles of in vitro fertilization (IVF) leading to 1 childbirth. The cumulative likelihood of live birth for couples receiving 3 publicly funded IVF treatments was analyzed.

Methods.—The study included 974 infertile couples undergoing their first cycle of IVF at 1 Swedish center during 1996-97. The women's mean age was 32.5 years. Most patients received 3 free completed cycles of IVF, defined as a stimulated IVF cycle with embryo transfer. The fertilization technique used in the first completed cycle was IVF in 47% of cases and intracytoplasmic sperm injection (ICSI) in 51%. The study end point was cumulative live birth rate.

Results.—Fresh, stimulated cycles had a pregnancy rate of 31% per started cycle and 37% per embryo transfer, whereas thawing cycles had a pregnancy rate of 27% per embryo transfer. Life-table analysis, performed with different sets of assumptions, indicated cumulative pregnancy rates after 3 completed cycles rated assumptions 65.2% "pessimistic," 66.2% "realistic," and 73.2% "optimistic." Cumulative pregnancy rates after 3 started cycles were 61.4%, 61.8%, and 67.1%, respectively. At least 1 IVF cycle was completed for 944 patients. After 3 completed cycles, the cumulative live birth rate was 55.5% under pessimistic assumptions, 63.1% under realistic assumptions, and 65.5% under optimistic assumptions. The rates per 3 started cycles were 50.9%, 56.3%, and 57.1%, respectively. "Realistic" estimates of live birth rate were similar for women aged 20 to 29 years and 30 to 34 years but significantly reduced for women aged 35 to 40 years (Fig 2). Live birth rate did not differ by infertility diagnosis. Live births from thawing cycles accounted for 10% of all live births, with a 20% change of live birth per completed thawing cycle. Sixty-five percent of couples without a live birth did not complete the entire program of 3 IVF cycles.

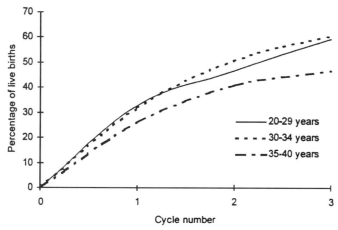

FIGURE 2.—Cumulative probability of live birth after IVF and ICSI for different age groups. P = .0178, 20 to 29 years versus 35 to 40 years, log-rank test. P = .0021, 30 to 34 years versus 35 to 40 years, log-rank test. (Courtesy of Olivius K, Friden B, Lundin K, et al: Cumulative probability of live birth after three in vitro fertilization/intracytoplasmic sperm injection cycles. *Fertil Steril* 77:505-510, 2002. Reprinted by permission from the American Society for Reproductive Medicine.)

Conclusions.—The Swedish data help to clarify the likelihood of live birth for infertile couples undergoing IVF/ICSI. Under realistic assumptions, 63% of couples will give birth after 3 treatment cycles. The high dropout rate in this study—despite the availability of subsidized treatment—is surprising and warrants further study.

▶ This study was performed in a large number of Swedish women who were able to have 3 cycles of IVF without cost to themselves. It was found that after 3 cycles of IVF about two thirds of the women had a live birth. Live birth rates were lower among women 35 years of age and older than women younger than 35. Live birth rates were also less after implantation of cryopreserved embryos than fresh embryos. The information obtained from this large study should be of use when counseling patients about their probability of having a live birth after 1 to 3 IVF procedures.

D. R. Mishell, Jr, MD

Prospective Evaluation of Blastocyst Stage Transfer vs Zygote Intrafallopian Tube Transfer in Patients With Repeated Implantation Failure

Levran D, Farhi J, Nahum H, et al (Edith Wolfson Med Ctr, Holon, Israel; Tel Aviv Univ, Israel)
Fertil Steril 77:971-977, 2002   15–11

Background.—Patients with repeated implantation failure (RIF) represent a challenge for the reproductive specialist. At the Wolfson Medical Center, patients who had experienced RIF have been offered in vitro fertilization

TABLE 3.—Cycle Outcome

Parameter	Blastocyst Stage Transfer (n = 32)	ZIFT (n = 32)	P
No. of cycles with embryo transfer (%)	27 (84.3)	31 (97)	.11
No. of embryos transferred	2.3 ± 1.4	5.5 ± 0.8	<.0001
No. of cycles with embryo cryopreservation	4	15	.0062
Clinical pregnancy rate per transfer, n (%)	1/27 (3.7)	13/31 (41.9)	.002
Clinical pregnancy rate per attempt, n (%)	1/32 (3.1)	13/32 (40.6)	.0009
Implantation rate (%)	1/73 (1.4)	24/177 (13.6)	.007
Live birth rate per transfer, n (%)	0	12/31 (38.7)	.0009
Live birth rate per attempt, n (%)	0	12/32 (37.5)	.0004

(Courtesy of Levran D, Farhi J, Nahum H, et al: Prospective evaluation of blastocyst stage transfer vs zygote intrafallopian tube transfer in patients with repeated implantation failure *Fertil Steril* 77:971-977, 2002. Reprinted by permission from The American Society for Reproductive Medicine.)

(IVF) with zygote intrafallopian transfer (ZIFT). The efficacy of ZIFT was compared with that of blastocyte stage transfer for patients with RIF.

Study Design.—The study group consisted of 64 women, aged 43 years or less, who came to the Wolfson Medical Center from 1996 through 1998 for IVF and had experienced RIF. After retrieval, oocytes were fertilized, and embryos cultured in P1 medium up to the stage of ZIFT or day 3, when embryos to be used for extended blastocyst culture were transferred to blastocyst medium. ZIFT was performed 24 or 48 hours after oocyte retrieval. Blastocyst transfer was performed 5 to 6 days after oocyte retrieval. The implantation rate, clinical pregnancy rate, and live birth rate for the ZIFT group was compared with the same variables for the blastocyte transfer group.

Findings.—The patient characteristics, the relative proportion of intracytoplasmic sperm injection (ICSI) cycles, and the fertilization rates were similar for both groups. In the blastocyst transfer group, the blastocyst formation rate was 31.3%, and 84.3% of patients had at least 1 blastocyst available for transfer. Significantly more embryos were transferred by ZIFT than blastocyst transfer, and more embryos were available for freezing. The implantation rate was significantly higher for the ZIFT group (Table 3). The clinical pregnancy rate/transfer was significantly higher in the ZIFT group. Only 1 pregnancy occurred in the blastocyst transfer group, and it ended in spontaneous abortion. In the ZIFT group, 13 pregnancies occurred, and only 1 ended in spontaneous abortion. In addition, there were 6 singleton deliveries, 5 twin deliveries, and 1 triplet delivery. For this group, the multiple pregnancy rate was 54%.

Conclusions.—This prospective study demonstrates that extended culture with transfer at the blastocyst stage does not increase implantation or pregnancy rates for patients with repeated implantation failure. ZIFT appears to offer these patients favorable implantation, clinical pregnancy, and live birth rates. ZIFT is an important clinical tool for the management of patients with RIF. Further studies are necessary to understand the etiologic factors that lead to RIF so that ZIFT may be used as soon as possible for those patients who are most likely to benefit.

▶ It is very disappointing to have an adequate number of embryos transferred after several cycles of IVF without the occurrence of an intrauterine pregnancy. In this study, after a mean of 7 cycles in which implantation failed to occur after embryo transfer, a 40% pregnancy rate was achieved with a single cycle of ZIFT. If these results are confirmed by other groups, clinicians should consider using ZIFT if pregnancy does not occur after 3 cycles of IVF and embryo transfer.

D. R. Mishell, Jr, MD

Progesterone Supplementation During Early Gestations After IVF or ICSI Has No Effect on the Delivery Rates: A Randomized Controlled Trial
Andersen AN; Popovic-Todorovic B, Schmidt KT, et al (Copenhagen Univ; Braedstrup Hosp, Denmark)
Hum Reprod 17:357-361, 2002   15–12

Introduction.—The practice of prescribing progesterone to women who achieve a pregnancy after either in vitro fertilization (IVF) or intracytoplasmic sperm injection (ICSI) is widespread, despite a lack of randomized clinical trials confirming its clinical benefit. In a study conducted at 2 centers in Denmark, 303 women who had become pregnant after IVF or ICSI were randomized to either withdrawal of all progesterone on the day of a positive human chorionic gonadotropin (HCG) test or the continuation of progesterone for another 3 weeks.

Methods.—The 2 randomized groups were comparable in age, distribution of causes of infertility, and number of earlier embryo transfers. The long protocol with GnRH agonists was used in all cases. After embryo transfer, all patients were treated with vaginal progesterone (200 mg, 3 times a day) until HCG measurement at a mean of 14 days later. Patients who fulfilled criteria for randomization had a serum or urinary HCG > 25 IU/L 14 days after transfer, with the absence or presence of slight vaginal bleeding. Transvaginal US was performed after 3 weeks, and women with a normal ongoing pregnancy followed usual antenatal care.

Results.—Miscarriage before week 7 of gestation occurred in 7 (4.6%) women who had progesterone withdrawn and in 5 (3.3%) who continued progesterone; miscarriage after week 7 occurred in 15 (10.0%) and 13 (8.5%) of these 2 groups, respectively. The number of deliveries did not differ significantly between women in the discontinued-progesterone and continued-progesterone groups (118 or 78.7% versus 126 or 82.4%, respectively). In addition, the 2 groups did not differ significantly in the distribution of single, twin, and triplet pregnancies and in number of deliveries or in the incidence of bleeding episodes.

Conclusion.—Because progesterone supplementation does not influence the miscarriage rate when pregnancy is achieved after IVF or ICIS, continuation of progesterone after a positive HCG test is not necessary. If a pregnancy occurs, rising endogenous HCG should support luteal function.

▶ Many therapies to treat the infertile couple have evolved because of perceived benefit without the scientific basis of a proven benefit as documented by randomized controlled trials. Administration of exogenous progesterone for several weeks in early pregnancy after in vitro fertilization (IVF) and embryo transfer is nearly always performed.

The results of this randomized controlled trial indicate that there is no benefit for continuing exogenous progesterone administration following IVF after the pregnancy test becomes positive. More randomized controlled trials such as this should be performed for many therapies given to the infertile couple, which are believed to be beneficial without evidence to substantiate their benefit.

D. R. Mishell, Jr, MD

16 Contraception

Body Weight and Risk of Oral Contraceptive Failure
Holt VL, Cushing-Haugen KL, Daling JR (Univ of Washington, Seattle; Fred Hutchinson Cancer Research Ctr, Seattle)
Obstet Gynecol 99:820-827, 2002   16–1

Introduction.—More than half a million unintended pregnancies occur each year in the United States among women using oral contraceptives (OCs). One biological factor that may be associated with OC failure is increased body weight. The relationship between a woman's body weight and her risk of pregnancy while using OCs was investigated by a retrospective cohort analysis.

Methods.—The cohort included 755 randomly selected women, aged 18 to 39 years, all of whom were enrolled in the Group Health Cooperative of Puget Sound. These women had previously served as control subjects for a case-control study of ovarian cysts and had completed in-person interviews and dietary questionnaires between 1990 and 1994. Data on body weight were used to categorize the study group according to weight quartile. Cox proportional hazards regression models were used to estimate the relative risk of pregnancy while using OCs. Length of follow-up averaged 12.5 years.

Results.—Women in quartile 1 (<56.5 kg) were more likely to be Asian, whereas women in quartiles 3 and 4 (62.5-≥70.5 kg) were more likely to be black. Women with a smoking habit were more common in quartile 4. During 2822 person-years of OC use, 106 confirmed pregnancies occurred. After controlling for parity, which was greater in quartile 4, the women in this highest weight quartile had a significantly greater risk of OC failure compared with the women in the other 3 quartiles combined. This increased risk was noted among both very low-dose OC users and low-dose OC users (Table 4), whereas high-dose OC use was not associated with an increased risk of failure.

Conclusion.—The risk of OC failure was 60% higher in women weighing 70.5 kg or more than in women of lower body weight. Very-low-dose and low-dose OCs were associated with the risk of OC failure in the heaviest women. The effect of body habitus on metabolism may need to be considered when prescribing OCs.

345

TABLE 4.—Risk of Oral Contraceptive Failure According to Body Weight Quartiles, by Oral Contraceptive Estrogen Dose

	Number of Failures	Person-Years OC Use	Failures per 100 Person-Years OC Use	RR (95% CI)*
Very low-dose OCs†				
Quartile 1	2	112.0	1.8	
Quartile 2	4	117.0	3.4	1.0 (reference)
Quartile 3	2	86.2	2.3	
Quartile 4	8	117.3	6.8	4.5 (1.4, 14.4)
Low-dose OCs‡				
Quartile 1	7	216.8	3.2	
Quartile 2	7	257.9	2.7	1.0 (reference)
Quartile 3	5	253.8	2.0	
Quartile 4	11	211.1	5.2	2.6 (1.2, 5.9)
High-dose OCs§				
Quartile 1	1	62.9	1.6	
Quartile 2	2	61.0	3.3	1.0 (reference)
Quartile 3	7	85.2	8.2	
Quartile 4	6	111.5	5.4	1.2 (0.4, 3.5)

*Multivariate model adjusted for parity, race, religion, menstrual cycle regularity, quartile 1-quartile 3 combined is reference group.

†Very low dose: monophasic OCs with <35 μg of ethinyl estradiol.

‡Low dose: monophasic OCs with <50 μg of ethinyl estradiol or <80 μg of mestranol (includes very low dose).

§High dose: monophasic OCs with 50 μg of ethinyl estradiol or ≥80 μg of mestranol.

Abbreviation: OC, Oral contraceptive.

(Courtesy of Holt VL, Cushing-Haugen, Daling JR: Body weight and risk of oral contraceptive failure. *Obstet Gynecol* 99:820-827, 2002. Reprinted with permission from The American College of Obstetricians and Gynecologists.)

▶ This interesting study indicates that the risk of pregnancy among users of OCs containing less than 50 μmg of ethinyl estradiol are several fold higher among women weighing more than 155 pounds than those of lower body weight. Among women using OCs with less than 35 μmg of estrogen, the risk of pregnancy among heavier women was greater than for those using OCs with less than 50 μmg of estrogen. It would be of great interest to know whether the increased risk of pregnancy was distributed equally among all weight groups greater than 70.5 kilograms or whether it was only increased in the most obese women, that is, those weighing more than 90 kilograms. In trials of the contraceptive patch, there was an increased risk of pregnancy failure only for women weighing 90 kilograms or more compared with women of lower body weight. If the findings of this retrospective study are confirmed by other studies, it may be advisable for heavy women, those weighing more than 155 pounds, to use oral contraceptives with 35 μmg of ethinyl estradiol instead of formulations with lower doses of estrogen to reduce the risk of an unwanted pregnancy.

D. R. Mishell, Jr, MD

Oral Contraceptives and Venous Thromboembolism: A Five-Year National Case-Control Study

Lidegaard Ø, Edström B, Kreiner S (Herlev Univ, Denmark)
Contraception 65:187-196, 2002   16–2

Background.—Many studies have investigated the influence of oral contraceptives (OCs) on the risk of venous thromboembolism (VTE), defined as deep venous thrombosis (DVT) plus pulmonary embolism (PE). Apparently, the risk of VTE is increased by OCs, but the differences in risk between OCs with second-generation progestins and those with third-generation progestins are questions that remain unresolved, as are also the clinical implications of these differences. The influence of different types of OCs on the risk of developing VTE was investigated in a 5-year case-control study conducted in Denmark.

Methods.—The study included all Danish women, aged 15 to 44 years, who experienced a first VTE or a first PE from 1994 through 1998. Control subjects were selected each year, with 600 per year selected in 1994 and 1995, and 1200 per year from 1996 through 1998. Women who were pregnant or had a history of thrombotic disease were excluded, thus, leaving 987 cases and 4054 control participants for analysis. In multivariate analysis, adjustment was made for the variables of age, year, body mass index (BMI), length of OC use, family history of VTE, cerebral thrombosis or myocardial infarction, coagulopathies, diabetes, years of schooling, and previous birth. Current users of OCs were categorized according to estrogen dose, progestin type, duration of use, and first-, second-, or third-generation OC use.

Results.—Slightly more than half (52.5%) of the women with VTE were current users of OCs, and 32.6% were former users; 50.0% of control subjects were users, and 29.8% were former users. Compared with nonusers of OCs, the risk of VTE among current users was primarily influenced by duration of use. Risk was greatest during the first year of use (odds ratio 7.0), then lessened with longer duration of OC use (odds ratio, 3.6 for 1 to 5 years and 3.1 for >5 years). After adjustment for progestin types and length of use, the risk of VTE decreased significantly with decreasing estrogen dose. The risk of VTE was also increased by smoking more than 10 cigarettes per day, a family history of VTE, BMI of more than 30, and coagulation disturbances.

Conclusion.—Use of OCs was significantly related to the risk of VTE, particularly during the first years of use. Among current users of OCs, VTE risk was influenced by length of use, estrogen dose, and progestin type. The difference in risk between users of third- and second-generation OCs was 33% (after correction for estrogen dose and duration of use).

▶ This well-done case-control study found that use of OCs containing gestodene and desogestrel (third generation) had a slightly increased risk (RR = 1.3) of venous thrombosis and/or pulmonary embolism (VTE) compared with agents containing 30- to 40-µg of ethinyl estradiol and levonorgestrel, norgestrel and norgestimate (second generation). Increasing duration of OC use and use of OCs containing 20-mg ethinyl estradiol were each associated with a decreased risk of VTE, whereas obesity, cigarette smoking and a family history of VTE were each associated with an increased risk of VTE. It is important to realize that VTE is an uncommon event (about 2 to 3 events per 10,000 women-years), and increasing the relative risk 2 to 3 times still results in a low attributable risk of developing a VTE.

D. R. Mishell, Jr, MD

Contraceptives and Cerebral Thrombosis: A Five-Year National Case-Control Study
Lidegaard Ø, Kreiner S (Herlev Univ, Denmark)
Contraception 65:197-205, 2002   16–3

Introduction.—Although the risk of ischemic stroke among current users of oral contraceptives (OCs) has been reduced with the introduction of low-dose (<50μg ethinyl estradiol) OCs, studies of the influence of different types of progestins have yielded conflicting results. The influence of estrogen dose and progestin types of OCs on young women's risk of developing cerebral thromboembolic attacks (CTAs) was assessed by a 5-year prospective case-control study initiated in Denmark in 1994.

Methods.—The study included all women, aged 15 to 44 years, who experienced a first-ever CTA during the study period. Age-matched control subjects were selected, with 600 selected each year for 1994 and 1995 and 1200 for each of the remaining 3 years. Both cases and control subjects completed questionnaires on use of OCs, smoking habits, medical history, and other factors potentially contributing to the risk of CTA. Current users of OC were categorized according to estrogen dose, progestin type, duration of OC use, and use of first-, second-, or third-generation products.

Results.—Among the 626 cases, 33.9% were current OC users and 48.1% were former users. Among the 1208 control participants, 29.8% were current OC users and 50.0% were former users. Crude estimates revealed a decreasing risk of CTA with length of OC use, a higher risk for second- than for third-generation OCs, and a decreasing risk with decreasing estrogen dose. Even with correction for length of use and estrogen dose, a significant difference remained; OCs with third-generation progestins carried a 38% lower risk. Additional factors that increased the risk of CTA included cigarette smoking, hypertension, a family history of thrombotic diseases, and a patient history of hyperlipidemia, coagulation disturbances, and heart disease.

Conclusion.—Both high-dose OCs and OCs with second-generation progestins were associated with the risk of CTA. An increase in estrogen dose from 20- to 50-μg ethinyl estradiol was associated with a 2.5 times increased risk of CTA, and women who used low-dose OCs with second-generation progestins had a 61% higher risk-association of CTA than those using OCs with third-generation progestins.

▶ This study evaluated the risk of thrombotic stroke as well as transient cerebral attacks, and use of various types of OCs. The use of OCs containing gestodene and desogestrel was associated with a lower risk of developing these cerebral vascular events than formulations containing levonorgestrel and norgestimate, when correlated for estrogen dose and duration of use. These 2 studies suggest that formulations containing gestodene and desogestrel have a decreased risk of developing arterial thrombotic events and an increased risk of developing venous thrombotic events compared with formulations containing levonorgestrel and norgestimate.

D. R. Mishell, Jr, MD

Oral Contraceptives and the Risk of Myocardial Infarction
Tanis BC, van den Bosch MAAJ, Kemmeren JM, et al (Leiden Univ, The Netherlands; Univ Med Ctr, Utrecht, The Netherlands)
N Engl J Med 345:1787-1793, 2001   16–4

Introduction.—The few studies directly comparing third- and second-generation progestagens, while examining the association between oral contraceptives (OCs) and myocardial infarction, have yielded conflicting results. A nationwide, population-based, case-control study assessed the effect of low-dose combined oral contraceptives on the risk of myocardial infarction.

Methods.—Subjects were 248 women aged 18 through 49 who had a first myocardial infarction from 1990 to 1995; 925 women without a myocardial infarction were control subjects, matched to the research subjects for age, calendar year of the index event, and area of residence. Both groups completed questionnaires on oral contraceptive use and major cardiovascular risk factors. Consent to undergo DNA analysis for factor V Leiden and the G20210A mutation in the prothrombin gene was given by 88% of the research subjects and 82% of the control subjects.

Results.—Compared with control subjects, research subjects had a higher prevalence of major risk factors for cardiovascular disease, including current smoking and a lower level of education. After adjustment for age, calendar year, and area of residence, the risk of myocardial infarction was twice as high among users compared with nonusers of any type of oral contraceptive. The adjusted odds ratio was higher among users of second-generation oral contraceptives compared with users of third-generation contraceptives (2.5 and 1.3, respectively). Factor V Leiden or a G20210A mutation in the prothrombin gene was detected in a similar proportion (8%) of research subjects and control subjects. Among users of oral contraceptives, the odds ratio was 2.1 for those without a prothrombotic mutation and 1.9 for those with such a mutation. The risk for myocardial infarction was highest among users of oral contraceptives with the cardiovascular risk factors of smoking, diabetes, and hypercholesterolemia (odds ratios, 13.6, 17.4, and 24.7, respectively).

Conclusion.—The use of currently available combined oral contraceptives increased the overall risk for a first myocardial infarction. Odds ratios did not differ significantly among age categories or among doses of estrogen, but the risk appears to be lower with third-generation oral contraceptives.

▶ There are substantial epidemiologic data indicating that OCs do not significantly increase the risk of myocardial infarction in nonsmoking, nonhypertensive women. Therefore, it is of interest that 84% of the women with myocardial infarction in this study were current smokers. Of the 99 women with a myocardial infarction who were using OCs, 84 were current smokers and only 15 were nonsmokers. The data in the article do not state how many of these 15 were hypertensive. Controversy exists as to whether OCs containing desogestrel or gestodene (3rd generation) increase the risk of venous thrombosis and/or pulmonary embolism more than OCs containing levonorgestrel (2nd generation). The information in this article suggests that the risk of myocardial infarction is not significantly increased among users of desogestrel- or gestodene-containing formulations but is increased among users of levonorgestrel-containing OCs. Since myocardial infarction is a greater health risk than venous thrombosis, the overall benefit/risk ratio may be better with use of gestodene or desogestrel formulations than levonorgestrel formulations.

D. R. Mishell, Jr, MD

Oral Contraceptives and the Risk of Breast Cancer
Marchbanks PA, McDonald JA, Wilson HG, et al (Ctrs for Disease Control and Prevention, Atlanta, Ga; Fred Hutchinson Cancer Research Ctr, Seattle; Univ of Southern California, Los Angeles; et al)
N Engl J Med 346:2025-2032, 2002   16–5

Background.—Large numbers of women who began taking oral contraceptives (OCs) early in their reproductive years are now reaching the age at which the incidence of breast cancer is increased. A population-based, case-control study was performed to examine the risk of breast cancer among former and current OC users, particularly among subgroups based on age, characteristics of OC use, and family history of breast cancer.

Methods.—The National Institute of Child Health and Human Development Women's Contraceptive and Reproductive Experiences (Women's CARE) Study examined the risk of breast cancer among OC users 35 to 64 years old. Subjects were enrolled from 5 large American cities; 65% were white and 35% were black. The cases comprised 4575 women (mean age, 49.7 years) with invasive breast cancer diagnosed between 1994 and 1998, and the controls were 4683 women without invasive or in situ breast cancer, matched for age, race, and city. All subjects were interviewed in person, and a standardized questionnaire was used to elicit detailed information about the use of OCs and other hormones, reproductive history, health, and family history. The relative risks (RRs) of breast cancer for the group as a whole and for subgroups based on race, current versus prior use, duration of use, age at initiation of use, estrogen dosage, and family history were estimated by conditional logistic regression.

Results.—OCs had been used by 77% of the cases and 79% of the controls. The risk of breast cancer was not significantly higher among the women who had ever used OCs (RR 0.9 compared with never-users). Among the subjects who had used or were using only 1 type of OC, the RRs of breast cancer were 0.6 for multiphasic formulations and 0.9 each for monophasic, sequential, and progestin-only formulations. The RRs of breast cancer were similar among white and black women. RRs generally hovered between 0.8 and 1.0 depending on the duration of OC use, the time since last use, and the age at initiation of use. The RR of breast cancer associated with prior or current use of high-dose estrogen (formulations with ≥540 µg of ethinyl estradiol or 75 µg of mestranol) was 0.8, whereas the RR of breast cancer for ever-users of lower-dose estrogen was 0.9. The RR of breast cancer was 0.9 for ever-uses of estrane progestins and 1.0 for ever-users of gonane progestins. The RRs of breast cancer associated with these variables did not differ significantly between women 35 to 44 years old and those 45 to 64 years old. In fact, the older women had a slightly reduced risk of breast cancer compared with the younger group. Finally, the RR of breast cancer associated with a family history of breast cancer among ever-users was 0.9.

Conclusion.—OC use was not associated with a significantly increased risk of breast cancer in women 35 to 64 years old. RRs were not significantly affected by race, duration of use, time since last use, age at initiation of use, or dose of estrogen; nor were results influenced by having a family history of breast cancer. These data support the belief that OC use does not increase the risk of breast cancer later in life.

▶ The results of this very large observational case-control study are very reassuring for the millions of current and past users of OCs. Analysis of the data indicated that current or prior use of oral contraceptives did not affect the risk of women developing breast cancer between the ages of 35 and 64. Furthermore, the risk of developing breast cancer was not increased among women who used OCs for long durations or who used formulations with high amounts of estrogen. Thus, these data indicate that ingestion of high amounts of exogenous estrogen and 19 testosterone progestins do not cause breast cancer while they are being ingested or after cessation of their use. Furthermore, women with a family history of breast cancer did not have an increased risk of developing breast cancer if they took OCs. Clinicians can reassure women with a family history of breast cancer that this and other studies have found that OC use does not increase their risk of developing breast cancer.

D. R. Mishell, Jr, MD

Family History of Cancer, Oral Contraceptive Use, and Ovarian Cancer Risk
Walker GR, Schlesselman JJ, Ness RB (Univ of Miami, Fla; Univ of Pittsburgh, Pa)
Am J Obstet Gynecol 186:8-14, 2002   16–6

Background.—Many factors have been reported as possibly increasing the risk of epithelial ovarian cancer. Whether women with a family history of ovarian cancer have a decreased risk of ovarian cancer associated with oral contraceptive (OC) use was determined in this population-based, case-control study.

Methods.—Between 1994 and 1998, 767 women with a diagnosis of epithelial ovarian cancer and 1367 control subjects were studied. The patients, aged 20 to 69 years, had been seen in 39 hospitals in 3 northeastern states. Personal interviews were conducted with all participants.

Findings.—Thirty-three case patients and 24 control subjects had a first-degree family history of ovarian cancer. In this subgroup, ovarian cancer risk declined with increasing duration of OC use. The risk reduction associated with short-term OC use did not significantly differ by family history. Risk reduction associated with long-term OC use was greater in women with a positive family history of ovarian cancer than in women with no such family history.

Conclusions.—These findings suggest that 4 to 8 years of OC use may markedly decrease the risk of ovarian cancer by age 70 years in women with a family history of this disease. The risk declined from about 4 in 100 non-users to only 2 per 100 OC users.

▶ Numerous studies have consistently reported that use of OC significantly reduces the risk of women developing epithelial ovarian cancer and that the reduction in risk is directly related to duration of use. The results of this study indicate that the reduction in risk of ovarian cancer with OC use for more than 4 years was much greater in women with a first-degree (mother or sister) family history of ovarian cancer than among women with a negative family history. Women whose mothers or sisters had ovarian cancer should be counseled that OC use for more than 4 years reduces their risk of developing ovarian cancer by nearly 90%.

D. R. Mishell, Jr, MD

Effect of Oral Contraceptives on Risk of Cervical Cancer in Women With Human Papillomarvirus Infection: The IARC Multicentric Case-control Study
Moreno V, for the International Agency for Research on Cancer (IARC) Multicentric Cervical Cancer Study Group (L'Hospitalet de Liobregat, Barcelona; et al)
Lancet 359:1085-1192, 2002   16–7

Background.—The use of oral contraceptives has been found to increase the risk of cervical cancer. However, the effects of human papillomavirus

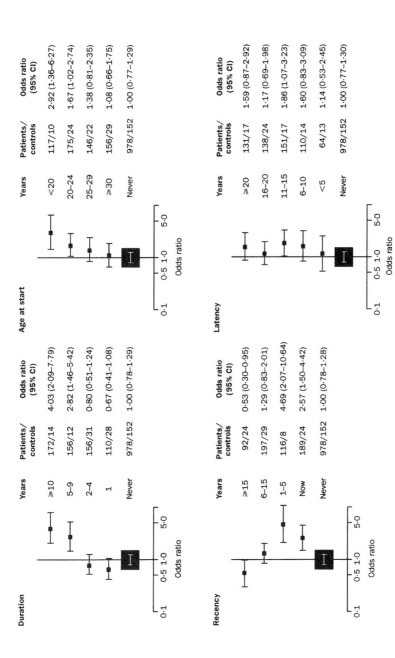

FIGURE 2.—Risk of cervical neoplasia associated with duration, age at start, recency, and latency of use of oral contraceptives. (Courtesy of Moreno V, for the International Agency for Research on Cancer [IARC] Multicentric Cervical Cancer Study Group: Effect of oral contraceptives on risk of cervical cancer in women with human papillomavirus infection: The IARC multicentric case-control study. *Lancet* 359:1085-1192, 2002. Reprinted by permission of Elsevier Science.)

(HPV), the main cause of cervical cancer, have often not been considered. The effects of oral contraceptive use in women testing positive for HPV DNA were investigated.

Methods.—Data from 8 case-control studies of patients with histologically verified invasive cervical carcinoma (ICC) and from 2 studies of patients with carcinoma in situ (ISC) were pooled. The studies included a total of 1561 patients with ICC, 292 with ISC, and 1916 control subjects.

Findings.—Overall, 94% of the patients with ICC, 72% with ISC, and 13% of control subjects tested positive for HPV DNA. Compared with women who had never used oral contraceptives, the odds ratio for cervical cancer in patients who had used oral contraceptives for fewer than 5 years was 0.73; for 5 to 9 years, 2.82; and for 10 or more years, 4.03 (Fig 2). These risks did not vary by time since first or last use.

Conclusion.—The long-term use of oral contraceptives appears to be a cofactor increasing the risk for cervical carcinoma by as much as 4-fold in women with HPV DNA positivity. Long-term oral contraceptive users need to be included in cervical screening programs.

▶ The results of this study indicate that long-term (more than 5 years) oral contraceptive (OC) use increases the risk of women who are infected with HPV to develop both ISU and ICC. For women not infected with HPV, long-term use of OCs does not affect the risk of developing cervical cancer. Thus, long-term use of oral contraceptives can have a promotional effect upon the carcinogenic action of HPV but not be an independent causative agent of cervical cancer. Because of this increased risk of ICC associated with long-term OC use in HPV-infected women, it is important to perform regular cytologic screening of the cervix in all OC users.

D. R. Mishell, Jr, MD

Oral Contraceptives and the Risk of Focal Nodular Hyperplasia of the Liver: A Case-Control Study
Scalori A, Tavani A, Gallus S, et al (Università degli Studi, Milan, Italy; Istituto di Ricerche Farmacologiche "Mario Negri", Milan, Italy; Istituto di Statistica Medica e Biometria di Milano, Italy)
Am J Obstet Gynecol 186:195-197, 2002   16–8

Introduction.—Focal nodular hyperplasia (FNH) of the liver is a rare benign lesion that occurs most often in young women, and approximately 50% to 75% of female patients with FNH use oral contraceptives (OCs). Although female hormones are thought to have a role in the development of FNH of the liver, the relationship between this lesion and OC use has not been confirmed. A hospital-based study conducted in Italy compared cases and control subjects for a number of potential risk factors, including age, age at menarche, menopausal status, number of children, age at first birth, and details of OC use.

Methods.—The cases were 23 women, aged from 22 to 58 years (median age, 41 years); the control subjects were 94 women of comparable age who resided in the same region as the patients and were admitted to the same hospitals for various acute diseases but not for hormonal, neoplastic, or liver diseases or for conditions related to smoking or alcohol use.

Results.—Diagnosis of FNH was obtained during US of the abdomen, performed to evaluate the onset of abdominal pain. Twenty patients had a single focal lesion (range, 1.5-9 cm in diameter) and 3 had more than 1 nodule. No relationship was found between FNH and age at menarche or menopausal status. Compared with nulliparae, the odds ratio (OR) of FNH was 2.18 in women with 1 child and 1.45 for women with 2 or more children. For women who first gave birth at age 30 years or older, the OR was 2.62. Current or previous use of OCs was more common in cases (83%) than in control subjects (59%), yielding an OR of 2.80 for OC use at any time. Longer duration of use and younger age at start of OC use were also associated with increased risk of development of FNH.

Conclusion.—The findings of this case-control study indicate that OC use is significantly, though moderately, associated with FNH of the liver. Menstrual and reproductive factors, however, do not appear to be relevant.

▶ Focal nodular hyperplasia (FNH) of the liver is a rare benign lesion that occurs much more commonly in women than men. The findings of this study provide support for an association between the use of oral contraceptives (OC) and the development of FNH. Because of the rarity of these tumors, there is little effect upon public health caused by this relation. The documented neoplastic benefits of OCs, mainly a substantial reduction of endometrial and ovarian cancer, far outweigh the increased risk of developing this rare tumor with OC use.

D. R. Mishell, Jr, MD

A Pooled Analysis of 10 Case–Control Studies of Melanoma and Oral Contraceptive Use
Karagas MR, Stukel TA, Dykes J, et al (Dartmouth Med School, Lebanon, NH; New South Wales Cancer Council, Kings Cross, Australia; Natl Cancer Control Initiative, Carlton Vic, Australia; et al)
Br J Cancer 86:1085-1092, 2002   16–9

Background.—Research findings on the effects of oral contraceptive (OC) use on women's risk of melanoma have been difficult to interpret. Whether the use of OC is associated with melanoma risk in women was investigated.

Methods.—A collaborative, pooled analysis of the original data of completed epidemiologic studies was performed. Ten case-control studies of melanoma in women, including a total of 2391 cases and 3199 control subjects, were reanalyzed. Unpublished data were also included. The study-specific odds ratios and standard errors were determined to obtain a pooled estimate that incorporated interstudy heterogeneity.

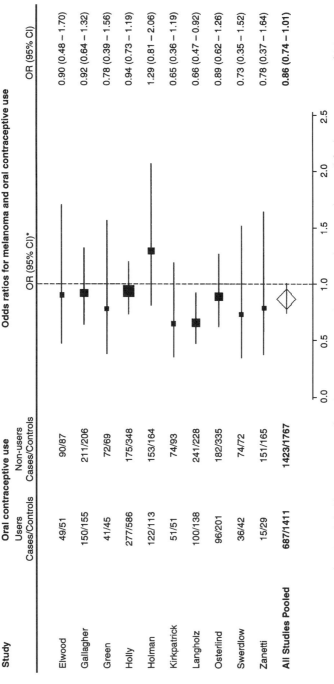

Odds ratios for melanoma and oral contraceptive use

Study	Oral contraceptive use		OR (95% CI)*	OR (95% CI)
	Users Cases/Controls	Non-users Cases/Controls		
Elwood	49/51	90/87		0.90 (0.48 – 1.70)
Gallagher	150/155	211/206		0.92 (0.64 – 1.32)
Green	41/45	72/69		0.78 (0.39 – 1.56)
Holly	277/586	175/348		0.94 (0.73 – 1.19)
Holman	122/113	153/164		1.29 (0.81 – 2.06)
Kirkpatrick	51/51	74/93		0.65 (0.36 – 1.19)
Langholz	100/138	241/228		0.66 (0.47 – 0.92)
Osterlind	96/201	182/335		0.89 (0.62 – 1.26)
Swerdlow	36/42	74/72		0.73 (0.35 – 1.52)
Zanetti	15/29	151/165		0.78 (0.37 – 1.64)
All Studies Pooled	**687/1411**	**1423/1767**		**0.86 (0.74 – 1.01)**

FIGURE 1.—Study-specific and pooled odds ratios (95% CIs) for melanoma in women in relation to use of OC. User of OC was defined as 1 or more years of OC use; nonuser was defined as never use or less than 1 year of use. Individual study odds ratios are shown as a *solid box* and pooled estimate as an *open diamond. Size of box is inversely proportional to SD for odds ratio. Lines* show 95% CIs. (Courtesy Karagas MR, Stukel TA, Dykes J, et al: A pooled analysis of 10 case-control studies of melanoma and oral contraceptive use. *Br J Cancer* 86:1085-1092, 2002.)

Findings.—Overall, there was no excess risk associated with OC use for 1 year or longer compared with use for less than 1 year or no use ever. There was no evidence of heterogeneity between studies. Melanoma incidence was unrelated to OC use duration, age at OC initiation, years of use, years since first or last use, and specifically current OC use (Fig 1).

Conclusions.—This analysis found no overall correlation between OC use and melanoma risk. The studies included in this analysis were the largest case-control studies of women completed by 1994 in which women were personally interviewed about their use of OCs and other melanoma risk factors.

▶ The incidence of melanoma in women exceeds that in men until about age 45 years. After that age, incidence rates increase in men but remain constant in women. For this reason it has been suggested that estrogen may have a causal relation to development of melanoma and that use of OC could increase the risk of development of this neoplasm. The results of epidemiologic studies have been conflicting. A few have reported an increased risk of melanoma in OC users compared with nonusers, but the majority have shown no excess risk of melanoma in OC users. This carefully performed pooled analysis of the original data from 10 large case-control studies found no relation between OC use for 1 year or longer and development of melanoma. Furthermore, no relation of risk of melanoma could be found with increased duration of OC use or current OC use. It appears that use of OCs, even for a long duration, does not affect the risk for melanoma development.

D. R. Mishell, Jr, MD

Evaluation of Interaction Between Fluconazole and an Oral Contraceptive in Healthy Women
Hilbert J, Messig M, Kuye O, et al (Pfizer Inc, Groton, Conn; Pfizer Inc, New York)
Obstet Gynecol 98:218-223, 2001   16–10

Background.—There have been reports of therapeutic failure of oral contraceptives (breakthrough bleeding or unexpected pregnancy) attributed to their interaction with other drugs. Several drugs lower the concentrations of oral contraceptives, including rifampicin, anticonvulsants, troglitazone, ritonavir, ABT-761 (a 5-lipoxygenase inhibitor), and broad-spectrum antibiotics. The most likely cause of decreases in oral contraceptive concentration is induction of metabolism or interference of enterohepatic recirculation of oral contraceptives by ABT-761, or antibiotics. The potential interaction between 2×150 mg fluconazole administered once weekly and an oral contraceptive containing ethinyl estradiol and norethindrone was investigated.

Methods.—Twenty-six healthy women aged 18 to 36 years took part in a placebo-controlled, double-masked, randomized, 2-way crossover study. The first cycle comprised 28 days, during which subjects received only the oral contraceptive. In the second cycle, the subjects were randomly assigned to oral contraceptive plus fluconazole or oral contraceptive plus placebo. The subjects then crossed over to the opposite treatment for the third cycle.

Results.—The study was completed by 21 subjects. The pharmacokinetic analysis included data only for those who completed the study; the safety analysis included data for all 26 subjects. A small but statistically significant increase in the 0- to 24-hour area under the plasma concentration–time curve was noted for treatment with oral contraceptive plus fluconazole with both ethinyl estradiol and norethindrone, compared with oral contraceptive plus placebo. The maximum plasma concentration for ethinyl estradiol was slightly but significantly higher for oral contraceptive plus fluconazole, compared with oral contraceptive plus placebo. The maximum plasma concentration for norethindrone was no different between the 2 groups. There were no adverse effects in the fluconazole treatment group.

Conclusion.—A slight increase in oral contraceptive concentration results from the concomitant administration of 300 mg fluconazole once weekly (twice the recommended dose for vaginal candidiasis) to women who are taking oral contraceptives. These findings suggest that concomitant fluconazole administration does not contribute to contraceptive failure.

▶ Ingestion of a single 150-mg dose of fluconazole is a safe, effective treatment for vaginal candidiasis. The results of this study indicate that with ingestion of 300 mg of fluconazole once per week for 3 weeks, there was no decrease in levels of ethinyl estradiol or norethindrone in women ingesting a combination oral contraceptive once a day for 3 weeks. Thus, women need not be concerned about contraceptive failure if they are taking oral contraceptives and also use fluconazole to treat vaginal candidiasis.

D. R. Mishell, Jr, MD

Efficacy and Safety of a Transdermal Contraceptive System
Creasy GW, for the ORTHO EVRA/EVRA 002 Study Group (Nashville, Tenn; et al)
Obstet Gynecol 98:799-805, 2001   16–11

Introduction.—The currently available contraceptive methods do not fully satisfy the needs of all women who desire safe, effective, easy-to-use, and reversible contraception. Until recently, the transdermal delivery of adequate amounts of progestin and estrogen for effective contraception has not been possible. The efficacy, cycle control, compliance, and safety of a transdermal contraceptive system that delivers norelgestromin 150 μg and ethinyl estradiol 20 μg daily was examined in an open-label, 73-center investigation.

Methods.—A total of 1672 healthy, ovulatory, sexually active women received ORTHO EVRA/EVRA for either 6 or 13 cycles (1171 and 501 participants, respectively). For each cycle, participants used 3 consecutive 7-day patches (21 days), followed by 1 patch-free week. Patches were applied on the buttocks, upper outer arm, lower abdomen, or upper torso.

Results.—The overall probability of pregnancy through 13 cycles was 0.7%; for method-failure probability, the rate was 0.4%. The overall Pearl Index and the method-failure Pearl Index were 0.71 and 0.59, respectively. The rate of breakthrough bleeding was low throughout the evaluation period. Perfect compliance (consisting of 21 consecutive days of dosing, followed by a 7-day drug-free interval, with no patch worn for more than 7 days) was observed in 90% of the participant cycles; 1.9% of patches detached completely. Adverse events were those typical of hormonal contraception. Most were mild to moderate in severity and not treatment limiting. The most frequently observed adverse events resulting in discontinuation were application site reactions (1.9%), emotional lability (1.5%), headache (1.1%), and breast discomfort (1.0%).

Conclusion.—The transdermal contraceptive patch offers combination hormonal contraception with convenient weekly dosing for a 21-day regimen. The excellent compliance observed in this and other trials may reflect the convenience of weekly dosing with the patch.

▶ Steroids are absorbed through the skin into the systemic circulation at a relatively constant rate. The results of this large multicenter study indicate that a transdermal contraceptive system that needs to be applied only once per week has effectiveness and side effects similar to those of oral contraceptives that need to be ingested once a day. It remains to be determined how many women will choose to use this convenient transdermal method of delivering contraceptive steroids once a week instead of taking a pill daily. Other new combination steroid contraceptives include an injection once a month and insertion of a steroid-delivering ring into the vagina once a month. Each of these long-acting effective contraceptive methods contains a progestin as well as an estrogen to control uterine bleeding and provide a woman with several different ways of administering contraceptive steroids.

D. R. Mishell, Jr, MD

Comparison of Cycle Control With a Combined Contraceptive Vaginal Ring and Oral Levonorgestrel/Ethinyl Estradiol
Bjarnadóttir RI, Tuppurainen M, Killick SR (Landspitalinn, Reykjavik, Iceland; Kuopio Univ, Finland; Princess Royal Hosp, Hull, England)
Am J Obstet Gynecol 186:389-395, 2002   16–12

Background.—The NuvaRing (NV Organon, Oss, The Netherlands) is a novel combined contraceptive vaginal ring. Cycle control and tolerability of the NuvaRing were compared with those of a standard combined oral contraceptive pill.

Methods.—Two hundred forty-seven healthy women, aged 18 to 40 years, requesting contraception were enrolled in the study. One hundred twenty-one women received the NuvaRing, and 126 received combined oral

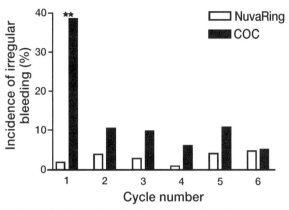

FIGURE 2.—Incidence of cycles with irregular bleeding with the NuvaRing or levonorgestrel/ethinyl estradiol (COC) (intention-to-treat analysis). The *double asterisk* represents *P* < .001 versus the respective NuvaRing group. (Courtesy of Bjarnadóttir RI, Tuppurainen M, Killick SR: Comparison of cycle control with a combined contraceptive vaginal ring and oral levonorgestrel/ethinyl estradiol. *Am J Obstet Gynecol* 186:389-395, 2002.)

contraceptive containing 30 µg ethinyl estradiol and 150 µg levonorgestrel. The women were monitored through 6 cycles, each consisting of 3 weeks of ring or pill use, followed by 1 week free of pills or rings.

Findings.—Both groups had withdrawal bleeding in virtually all cycles. The incidence of irregular bleeding with the NuvaRing was 5% or less in all cycles. The incidence with oral contraceptives was 5.4% to 38.8% (Fig 2). The incidence of a normal intended bleeding pattern was significantly greater in the NuvaRing than in the oral contraceptive group. Women tolerated both contraceptive approaches well.

Conclusions.—The NuvaRing appears to have excellent cycle control. In addition, this contraceptive approach was tolerated as well as oral contraceptives.

▶ The new contraceptive vaginal ring, which releases only 15 mg of ethinyl estradiol per day, maintains the endometrium very well. Despite this low dose of estrogen, the incidence of bleeding during the time the ring is in place—exclusive of bleeding contiguous with withdrawal bleeding—is very low, occurring less than 5% of treatment cycles. In this comparison study, intermenstrual bleeding was significantly higher than with the ring in the first cycle of use of an oral contraceptive containing 30 mg of ethinyl estradiol and ranged between 5% and 10% in the next 5 cycles of use of the oral contraceptive. The low rate of intermenstrual bleeding with the vaginal ring is probably due to the constant level of circulating ethinyl estradiol that occurs with ring use, in contrast to the peaks and troughs that occur with use of oral contraceptives.

D. R. Mishell, Jr, MD

Comparison of Weight Increase in Users of Depot Medroxyprogesterone Acetate and Copper IUD up to 5 Years

Bahamondes L, Del Castillo S, Tabares G, et al (Universidade Estadualide de Campinus (UNICAMP), Brazil)
Contraception 64:223-225, 2001   16–13

Background.—Weight gain is a common concern of women starting depot medroxyprogesterone (DMPA) for contraception and is frequently cited as a reason for discontinuing this safe and effective form of birth control. However, the relation between DMPA and weight gain remains a topic of debate. Changes in weight were compared for women starting DMPA contraception compared with users of an intrauterine device (IUD).

Methods.—The retrospective study included 103 women who started using DMPA for contraception and a matched group of 103 women who used a TCu380A IUD. Women in the IUD group had never received any form of hormonal contraception. The 2 groups were matched for baseline age (mean 33 years in both groups) and body weight (about 60 kg in both groups). They were followed up for changes in body weight at up to 5 years.

Findings.—The 2 groups were similar in terms of body weight at baseline and at the end of the first year's follow-up. However, from year 2 to year 5, women using DMPA had significantly greater weight gain. At the end of the observation period, weight gain was significant for both groups but greater in the DMPA group (Fig 1).

Conclusions.—This retrospective study suggests that women using DMPA for birth control have greater long-term weight gain than women using a nonhormonal method of contraception. Weight gain may not be-

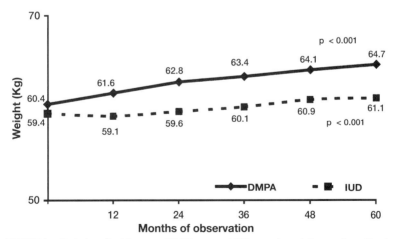

FIGURE 1.—Evolution of weight among DMPA users and IUD users through 5 years of use. (Reprinted from Bahamondes L, Del Castillo S, Tabares G, et al: Comparison of weight increase in users of depot medroxyprogesterone acetate and copper IUD up to 5 years. *Contraception* 64:223-225. Copyright 2001, with permission from Elsevier Science.)

come apparent until after 2 years of DMPA use. Women considering DMPA should receive appropriate counseling about the possibility of weight gain.

▶ This study found that there was an increase in body weight over time among 2 similar groups of women who used either an IUD or DMPA for contraception. It was found that the DMPA users gained significantly more weight than IUD users. Prior studies have yielded conflicting data about weight gain with DMPA use, with some reporting a significant increase and others no significant increase. It is possible that the use of DMPA increases appetite. Therefore, women using DMPA as a contraceptive should be counseled to restrict their caloric intake to prevent excessive weight gain.

D. R. Mishell, Jr, MD

Overview of the Relationship Between Use of Progestogen-only Contraceptives and Bone Mineral Density

Banks E, Berrington A, Casabonne D (Univ of Oxford, England)
Br J Obstet Gynaecol 108:1214-1221, 2001   16–14

Background.—The use of progestogen-only contraceptives may reduce bone mineral density, thereby increasing the risk of osteoporotic fracture. The evidence to date on the relationship between the use of such contraception and bone mineral density was summarized.

Methods and Findings.—Seventeen studies of the use of progestogen-only contraceptives and bone mineral density were identified for the analysis. A total of 1529 women exposed to progestogen-only contraceptives and 2086 control subjects were included. Mean bone mineral density was decreased in current users of depot medroxyprogesterone acetate compared with nonusers (Figs 1 and 2). However, users' density was within 1 standard deviation of the mean in nonusers. Significant heterogeneity was noted between the results of the different studies. The bone mineral density reduction appeared to be more pronounced at the lumbar spine, femoral neck, and ultradistal forearm than at the midshaft of the ulna. Studies of women who used depot medroxyprogesterone acetate for longer than average showed greater decreases in bone mineral density compared with studies of women with shorter use durations. The limited data indicated no difference in bone mineral density between former and never users of depot medroxyprogesterone acetate. The effects of levonorgestrel implants were unclear.

Conclusions.—Current depot medroxyprogesterone acetate users appear to have a lower mean bone mineral density than nonusers. The magnitude of this effect is not known. However, it appears to be greater with longer durations of use.

▶ This review of published studies of progestin-only contraceptives showed that nearly all studies found there was a modest decrease in bone mineral density (BMD) while women were using injectable depot medroxyprogesterone acetate (DMPA) for contraception. Two small studies have reported no signif-

Chapter 16–Contraception / 363

Study	Current DMPA users	Non-users	Duration of use (years)	Z score & 95%CI
Lumbar spine				
Scholes et al 1999[5]	183	274	<1*	
Paiva et al 1998[4]	47	47	3.5	
Gbolade et al 1998[9]	181	-	5*	
Tang et al 1999[2]	67	218	6	
Cundy et al 1998[+10]	200	350	12*	
Femoral neck				
Scholes et al 1999[5]	183	274	<1*	
Paiva et al 1998[4]	47	47	3.5	
Gbolade et al 1998[9]	181	-	5*	
Tang et al 1999[2]	67	218	6	
Distal radius/Ultradistal Forearm				
Petitti et al 2000[7]	133	652	3*	
Bahamondes et al 1999[11]	50	50	3.9	
Taneepanichskul et al 1997[8]	50	50	4.9	
Midshaft ulna/Distal forearm				
Petitti et al 2000[7]	133	652	3*	
Bahamondes et al 1999[11]	50	50	3.9	
Taneepanichskul et al 1997[8]	50	50	4.9	

* Median duration of DMPA use. All other figures are mean durations.
† Incorporating data from Cundy et al 1991.

-1.5 -1.0 -0.5 0.0 0.5

FIGURE 1.—Cross-sectional studies of current use of depot-medroxyprogesterone acetate (DMPA) and bone mineral density. The figure shows Z score and 95% CI for the difference in mean bone mineral density between current users of depot medroxyprogesterone acetate and nonusers. *Note:* Reference numbers listed are from the original journal in which this figure appeared. (Reprinted from Banks E, Berrington A, Casabonne D: Overview of the relationship between use of progestogen-only contraceptives and bone mineral density. *Br J Obstet Gynaecol* 108:1214-1221. Copyright 2001, with permission from Elsevier Science.)

icant decrease in BMD in past users of DMPA, suggesting that the effect of decreased BMD may be transient. Loss of BMD occurs only while using DMPA and is reversible after stopping. There are no published data other than case reports regarding fracture risk in current or past DMPA users. Such studies should be performed in order to counsel women appropriately regarding the

Study	Site of BMD measurement	Past DMPA users	Non-users	Median duration in users (years)	Z score & 95%CI
Petitti et al 2000[7]	Distal radius	32	652	<3	
	Midshaft ulna				
Orr-Walker et al 1998[12]	Lumbar spine	34	312	3	
	Femoral neck				

-0.5 -0.25 0.25 0.5

FIGURE 2.—Cross-sectional studies of past use of depot medroxyprogesterone acetate and bone mineral density. *Note:* Reference numbers listed are from the original journal in which this figure appeared. (Reprinted from Banks E, Berrington A, Casabonne D: Overview of the relationship between use of progestogen-only contraceptives and bone mineral density. *Br J Obstet Gynaecol* 108:1214-1221. Copyright 2001, with permission from Elsevier Science.)

benefits and risks of DMPA. Despite higher endogenous estradiol levels with levonorgestrel-releasing implants than with DMPA, 1 of 2 studies also reported lower BMD with use of the implants.

D. R. Mishell, Jr, MD

Menopausal Bone Loss in Long-term Users of Depot Medroxyprogesterone Acetate Contraception

Cundy T, Cornish J, Roberts H, et al (Univ of Auckland, New Zealand; Family Planning Assoc of New Zealand, Auckland)
Am J Obstet Gynecol 186:978-983, 2002   16–15

Background.—In several cross-sectional studies, depot medroxyprogesterone acetate (DMPA) users have been found to have decreased bone mineral density compared with nonusers. In addition, a longer duration of use and younger age at DMPA initiation have been associated with a greater def-

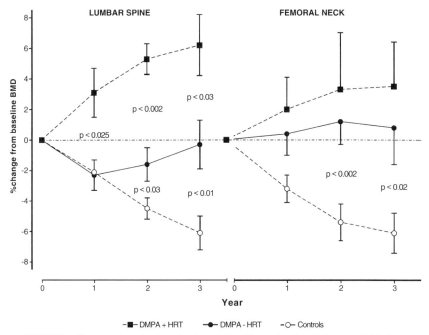

FIGURE 1.—Change in bone density at lumbar spine and femoral neck over 3-year period in 3 groups that were studied. Results are expressed as percentage difference from baseline scan. Mean and SEM are indicated. Probability values refer to the statistical significance of between-group differences that compared the former users of DMPA who did not undergo HRT with the other 2 groups, as indicated. *Open circles* indicate control subjects who reached a natural menopause (control subjects); *closed circles with solid lines* indicate former users of DMPA who did not undergo HRT; *closed squares with broken lines* indicate former users of DMPA who subsequently underwent HRT. (Courtesy of Cundy T, Cornish J, Roberts H, et al: Menopausal bone loss in long-term users of depot medroxyprogesterone acetate contraception. *Am J Obstet Gynecol* 186:978-983, 2002.)

icit. Whether DMPA-associated bone loss and early menopausal bone loss are the same phenomenon was investigated.

Methods.—Fifteen women reaching a natural menopause and who had not had hormone replacement therapy (HRT) were studied, along with 16 long-term DMPA users who stopped use only on reaching menopause. Five women in the latter group eventually took HRT. Bone mineral density at the lumbar spine and femoral neck was determined prospectively over a 3-year period.

Findings.—In the control group, early menopausal bone loss was rapid at 6% in both sites over a 3-year period. However, DMPA users not taking HRT had little change in bone mineral density (Fig 1). Differences between groups were significant at 2 and 3 years at both sites. Bone mineral density significantly increased at the lumbar spine in DMPA users undergoing HRT. At the femoral neck, it was static.

Conclusions.—Women using DMPA up to menopause have attenuated rates of bone loss from the lumbar spine and femoral neck. This is probably because they have already lost the estrogen-sensitive component of the bone.

▶ The results of this study confirm the fact that the use of DMPA for contraception results in about a 10% decrease in bone mineral density of the lumbar spine and femoral neck. Women who use DMPA and reach menopause and stop DMPA but do not take estrogen replacement do not have a further decrease in bone mineral density, as do women who have not taken DMPA and do not take estrogens. There are no data published that report postmenopausal fracture incidence in former DMPA users. The findings of this study suggest the incidence of fractures in former DMPA users may not be increased compared with postmenopausal women who did not use DMPA and do not take estrogen replacement.

D. R. Mishell, Jr, MD

Use of Copper Intrauterine Devices and the Risk of Tubal Infertility Among Nulligravid Women

Hubacher D, Lara-Ricalde R, Taylor DJ, et al (Family Health Internatl, Research Triangle Park, NC; Natl Perinatology Inst, Mexico City)
N Engl J Med 345:561-567, 2001   16–16

Introduction.—Earlier trials evaluating the use of intrauterine devices (IUDs) indicated that they may cause tubal infertility. There is concern that IUDs that contain copper, which most in current use do, may increase the risk of infertility in nulligravid women. This has limited the use of this highly effective birth control method. Three hundred fifty-eight women with primary infertility who had tubal occlusion documented by hysterosalpingography, 953 women with primary infertility who did not have tubal occlusion (infertile controls), and 584 primigravid women (pregnant controls) participated in a case-control investigation.

Methods.—Data were collected regarding participants' past use of contraceptives, including copper IUDs, previous sexual relationships, and a history of genital tract infections. Serum samples were tested for antibodies to *Chlamydia trachomatis.* The relationship between the previous use of copper IUD and tubal occlusion was examined.

Results.—The prevalence of the possible risk factors for tubal occlusion was similar in women with tubal occlusion and the infertile controls. The odds ratio (OR) for tubal occlusion associated with the previous use of a copper IUD was 1.0 (95% CI, 0.6-1.7). When primagravid women served as controls, the corresponding OR was 0.9 (95% CI, 0.5-1.6). Tubal infertility was not correlated with the duration of IUD presence or the absence of gynecologic problems related to its use. The presence of antibodies to *Chlamydia* was correlated with infertility.

Conclusion.—The findings that the use of a copper IUD was not a risk factor for tubal occlusion among nulligravid women contradicts some earlier reports that suggested that there is reason for concern about future fertility in women who use copper IUDs. Contemporary copper IUDs may be among the safest, most effective, and least expensive reversible contraceptives available.

▶ A large body of evidence indicates that an IUD with a monofilament tail string does not increase the risk of developing salpingitis, also called pelvic inflammatory disease, more than 1 month after insertion of the device. Nevertheless, concern still exists that an IUD can cause salpingitis and result in tubal occlusion.

For this reason, IUDs are not commonly used in nulliparous women. This well-done study found that copper IUDs do not increase the risk of developing tubal occlusion in nulliparous women. Thus, this effective, convenient, reversible method of contraception can be used by nulliparous as well as multiparous women who are not at risk of contacting sexually transmitted infections.

D. R. Mishell, Jr, MD

Insertion of an Intrauterine Contraceptive Device After Induced or Spontaneous Abortion: A Review of the Evidence
Stanwood NL, Grimes DA, Schulz KF (Univ of North Carolina, Chapel Hill; Family Health Internatl, Research Triangle Park, NC)
Br J Obstet Gynaecol 108:1168-1173, 2001   16–17

Background.—Immediate insertion of an IUD after abortion (spontaneous or induced) has many advantages but may be associated with increased rates of expulsion, infection, or perforation. The efficacy and safety of immediate postabortal insertion of IUDs was evaluated in a retrospective review.

Study Design.—MEDLINE, Embase, and Popline computer searches were performed along with the Cochrane Controlled Trials Register. Randomized, controlled trials with at least 1 arm with immediate postabortal IUD insertion were included. The primary outcome measures were rates of perforation, expulsion, pelvic inflammatory disease (PID), contraceptive failure and continuation.

Findings.—The review included 8 clinical trials. Complication rates were low, with a rate of about 1 perforation per 1000 insertions. Across the 8 included studies, gross cumulative expulsion rates ranged from 1.8% to 12.6%, pregnancy rates from 0.6% to 2.1%, and continuation rates ranged from 54% to 90%. The net discontinuation rate because of PID ranged from 0 to 0.8 per 1000 women per year. Women using IUDs with copper had lower pregnancy rates than those who did not use such IUDs. "T"-shaped IUDs had the lowest expulsion rates. Increasing gestational age was associated with increased expulsion rates. The expulsion rate was slightly higher when the IUD was inserted in the immediate postabortal period than when insertion was delayed.

Conclusions.—Insertion of an IUD in the immediate postabortal period appears to be safe and efficacious. Although immediate insertion is associated with a slightly increased rate of spontaneous expulsion, especially after a second-trimester abortion, these risks may be outweighed by the benefits of immediate contraception.

▶ If a woman wishes to use an IUD for contraception following a spontaneous or induced abortion, it is safe and effective to insert the IUD immediately after the uterus is evacuated. In 2 large trials performed by the World Health Organization, the incidence of uterine perforation and pelvic infection were very low when an IUD was inserted immediately after a spontaneous or induced abortion. The risk of expulsion of the IUD was low when it was inserted immediately after a first-trimester abortion but increased slightly when the IUD was inserted immediately after a second-trimester abortion.

D. R. Mishell, Jr, MD

Immediate Post-Partum Insertion of Intrauterine Devices: A Cochrane Review
Grimes D, Schulz K, van Vliet H, et al (Family Health Internatl, Research Triangle Park, NC; Leiden Univ, The Netherlands; Univ of Rochester, NY)
Hum Reprod 17:549-554, 2002   16–18

Background.—Insertion of an intrauterine device immediately after delivery is convenient for both patient and physician, but may be associated with higher spontaneous expulsion or uterine perforation rates. The safety and efficacy of immediate postpartum IUD insertion was retrospectively investigated.

Study Design.—MEDLINE, Embase, and Popline computer searches were performed along with the Cochrane Controlled Trials Register. Randomized, controlled trials with at least 1 arm with immediate postpartum IUD insertion were included.

Findings.—No randomized, controlled trials that compared immediate postpartum IUD insertion with later insertion were found, but 8 clinical trials were included in this review. Modifications of existing IUDs did not appear beneficial in any way. No differences were between hand or instrument insertion. Immediate postpartum IUD expulsion rates appeared to be higher when the IUD was inserted at this time.

Conclusions.—Immediate postpartum insertion of intrauterine devices appears to be safe and effective, in addition to being convenient. Spontaneous expulsion rates are higher when the device is inserted at this time, but the convenience may outweigh the disadvantage in some situations. Randomized, controlled clinical trials are needed to directly compare immediate and delayed insertion of IUDs.

▶ Immediate postpartum insertion of an IUD is convenient for both the clinician and the patient. The procedure appears to be safe and effective. No randomized trials have been published comparing immediate postpartum insertion with delayed postpartum insertion or interval insertion. Nevertheless, in observational studies, the expulsion rate appears to be higher when the IUD is inserted immediately postpartum instead of after the uterus has involuted. Immediate postpartum insertion of an IUD may be useful in certain areas of the world where women are unable or unwilling to return to the clinic for a postpartum visit. Otherwise, it is probably better to perform IUD insertion after the uterus has involuted instead of immediately after delivery to lower the rate of expulsion of the IUD.

D. R. Mishell, Jr, MD

Emergency Contraception With Multiload Cu-375 SL IUD: A Multicenter Clinical Trial
Liying Z, Bilian X (Natl Research Inst for Family Planning, Beijing, People's Republic of China)
Contraception 64:107-112, 2001   16–19

Background.—Emergency contraception may be required in cases of unprotected intercourse, and insertion of a copper intrauterine device (IUD) can be a very effective method. The efficacy, side effects, and menstrual changes that occur after insertion of a copper IUD—specifically the Multiload (ML) Cu-375 SL IUD—within 5 days after unprotected intercourse were assessed, as was the acceptability of this device by women who desired emergency contraception.

Methods.—The women had good general health, experienced regular menstrual cycles, had had at least 1 spontaneous menstrual cycle of normal length after discontinuing hormonal contraception or after abortion or delivery, came to the clinic within 120 hours of unprotected coitus, and were available for follow-up as required. Each had a general physical and pelvic examination, as well as a urine pregnancy test to exclude possible preexisting pregnancy. The copper IUD was inserted and the woman received 600 mg/d of metronidazolum for 3 days.

Results.—The 1013 women were divided into 2 groups based on parity (parous, 843 women; nulliparous, 170 women). For 60.5% of the women, condoms were the primary mode of contraception; for 26.7%, periodic abstinence was used. Only 3.0% to 8.2% had used emergency contraception previously. It was requested because of contraceptive failure or withdrawal failure for 54.7% and because no other contraceptive method had been used by 45.3%.

More than 87% of the women overall had only 1 incidence of unprotected intercourse before insertion of the IUD. The mean time to insertion from intercourse was 42.9 hours for parous women and 45.2 hours for nulliparous women; the range was 1.5 to 119 hours. The IUD was easily inserted in 96% of the parous women and 82% of the nulliparous women. At follow-up, 2 pregnancies were confirmed in each group, for a pregnancy rate of 0.20 per 100 women. The total expected pregnancy was 56.8, based on the probability of pregnancy on each cycle day. Thus, the total efficacy of the IUD in preventing pregnancy was 96.9% (98.1% for parous women and 92.4% for nulliparous women).

After IUD insertion, 644 women had further intercourse, but the risk of pregnancy was not increased. Two complete and 3 partial expulsions of the IUD were reported. Menstrual cycle length was shortened in 12.4% of nulliparous women and prolonged in 20.4%; these figures were 6.5% and 11.4% for the parous group. More than 32% of the nulliparous women experienced some disruption of their normal cycle. Most parous women desired to continue using the IUD for long-term contraception, with only 30 of them asking for its removal after menstruation returned. Of the 170 nulliparous women, 26 requested that the IUD be removed.

Conclusion.—The ML Cu-375 SL proved to be highly effective in providing emergency contraception for both parous and nulliparous women. One advantage of this method is its long-term effect, even when unprotected intercourse had taken place 120 hours previously. The IUD also proved highly acceptable to both nulliparous and parous women who desired to continue its use for long-term contraception.

▶ Insertion of a copper-bearing IUD for emergency contraception is infrequently performed because of concern of causing pelvic infection and the high initial cost of the IUD. Nevertheless, insertion of a copper IUD for emergency contraception has several advantages compared with ingestion of contraceptive steroids. The copper IUD is more effective than contraceptive steroids, and insertion of the IUD is effective for at least 5 days after a single act of unprotected sexual intercourse compared with less than 3 days for contraceptive steroids. In addition, once the copper IUD is inserted, it provides continued effective contraception for at least 10 years. Clinicians should be aware of the advantage of inserting a copper IUD for emergency contraception and counseling patients about its use.

D. R. Mishell, Jr, MD

Tubal Sterilization in the United States, 1994-1996

MacKay AP, Kieke BA Jr, Koonin LM, et al (Ctrs for Disease Control and Prevention, Hyattsville, Md; Ctrs for Disease Control and Prevention, Atlanta, Ga; EngenderHealth, New York)
Fam Plann Perspect 33:161-165, 2001   16–20

Background.—Tubal sterilization has been used for birth control or permanent termination of reproductive ability. The characteristics of women who request tubal sterilization, the number and rate of tubal sterilizations that are being performed, and the settings in which they are performed were estimated for 1994 through 1996.

Methods.—Data were obtained from the National Hospital Discharge Survey (NHDS) and the National Survey of Ambulatory Surgery (NSAS) for 1994, 1995, and 1996, which are the years from which the most recent data are derived. Classifications were developed for clinical settings, including hospital inpatient facilities, hospital ambulatory surgery centers, and freestanding surgery centers. Rates were assessed as the number of procedures done for every 1000 women of reproductive age in the United States between the ages of 20 and 49 years, using the population estimates for 1994, 1995, and 1996.

Results.—An estimated 200 million plus women between ages 20 and 49 years in the United States had a tubal sterilization procedure between 1994 and 1996. For each of these years, an average of 684,000 women had tubal sterilizations. The rate calculated was 11.5 tubal sterilizations per 1000 women, with little variance in the annual rate over the 3 years studied. Half of the procedures were done postpartum; half were interval procedures. Only 4% of the interval procedures were performed with the woman as a hospital inpatient; most were performed as outpatient procedures in either hospital ambulatory surgery centers or freestanding surgery centers.

The postpartum sterilization rates for women aged 20 to 29 years were higher than the interval rates; for women aged 35 to 49 years, the reverse was true. In 1995, 50% of the contraceptive users aged 40 to 44 years had had sterilization procedures. The rates for postpartum sterilization among black women were twice as high as for white women. Both inpatient and outpatient interval sterilization rates for women with stated race were higher for black women than for white women. The highest rates were found in the South, with the other regions having approximately the same rates. Of those who had postpartum sterilization, 58% had a vaginal delivery and 42% a cesarean delivery. Laparoscopic procedures were used for interval sterilization in 89% of the outpatient cases and 53% of the inpatient cases. For tubal sterilization done on an outpatient basis, general anesthesia was used for 93% of the patients.

Conclusion.—The NHDS and NSAS offer the most comprehensive data on tubal sterilizations for the time period studied, and based on these data, the highest rates for tubal sterilization were among women aged 25 to 34 years. A significant change has occurred in the setting of these procedures, with the rate and number of procedures performed in the hospital falling significantly and the rate and number done in either outpatient or freestanding clinics rising dramatically. Black women have tubal sterilization rates more than twice those of white women.

▶ Tubal sterilization is the most commonly used method of contraception in the United States. In this country, 28% of women aged 14 to 44 using contraception have had a tubal sterilization procedure, and 50% of women aged 40 to 55 using contraception have had tubal sterilization. This article provides much additional useful information about postpartum and interval tubal sterilization procedures performed in the United States between 1994 and 1996.

D. R. Mishell, Jr, MD

17 Abortion

Outcome of Expectant Management of Spontaneous First Trimester Miscarriage: Observational Study
Luise C, Jermy K, May C, et al (St George's Hosp, London; King's College Hosp, London)
BMJ 324:873-875, 2002   17–1

Background.—Expectant management with serial monitoring may be used to identify women with miscarriage who do not need surgery. The outcome of expectant management of spontaneous first trimester miscarriage was reported.

Methods.—A total of 1096 consecutive patients diagnosed as having spontaneous first trimester miscarriage in an early pregnancy assessment unit were included in the study. Two patients with molar pregnancies were excluded. Of the remainder, 37% were classified as having had a complete miscarriage. Seventy percent of those with retained products of conception chose expectant management, 6% of whom were lost to follow up.

Findings.—Eighty-one percent of patients obtained a successful outcome without surgical intervention. The rate of spontaneous completion was 91% among women classified as having incomplete miscarriages, 76% for missed miscarriage, and 66% for anembryonic pregnancy. Miscarriages were completed in 70% of women within 14 days after classification.

Conclusion.—In this series, most women with retained products of conception preferred expectant management. Clinicians can use US to advise patients on the likelihood that nonsurgical outcomes will be successful.

▶ Pelvic sonography can be used to determine whether women with an incomplete abortion, early embryonic demise, or an anembryonic gestation have completely expelled the gestational contents from the uterine cavity without the need for curettage. If patients without a great amount of blood loss have 1 of these problems, there is a high likelihood of spontaneous complete evacuation of the uterine contents with expectant management, so the patients can be counseled accordingly. Medical abortion agents such as misoprostol can also be given to hasten the abortion process in women with early pregnancy failure.

D. R. Mishell, Jr, MD

The Role of Ultrasound in the Expectant Management of Early Pregnancy Loss

Sairam S, Khare M, Michailidis G, et al (Homerton Hosp, London; St Bartholomew's and The Royal London Hosps School of Medicine and Dentistry, London)

Ultrasound Obstet Gynecol 17:506-509, 2001   17–2

Background.—Early pregnancy loss is the most common complication of pregnancy and a major source of clinical workload for gynecologists. The treatment of choice since the 1930s has been surgical evacuation of the uterus. However, recent studies have supported the role of expectant and medical management in early pregnancy loss. The clinical and sonographic criteria that best determined the likelihood of successful expectant management and early pregnancy failure (EPF) were evaluated.

Methods.—Over 12 months, a total of 1307 women with complications of early pregnancy were seen. Early pregnancy loss was diagnosed on the basis of clinical history and examination, positive urinary β–human chorionic gonadotropin (βhCG), and US findings. The diagnosis of incomplete miscarriage was made on the basis of endometrial thickness of more than 5 mm with loss of midline echo suggestive of retained products. Missed miscarriage was diagnosed when either the mean diameter of the empty gestation sac was 20 mm or greater (anembryonic gestation) or the crown rump length was 7 mm or greater without a detectable heart beat.

All women with a diagnosis of EPF at 7 to 14 weeks' gestation were offered the option of either expectant management or surgical evacuation. Women were excluded if they had heavy vaginal bleeding or severe abdominal pain, clinical evidence of intrauterine infection, suspected molar/ectopic pregnancy, other medical complication, or gestation of more than 14 weeks.

Results.—There were 545 women with a diagnosis of EPF. Incomplete miscarriage was diagnosed in 298 women, and 247 women had missed miscarriage or anembryonic pregnancy. Expectant management was chosen by

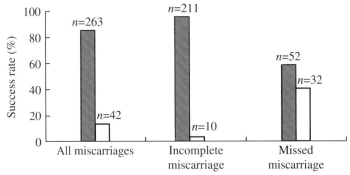

FIGURE 1.—The overall success rate of expectant management of miscarriages compared with the individual success (*black bars*) and failure (*white bars*) rates of incomplete and missed miscarriages. (Courtesy of Sairam S, Khare M, Michailidis G, et al: The role of ultrasound in the expectant management of early pregnancy loss. *Ultrasound Obstet Gynecol* 17:506-509, 2001. Reprinted by permission of Blackwell Science Inc.)

305 women, with an overall success rate of 86% (Fig 1). The success rate for incomplete miscarriage was 96%, compared with a success rate of 62% for missed miscarriage.

Conclusion.—Early pregnancy failure can be safely managed expectantly. US is a vital tool for predicting the success of expectant management, which facilitates informed choices by patients.

▶ The results of this study indicate that more than 95% of women who had a first trimester incomplete abortion without heavy uterine bleeding could be successfully managed expectantly without a curettage. However, only 62% of women with EPF caused by an anembryonic gestation or embryonic death were successfully managed expectantly during the 2-week time after diagnosis. More studies need to be performed in which women with EPF are treated medically with misoprostol with and without mifepristone (RU 486).

D. R. Mishell, Jr, MD

Medical Management of Missed Abortion: A Randomized Clinical Trial
Wood SL, Brain PH (Univ of Calgary, Alta, Canada)
Obstet Gynecol 99:563-566, 2002   17–3

Background.—Missed abortion is common in early pregnancy and is usually treated with dilation and curettage (D&C). The effectiveness of treatment with misoprostol was compared with that of expectant management to determine if medical management can reduce the D&C rate in a randomized, blinded trial.

Study Design.—The study included 50 women with a US diagnosis of a nonviable pregnancy, who were not experiencing cramping and bleeding, and were randomized to either misoprostol treatment or placebo. Follow-up occurred at 1 day, 2 days, and 1 week. Hemoglobin and serum β-human chorionic gonadotropin (βhCG) levels were assessed. A patient satisfaction questionnaire and symptom log were completed. Complete abortion was defined as expulsion of conception products without D&C and a negative follow-up urine βhCG test. At 48 hours, if abortion was incomplete, participants were offered a D&C. The primary patient outcomes were rates of complete abortion and D&C.

Findings.—The complete abortion rate was 80% in the misoprostol group and 16% in the placebo group. The D&C rate was 28% in the misoprostol group and 84% in the placebo group. One participant in the misoprostol group had an emergency D&C for heavy bleeding. None of the study participants required blood transfusions. The average hemoglobin reduction from day 1 to day 7 was 3.2 g/L in the misoprostol group and 4.3 g/L in the placebo group (Table 2). Vaginal misoprostol treatment appeared to be well tolerated and patient satisfaction was high.

Conclusions.—Medical management of missed abortion with misoprostol appears to be safe and effective and reduces the D&C rate significantly. It is also associated with a high rate of patient satisfaction. A large prospec-

TABLE 2.—Results

	Misoprostol (n = 25)	Placebo (n = 25)	P
Complete abortion	80% (20)	16% (4)	<.001
Dilation and curettage	28% (7)	84% (21)	<.001
Hemoglobin Δ day 1-7 (u, SD)	3.2 (7.9) g/L	4.3 (10.1) g/L	.72
Hemoglobin Δ day 1-7 > 10 g/L	10% (5)	8% (4)	.71

Abbreviations: u, Mean; *SD,* standard deviation.
(Courtesy of Wood SL, Brain PH: Medical management of missed abortion: A randomized clinical trial. *Obstet Gynecol* 99:563-566, 2002. Reprinted by permission of The American College of Obstetricians and Gynecologists.)

tive study should be performed to confirm these findings, but misoprostol appears to be a useful alternative to D&C for the treatment of missed abortion.

▶ Vaginal administration of 1 or 2 doses of 800 mg of misoprostol is an effective and safe method to terminate pregnancies with early pregnancy failure due to either absence of an embryo or embryonic demise. Clinicians and patients may wish to use this method of treating early pregnancy failure instead of performing a dilatation and curettage. Studies should be performed to determine whether the addition of mifepristone to misoprostol results in a greater success rate than the use of misoprostol alone for treatment of early pregnancy failure.

D. R. Mishell, Jr, MD

Medical Management of Early Fetal Demise Using Sublingual Misoprostol
Wagaarachchi PT, Ashok PW, Smith NC, et al (Univ of Aberdeen, Scotland)
Br J Obstet Gynaecol 109:462-465, 2002   17–4

Background.—The advent of routine early pregnancy scanning has been associated with an increasingly common diagnosis of early pregnancy demise. Surgical evacuation, the standard treatment for many years, carries well-documented risks. A pilot study was done to determine the efficacy, adverse effects, and acceptability of sublingual misoprostol in the management of early fetal demise.

Methods and Findings.—The prospective study included 56 women. At the diagnosis of fetal demise, the mean gestation was 9.6 weeks. Participants were first given oral mifepristone, 200 mg. This was followed 36 to 48 hours later by sublingual misoprostol, 400 µg, given sequentially at 3-hourly intervals. Complete miscarriage was obtained with mifepristone alone in 4 women. Overall, the success rate was 83.9%. The median induction-miscarriage interval was 8.19 hours. Among women with successful outcomes, 91.5% were satisfied with their treatment.

Conclusion.—Sublingual misoprostol combined with mifepristone appears to be a safe, effective alternative to vaginal or oral misoprostol in managing early fetal demise. Sublingual misoprostol administration may be useful for home medical management.

▶ With increasing use of US, the diagnosis of early pregnancy failure due to anembryonic gestation or intrauterine embryonic death is being made more frequently. Early pregnancy failure is usually treated by surgical curettage, although expectant management is also utilized. Several small studies have reported that medical management of early pregnancy failure with oral or vaginal misoprostol is an effective therapy.

This study indicated that a single 200-mg dose of mifepristone followed by 3 doses of 400-μg sublingual misoprostol every 3 hours resulted in an 84% success rate for treatment of early pregnancy failure. Additional studies need to be performed to determine the best dose, dosing interval, and route of administration of misoprostol for the treatment of early pregnancy failure. Studies also need to be performed to determine whether initial use of mifepristone enhances the incidence of successful treatment of early pregnancy failure with misoprostol.

D. R. Mishell, Jr, MD

Medical Management of Early Fetal Demise Using a Combination of Mifepristone and Misoprostol
Wagaarachchi PT, Ashok PW, Narvekar N, et al (Aberdeen Maternity Hosp, Scotland)
Hum Reprod 16:1849-1853, 2001   17–5

Introduction.—For most women with miscarriage, management consists of surgical evacuation of the uterus. Regimens consisting of the antiprogesterone agent mifepristone and a prostaglandin analog have been evaluated, with mixed success rate. A new regimen of mifepristone and misoprostol for the management of early fetal death was evaluated.

Methods.—The prospective study included 2220 consecutive women with "delayed miscarriage" diagnosed at 6 to 13 weeks' gestation. All had opted for medical rather than surgical management. US confirmed the diagnosis of missed miscarriage in 63% of women and anembryonic pregnancy in 37%. Consenting women received a single oral dose of mifepristone, 200 mg, in the hospital. If miscarriage did not occur within 36 to 48 hours, the women received vaginal misoprostol (4 tablets, 800 μg) inserted into the posterior vaginal fornix, followed by another 2 tablets every 3 hours. Women with heavy bleeding received oral misoprostol instead. If the uterus was not emptied overnight, the patients were offered repeat medical treatment or surgical evacuation.

Results.—Twenty percent of women had heavy bleeding within 48 hours after treatment with mifepristone alone. Forty of these 44 women had US confirmation of complete miscarriage, although 4 required emergency curettage because of heavy bleeding. One hundred seventy-six women proceeded to misoprostol treatment, of whom 145 had complete miscarriage without surgery. The overall success rate of the mifepristone/misoprostol regimen was 84%. Although 7 women had blood loss of greater than 500 mL, none needed blood transfusion.

The treatment failure rate was 21% among 142 women who were initially symptomatic compared with 6% of asymptomatic women in whom nonviable pregnancy was diagnosed on routine US. Overall, the women received a median of 3 doses of misoprostol. Fifty percent of women proceeding to this phase of treatment had completed miscarriage within 6 hours of the first misoprostol dose. The median interval from induction to miscarriage was 8 hours.

Conclusions.—Oral mifepristone followed by vaginal or oral misoprostol is a potentially useful medical alternative for management of early fetal demise. The overall success rate was 84%, with an emergency surgery rate of only 4%.

▶ This large series of women with early pregnancy failure treated with mifepristone followed by vaginally administered misoprostol had a success rate of 84%. The success rate in asymptomatic women, those without bleeding and/or pain, was greater than 90%. Thus clinicians can offer this medical therapy to women with early pregnancy failure, either anembryonic gestation or early embryonic demise, as an alternate to surgical curettage or expectant management.

D. R. Mishell, Jr, MD

Pilot Study on the Use of Sublingual Misoprostol for Medical Abortion
Tang OS, Ho PC (Univ of Hong Kong, People's Republic of China)
Contraception 64:315-317, 2001   17–6

Background.—A new route in which misoprostol is given by sublingual administration has been developed. The use of sublingual misoprostol for medical abortion was reported.

Methods.—Twenty-five women with first-trimester, nonviable intrauterine gestations and 18 seeking mid-trimester pregnancy terminations were included in the study. The former group received 600 μg of misoprostol sublingually every 3 hours for up to 3 doses. The latter group received 400 μg of misoprostol sublingually every 3 hours for up to 5 doses.

Findings.—Ninety-two percent of the women with nonviable gestations had complete abortion after sublingual treatment. All women requesting abortion in the second trimester had an abortion. The median interval between induction and abortion was 11.6 hours.

Conclusion.—Sublingual misoprostol is a promising technique for performing medical abortion. Prospective randomized trials are now needed to compare the efficacy and safety of this approach with that of vaginal misoprostol. Optimal dosage and dosing intervals also need to be established.

▶ The results of this preliminary study suggest that placing misoprostol under the tongue is an effective means to terminate nonviable first trimester pregnancies as well as viable pregnancies before 14 and 20 weeks gestational age. Others have shown that vaginal administration of misoprostol is also an effective means to terminate both first and second trimester pregnancy. Prospective, randomized studies should be performed to compare the effectiveness and side effects of these 2 ways to administer misoprostol to terminate pregnancies of up to 20 weeks' gestational age.

D. R. Mishell, Jr, MD

Double-blind Randomized Trial of Mifepristone in Combination With Vaginal Gemeprost or Misoprostol for Induction of Abortion Up to 63 Days Gestation
Bartley J, Brown A, Elton R, et al (Univ of Edinburgh, Scotland)
Hum Reprod 16:2098-2102, 2001   17–7

Background.—Gemeprost and misoprostol are among the most-used prostaglandins in combination with mifepristone for induction of abortion in early pregnancy. However, there have been no previous assessments of the safety and efficacy of these 2 prostaglandins in a randomized trial. The clinical efficacy and side-effects of low-dose mifepristone in combination with gemeprost and with misoprostol were compared.

Methods.—A randomized, double-blind, controlled trial enrolled 999 women undergoing an abortion at gestational age of 63 days or less. All of the women received either 0.5 mg gemeprost (499 women) or 800 μg misoprostol (500 women) vaginally about 48 hours after taking 200 mg oral mifepristone. The main outcome measures were comparison of the rates of complete abortion and the side effects between the groups.

Results.—Eighty-nine women were excluded from full analysis of outcome because of abortion after mifepristone alone (2 women), ectopic pregnancy (1 woman), or uncertain outcome from failure to attend the follow-up appointment (86 women). Both groups had very high rates of complete abortion (>95%); however, these rates were significantly higher after treatment with misoprostol (98.7%) compared with gemeprost (96.2%), and there were fewer ongoing pregnancies. The incidence of surgical intervention rose significantly with gestation in women who received gemeprost, but not in women who received misoprostol. The 2 groups had similar incidences of side effects such as diarrhea (16.4% for group 1 vs 13.7% for group 2) and vomiting (27.8% and 29.7%, respectively). The duration and amount of bleeding were also similar between groups.

Conclusion.—Both vaginal gemeprost and vaginal misoprostol with a reduced dose of mifepristone are highly effective for induction of abortion in early pregnancy. However, vaginal misoprostol is preferred over gemeprost because it is associated with fewer failures, particularly at 49 days or less gestation.

▶ The regimen for medical abortion approved for use in the United States is 600 mg of mifepristone (RU = 486) followed 48 hours later by 400 pg of misoprostol orally. This regimen is approved only for pregnancies of less than 49 days' gestational age. Several studies have shown that 200 mg of mifepristone is as effective as 600 mg and that vaginal administration of 800 pg of misoprostol is more effective than 400 pg misoprostol given orally. The success rate of 98.7% when 200 mg mifepristone orally is followed by 800 pg misoprostol vaginally for pregnancies less than 63 days' gestational age reported in this large trial is very impressive. Only 1 of 457 women treated with this regimen had an ongoing pregnancy. Mifepristone is available in many countries and misoprostol is also widely available. With the use of the regimen reported in this article, clinicians can offer medical abortion to women with a gestational age of 63 days or less.

D. R. Mishell, Jr, MD

Comparison of Abortions Induced by Methotrexate or Mifepristone Followed by Misoprostol
Wiebe E, Dunn S, Guilbert E, et al (Univ of British Columbia, Vancouver, Canada; Univ of Toronto; Univ of Laval, PQ, Canada; et al)
Obstet Gynecol 99:813-819, 2002   17–8

Background.—The demand for medical abortion is increasing. The 2 most commonly used regimens are misoprostol in combination with either mifepristone or methotrexate. Mifepristone is more expensive and less widely available than methotrexate. The efficacy, acceptability, and side effects of these 2 medical abortion methods were compared in a multicenter, randomized, controlled study.

Study Design.—The study group consisted of 1042 pregnant women, at a short period of gestation ($\leq$49 days), who desired an elective abortion at 5 Canadian clinics. Patients were randomized to 1 of the 2 medical abortion methods. At 7-day follow-up, US was performed. Women who still had a gestational sac in the uterus received a second dose and returned 1 week later. At the 2-week visit, those with ongoing pregnancies were scheduled for surgical abortion. Those with a delayed response were asked to return on day 36. Pain, bleeding, side effects, and patient satisfaction were evaluated.

Findings.—Abortions induced with the methotrexate combination took longer to complete than those induced using mifepristone. At the 8-day follow-up, 75% of the women in the methotrexate group and 91% of the women in the mifepristone group had completed the abortion. The average day of abortion was 7.1 days in the methotrexate group and 3.3 days in the mifepristone group. The average total number of bleeding days was 13 for methotrexate and 14.5 for mifepristone. The rates of surgical abortion were not significantly different between these 2 treatment groups. Side effects also were similar between the 2 groups. Acceptance was high for both groups, but slightly higher for the mifepristone treatment group.

Conclusions.—Although medical abortion induced with either methotrexate or mifepristone is safe, effective and accepted by patients, mifepristone-induced abortions occur much more rapidly. Most clinicians and patients would choose mifepristone if offered the choice.

▶ Administration of mifepristone followed by misoprostol, or methotrexate followed by misoprostol are both very effective medical methods of electively terminating pregnancies less than 7 weeks' gestational age. Methotrexate is less expensive than mifepristone, but complete abortion occurs later following methotrexate and misoprostol than following mifepristone and misoprostol. The mean day of abortion after initial medication with the former regimen was 7.1 days and with the latter regimen, 3.3 days. By day 8, 92% of the abortions were completed after mifepristone plus misoprostol compared with 75% with methotrexate and misoprostol. The mean total days of bleeding were slightly, but significantly, greater with mifepristone than methotrexate. For these reasons, it appears preferable to induce early abortion with mifepristone and misoprostol instead of methotrexate and misoprostol unless the increased cost and decreased availability of mifepristone restricts its use.

D. R. Mishell, Jr, MD

A Randomised Trial of Oral Versus Vaginal Administration of Misoprostol for the Purpose of Mid-Trimester Termination of Pregnancy
Gilbert A, Reid R (Univ of Otago, Christchurch, New Zealand)
Aust N Z J Obstet Gynaecol 41:407-410, 2001   17–9

Background.—Among the reasons for mid trimester terminations of pregnancy is threat to maternal mental health. The use of the 18-week anomaly US scan has led to an increasing number of fetal anomalies detected antenatally and an increase in the number of women undergoing termination of pregnancy at this stage. In the latter part of the second trimester, medical methods are a safer option than surgical suction or dilation and evacuation. Misoprostol has long been recognized as an agent for induction of abortion; recently it has also been investigated for use in both induction of labor and management of postpartum hemorrhage. Recent studies have indicated that oral administration of misoprostol may be effective. The efficacy of oral and vaginal administration of misoprostol for termination of pregnancy in the mid trimester was investigated.

Methods.—A total of 55 women took part in the trial. Misoprostol was administered vaginally to 29 women and orally to 26 women. The dosing regimen was 440 µg as the initial dose, followed by a second dose of 200 µg 2 hours later, and then 200-µg doses every 4 hours until delivery or 32 hours from initiation of treatment. A Syntocinon infusion was started synchronously if delivery was not effected by the last dose of misoprostol.

Results.—Vaginal administration of misoprostol was significantly more effective than oral administration on the basis of induction-to-delivery interval and the need to augment therapy with a Syntocinon infusion. The vaginal administration group had an average induction-to-delivery interval of 17.5 hours, compared with 33 hours for the oral administration group. The percentages of women who delivered at 24 and 48 hours were 93% and 100%, respectively, in the vaginal administration group, compared with 19% and

70%, respectively, in the oral administration group. There were no significant differences between the 2 groups in complication rates or side effects.

Conclusions.—The findings suggest that misoprostol is more effective when administered vaginally rather than orally. Further studies are recommended to assess whether alternative dose regimens for oral misoprostol are as effective as vaginal administration. These studies should factor in parity and women's preferences for route of administration, as well as their attitude regarding the importance of the induction-to-delivery interval.

▶ Several studies have shown that vaginal administration of 200 µg of misoprostol at intervals of 2 to 6 hours is an effective method of terminating second trimester pregnancies. The results of this randomized trial provide evidence that vaginal administration of misoprostol is more effective than when the same dose is administered orally. Misoprostol is widely available, inexpensive, and does not require refrigeration. When administered vaginally, there is a very high rate of successful termination of second-trimester pregnancies. Clinicians should consider the use of this agent for terminating pregnancies in the second trimester.

D. R. Mishell, Jr, MD

The Optimization of Intravaginal Misoprostol Dosing Schedules in Second-Trimester Pregnancy Termination

Dickinson JE, Evans SF (Univ of Western Australia, Perth)
Am J Obstet Gynecol 186:470-474, 2002   17–10

Introduction.—Prostaglandin agents are commonly used in the termination of second-trimester pregnancy. At the study institution, misoprostol has become the primary medical therapy for second-trimester pregnancy interruption. The clinical efficacy and the incidence of maternal side effects of 3 different regimens of intravaginal misoprostol were compared in a prospective study.

Methods.—The study included 150 women who underwent pregnancy termination between 14 and 30 weeks of gestation. In a double-blind manner, women were randomized to 1 of 3 intravaginal misoprostol regimens: 200 µg at 6-hour intervals (group 1); 400 µg at 6-hour intervals (group 2); and a loading dose of 600 µg misoprostol followed by 200 µg at 6-hour intervals (group 3). The maximum duration of misoprostol treatment was 48 hours. Women who were undelivered after 48 hours received a transcervical Foley catheter with extra-amniotic prostaglandin F2α instillation or high-concentration IV oxytocin.

Results.—Indications for pregnancy interruption were severe fetal anomaly (61%), fetal death in utero (24%), and maternal indications (15%). The median time to achieve delivery differed significantly among the 3 groups: 18.2 hours for group 1, 15.1 hours for group 2, and 13.2 hours for group 3. Delivery within 24 hours occurred in 59% of the women in group 1, 76% of the women in group 2, and 80% of the women in group 3. After 48 hours,

TABLE 2.—Delivery Interval Characteristics

Characteristic	Group 1 (n = 51)	Group 2 (n = 50)	Group 3 (n = 49)	P Value
Median abortion interval (hr)	18.2 (IQ 13.3-32.5)	15.1 (IQ 10.9-23.7)	13.2 (IQ 11.2-21.7)	.035
Delivery <24 hrs (n)	30 (58.8%)	38 (76%)	39 (79.6%)	.013
Delivery >48 hrs (n)	4 (7.8%)	0 (0%)	1 (2.0%)	.021

Abbreviation: IQ, Interquartile range.
(Courtesy of Dickinson JE, Evans SF: The optimization of intravaginal misoprostol dosing schedules in second-trimester pregnancy termination. *Am J Obstet Gynecol* 186:470-474, 2002.)

7.8% of women in group 1 and 2% of those in group 3 had not delivered; all group 2 women delivered within 48 hours (Table 2). Significantly more women in group 3 experienced vomiting at 3 hours, and fever was also significantly more common in these women during the first 12 hours of induction. Placental retention occurred at similar rates in the 3 groups. No cases of uterine rupture occurred. Pain scores and analgesic usage did not differ significantly among treatment groups.

Conclusion.—Regardless of the actual dose administered, more than 90% of women undergoing second-trimester medical termination of pregnancy delivered in 48 hours with a 6-hour misoprostol dosing interval. The regimen of 400 µg of misoprostol at 6-hour intervals achieves delivery faster than the 200-µg regimen with fewer maternal side effects than the 600 µg loading dose.

▶ Several studies including this one, have demonstrated that vaginal administration of misoprostol is an effective method to terminate pregnancy in the second trimester. Many different dosages and dosing intervals of misoprostol have been used in the various studies, and the optimal dose and dosing interval remain to be determined. In this study, when the fetus was alive, vaginal administration of 400 µmg of misoprostol every 6 hours was more effective than 200 µmg of misoprostol every 6 hours, and the induction to delivery interval was shorter with the higher dose. At present, it appears that the preferred regimen of vaginal misoprostol for second-trimester pregnancy termination is 400 µmg of misoprostol every 6 hours.

D. R. Mishell, Jr, MD

Factor V Leiden and G20210A Prothrombin Mutations Are Risk Factors for Very Early Recurrent Miscarriage

Reznikoff-Etiévant MF, Cayol V, Carbonne B, et al (Saint Antoine Hosp, Paris; Tenon Hosp, Paris)
Br J Obstet Gynaecol 108:1251-1254, 2001   17–11

Background.—Research has shown an association between late recurrent fetal loss and activated protein C resistance and factor V Leiden mutation. Hereditary and acquired activated protein C resistance may cause vascular placental insufficiency. The relationship between early recurrent miscarriage and factor V Leiden and G20210A prothrombin mutations was further investigated in a prospective study .

Methods.—Two hundred sixty women with early unexplained recurrent miscarriage (before 10 weeks of pregnancy) and 240 women with no previous history of thromboembolism were studied. Women were screened for defects in the protein C anticoagulant pathway using the anticoagulant response to agkistrodon confortrix venom (ACV test). When ACV levels were low, protein C and factor V Leiden mutation testing was done. All samples were assessed for the G20210A prothrombin mutation.

Findings.—Early recurrent spontaneous miscarriage correlated with factor V Leiden and G20210A mutations. The odds ratios were 2.4 and 2.7, respectively. Findings were comparable whether or not patients had previously had a live birth.

Conclusion.—Early recurrent miscarriage is significantly correlated with factor V or G20210A prothrombin mutations. Anticoagulant prevention may play a role in early miscarriages.

▶ Most previous studies have reported that activated protein C resistance and/or factor V Leiden mutation are associated with second, but not first, trimester recurrent spontaneous abortion. The results of this study suggest that 2 thrombophillic conditions, factor V Leiden as well as G20210A prothrombin mutations, are found more frequently in women having unexplained recurrent abortion before 10 weeks' gestation, compared with normal controls. If these results are confirmed by others, measurement of these 2 factors should be performed with both early and late recurrent abortions without a defined cause. It remains to be determined whether treating women with these thrombophillic conditions and recurrent spontaneous abortion with aspirin and heparin improves the viable pregnancy rate.

D. R. Mishell, Jr, MD

Factor V Leiden and Recurrent Miscarriage—Prospective Outcome of Untreated Pregnancies
Rai R, Backos M, Elgaddal S, et al (Imperial College of Science, Technology and Medicine, London; St Mary's Hosp, London)
Hum Reprod 17:442-445, 2002   17–12

Introduction.—Factor V Leiden, a common thrombophilic mutation, has been reported in association with placental thrombosis. Although some cases of recurrent miscarriage and later pregnancy complications have a thrombotic basis, existing data on the association between Factor V Leiden and pregnancy outcome is limited. The pregnancy outcome of women with recurrent miscarriage who carry the Factor V Leiden allele was investigated in a prospective observational study.

Methods.—The study included 25 consecutive white women heterozygous for the Factor V Leiden allele with a history of either recurrent early miscarriage or a history of at least 1 late (>12 weeks of gestation) miscarriage. Control subjects were 198 consecutive white women with similar histories of miscarriage but with a normal Factor V genotype. None of the women in the study had a personal history of systemic venous thrombosis, and all had persistently negative tests for antiphospholipid antibodies. The only pharmacologic treatment during pregnancy was folic acid (400 mg/d).

Results.—Among women who carried the Factor V Leiden allele and had a history of early miscarriage, the live birth rate was 37.5%, a figure significantly lower that the live birth rate in the early miscarriage control group (69.3%). Among women with a history of late miscarriage, the live birth rate was 11.1% in those carrying the Factor V Leiden allele and 48.9% in those with a normal Factor V genotype. None of the women with or without the Factor V Leiden allele had a symptomatic venous thrombosis during the antenatal, intra-partum, or postpartum periods.

Conclusion.—Women with recurrent miscarriage who carry the Factor V Leiden allele are at significantly increased risk for subsequent miscarriage, although some have successful pregnancies with a live birth at term. The challenge is to identify and treat those women with Factor V Leiden who are at increased risk for future pregnancy loss.

▶ The results of this prospective cohort analysis of women with either unexplained recurrent first-trimester miscarriage or at least 1 second-trimester miscarriage indicate that the presence of the Factor V Leiden allele is an independent risk factor for further pregnancy loss. It remains to be determined whether treatment with heparin will improve the prognosis for a viable birth among women with unexplained recurrent miscarriage and Factor V Leiden.

D. R. Mishell, Jr, MD

High Serum Luteinizing Hormone and Testosterone Concentrations Do Not Predict Pregnancy Outcome in Women With Recurrent Miscarriage
Nardo LG, Rai R, Backos M, et al (Imperial College School of Medicine, London)
Fertil Steril 77:348-352, 2002   17–13

Purpose.—Hypersecretion of luteinizing hormone (LH), hyperandrogenemia, obesity, and other endocrine conditions have been associated with pregnancy loss. However, no prospective studies have examined the outcomes of women with recurrent miscarriage who have any of these endocrine conditions. The effects of certain endocrine factors on the pregnancy outcomes in women with recurrent miscarriage were investigated.

Methods.—The prospective, observational study included 344 women with recurrent first trimester miscarriage. The women, median age 32 years, had had a median of 4 miscarriages before 12 weeks' gestation. For the current study, all women had conceived spontaneously and had received no pharmacologic therapy during pregnancy. None of the women tested positive for antiphospholipid antibodies. All women and their partners were karyotypically normal. Each patient underwent measurement of serum LH and testosterone levels on day 8 of the menstrual cycle. The effects of these hormonal factors and of the women's body mass index (BMI) on pregnancy outcome were evaluated.

Results.—The women had a live birth rate of 56% and a miscarriage rate of 44%. Fifty-one percent of women met US morphologic criteria for polycystic ovary (PCO). However, the live birth rate was not significantly different for women with or without PCO: 57% and 50%, respectively. Serum LH measurements were low in 20% of women, normal in 70%, and high in 9%; live birth rates in these groups were 54%, 58%, and 41%, respectively. These differences were nonsignificant. Testosterone level and BMI also had no significant association with pregnancy outcome.

Conclusions.—For women with a history of unexplained recurrent miscarriage, none of the endocrine factors evaluated was significantly related to the outcome of a new spontaneous pregnancy. There remains no causative link between PCO, LH, or testosterone level, or BMI and recurrent miscarriage.

▶ Other studies have found that PCO and high levels of LH in the follicular phase of the cycle are associated with a high rate of miscarriage. The results of this study confirm these findings. However, when studying a group of women with unexplained recurrent miscarriage, the presence of either PCO, high follicular phase LH, or testosterone as well as high BMI was not associated with a higher rate of miscarriage compared with women with normal ovaries, BMI, or LH or testosterone levels. Thus, whether PCO and/or elevation of LH and/or testosterone are causes of recurrent miscarriage remains to be established.

D. R. Mishell, Jr, MD

Thrombophilia Is Common in Women With Idiopathic Pregnancy Loss and Is Associated With Late Pregnancy Wastage
Sarig G, Younis JS, Hoffman R, et al (Rambam Med Ctr, Haifa, Israel)
Fertil Steril 77:342-347, 2002   17–14

Purpose.—Recent studies have shown that various forms of inherited thrombophilia may play a role in pregnancy loss. However, the impact of specific thrombophilic defects on specific types of pregnancy loss remains unclear. The relative importance of the various thrombophilic factors as causative agents of pregnancy loss was evaluated in a prospective study.

Methods.—The study included 145 consecutive women with pregnancy loss of unknown cause occurring at various stages of pregnancy. All patients had 3 or more pregnancy wastages in the first trimester (7 to 12 weeks), 2 or more losses in the second trimester (13 to 24 weeks), or at least 1 intrauterine fetal demise after 24 weeks. These criteria excluded first trimester preclinical and blighted ovum miscarriages; all subjects had postembryonic losses after disappearance of the fetal pulse on ultrasound. The cases were matched for age and ethnicity to 145 women with at least 1 successful gestation and no more than 1 first trimester pregnancy loss. In both groups, the presence of thrombophilic factors was tested in blood samples taken when the women were not pregnant.

Results.—Twenty-five percent of gestations in the study group resulted in delivery of a live newborn compared with 94% in the control group. One or more thrombophilic defects was detected in 66% of the women with a history of pregnancy loss versus 28% of control subjects. Within the pregnancy loss group, the live birth was similar for women with versus without thrombophilic factors. However, women with thrombophilia were more likely to have second or third trimester pregnancy loss (37% vs 24%).

On analysis of specific thrombophilic polymorphisms, 25% of the pregnancy loss group had factor V G1691A compared with 8% of the control group. The 2 groups had similar prevalences of factor II G20210A and MTHFR C677T. Women in the pregnancy loss group were more likely to have antiphospholipid antibodies (14% vs 3%); both groups had low rates of antithrombin III and protein C deficiency. The single most common thrombophilic factor was activated protein C resistance, found in 39% of the pregnancy loss group compared with 3% of the control group. Fifty-four percent of women with activated protein C resistance also had factor V Leiden mutation. The rate of late pregnancy wastage was 44% for women with factor V Leiden mutation compared with 25% for those with antiphospholipid antibodies as their sole thrombophilic defect.

Conclusions.—Two thirds of women with pregnancy loss of unknown cause have at least 1 thrombophilic defect; more than one fifth have 2 or more defects. activated protein C resistance without factor V Leiden mutation is a commonly identified defect in this group of patients, along with factor V Leiden mutation and antiphospholipid antibodies. Thrombophilia may be particularly associated with late pregnancy wastage.

▶ The results of this study confirm the fact that antiphospholipid antibodies are present in about 15% of women with no other causes for recurrent pregnancy loss. In this population of women who had no diagnosed cause for recurrent pregnancy loss, thrombophilic abnormalities were found in two thirds. It remains to be determined whether this high incidence is found in other ethnic groups and whether treating these women with anticoagulants will increase their rate of viable birth.

D. R. Mishell, Jr, MD

Effects of Metformin on Early Pregnancy Loss in the Polycystic Ovary Syndrome
Jakubowicz DJ, Iuorno MJ, Jakubowicz S, et al (Central Univ of Venezuela, Caracas; Virginia Commonwealth Univ, Richmond)
J Clin Endocrinol Metab 87:524-529, 2002   17–15

Background.—Polycystic ovarian syndrome (PCOS) affects 5% to 10% of women of reproductive age in the United States. Not only is PCOS associated with difficulty conceiving, it also increases the risk of miscarriage. Factors that increase the risk of miscarriage in PCOS include obesity, hyperandrogenemia, and hyperinsulinemic insulin resistance. Metformin has beneficial effects on all 3 of these factors. The pregnancy outcomes of patients with PCOS who did or did not take metformin during their pregnancy were compared in an observational study.

Methods.—The subjects were 96 women with PCOS being treated at an academic endocrinology clinic who became pregnant during a 4½-year period. None of the patients had diabetes mellitus, and all had PCOS confirmed by US. Thirty-one patients did not take metformin at any time during their pregnancy and served as controls. The remaining 65 patients became pregnant while taking metformin and continued the drug throughout their pregnancy at a dosage of 1000 to 2000 mg/d. The rates of pregnancy loss during the first trimester were compared between the groups as a whole and between the subset of patients within each group who had a prior history of early pregnancy loss.

Results.—Of the 65 patients in the metformin group, 17 were nulliparous and 48 had a history of early pregnancy loss. Among these 48 patients, there had been 75 pregnancies, including 22 live births and 53 miscarriages. Thus, the miscarriage rate in this group at study entry was 70.7%. Of the 31 patients in the control group, 10 were nulliparous and 21 had a history of early pregnancy loss. Among these 21 patients, there had been 24 pregnancies, including 11 live births and 13 miscarriages. Thus, the miscarriage rate in this group at study entry was 54.2%.

During the study period, there were 68 pregnancies among the 65 patients in the metformin group. Early pregnancy loss occurred in only 6 pregnancies (8.8%). In contrast, there were 31 pregnancies among the 31 patients in the control group, and early pregnancy loss occurred in 13 pregnancies (41.9%). The incidence of early pregnancy loss was significantly lower in the metformin group than in the control group, both for the groups as a whole (8.8% and 41.9%, respectively) and for the subgroup of patients with a prior history of early pregnancy loss (11.1% vs 58.3%). The incidence of early pregnancy loss in the metformin group was eightfold lower with metformin treatment than at study entry (8.8% vs 70.7%), while the incidence of early pregnancy loss in the control group did not change over time (54.2% at study entry, 41.9% at study end).

The serum insulin area under the curve (AUC) at study entry was significantly higher in the metformin group than in the controls (14.2 vs 11.2 mU/mL/min). During the study, the serum insulin AUC increased during the first trimester by 1.8 mU/mL/min in the control group but decreased by 4.9 mU/mL/min in the metformin group. This between-group difference was statistically significant. The serum glucose AUC at study entry was similar in the metformin and control groups. During the study, the serum glucose AUC decreased in the metformin group (from 15,593 to 13,346 mg/dL/min) but increased in the control subjects (from 14,505 to 15,803 mg/dL/min). Again, this between-group difference was statistically significant.

As for fetal outcomes, 62 pregnancies in the metformin group and 18 in the control group resulted in live births. This included 53 term and 8 preterm deliveries in the metformin group, and 12 term and 6 preterm deliveries in the control group. All neonates were normal, except for 1 term baby in the metformin group who was born with achondrodysplasia.

Conclusions.—In patients with PCOS, metformin treatment throughout pregnancy dramatically decreased the rate of early pregnancy loss, even in patients with a prior history of miscarriage. The only adverse fetal outcome that occurred in the metformin group was 1 case of achondrodysplasia.

▶ Women with PCOS who conceive have a high rate of spontaneous abortion in the first trimester, ranging from about 30% to 50%. Results of a small observational study published in 2001[1] as well as this larger observational study indicate that continuing metformin therapy throughout pregnancy for women with PCOS in a dosage of 1000 to 2500 mg/d reduces the rate of early spontaneous abortion to about 10%. The mechanisms whereby metformin reduces the rate of miscarriage have not been determined but may include reducing testosterone levels, increasing insulin sensitivity, and/or reducing plasminogen activator inhibitor–1 activity. A randomized controlled trial utilizing metformin and placebo in women with PCOS who become pregnant should be performed to confirm that metformin reduces the high rate of miscarriage for these women.

D. R. Mishell, Jr, MD

Reference

1. 2002 YEAR BOOK OF OBSTETRICS, GYNECOLOGY, AND WOMEN'S HEALTH, p 323.

Recurrent Pregnancy Loss With Antiphospholipid Antibody: A Systematic Review of Therapeutic Trials
Empson M, Lassere M, Craig JC, et al (Auckland Hosp, New Zealand; Westmead Hosp, Sydney, Australia; St George Hosp, Sydney, Australia; et al)
Obstet Gynecol 99:135-144, 2002   17–16

Background.—An association between circulating maternal antiphospholipid (APL) antibodies and recurrent pregnancy loss has been recognized for many years, and a number of interventions have been proposed to aid in maintenance of the pregnancy until successful delivery. The effects of these various interventions to improve pregnancy outcome in women with APL antibodies were explored in a systematic review.

Methods.—Randomized and quasi-randomized controlled trials of therapy for pregnancy loss associated with APL antibodies were identified through searches of the Cochrane Controlled Trials Register, the Cochrane Collaboration Pregnancy and Childbirth Group's Specialized Register of Controlled Trials, EMBASE, and MEDLINE. The searches were conducted in December 1999.

Results.—From a total of 565 studies initially identified, 10 studies involving 627 subjects were included in the final analysis. Quantitative analysis of summary data was performed by means of the fixed- and random-effects models with heterogeneity assessments. The main outcome measures were pregnancy loss and adverse neonatal outcomes. Three trials compared aspirin alone and showed no significant reduction in pregnancy loss. In 2 trials, heparin combined with aspirin significantly reduced pregnancy loss compared with aspirin alone. The combination of aspirin and prednisone resulted in a significant increase in prematurity, but there was no significant reduction in pregnancy loss.

Conclusion.—This review of treatment for pregnancy loss associated with antiphospholipid antibodies found that combination therapy with aspirin and heparin could reduce pregnancy loss in these patients by 54%. More large, randomized, controlled trials are needed to exclude significant adverse effects.

▶ Many therapies have been utilized for the treatment of recurrent pregnancy loss (RPL) in women with APLs, particularly anticardiolipin antibody and lupus anticoagulant. The results of this review of randomized trials of various therapies used to treat RPL with APL found that only the combination of heparin and aspirin resulted in a significant decrease of RPL. Thus, at present, the treatment of RPL with APL should be the use of 5000 U of heparin twice daily subcutaneously plus 81 mg aspirin daily. At present, there are no data to show that low molecular weight heparin has the same benefit as use of unfractionated heparin. Therefore, it remains to be determined whether low molecular weight heparin can be used to treat RPL with APL.

D. R. Mishell, Jr, MD

A Randomized, Double-Blind, Placebo-Controlled Trial of Intravenous Immunoglobulin in the Prevention of Recurrent Miscarriage: Evidence for a Therapeutic Effect in Women With Secondary Recurrent Miscarriage
Christiansen OB, Pedersen B, Rosgaard A, et al (Aalborg Hosp, Denmark; Copenhagen Univ)
Hum Reprod 17:809-816, 2002   17–17

Introduction.—Fetal aneuploidy is a common cause of miscarriage, but women who experience recurrent miscarriage (RM) are likely to have other causes of pregnancy loss. In many cases of RM, immunologic disturbances can be a risk factor. Because IV immunoglobulin (IVIG) has been documented to be effective for many disorders caused by immunologic abnormalities, IVIG was evaluated in a placebo-controlled trial for the treatment of patients with at least 4 previous miscarriages.

Methods.—Women eligible for the trial had regular menstruations with cycle length between 21 and 35 days and were free of uterine or parental chromosomal abnormality. Excluded were women with total IgA deficiency, insulin-dependent diabetes mellitus, and women whose pregnancy was obtained by in vitro fertilization or controlled ovarian stimulation. All couples had normal chromosomes. The 58 trial participants were randomized to receive either infusions of high doses of IVIG (Nordimmun) or placebo, start-ing as soon as the pregnancy test was positive. A total of 14 infusions in suc-cessful pregnancies were given until week 26 of gestation.

Results.—Enrollment in the study continued from June 1994 to June 1999. All participants complied with the infusion schedule until the preg-nancy was concluded by a birth, miscarriage, or an ectopic pregnancy. No other therapies used in the management of RM were administered. In the intention-to-treat analysis, the live birth rate was 45% in both IVIG and pla-cebo groups. Among patients with secondary RM (RM after a pregnancy continued to at least week 26), the success rate was 27% higher for the IVIG group; this difference, however, was not statistically significant. Adverse ef-fects were more common, however, in the IVIG group, although generally mild or moderate. Only 7% of karyotyped abortuses were abnormal. Com-bining data from this trial and a previous placebo-controlled trial of the same treatment, a significant advantage of IVIG over placebo (58% vs 24% successful outcome) was noted for patients with secondary RM.

Conclusion.—Treatment with IVIG may be beneficial in a subset of wom-en with secondary RM. An unexpected finding was a highly significant ex-cess of both female infants and female abortuses.

▶ Many clinicians are treating patients with recurrent miscarriage without an etiology with IVIG at frequent intervals throughout gestation. A beneficial ef-fect of such therapy has been previously reported in 2 placebo-controlled trials, but no benefit was found in 4 other controlled trials. Overall, no benefit for IVIG therapy was found in this large trial in which the therapy was started early in pregnancy and used large doses of IVIG. Although a benefit of IVIG was shown in the subset of women with recurrent miscarriage who also had a prior preg-nancy advancing beyond 20 weeks, the beneficial effect was not statistically significant. At present, a beneficial effect for IVIG therapy of women with re-current miscarriage has not been substantiated. IVIG therapy is costly and is associated with side effects. Therefore, IVIG should only be given under the conditions of an approved investigational protocol with full informed consent of the subject.

D. R. Mishell, Jr, MD

18 Ectopic Pregnancy

Human Chorionic Gonadotropin Patterns After a Single Dose of Methotrexate for Ectopic Pregnancy
Natale A, Busacca M, Candiani M, et al (Univ of Milan, Italy; Istituti Clinici di Perfezionamento, Milan, Italy)
Eur J Obstet Gynecol Reprod Biol 100:227-230, 2002   18–1

Introduction.—Ectopic pregnancies have been managed successfully with a single dose of methotrexate (MTX), but a potential complication is the persistence of trophoblastic tissue. The human chorionic gonadotropin (HCG), an accurate marker of trophoblastic tissue vitality, is widely used to identify persistences. Different patterns of HCG levels after a single dose of MTX for ectopic pregnancy were analyzed prospectively, with special emphasis on cases showing an initial rise of the HCG curve before resolution.

Methods.—Patients eligible for the study had confirmation of an ectopic pregnancy, exclusion of an intrauterine or tubal spontaneous abortion, an absence of embryonic cardiac activity, HCG levels less than 4000 mIU/mL, a US diameter less than 4 cm, and no contraindication to MTX therapy. Blood samples to measure HCG levels were obtained on the day of MTX therapy, at 3, 7, and 14 days after MTX administration, then once a week until values were completely undetectable.

Results.—Patients were classified as persistent pathology (group 1, 11 women), complete resolution with a decrease of HCG levels at day 3 (group 2, 30 women), or complete resolution after a rise of HCG values at day 3 (group 3, 9 women). The HCG values of day 1 were statistically similar for all 3 groups. In group 3, HCG levels fell rapidly after day 3 and were significantly different from those of group 1 at day 7. Differences in HCG levels between groups 2 and 3 became indistinguishable from day 21 (Fig 1).

Conclusion.—Medical treatment can be a safe and effective alternative to surgical conservative treatment for patients with ectopic pregnancy. Persistence of trophoblastic tissue can occur after various types of therapy and can be monitored by HCG curves. Because a high variability in HCG levels is present after medical therapy, expectant management should continue for 1 week. After 21 days, HCG values are similar for all patients undergoing resolution.

▶ Injections of methotrexate are being used with increased frequency to treat unruptured ectopic pregnancy. It is important for clinicians to measure

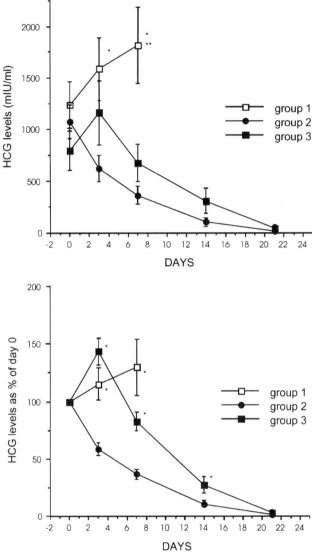

FIGURE 1.—HCG value profiles in patients treated with 50 mg/m^2 MTX IM for ectopic pregnancy. Day 0 represents the day on which the therapy was administered. Data for patients undergoing persistence of trophoblastic tissue (group 1) were compared to those for patients undergoing resolution with an immediate decrease of the hormonal parameter (group 2) and to those for patients undergoing resolution with an immediate increase of HCG levels at day 3 (group 3). *Top*, HCG real values; *bottom*, levels of HCG as a percentage of day 0 measurement. Statistical significance, when present, is indicated as follows: *significantly different vs correspondent group 2 values ($P < .01$); **significantly different vs correspondent group 3 values ($P < .05$). (Courtesy of Natale A, Busacca M, Candiani M, et al: Human chorionic gonadotropin patterns after a single dose of methotrexate for ectopic pregnancy. *Eur J Obstet Gynecol Reprod Biol* 100:227-230. Copyright 2002 from Elsevier Science.)

circulating HCG levels in patients on the day of treatment, 3 and 7 days later, and weekly thereafter until HCG is no longer detected. The level of HCG frequently increases between the day of treatment and day 3, but by day 7, levels should decline at least 15% from the day 3 levels if resolution of the ectopic pregnancy is going to occur. In this study, about half the patients who had an initial rise in HCG levels between the day of methotrexate treatment and day 3 had resolution of their ectopic pregnancies. If HCG levels on day 7 do not decline at least 15% from the level on day 3, an additional injection of methotrexate should be given.

D. R. Mishell, Jr, MD

Intramuscular Methotrexate for Tubal Pregnancy
El-Lamie IK, Shehata NA, Kamel HA (Ain Shams Univ, Cairo)
J Reprod Med 47:144-150, 2002   18–2

Background.—The incidence of tubal pregnancy has increased markedly in the past 3 decades. A study was undertaken to determine the safety and efficacy of medical treatment for tubal pregnancy in hemodynamically stable women who were using intramuscular methotrexate, even when adnexal masses were as large as 5 cm in diameter.

Methods.—Thirty-five patients who met eligibility criteria were included in the prospective, observational study. Seventeen had an adnexal mass 3.6 to 5 cm in diameter. All women received methotrexate, 50 mg/m^2, intramuscularly.

Findings.—Cure was documented in 94.3% of the women. A single methotrexate dose was needed in 75.8%, 2 doses in 21.2%, and 3 doses in 3%. Treatment failure occurred in 2 women (5.7%), both of whom had masses larger than 3.5 cm. Mean time to human chorionic gonadotropin (hCG) normalization was 34.8 days. Of the 33 patients cured, 60.6% were treated as outpatients, 21.2% with a brief admission indicated by severe separation pain, and 18.2% as inpatients for logistic reasons. The serum hCG differed significantly when a cutoff level of 1000 mIU/mL was used to compare those with an adnexal mass of 3.5 cm or smaller and those with a mass of 3.6 to 5 cm, as well as those requiring more than 1 dose and those needing 1. Number of doses needed differed significantly between those with smaller masses and those with larger masses. However, because of the small sample size and the limited number of events, a multivariate analysis did not show any significant relationship between treatment failure, hCG level, mass size, gestational age, or number of doses.

Conclusions.—IM methotrexate appears to be effective and safe in hemodynamically stable women with tubal pregnancy, even when adnexal masses are as large as 5 cm. Larger studies are needed to verify these findings.

▶ Medical treatment of unruptured ectopic pregnancy with methotrexate is becoming more frequently used worldwide because it is less expensive than laparoscopic surgery. Most centers use methotrexate therapy only in women with an unruptured ectopic pregnancy, a serum hCG level less than 10,000 mIU/mL, and an adnexal mass less than 3.5 to 4 cm in diameter without the presence of fetal cardiac activity. In this series, women with an adnexal mass diameter as large as 5 cm and hCG levels as high as 32,000 mIU/mL were treated with methotrexate. Among 35 women treated with methotrexate, there were only 2 treatment failures. Additional trials are needed to determine whether methotrexate is effective therapy for women with an unruptured ectopic pregnancy and an adnexal mass between 3.5 and 5 cm in diameter.

D. R. Mishell, Jr, MD

Clinical and Pregnancy Outcome Following Ectopic Pregnancy; A Prospective Study Comparing Expectancy, Surgery and Systemic Methotrexate Treatment
Olofsson JI, Poromaa IS, Ottander U, et al (Umeå Univ, Sweden)
Acta Obstet Gynecol Scand 80:744-749, 2001   18–3

Background.—Now that ectopic pregnancy (EP) can be diagnosed earlier by the measurement of serial quantitative β-subunit human chorionic gonadotropin (hCG) levels and the use of transvaginal US, the options for conservative treatment have expanded. Methotrexate (MTX) has been used as an alternative to surgical options. Its use avoids the need for surgical intervention and costs less. The effectiveness of MTX treatment and pregnancy outcome in routine clinical practice were assessed.

Methods.—Over the course of 3 years (January 1, 1995, to December 31, 1997), all patients coming for treatment who had signs and symptoms of EP were included. Treatment options were MTX, laparoscopic surgery, open surgery, and expectant management. Randomization was not done, but patients were handled as conservatively as possible. Those who were eligible for MTX treatment had to be hemodynamically stable, have no incapacitating pain, and have β-hCG levels under 7500 IU/L. The 50 mg/m^2 dose of systemic MTX was given IM. If the β-hCG level fell less than 15% between the fourth and seventh days, an additional dose of MTX (50 mg/m^2) was administered. Patients were followed up weekly until the ectopic mass completely resolved. The primary outcome measure was the ability of MTX to nonsurgically eliminate the EP. All patients were followed up with careful documentation of clinical findings and laboratory data.

Results.—Eighty-nine patients had EP, and of these, 25 received MTX, 46 had laparoscopy or laparotomy, and 17 had expectant management. The MTX group had lower initial β-hCG levels than the other patients, but other factors were similar. For 77% of these patients, MTX treatment was successful within a mean of 24 days. No correlation was found between β-hCG levels before treatment and length of time to resolution. Only 2 patients needed the second dose of MTX. For 6 patients who initially received MTX, surgery was eventually required. By August 2000, intrauterine pregnancies were achieved in 63.6% of the eligible patients who had MTX treatment, 52.4% of the surgery patients, and 30.8% of the conservatively treatment patients.

Conclusion.—The number of patients who required surgical intervention was lowered to 62% by the use of MTX treatment. MTX achieved resolution of the EP in 77% of cases. Pregnancy rates were not adversely affected by MTX, with the levels achieved at least equal to those noted with surgery. Thus, single-dose MTX treatment appears safe and effective for EP, but careful monitoring must accompany its use.

▶ With the use of pelvic sonography and serial measurements of hCG, EP is more frequently diagnosed before tubal rupture than occurred previously. Unruptured EP can be treated expectantly, with MTX, or by surgical excision. The results from this nonrandomized study show a similar rate of subsequent intrauterine pregnancy after MTX as occurred after surgical treatment of the EP. Sufficient experience has now been obtained with MTX treatment of EP for clinicians to consider offering the use of this treatment of unruptured tubal pregnancy as an effective alternative to surgical excision.

D. R. Mishell, Jr, MD

19 Premenstrual Syndrome

Efficacy of Progesterone and Progestogens in Management of Premenstrual Syndrome: Systematic Review
Wyatt K, Dimmock P, Jones P, et al (Keele Univ, England)
BMJ 323:1-8, 2001   19–1

Background.—Premenstrual syndrome is the recurrence of psychological and physical symptoms in the luteal phase, which remit in the follicular phase of the menstrual cycle. An estimated 1.5 million women in the United Kingdom have symptoms severe enough to affect their quality of life and interpersonal relationships. Over 35% of these women will seek medical treatment. Progesterone and progestogens have been used in the management of premenstrual syndrome on the premise that progesterone deficiency is the cause; however, this premise has not been substantiated. The efficacy of progesterone and progestogens in the management of premenstrual syndrome was evaluated.

Methods.—A systematic review of 10 trials of progesterone therapy and 4 trials of progestogen therapy was conducted. All of the studies were randomized placebo-controlled trials. The progesterone trials involved a total of 531 women, and the progestogen trials involved a total of 378 women. The main outcome measure was the proportion of women whose symptoms showed improvement with progesterone preparations or progestogens. The efficacy of progesterone and progestogens in managing physical and behavioral symptoms was also assessed.

Results.—There was no clinically significant difference between progesterone and placebo. The standardized mean difference in efficacy for all the progesterone trials was −0.028, with an odds ratio of 1.05 in favor of progesterone. For progestogens, the overall standardized mean difference was −0.036, with an odds ratio of 1.07, a statistically but not clinically significant improvement.

Conclusion.—The findings in this meta-analysis do not support the use of progesterone and progestogens in the treatment of premenstrual syndrome.

▶ There is an unsubstantiated belief that progesterone deficiency is the cause of the premenstrual syndrome (PMS). For this reason, many clinicians treat women with PMS with progesterone or progestins. The results of this meta-analysis indicate that there is a slight statistical benefit but not a substantial clinical benefit for the use of progesterone or progestins in the treatment of PMS. Management with one of the selective serotonin reuptake inhibitors provides much better improvement of the symptoms of PMS than progesterone. Therefore, one of these agents should be used to treat PMS instead of progesterone.

D. R. Mishell, Jr, MD

A New Monophasic Oral Contraceptive Containing Drospirenone: Effect on Premenstrual Symptoms
Brown C, Ling F, Wan J (Univ of Tennessee, Memphis)
J Reprod Med 47:14-22, 2002   19–2

Introduction.—Some women report reduced premenstrual symptoms when taking combined hormonal oral contraceptives (OC), although certain symptoms—those related to water retention and mood swings—may be increased in OC users. A new monophasic OC formulation containing drospirenone in combination with ethinyl estradiol (DRSP/EE) has been described. Because DRSP has direct as well as indirect antiandrogenic activity, it may improve some types of premenstrual symptoms. The effects of the new DRSP/EE preparation on premenstrual symptoms were evaluated.

Methods.—The multicenter, open-label trial included 326 healthy women, aged 18 to 35 years, including 150 new users of hormonal contraceptives and 176 previous users of other OC. The women were to take DRSP/EE for 13 menstrual cycles. Before treatment and after 6 cycles, the women rated their premenstrual symptoms with the Women's Health Assessment Questionnaire (WHAQ). This instrument addressed specific symptoms of negative affect, water retention, impaired concentration, increased appetite, well-being, and undesirable hair changes.

Results.—Two thirds of women completed all 13 cycles. Mean baseline scores for negative affect were significantly increased during the premenstrual and menstrual phases of the cycle compared with the postmenstrual phase. After 6 cycles of treatment, mean negative affect score during the premenstrual and menstrual phases was significantly decreased. On assessment of negative affect T scores, which compared with raw scores with a normative sample, significant reductions were confirmed among both new OC users and women who switched from other OC. During the menstrual phase, nearly all components of the negative affect scale were significantly improved, including anxiety, mood swings, crying, irritability, tension, sadness, and restlessness. Most items were reduced during the menstrual phase as well.

The use of DRSP/EE was also associated with significant reductions in water retention during the premenstrual and menstrual phases. Again, analysis of T scores confirmed these changes. Scores for impaired concentration improved during all 3 phases, with the greatest change during the menstrual phase.

Conclusions.—In a group of women with relatively mild premenstrual symptoms, the use of DRSP/EE is associated with significant improvement in mood symptoms. Substantial improvements in irritability and mood swings during the premenstrual and menstrual phases were noted both in new OC users and women who have switched from other OC. The new DRSP-containing OC appears to improve other premenstrual symptoms as well, such as water retention and increased appetite.

▶ This study found that women receiving a new OC containing a nonandrogenic antimineralocorticoid progestin for 6 cycles had a reduced frequency of many adverse symptoms that were previously increased premenstrually. The study population was a group of normal women, not those with severe premenstrual symptoms. Unfortunately, this was not a randomized, placebo-controlled trial. Therefore, all or part of the improvement in symptoms could be a placebo effect and not drug related. A more valid approach would have been to have the women rate symptoms prospectively by a diary instead of retrospectively, as was done in this study. Nevertheless, the results of this study warrant the performance of a placebo-controlled trial using this OC in a group of women with severe premenstrual symptoms.

D. R. Mishell, Jr, MD

Venlafaxine in the Treatment of Premenstrual Dysphoric Disorder
Freeman EW, Rickels K, Yonkers KA, et al (Univ of Pennsylvania, Philadelphia; Univ of Texas, Dallas; Wyeth-Ayerst Research, Radnor, Pa)
Obstet Gynecol 98:737-744, 2001   19–3

Background.—Approximately 3% to 5% of menstruating women experience premenstrual dysphoric disorder (PMDD). It is thought that abnormalities in central serotonergic activities have a role in the pathophysiology of PMDD because of the associated alterations in mood, behavior, and appetite. Antidepressants with serotonin reuptake–inhibiting properties have been found to provide relief of PMDD symptoms in a number of trials. However, many women did not respond to such treatment for unknown reasons. The efficacy and safety of venlafaxine, a new-generation serotonin reuptake–inhibiting antidepressant, was evaluated in the treatment of PMDD.

Methods.—A randomized, double-blind, placebo-controlled, parallel-group, flexible-dose trial was conducted. A total of 164 women participated in 3 screening cycles before being randomly assigned to treatment with either venlafaxine (50 to 200 mg/d) or placebo for 4 menstrual cycles. Primary outcome measures were the total premenstrual symptom scores according to a daily symptom report and the Hamilton Rating Scale for Depression.

Results.—The daily symptom reports scores indicated that venlafaxine was significantly more effective than placebo in reducing PMDD symptoms.

Improvement of more than 50% was reported in 60% of venlafaxine subjects compared with 35% of placebo subjects. Improvement was rapid, with a reduction in symptoms of about 80% in the first treatment cycle. The mean doses for venlafaxine ranged from 50 mg/d in the first treatment cycle to 130 mg/d in the fourth treatment cycle. Mild, transient adverse effects were reported, including nausea, insomnia, and dizziness.

Conclusion.—Venlafaxine was significantly more effective than placebo in the treatment of PMDD. Response to treatment may occur in the first treatment cycle. Further studies are needed to investigate the potential for luteal phase dosing of venlafaxine and its efficacy in long-term maintenance treatment.

▶ Several serotonergic antidepressants have been shown in placebo-controlled trials to be effective agents for the treatment of PMDD. This well-done study shows that daily administration of a recently developed serotoningeric antidepressant called venlafaxine—an agent that selectively inhibits the reuptake of both serotonin and norepinephrine—provides better therapy than placebo for PMDD. Side effects were mild and response to treatment was rapid with this agent. Additional studies should be done to determine whether intermittent luteal phase dosing is also effective.

D. R. Mishell, Jr, MD

20 Uterus

Tumor Makers

Serum CA-125 in Preoperative Patients at High Risk for Endometriosis
Cheng Y-M, Wang S-T, Chou C-Y (Natl Cheng King Univ, Tainan, Taiwan)
Obstet Gynecol 99:375-380, 2002   20–1

Introduction.—Bowel injury is a risk of laparoscopically assisted vaginal hysterectomy in patients with endometriosis. Several trials and a meta-analysis have reported the performance of serum CA-125 assay in the detection of endometriosis and have shown a specificity of 85% and sensitivity ranging between 20% and 50%. These trials have focused on infertile women, and the number of patients was small. The factors related to an increased level of CA-125 in endometriosis were examined, along with the usefulness of preoperative CA-125 assay in identifying women at risk who would require bowel preparation preoperatively.

Methods.—Six hundred eighty-five women undergoing surgery for endometriosis between July 1988 and June 1999 underwent determination of preoperative serum CA-125 levels. The levels were compared with various pelvic conditions. Multiple regression was used to ascertain significant correlates of elevated serum CA-125. The receiver operating characteristic curve was used to examine the utility of serum CA-125 in preoperative preparation. The sample size needed to identify a difference in mean serum CA-125 levels of ½ of 1 standard deviation with a power of 90% when the sample size ratio of the 2 groups was 1:50 was 675.

Results.—The mean serum CA-125 levels (IU/mL) for American Society of Reproductive Medicine stages I, II, III, and IV endometriosis were 18.8, 40.9, 77.1, and 182.4, respectively, and the CA-125 levels were significantly elevated with advanced stages ($P < .001$). The serum CA-125 levels were significantly increased in patients with more extensive adhesions to the peritoneum, omentum, ovary, fallopian tube, colon, and cul-de-sac, or those with ruptured endometrioma ($P < .001$). Patients with at least 1 of the 3 factors, including dense omentum adhesion, ruptured endometrioma, and complete cul-de-sac obliteration, were classified as the high-risk group that needed preoperative bowel preparation, and the others were classified as the low-risk group. Receiver operating characteristic curve analyses set a cutoff point of 65 IU/mL, which yielded a sensitivity of 76%, a specificity of 71%, a positive predictive value of 76%, and a negative predictive value of 93.2%.

Conclusion.—Preoperative CA-125 assay is helpful in determining which patients should undergo preoperative bowel preparation. Patients with endometriosis who have preoperative CA-125 levels higher than 65 IU/mL are at high risk of severe pelvic adhesions that necessitate thorough preoperative bowel preparation.

▶ The preoperative assessment of women presumed to have endometriosis should include those tests that will help distinguish the cases with more severe disease. It is easier for the patient to understand the need for bowel preparation if clinical or laboratory findings suggest advanced disease. The surgeon, as well, can allot appropriate time for the case and assure the availability of a good assistant. This article correlates higher (>65 IU/mL) CA 125 with an increased probability of extensive peritoneal adhesions. This laboratory finding, along with a history and examination findings consistent with extensive endometriosis, suggests that the surgeon prepare for a more challenging dissection, whether the procedure planned is laparoscopic or open, extirpative or fertility-enhancing.

R. D. Arias, MD

Falsely Elevated Human Chorionic Gonadotropin Leading to Unnecessary Therapy
Olsen TG, Hubert PR, Nycum LR (David Grant Med Ctr, Travis Air Force Base, Calif)
Obstet Gynecol 98:843-845, 2001   20–2

Introduction.—Serum analysis of β–human chorionic gonadotropin (β-hCG) is important in the diagnosis and treatment of abnormal intrauterine pregnancies, ectopic gestations, and gestational trophoblastic neoplasia. The validity of serum β-hCG concentrations is rarely questioned because of its greater sensitivity and specificity for trophoblastic tissue. The cases of 2 patients who received treatment based on incorrect findings of elevated β-hCG were reported.

Case 1.—Woman, 18, nulliparous, with a history of Evans syndrome, had a history of multiple transfusions at the time of menarche. The Evans syndrome had been in spontaneous remission for several years and the patient was otherwise healthy. After reporting that she was late for her menses, a qualitative β-hCG was found to be 36.5 mIU/mL. She was seen in the emergency department for vaginal bleeding 12 days later. Her serum β-hCG was 14 mIU/mL and US showed no evidence of intrauterine or ectopic pregnancy. She passed tissue and the bleeding ceased. At follow-up, her β-hCG was 39.6 mIU/mL. The level was 35.7 mIU/mL 2 days later and a nonviable intrauterine pregnancy or ectopic pregnancy was diagnosed. Dilation and curettage yielded secretory endometrium without products of conception. The serum β-hCG remained elevated despite the dilation and curettage and 3 courses of methotrexate. Her serum was forwarded to a reference laboratory, which reported a β-hCG of less than 3.0 mIU/mL on the same sample that the authors' laboratory had measured at 21.1 mIU/mL. Urine β-hCG was also negative.

Case 2.—Woman, 31, nulliparous, was seen at 6 weeks gestation for vaginal bleeding. Quantitative β-hCG measured 4932 mIU/mL. US showed a single intrauterine pregnancy with cardiac activity. The β-hCG did not rise appropriately, and the patient passed tissue containing decidua without products of conception. The β-hCG initially dropped, then reached a nadir of 56 mIU/mL; it rose again to 105 mIU/mL. The patient denied symptoms of pregnancy. She reported normal menses several weeks after passing tissue. The serum β-hCG remained elevated. The urine and reference laboratory serum assay for β-hCG tested negative.

Conclusion.—These 2 case reports are a reminder that, although laboratory evaluation of β-hCG is usually reliable, it is not perfect. Unnecessary therapy was based on a false elevation of β-hCG in both cases.

▶ As this article was published, I received a letter from the diagnostics division of Abbott Laboratories stating that the intended use of their hCG assay "is the quantitative or qualitative determination of human chorionic gonadotropin in human serum and plasma for the early detection of pregnancy." They further stated: "These assays should not be used to diagnose any condition unrelated to pregnancy." These were exculpatory qualifiers not prominently mentioned in any of their advertising. Perhaps the most important use of an hCG test is making the diagnosis of abnormal gestation, be it ectopic pregnancy or an anembryonic gestation as seen in the gestational trophoblastic diseases. As discussed in the previous edition of the YEAR BOOK, this article reminds us that no laboratory test is perfect and no morbid intervention, such as chemotherapy or sterilizing surgery, should be applied based on a laboratory test alone.[1] A false positive hCG should be suspected whenever hCG levels are not confirmed by clinical findings. Such laboratory results can be easily confirmed or disproved with the use of alternative assays, serial dilution of the specimen, or measurements for urinary hCG levels.

D. S. Miller, MD

Reference

1. 2001 YEAR BOOK OF OBSTETRICS, GYNECOLOGY, AND WOMEN'S HEALTH, pp 477.

Corpus Uteri

Pyometra: What Is Its Clinical Significance?
Chan LY, Lau TK, Wong SF, et al (Chinese Univ of Hong Kong; Princess Margaret Hosp, Shatin, Hong Kong)
J Reprod Med 46:952-956, 2001   20–3

Introduction.—Most incidents of pyometra are linked to malignant lesions of the genital tract or to previous radiotherapy. New data concerning pyometra have been sparse since the 1960s. The clinical significance of pyometra, particularly its relationship with malignant diseases, was examined retrospectively, along with the rate of spontaneous perforation and the risk of recurrent disease.

Methods.—The medical records of all patients admitted to 2 large regional hospitals in Hong Kong, China, between January 1993 and December 1999 with a diagnosis of pyometra were reviewed. Data were gathered concerning patient age, other demographic characteristics, presenting symptoms, methods of treatment, and recurrent disease.

Results.—There were 29 cases of pyometra out of a total of 76,118 gynecologic admissions (0.038%) during the evaluation period. Medical records were not available for 2 cases. Mean patient age was 72.7 years (range, 22-92 years). Three women were nulliparous, and all but 1 were postmenopausal. Pyometra in the premenopausal woman was secondary to uterus didelphys with a blind hemivagina. Six cases (22%) were associated with malignant disease, 1 was associated with genital tract abnormality, and 20 (74%) were idiopathic. Patients with idiopathic pyometra tended to be older and had a higher rate of concurrent medical conditions. Five women (18%) had spontaneous perforation. A preoperative diagnosis of pyometra was correct in 17 of 22 patients without spontaneous perforation (77%). Most women were treated with dilatation of the cervix and drainage. Nine patients (33%) had persistent or recurrent pyometra; 3 had no symptoms.

Conclusion.—Pyometra is a rare condition. It involves a considerable rate of associated malignancy and a risk of spontaneous perforation that is higher than previously believed. Dilatation and drainage is the treatment of choice. Regular monitoring after initial treatment is recommended to identify persistent and recurrent disease.

▶ Pyometra is an uncommon manifestation of cervical stenosis. The overmanagement of pyometra is probably because of the perception that it is strongly associated with malignant disease. In this review of 27 cases, 4 cases were associated with an intercurrent cancer; 2 more were associated with postradiation stenosis. Cervical dilation and drainage is appropriate management for this condition along with postdilation monitoring for recurrence, which most commonly occurs in the first year after initial drainage. Spontaneous perforation was much more likely to be associated with a new diagnosis of cervical cancer or a late finding after previous irradiation for the treatment of cervical cancer.

R. D. Arias, MD

Is Pelvic Organ Prolapse a Cause of Pelvic or Low Back Pain?
Heit M, Culligan P, Rosenquist C, et al (Univ of Louisville, Ky; Rush Presbyterian-St Luke's Med Ctr, Chicago)
Obstet Gynecol 99:23-28, 2002   20–4

Background.—Many references cite pelvic organ prolapse as a possible cause of pelvic pain. However, little empiric evidence exists for including prolapse as part of a workup for pelvic or low back pain. Whether pelvic organ prolapse is associated with pelvic or low back pain was investigated in a cross-sectional study.

Methods.—The study included 152 consecutive patients (mean age, 62 years) with symptoms of pelvic organ prolapse. Each patient rated her level of pelvic or low back pain on separate 6-point "visual faces" scales (0 = happy face, indicating no pain, 5 = crying face, indicating worst pain). Prolapse severity was assessed by the following 3 methods: (1) a pelvic organ prolapse quantification system was used to compare the position of 6 points along the vagina in relation to the hymenal ring during strain; (2) the leading edge of the prolapse beyond the introitus during strain was measured; and (3) dynamic cystoproctography was performed to determine which pelvic organ descended maximally. Data were analyzed to determine any linear or nonlinear associations between prolapse severity and pain.

Results.—No significant associations were found between the severity of pelvic organ prolapse and pelvic pain. A significant linear relationship was noted between the descent of the leading edge of prolapse with low back pain, in that patients with greater descent reported less pain ($r = .176$, $P = .034$). A nonlinear relationship was noted between bladder descent during dynamic cystoproctography and low back pain ($P = .037$). However, after controlling for possible confounders (age, vaginal parity, body mass index, presence of uterus or ovaries, prior continence surgery, and prior prolapse surgery), neither of these associations remained significant. Both age ($P = .021$) and prior prolapse surgery ($P = .035$) were significantly related to low back pain.

Conclusions.—Many factors can cause pelvic or low back pain; pelvic organ prolapse does not appear to be 1 of them. Thus, clinicians should not counsel a patient that reconstructive pelvic surgery will relieve pelvic or low back pain, and other causes for the pain should be sought.

▶ Chronic pelvic pain is a nonspecific symptom for which causes can be elusive. It does not appear from this study that pelvic organ prolapse distinguishes those women more likely to report pelvic pain. The degree to which patients with both pelvic organ prolapse and pelvic pain can expect reduction in their pain from surgery has yet to be established. Therefore, in the preoperative counseling of women complaining of pelvic/lower back pain, it should be clear that pain relief cannot be reliably expected from surgical correction of prolapse.

R. D. Arias, MD

21 Cervix

Screening

Randomized Clinical Trial of PCR-Determined Human Papillomavirus Detection Methods: Self-Sampling Versus Clinician-Directed–Biologic Concordance and Women's Preferences

Harper DM, Noll WW, Belloni DR, et al (Dartmouth Med School, Hanover, NH)
Am J Obstet Gynecol 186:365-373, 2002   21–1

Introduction.—For many women, clinician-directed speculum screening for human papillomavirus (HPV) is not acceptable. Prior self-sampling techniques for HPV detection have included cervicovaginal lavage, cytobrushes, Dacron swabs, and tampons. The acceptability of these self-sampling approaches has not been thoroughly examined and was thus evaluated in 103 women who required a colposcopy.

Methods.—All of the women participated in 5 HPV screens: clinician-directed ectocervical, clinician-directed endocervical, 1 self-sampled Dacron swab, a second self-sampled Dacron swab, and a self-sampled tampon. The gold standard for high-risk HPV identification was ascertained as any presence of high-risk HPV in the composite of all sampling techniques. Agreement between clinician-directed and self-sampling was examined. Clinicians were blinded to the order of the sampling. After sampling, participants were asked to complete an acceptability questionnaire before leaving the clinic.

Results.—All self-directed samplings were comparable to clinician sampling for all cervical intraepithelial neoplasia disease states. High-risk HPV was identified by self-sampling and clinician-directed methods in 83% of women with cervical intraepithelial neoplasia, grade 2/3. The 2 sequential swabs had a trend toward better identification of high-risk types of HPV versus other approaches in women with normal histologic factors ($P = .736$). Ninety-four percent of the women indicated that they would accept self-sampling for their yearly cervical screen.

Conclusion.—Self-sampling is comparable to clinician sampling in the identification of high-risk HPV and is acceptable to women as a yearly screen.

▶ Most women who develop cervical cancer have not been screened. It is the hypothesis of some that screening in developing and developed countries could be improved if there were a patient-controlled method of identifying women at risk of cervical cancer. This study showed that patient-collected sampling done with tampons was as good as clinician-directed sampling for detecting high-risk HPV types and that this method was very acceptable to patients. It remains to be seen in a population-based study whether self-sampling will reach more women than clinician-directed sampling, much less decrease the incidence of cervical cancer.

D. S. Miller, MD

Does Liquid-Based Technology Really Improve Detection of Cervical Neoplasia? A Prospective, Randomized Trial Comparing the ThinPrep Pap Test With the Conventional Pap Test, Including Follow-up of HSIL Cases
Obwegeser JH, Brack S (Cytology Lab of Jörg H Obwegeser, Zurich, Switzerland)
Acta Cytol 45:709-714, 2001   21–2

Background.—The detection of precursors to cervical cancer has reportedly been improved using liquid-based preparation technologies rather than conventional technique. However, no randomized evaluation of the 2 techniques was conducted. The sensitivity, specificity, and specimen adequacy of the ThinPrep Pap Test (TP) were assessed with respect to the conventional Pap smear (CV).

Methods.—The patients chosen were at low risk and were randomly placed in either the TP group (997 patients) or the CV group (1002 patients). All mucus and debris was removed from the surface of the cervix using a cellulose swab before the TP and CV groups had Pap smears obtained.

Results.—The detection of low-grade squamous intraepithelial lesions (LSIL), of high-grade squamous intraepithelial lesions (HSIL), of atypical squamous cells of undetermined significance/atypical glandular cells of undetermined significance (ASCUS/AGUS), of LSIL+ (which is cervical intraepithelial neoplasm [CIN] 2 or more severe), and of ASCUS/AGUS+ (which includes all abnormal cells) was essentially the same regardless of method (Table 1). The TP group had a significantly higher specimen adequacy finding than the CV group (5.5% vs 2.5%). Scant cellularity resulted in an unsatisfactory rate in the TP group of 1.4%; none was noted in the CV group. Ninety-one percent of the TP group and 100% of the CV group had cytologic diagnoses of HSIL that correlated with the available diagnosis on histology.

Conclusions.—Because the methods themselves do not show significant differences in their ability to detect disease, a better sampling technique may be responsible for the improved accuracy with liquid-based preparations. The act of removing all mucus and cellular debris from the cervical surface before sampling and the use of a proper sampling device may account for the difference in outcome, meaning that the less expensive conventional technique can achieve results comparable to those of the liquid-based method.

TABLE 1.—Concurrent Results: TP vs. CV

Results	CV (1,002 Patients)		TP (997 Patients)		P Value
	n	%	n	%	
WNL	931	92.9	924	92.7	NS
LSIL	37	3.7	47	4.7	NS
HSIL	19	1.8	16	1.6	NS
Carcinoma	1	0.1	0	0.0	NS
ASCUS/AGUS	14	1.4	10	1.0	NS
LSIL +		5.6		6.3	NS
ASCUS/AGUS +		7.0		7.3	NS
SBLB	25	2.5	55	5.5	<.001
US	0	0	14	1.4	<.001

Abbreviations: WNL, Within normal limits; *LSIL,* mild dysplasia, including human papilloma virus changes; *HSIL,* cervical intraepithelial neoplasm (CIN) 2 and CIN 3 and CIS; *US,* unsatisfactory; *LSIL +* CIN 1 and more severe; *ASCUS/AGUS+,* all abnormal cells.
(Courtesy of Obwegeser JH, Brack S: Does liquid-based technology really improve detection of cervical neoplasia? A prospective, randomized trial comparing the ThinPrep Pap Test with the conventional Pap test, including follow-up of HSIL cases. *Acta Cytol* 45:709-714, 2001.)

▶ The liquid-based cervical cytology method known as ThinPrep (Cytyc Corp, Boxborough, Massachusetts) has been approved by the U.S. Food and Drug Administration to claim a higher detection rate for high-grade as well as low-grade squamous intraepithelial lesion cases. The data supporting this indication were generated by 2 types of studies. The first were "split sample" in which the specimen was placed on a conventional slide and then the residual was placed in the ThinPrep Media. This was then followed by "direct to vial" trials where laboratories compared their historical data on conventional slides with their experience after adopting ThinPrep in what were presumed to be similar populations. Roughly half the cervical cytology done in the United States uses the ThinPrep technology. This is the first study I know of that appears to be a randomized controlled trial comparing the 2 methods. Interestingly, no significant difference was seen. The authors attribute this to cleaning of the cervix before specimen collection with the szalay spatula. We await with interest further trials evaluating this technological advance.

D. S. Miller, MD

ASCUS

Cervicography for Triage of Women With Mildly Abnormal Cervical Cytology Results
Ferris DG, for the ALTS Group (Med College of Georgia, Augusta; Natl Cancer Inst, Bethesda, Md)
Am J Obstet Gynecol 185:939-943, 2001   21–3

Background.—Cervicography is the standardized photography of the cervix after 5% acetic acid application. A specialized 35-mm camera is used, and the images are interpreted by experts. Quality control measures are provided by a qualified evaluator. The sensitivity and specificity of cervicography in detecting cervical cancer precursor lesions in women were determined.

Methods.—Cervigrams were obtained from 3134 women participating in the National Cancer Institute's multicenter study of atypical squamous cells of undetermined significance (ASCUS) and low-grade squamous intraepithelial lesion (LSIL) triage study (ALTS). All women undergoing cervicography had a referral Papanicolaou smear diagnosis of ASCUS or LSIL. Cervigram and cervical histologic findings were compared by using cervical intraepithelial neoplasia (CIN) 2 and CIN 3 disease end points.

Findings.—Four hundred forty-four women had histologic findings of CIN 2 or more, and 222 had CIN 3. When a threshold of greater than or equal to atypical was used, cervicography interpretation had a sensitivity of 79%, a specificity of 61%, and positive and negative predictive values of 13% and 97%, respectively, for identifying CIN 3 or greater. Cervicography had a sensitivity and specificity of 81% and 56%, respectively, for detecting CIN in women younger than 35 years, compared with 57% and 82%, respectively, in women aged 35 years or older.

Conclusions.—Cervicography was moderately good at identifying CIN 2 or 3 in women with ASCUS and LSIL Papanicolaou smear findings. The sensitivity of cervicography was higher in younger women.

▶ Cervicography, which is a photographic record of the cervix after the application of 5% acetic acid, has been touted as a screening test for cervical cancer. The authors report preliminary data from the ALTS trial on the triage of LSIL and ASCUS Pap smears by cervicography. Unfortunately, a statistical comparison with repeat Pap smear or human papillomavirus (HPV) testing was not reported. But, it does appear that cervicography is slightly less helpful than a repeat Pap smear or HPV testing in the triage of minimally abnormal Pap smears.[1,2]

D. S. Miller, MD

References

1. Koutsky LA: Human papillomavirus testing for triage of women with cytologic evidence of low-grade squamous intraepithelial lesions: Baseline data from a randomized trial. *J Natl Cancer Inst* 92:397-402, 2000.
2. Solomon D, for the ALTS Group: Comparison of three management strategies for patients with atypical squamous cells of undetermined significance: Baseline results from a randomized trial. *J Natl Cancer Inst* 93:293-299, 2001.

Management of Women With Atypical Papanicolaou Tests of Undetermined Significance by Board-Certified Gynecologists: Discrepancies With Published Guidelines
Smith-McCune K, Mancuso V, Contant T, et al (Univ of California, San Francisco)
Am J Obstet Gynecol 185:551-556, 2001   21–4

Background.—The Bethesda System, introduced in 1988 to simplify the classification of Papanicolaou test results and establish uniform reporting and management guidelines, created 2 categories of atypia: atypical glandular cells of undetermined significance (AGUS) and atypical squamous cells of undetermined significance (ASCUS). The extent to which clinicians agree on the management of ASCUS and AGUS was investigated.

Methods.—A survey was mailed to a random sample of 491 fellows of the American College of Obstetricians and Gynecologists. The response rate was 50.6%.

Findings.—Twenty-three percent of the 241 respondents said they would perform colposcopy for first-time ASCUS, and 24.4% would repeat the Papanicolaou test within 3 months. For recurrent ASCUS, 88.7% reported that they would follow recommendations to manage with colposcopy. In the management of AGUS, 23% said they would repeat the Papanicolaou test. Only 23% would manage the condition appropriately. For recurrent AGUS, only 25% said they would perform surgical excision.

Conclusions.—Physicians appear to undermanage AGUS and overmanage ASCUS. In the current study, 47.4% of respondents would have managed ASCUS aggressively. Additional physician education is needed.

▶ The overmanagement of ASCUS Pap smears revealed in this survey of board-certified gynecologists is perhaps understandable given the variety of patient preferences and payment methods in this country. The underevaluation of AGUS by a majority of respondents is, however, both remarkable and disturbing. Perhaps the similarity in nomenclature has falsely led physicians to believe that they have similar clinical significance. Perhaps, too, the recent publication of the revised Bethesda treatment recommendations will provide clarification.[1]

R. D. Arias, MD

Reference

1. Wright TC, Cox JT, Massad LS, et al: 2001 consensus guidelines for the management of women with cervical cytological abnormalities. *JAMA* 287:2120-2129, 2002.

Empiric Vaginal Metronidazole in the Management of the ASCUS Papanicolaou Smear: A Randomized Controlled Trial

Connor JP, Elam G, Goldberg JM (Univ of Illinois, Chicago)
Obstet Gynecol 99:183-187, 2002   21–5

Introduction.—Since introduction of the Bethesda System for Papanicolaou smear reporting, the optimal management of the atypical squamous cells of undetermined significance (ASCUS) is uncertain. Empiric vaginal metronidazole treatment of ASCUS on Papanicolaou smear was assessed in a prospective, double-masked, randomized trial.

Methods.—Patients were randomly assigned to treatment with either vaginal metronidazole 37.5 mg twice daily or placebo gel twice daily for 5 days. The major end point was normalization of repeated Papanicolaou smear at 3 months. Regression to normal between the 2 groups was compared by means of χ^2 analysis. Power analysis required 45 women per study arm to demonstrate a 50% improvement in regression to normal among metronidazole-treated women at $\alpha = 0.05$ and 80% power.

Results.—Of 106 tubes of gel that were dispersed, 54 were from the metronidazole group and 52 were from the placebo group. Eighty-four women (79%) returned for repeated cytologic examination at a mean of 6.5 months. Overall, 50 women (60%) had normal findings on repeated cytologic evaluation. Thirty-four patients had repeated ASCUS and 11 had squamous intraepithelial lesions (SIL) on repeated cytologic examinations. Regression to normal was observed in 22 metronidazole-treated women (54%) and 28 controls (65%). The number of repeated ASCUS (31% vs 25%) or SIL (15% vs 10%) were similar for both groups.

Conclusion.—Empiric vaginal metronidazole does not improve the management of women with ASCUS on Papanicolaou smear and is not recommended.

▶ Vaginal metronidazole is an effective treatment for bacterial vaginosis. Laboratory and clinical data have linked anaerobic bacterial vaginitis with cervical dysplasia. Many ASCUS Pap smears are attributed to reactive or inflammatory changes in the cervical epithelium. Technologically elaborate evaluation and treatment algorithms have been proposed.[1] This straightforward randomized trial evaluated a potentially low-tech solution to the problem. Fortunately, most patients cleared their ASCUS Pap smear. Unfortunately, vaginal metronidazole was no better than placebo in clearing ASCUS Pap smears.

D. S. Miller, MD

Reference

1. Wright TC, Cox JT, Massad LS, et al: 2001 Consensus Guidelines for the Management of Women with Cervical Cytological Abnormalities. *JAMA* 287:2120-2129, 2002.

The Bethesda System

The 2001 Bethesda System: Terminology for Reporting Results of Cervical Cytology
Solomon D, for the Forum Group Members and the Bethesda 2001 Workshop (Natl Cancer Inst, Bethesda, Md; et al)
JAMA 287:2114-2119, 2002   21–6

Background.—In 2001, the Bethesda Workshop was convened to assess and update the 1991 terminology for reporting the findings of cervical cytology. A new approach was developed to broaden participation in the consensus process. This process and the conclusions reached are described.

Methods and Findings.—The National Cancer Institute and 44 professional societies sponsored the Bethesda 2001 Workshop. More than 400 cytopathologists, cytotechnologists, histopathologists, family practitioners, gynecologists, public health physicians, epidemiologists, patient advocates, and attorneys from more than 20 countries participated. Recommendations were based on a literature review, expert opinion, and input from an Internet bulletin board. The year-long iterative review process involved an Internet bulletin board discussion of issues and drafts of recommendations. The workshop's final draft of recommendations was posted for a last round of critical review before the terminology was finalized.

Conclusions.—The Bethesda 2001 Workshop developed management guidelines for women with abnormal cytology results by using a collaborative process. This collaborative and integrated development of terminology and management guidelines may be expected to result in more uniform, evidence-based care of women with cervical abnormalities.

▶ Despite the stunning success of cervical cytology screening in decreasing the incidence of and number of deaths caused by cervical cancer over the last 50 years in North American and other developed countries, it was believed by some that there was a problem with cervical cytology nomenclature. In 1988, The National Cancer Institute convened a group of cytologists and a few gynecologists who proposed the Bethesda system, a previously untested, much less validated, classification system.[1] There is no evidence that I am aware of that the Bethesda system has resulted in a cancer prevented or a life saved. However, it did bring relative uniformity to cervical cytology result reporting.

Some improvements appear to have been made. The previously vague category of "benign cellular changes" should now be correctly classified as negative. The most significant change is to the former category of atypical squamous cells of uncertain significance (ASCUS). That category is now termed atypical squamous cells—of uncertain significance (ASC-US) or atypical squamous cells—cannot exclude a high-grade lesion (ASC-H). I am concerned that this classification will be of dubious value because even the most expert cytologists recently and in the past have not been able to agree or reproducibly confirm the diagnosis of ASC.[2] Nonetheless, these recommendations have been adopted by most of our major gynecologic and pathologic organizations. Unlike a decade ago when the original Bethesda classification was instituted and management guidelines did not follow for another 4 years, this report is accompanied by an article with management guidelines.[3]

D. S. Miller, MD

References

1. National Cancer Institute Workshop: The 1988 Bethesda system for reporting cervical/vaginal cytologic diagnoses. *JAMA* 262:931-934, 1989.
2. Stoler MH, Schiffman M: Atypical squamous cells of undetermined significance-low-grade squamous intraepithelial lesion triage study (ALTS) group. *JAMA* 285:1500-1505, 2001.
3. Wright TC, Cox JT, Massad LS, et al: 2001 consensus guidelines for the management of women with cervical cytological abnormalities. *JAMA* 287:2120-2129, 2002.

2001 Consensus Guidelines for the Management of Women With Cervical Cytological Abnormalities

Wright TC Jr, for the 2001 ASCCP-Sponsored Consensus Conference (Columbia Univ, New York; et al)

JAMA 287:2120-2129, 2002   21–7

Background.—About 7% of the 50 million women undergoing Papanicolaou testing annually in the United States are diagnosed as having a cytologic abnormality. The current study provides evidence-based consensus guidelines for the management of women with cervical cytologic abnormalities and cervical cancer precursors.

Methods.—One hundred twenty-one experts in diagnosing and managing cervical cancer precursors participated in a consensus conference sponsored by the American Society for Colposcopy and Cervical Pathology (ASCCP). Participants represented 29 professional organizations, federal agencies, and national and international health organizations. The guidelines were developed through a multistep process.

Guidelines.—The management of atypical squamous cells (ASC) relies on whether the Papanicolaou test is subclassified as "of undetermined significance" (ASCUS) or as "cannot exclude high-grade squamous intraepithelial lesion" (ASC-H). The management of ASCUS includes a program of 2 repeat cytology tests, immediate colposcopy, or DNA testing for high-risk types of human papillomavirus. Testing for human papillomavirus DNA is preferred when liquid-based cytology is used for screening. Most women with ASC-H, low-grade or high-grade squamous intraepithelial lesion, and atypical glandular cells need to be referred for immediate colposcopic assessment.

Conclusions.—The methods and recommendations of the ASCCP Consensus Conference in Bethesda were reported. The guidelines were established only after extensive discussion and revision.

▶ When the first Bethesda classification was instituted in 1988, clinicians were left with little guidance as to the best management for the categories described, especially for that of ASCUS.[1] It was not until 1992 that a treatment recommendation conference was convened and another 2 years until its consensus was published.[2] Fortunately, this time concomitant management guidelines have been published with the new Bethesda system. The most significant change is that involving the category of ASC. It is now recommended that patients with ASCUS undergo human papillomavirus testing or a repeat Pap smear to differentiate those who are at risk for an occult high-grade lesion that should be evaluated by colposcopy (Table 2 in the original journal article). That HPV evaluation is most efficiently done by reflex testing of a liquid cytology sample. Thus, a diagnosis of ASCUS generates another test and gives rise to the concern that the number of cases diagnosed as ASCUS may increase. Those diagnosed as ASC-H are recommended to proceed straight to colposcopy. Further validation of these recommendations will be required to determine if any cancers will be prevented or lives saved by this new algorithm.

D. S. Miller, MD

References

1. National Cancer Institute Workshop. The 1988 Bethesda System for reporting cervical/vaginal cytologic diagnoses. *JAMA* 262:931-934, 1989.
2. Kurman RJ, Henson DE, Herbst AL, et al: Interim guidelines for management of abnormal cervical cytology. *JAMA* 271:1866-1869, 1994.

Treatment

Loop Diathermy Excision Compared With Cervical Laser Vaporisation for the Treatment of Intraepithelial Neoplasia: A Randomised Controlled Trial

Dey P, Gibbs A, Arnold DF, et al (Centre for Cancer Epidemiology, Manchester, England; Hope Hosp, Salford, England; Withington Hosp, West Didsbury, England)

Br J Obstet Gynaecol 109:381-385, 2002   21–8

Background.—In recent years, loop diathermy excision of the cervical transformation zone has replaced laser vaporization as the most commonly used outpatient treatment for cervical intraepithelial neoplasia. Loop diathermy excision is simple and quick, and allows a more precise histologic and topographic characterization of the cervical lesion. Because the transformation zone was excised and not simply destroyed, many clinicians believed

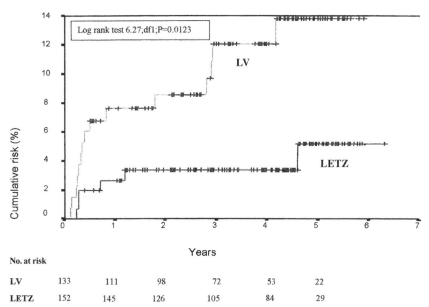

No. at risk

LV	133	111	98	72	53	22
LETZ	152	145	126	105	84	29

FIGURE 2.—Cumulative risk of a smear reported as moderate dyskaryosis or worse. *Abbreviations: LV,* Laser vaporization; *LETZ,* loop excision diathermy of the transformation zone. (Courtesy of Dey P, Gibbs A, Arnold DF, et al: Loop diathermy excision compared with cervical laser vaporisation for the treatment of intraepithelial neoplasia: A randomised controlled trial. *Br J Obstet Gynaecol* 109:381-385. Copyright 2002, with permission from Elsevier Science.)

that it was safe to examine and treat the patient in the same visit. There have been concerns expressed that the simplicity of loop diathermy excision of the transformation zone may result in the overtreatment of some women. In response, the National Health Service (United Kingdom) recommended that at least 90% of women treated at their initial visit should have histologic evidence of cervical intraepithelial neoplasia. Whether loop diathermy excision of the transformation zone and laser vaporization are equally effective in these patients was determined.

Methods.—In a randomized controlled trial, women referred for evaluation of cytologic abnormality and considered candidates for outpatient local destructive treatment were treated with loop diathermy excision of the transformation zone or laser vaporization. The main outcome measure was a smear reported as moderate dyskaryosis or worse after treatment.

Results.—Of the 289 women randomly assigned to treatment, 285 women had 1 or more smears after treatment. Women were more likely to have a smear reported as moderate dyskaryosis or worse after laser vaporization than after loop diathermy excision. The cumulative risk of a smear reported as moderate dyskaryosis or worse was 6.0% at 6 months and 12.1% at 3 years in patients who underwent laser vaporization, compared with 2.0% at 6 months and 3.3% at 3 years in patients who underwent loop diathermy excision of the transformation zone (Fig 2).

Conclusions.—Loop diathermy excision is more effective than laser vaporization in the treatment of cervical intraepithelial neoplasia.

▶ More than 20 years ago, carbon dioxide lasers were introduced and became accepted as standard treatment for the destruction of intraepithelial neoplasia even though they were technically cumbersome to maintain and operate. Even more rapidly in the 1990s, loop diathermy replaced laser as the preferred treatment, not because loop, LEEP, or LLETZ produced better results but because the equipment and certification required for use were much less cumbersome. This study supports that popular trend. With the advantage of longer follow-up than most of the prior trials, the authors found a small but significant benefit to loop excision of the transformation zone over laser vaporization.

D. S. Miller, MD

A Randomized, Double Blind, Phase III Trial Using Oral β-Carotene Supplementation for Women With High-Grade Cervical Intraepithelial Neoplasia

Keefe KA, Schell MJ, Brewer C, et al (Univ of California, Irvine; Brown Univ, Providence, RI; Univ of North Carolina, Chapel Hill; et al)
Cancer Epidemiol Biomarkers Prev 10:1029-1035, 2001   21–9

Background.—The primary mechanism of action of β-carotene has not been clearly defined. Its chemoprotective effect may be mediated through an effect on epithelial cell proliferation and differentiation. Also, β-carotene inhibits tumor cell proliferation by decreasing epidermal growth factor receptor concentrations on keratinocytes immortalized with human papillomavirus (HPV)-16. Recent randomized studies of β-carotene as a possible chemopreventive agent for cervical cancer have yielded mixed findings. The effect of β-carotene in the treatment of high-grade cervical intraepithelial neoplasia (CIN) was examined.

Methods.—A total of 124 women with CIN 2 or 3 lesions were enrolled in the 2-year, randomized, placebo-controlled study. The patients received 30 mg of β-carotene daily or placebo. All underwent HPV typing to determine whether lesion regression was associated with HPV. In addition, miconutrient levels were assessed to determine whether the concentrations predicted regression. Cytology and colposcopy were performed every 3 months. Cervical biopsies were done before and 6 and 24 months after treatment. Patients in whom CIN persisted or progressed were removed from the study. For various reasons, 21 women did not undergo randomization.

Findings.—Thirty-three of the 103 randomized women had lesion regression, 45 had persistent or progressive disease, and 25 were nonresponders. Overall, the regression rate, at 32%, was similar between groups after stratification for CIN grade. Among 99 women with HPV typing, 77% were HPV positive at enrollment and 23%, HPV negative. After HPV-positive lesions were stratified as indeterminate, low, or high risk, analysis showed that women with no HPV detected had the highest response rate (61%), followed by those with indeterminate and low-risk lesions (30%), and those with high-risk lesions (18%). Retinol concentration was associated negatively with CIN regression.

Conclusions.—β-Carotene supplementation was not associated with regression in women with high-grade, biopsy-proved cervical lesions. Regression was more likely to occur in women with biopsy-proved CIN 2 or 3 lesions but with no HPV in their cervical scarpings at study enrollment. A higher regression rate at 6 months was observed in women whose pretreatment retinol concentrations were lower.

▶ Epidemiologic studies have shown that diets deficient in fruits and vegetables or having a low intake of β-carotene are associated with an increased risk of cervical dysplasia. Other studies have shown that carotenes can interfere with the various steps of HPV oncogenesis. This study illustrates to us the peril of drawing clinical conclusions from epidemiologic studies. Factors that are involved in the development of a disease when later corrected do not result in cure of the already present disease. This study was a necessary step to which "nutritional" strategies should be required to take before they are promulgated on the public.

D. S. Miller, MD

22 Vulva and Vagina

Self-Reported Papanicolaou Smears and Hysterectomies Among Women in the United States
Saraiya M, Lee NC, Blackman D, et al (Ctrs for Disease Control and Prevention, Atlanta, Ga; Klemm Analysis Group, Atlanta, Ga)
Obstet Gynecol 98:269-278, 2001
22–1

Background.—The decline in incidence of and death from cervical cancer over the past 40 years is due primarily to the detection of early cancer and precancerous lesions by means of the Papanicolaou smear. However, concern has been growing that the Papanicolaou smear is often used inappropriately in certain populations of women. The United States Preventive Services has recommended that women who have had hysterectomies in which the cervix was removed should not be screened for cervical cancer with a Papanicolaou smear unless they have a history of cervical cancer or its precursors. The potential overuse of Papanicoloau smears among women who have undergone hysterectomy was evaluated.

Methods.—Two surveys of women 18 years of age or older—the Behavioral Risk Factor Surveillance System (1992-1997) and the National Health Interview Survey (1993-1994)—were analyzed, along with 1 survey of hospitals, the National Hospital Discharge Survey, 1980-1997. The number of women who underwent hysterectomy and who had a recent Papanicolaou smear (within 3 years) was examined. Included in this study was an evaluation of trends in the proportions and rates of hysterectomies by diagnoses and type of procedure that could require a Papanicolaou smear.

Results.—According to the Behavioral Risk Factor Surveillance System, about 21.2% of women in the United States have had a hysterectomy. Among these women, 78.3% also had a recent Papanicolaou smear. Among the women who reported not having had a hysterectomy, 82.1% had a recent Papanicolaou smear. These findings were similar to estimates from the National Health Interview Survey. According to the National Hospital Discharge Survey, 6.7% to 15.4% of women who had undergone a hysterectomy would require a subsequent Papanicolaou smear because they received a diagnosis related to cervical neoplasia or had undergone a supracervical hysterectomy. That test could be considered unnecessary in 10.6 to 11.6 million of the approximately 12.5 million women who had both a hysterectomy and a recent Papanicoloau smear.

Conclusions.—The continued use of the Papanicolaou smear in women without intact uteri may result in overuse of resources with minimal effects on the reduction of the incidence of and death from cervical cancer.

▶ Most vaginal cancers will occur in patients who have had hysterectomies (usually for cervical dysplasia) and will be found beneath the blades of the examining speculum. No effective screening test has yet been identified, including vaginal cytology screening.[1] This is probably because of the very low incidence of vaginal cancer. Yet, as this study reports, Pap smears continue to be performed in women without a cervix at a rate almost equal to that of women who have a cervix. Several of our learned organizations have recommended against this practice because it is clearly not cost effective.[2,3] Unfortunately, the implementation of this is problematic because many patients, and not a few practitioners, equate Pap smears with the annual exam and may not make this visit and miss the benefits of breast examination, mammography, bimanual pelvic examination, and rectal exam with evaluation for fecal occult blood.

D. S. Miller, MD

References

1. Pearce KF, Haefner HK, Sarwar SF, et al: Cytopathological findings on vaginal Papanicolaou smears after hysterectomy for benign gynecologic disease. *N Engl J Med* 335:1559, 1996.
2. United States Preventive Services Task Force. Guide to clinical preventive services. 2nd ed Baltimore: Williams & Wilkins, 1996.
3. American College of Obstetricians and Gynecologists. Routine cancer screening. ACOG committee opinion no 247. Washington DC: American College of Obstetricians and Gynecologists, 2000.

A Double-Blind Placebo-Controlled Study of ArginMax, a Nutritional Supplement for Enhancement of Female Sexual Function
Ito TY, Trant AS, Polan ML (Univ of Hawaii, Honolulu; Daily Wellness Company, Mountain View, Calif; Stanford Univ, Calif)
J Sex Marital Ther 27:541-549, 2001   22–2

Background.—The incidence of sexual dysfunction was recently reported to be greater in women than in men, at 43% and 31%, respectively. However, no effective pharmacotherapy for women is available. The efficacy of ArginMax, a nutritional supplement for enhancing female sexual function, was investigated.

Methods.—Seventy-seven women aged 21 years and older who wished to improve their sexual function were enrolled in the study. Thirty-four received ArginMax; 43 received placebo. Active treatment, ArginMax for Women, is a proprietary nutritional supplement composed of extracts of ginseng, ginkgo, and damiana as well as L-arginine, multivitamins, and minerals.

Findings.—After 4 weeks, satisfaction with overall sex life was improved in 73.5% of ArginMax recipients and only 37.2% of placebo recipients. Improvements were notable in sexual desire, vaginal dryness, frequency of sexual intercourse and orgasm, and clitoral sensation. There were no significant adverse effects.

Conclusions.—In this study, active treatment increased lubrication, clitoral sensitivity, frequency of orgasm, and sexual desire. Further research on ArginMax is warranted.

▶ There are few studies in the sexology literature that are double blind and placebo controlled. Thus, this study deserves some attention. ArginMax is a concoction purported to contain ginseng, ginkgo, damiana, arginine, multivitamins, and minerals. It is sold as a nutritional supplement and as such is not regulated by the Food and Drug Administration. Nonetheless, it was better than placebo for improving overall sex life. The postulated mechanism of this is vasodilation, although the active ingredient is not identified. This study is also a reminder to physicians of the frequent use by our patients of alternative therapies, some of which may not have the desired effect.[1]

D. S. Miller, MD

Reference

1. vonGruenigen VE, White LJ, Kirven MS, et al: A comparison of complementary and alternative medicine use by gynecology and gynecologic oncology patients. *Int J Gynecol Cancer* 11:205-209, 2001.

Vulvar Vestibulitis Syndrome: Reliability of Diagnosis and Evaluation of Current Diagnostic Criteria
Bergeron S, Binik YM, Khalifé S, et al (McGill Univ, Montreal; Cornell Univ, New York)
Obstet Gynecol 98:45-51, 2001   22–3

Introduction.—Diagnostic criteria for vulvar vestibulitis as defined by Friedrich includes (1) severe pain on vestibular touch or attempted vaginal entry, (2) tenderness to pressure localized within the vulvar vestibule, and (3) physical findings confined to vestibular erythema of various degrees. It has not been determined whether Friedrich's criteria are sufficient to differentiate vulvar vestibulitis from other vulvar and coital pain syndromes. The reliability of the diagnosis of vestibulitis as defined by Friedrich was examined, along with the usefulness of Friedrich's criteria in the diagnostic process.

Methods.—One hundred forty-six women with dyspareunia had 2 sets of gynecologic examinations involving vulvar pain ratings. They participated in structured interviews and completed the McGill-Melzach Pain Questionnaire.

Results.—Kappa values for the vulvar vestibulitis diagnosis ranged from 0.66 to 0.68 for interrater agreement. They ranged from 0.49 to 0.54 for test-retest reliability. The mean vestibular pain ratings ranged from 2.45 at the 12 o'clock site to 7.58 at the 9-12 o'clock site. There was a significant correlation between gynecologists for ratings at sites. Pain in the labia majora and labia minora was minimal for both evaluation methods (mean participant pain rating ranged from 0 to 1.49). Gynecologists' erythema ratings were not significantly correlated with regard to either interrater agreement or test-retest reliability. Of the 3 criteria defined by Friedrich, only tenderness to pressure within the vulvar vestibule differentiated patients with dyspareunia with and without vulvar vestibulitis. Regarding coital pain, 88.1% of the women with vulvar vestibulitis chose adjectives from the McGill-Melzach Pain Questionnaire that described a thermal quality and 86.6% chose adjectives that described an incisive pressure sensation.

Conclusion.—Vulvar vestibulitis can be reliably diagnosed in women with dyspareunia. Pain is limited to the vulvar vestibule and can be rated and described in a consistent manner by these women. Erythema does not seem to be useful as a diagnostic criterion.

▶ One of the challenges in the emerging field of vulvology is developing reproducible diagnoses so that treatment results from various centers can be compared and evaluated. Dr Friedrich attempted to contribute to this by describing the vulvar vestibulitis syndrome in 1987.[1] This study is 1 of the few attempts to validate the diagnostic criteria of severe vulvar pain on vestibular touch or attempted vaginal entry, tenderness to pressure localized within the vulvar vestibule, and vestibular erythema. Tenderness to pressure within the vulvar vestibule best differentiated dyspareunia patients with and without vulvar vestibulitis based on the examination of separate experienced gynecologists.

D. S. Miller, MD

Reference

1. Friedrich EG: Vulvar vestibulitis syndrome. *J Reprod Med* 32:110, 1987.

Vulvar Intraepithelial Neoplasia Treated With Cavitational Ultrasonic Surgical Aspiration
Miller BE (Wake Forest Univ, Winston-Salem, NC)
Gynecol Oncol 85:114-118, 2002   22–4

Background.—The incidence of vulvar intraepithelial neoplasia (VIN) has been increasing with that of cervical and vaginal intraepithelial neoplasia. The cavitron ultrasonic surgical aspirator (CUSA) combines the advantages of laser removal of the superficial dermal layers without scarring and those of resection with collection of a pathologic specimen. The value of CUSA in the treatment of VIN was investigated.

Methods.—Thirty-seven patients with VIN underwent CUSA treatment between 1992 and 1998. The median patient age at diagnosis was 40 years. Eleven had received previous treatment for VIN. Diagnosis was established by inspection before and after ascitic acid application, colposcopy, and multiple biopsies. Twenty-two percent of the patients had VIN II; 78% had VIN

III. Two or more quadrants of the vulva were involved in 43% of patients and 3 of 4 in 33%. All lesions with a 1-cm margin were removed with CUSA under anesthesia.

Findings.—Healing was complete in 4 to 6 weeks. No scarring developed. The only complication was 1 hospital admission for pain control. Final pathologic examination verified preoperative diagnostic grade in 65% of the patients. In 11%, dysplasia was upgraded. Three patients with widespread disease needed a second treatment. Mean follow-up was 33 months. Recurrences developed in 35% of the patients after a median 16 months. Recurrences were significantly more frequent when VIN involved hair-bearing tissue.

Conclusions.—Treatment with CUSA can be effective for VIN in the non–hair-bearing areas of the vulva. Careful patient selection is essential. Invasive disease must be excluded, and excisional therapy is the preferred treatment when there is an ulceration or mass.

▶ CUSA conjures up visions of the Memorex tape commercial with Ella Fitzgerald's voice shattering a champagne glass. Such are not the physics of this device. Tissue is not obliterated by ultrasonic sound waves. In fact, it is a surgical jackhammer. Tissue is pulverized by an oscillating cylinder vibrating at a very high frequency tuned to pulverize tissue with a high water content, such as epithelium or tumor, and relatively spare that with a high collagen content, such as dermis, vessels, ducts, and nerves. Thus, it can be used to remove abnormal epidermis and spare the dermis, making it quite suitable for the destructive treatment of VIN or even vaginal intraepithelial neoplasm. This study also reminds us of the high recurrence rate typical of series in this disease reporting more than short-term follow-up. Two confounding factors for outcome of VIN treatment found in our practice—smoking and HIV—but not discussed in this article appear to have a significant impact on prognosis. We have modified our approach to VIN to that of treating a chronic disease that is unlikely to be successfully resolved unless the patient stops smoking or has her HIV under control.

D. S. Miller, MD

23 Operative Gynecology

Adnexa

Ovarian and Adnexal Torsion: Spectrum of Sonographic Findings With Pathologic Correlation
Albayram F, Hamper UM (Johns Hopkins Univ, Baltimore, Md)
J Ultrasound Med 20:1083-1089, 2001   23–1

Background.—Diagnosing adnexal torsion is challenging. The range of gray scale and color Doppler sonographic findings of ovarian and adnexal torsion were studied.

Methods.—Fifteen patients with surgically confirmed ovarian or adnexal torsion who underwent sonographic examination before surgery were included. All sonograms were analyzed retrospectively.

Findings.—Gray scale abnormalities included complex masses in 73% of the patients, cystic masses in 20%, and a solid mass in 7%. Eighty-seven percent had cul-de-sac fluid. Adnexal neoplasms were seen in 27% of the patients on pathologic assessment. Doppler findings were abnormal in 93% of the patients and normal in 7%. Abnormal findings included an absence of arterial and venous flow in 40% of patients, reduced venous flow with no arterial flow in 33%, decreased venous and arterial flow in 13%, and reduced arterial flow with no venous flow in 7%. Eighty-seven percent had small amounts of cul-de-sac fluid.

Conclusions.—The diagnosis of ovarian and adnexal torsion cannot be based only on the absence or presence of flow on color Doppler sonography because these findings do not exclude the diagnosis of adnexal torsion. Comparing the morphologic appearance and flow patterns of the contralateral ovary is helpful in establishing diagnosis.

▶ Although abnormalities of arterial and venous ovarian blood flow were seen in the majority of women with adnexal torsion, a wide variety of findings were noted in this retrospective evaluation of 15 cases. No single blood flow pattern was characteristic of torsion. Indeed, 1 case appeared to have normal flow studies. The mere presence of blood flow does little to rule out adnexal torsion. The presence of acute pelvic pain and an enlarged adnexa should raise suspicion of the diagnosis; the additional findings of abnormal color Doppler flow and cul-de-sac fluid should hasten surgical intervention, but the mere presence of blood flow should not unduly delay surgery if ovarian preservation is important.

R. D. Arias, MD

Pregnancy Rates Following Fimbriectomy Reversal Via Neosalpingostomy: A 10-Year Retrospective Analysis

Tourgeman DE, Bhaumik M, Cooke GC, et al (Univ of Southern California, Los Angeles)

Fertil Steril 76:1041-1044, 2001   23–2

Background.—While it is not recommended that women have reconstructive surgery for all causes of tubal infertility, the reversal of tubal sterilization procedures has been done with substantial success. Fecundability and cumulative pregnancy rate determinations were made after fimbriectomy reversal. Factors influencing the outcome of fimbriectomy reversal were noted.

Methods.—Fimbriectomy reversal was performed in 41 women (mean age, 33.8 years) who had either unilateral or bilateral neosalpingostomies. Three months after the procedure, medical charts, radiologic results, and patient interviews were assessed for the following: time from fimbriectomy sterilization to reversal, laparoscopy or laparotomy for reversal, unilateral or bilateral neosalpingostomies, Bruhat or suture technique for the neosalpingostomy, tubal length, results of the postoperative hysterosalpingogram, the use of ovulation induction agents after surgery, the length of follow-up, and the outcome of pregnancy.

Results.—The mean gravidity was 3.1 and the mean parity 3.0. A mean of 11.5 years elapsed between the sterilization and reversal procedures. Six women conceived at least once. Higher pregnancy rates accompanied laparotomy than laparoscopy, but the difference was not statistically significant. No statistically significant differences in success accompanied unilateral versus bilateral neosalpingostomy or use of the Bruhat versus the suture technique. Of those who conceived, the mean tubal length was 8.0 cm; of those who did not conceive, it was 6.7 cm. Women who conceived had at least 1 tube that was a minimum of 7 cm in length; only 18 of those not conceiving had a tube of this length.

Twenty-six women were given clomiphene citrate to induce ovulation and 1 conceived, whereas 5 of those not receiving clomiphene citrate conceived. Considering those women who had at least 1 tube measuring over 7 cm, the pregnancy rate for spontaneously ovulatory women was 45%. The monthly fecundability rate was .0097, which translated to a cumulative conception rate of 9.76% after 1 year, 14.8% after 2 years, 20.9% after 3 years, 26.5% after 4 years, and 31.2% after 5 years. None of the women conceived more than 5 years after the fimbriectomy reversal.

Conclusion.—The best candidates for fimbriectomy reversal are spontaneously ovulatory and have a tubal length exceeding 7 cm. The monthly fecundability and cumulative pregnancy rates are low in women who do not meet these criteria. These women should be counseled to consider in vitro fertilization as the most efficient way to achieve conception.

▶ The place for tubal reconstructive surgery is becoming less obvious in light of the enhanced success with assisted reproductive technologies. Although tubal sterilization is intended to be permanent, a percentage of patients desire surgical reversal. Fimbriectomy by the Kroener method, however, is thought to have the lowest chance of reversal success.

This article provides an excellent review of the literature to date for fimbriectomy reversal success. This retrospective study is the largest series in the literature and demonstrates a 1% monthly fecundability with a cumulative conception rate of 31% after 5 years. It also shows that the pregnancy rate for a spontaneously ovulatory patient with at least 1 fallopian tube measuring more than 7 cm after neosalpingostomy is 45%. Therefore, prudent selection and counseling is warranted in patients who have undergone fimbriectomy. But for the appropriate candidate, fimbriectomy reversal is a viable option.

R. D. Arias, MD

Prophylactic Methotrexate After Linear Salpingostomy: A Decision Analysis
Gracia CR, Brown HA, Barnhart KT (Univ of Pennsylvania, Philadelphia; Yale Univ, New Haven, Conn)
Fertil Steril 76:1191-1195, 2001   23–3

Introduction.—Persistent ectopic pregnancy after linear salpingostomy occurs in 3% to 20% of patients. There is no effective way to predict when persistent ectopic pregnancy will develop. Two strategies for managing patients after linear salpingostomy were examined in the treatment of tubal pregnancy.

Methods.—A clinical decision analysis was performed to compare prophylactic methotrexate with observation after laparoscopic linear salpingostomy. In the decision analysis, a patient treated for tubal pregnancy with laparoscopic linear salpingostomy is either given a single dose of methotrexate 1 mg/kg or observed. Biweekly serial HCG levels are followed postoperatively in both algorithms to identify persistent ectopic pregnancy. The primary outcome measures are the number of ruptured ectopic pregnancies, surgical procedures, complications, and cost for each group (observation vs prophylaxis).

Results.—Prophylactic methotrexate resulted in fewer instances of tubal rupture (0.4% vs 3.7%) and fewer procedures (1.9% vs 4.7%) at a lower cost ($67.55 less/patient) than observation alone. Methotrexate-related complications occurred more frequently with prophylaxis (5.5% vs 0.8%). Certain conditions changed the strategy that was preferred. Observation was the best strategy when the persistent ectopic pregnancy rate was under 9%; the success of prophylaxis was below 95%, the complication rate linked with methotrexate was above 18%, or the rupture rate of persistent ectopic pregnancies was under 7.3%.

Conclusion.—Prophylactic methotrexate at the time of linear salpingostomy for treatment of ectopic pregnancy was preferable to observation as long as certain conditions existed.

▶ Surgeons (or training facilities) with a rate of persistent ectopic rate greater than 9% might well consider the use of prophylactic methotrexate at the time of initial surgery. The number of repeat operations (and salpingectomies) is reduced by the use of prophylactic methotrexate at the time of linear salpingostomy for ampullary ectopic pregnancy. With a persistent ectopic rate of greater than 9%, the initial financial impact of methotrexate (and complications) is less than the loss associated with expectant management. To make informed use of the recommendations in this review, an analysis of both the persistent ectopic rate and the complication rate with methotrexate would have to be evaluated for each institution (or surgeon). This decision analysis serves as a reminder of the importance of a careful preoperative review with the patient of treatment options, including risks and benefits of the recommended therapy as well as the alternatives.

R. D. Arias, MD

Transcervical

Dilatation and Curettage Fails to Detect Most Focal Lesions in the Uterine Cavity in Women With Postmenopausal Bleeding
Epstein E, Ramirez A, Skoog L, et al (Univ of Lund, Malmö, Sweden)
Acta Obstet Gynecol Scand 80:1131-1136, 2001   23–4

Background.—Because 5% to 15% of women with postmenopausal bleeding have endometrial carcinoma and 60% of women with postmenopausal bleeding and an endometrium of at least 5 mm have pathologic conditions, an endometrial sample must be obtained to check for these more-serious conditions. Usually, dilatation and curettage (D&C) is the chosen procedure, but up to 90% of polyps and 66% of hyperplasias reportedly have been missed with this method. Since both polyps and hyperplasia are potential risk factors for developing endometrial carcinoma, a better method is desirable. The prevalence of focally growing lesions in the uterine cavity was assessed, as well as whether they can be diagnosed and removed using conventional D&C in women with postmenopausal bleeding and an endometrium of at least 5 mm on transvaginal US examination.

Methods.—Diagnostic hysteroscopy, D&C, and hysteroscopic resection were performed in 105 women who had postmenopausal bleeding and an endometrium of at least 5 mm on transvaginal US, removing any focally growing lesion that was still left in the uterine cavity. Subsequent hysterectomy was performed in 24 women. When differing diagnoses were obtained from the specimens, the most relevant one was chosen.

Results.—Hysteroscopy revealed that 83% of the women had focally growing lesions, and 87% had whole or parts of the focal lesion remaining after the D&C. Hysteroscopy was less than optimal in 6 women, and technical problems led it to fail in 1 woman, but it succeeded in 98 women. Of the 24 women undergoing hysterectomy, 22 of the procedures were done because of malignant or premalignant findings on the D&C or hysteroscopic resection. Eighty percent of the women had endometrial pathology, yet the D&C uncovered only 50%, failing to diagnose 58% of the polyps, 50% of the hyperplasias/focal hyperplasias, 60% of the complex atypical hyperplasias, 11% of the endometrial cancers, and the 1 adenosarcoma in the group. Those women who had polyps removed at D&C had a median endometrial thickness of 8.5 mm; those whose polyps were missed had a median endometrial thickness of 10.0 mm. The agreement between diagnoses on D&C and final diagnoses was 59% in women who had focally growing lesions and 94% in women lacking these lesions. At hysteroscopy, 96% of the premalignant or malignant conditions, 98% of the polyps, all the submucous myomas, all the hyperplasias, and 29% of the normal endometria were identified; none of the 4 insufficient samples was useful. Using the area under the receiver operating characteristic curve, the best cutoff value that predicts the presence of focally growing lesions at hysteroscopy was 10 mm, with values of 10 or more indicating focal lesions and 57 of 59 women having focally growing lesions, versus 30 of 46 women having such lesions when the endometrial thickness was 5 to 9 mm.

Conclusions.—Most pathologic lesions found in the uterine cavity have a pattern of focal growth that is detected more readily on hysteroscopic resection than on D&C. While office hysteroscopy or hydrosonography may be used to screen patients, operative hysteroscopy should be used for all women with postmenopausal bleeding and an endometrium of 5 mm or greater who have focal lesions.

▶ The prospective evaluation of D&C compared with D&C plus hysterectomy revealed the superiority of hysteroscopy in the diagnosis of focal endometrial lesions. The blind procedure failed to diagnose about half the benign conditions and a significant proportion of the malignancies and premalignancies. The combination of a thick endometrium and an insufficient specimen from the D&C correlated with a focal lesion that was then accurately diagnosed at hysteroscopy. It would, therefore, appear that hysteroscopic biopsy or resection of focal endometrial pathology is a more-precise diagnostic tool than D&C. The question of the potential for peritoneal dissemination of malignant cells remains. It would appear that the known risks associated with a failure to diagnose are greater than the as-yet-theoretical risks associated with iatrogenic positive peritoneal cytology.

R. D. Arias, MD

Is It Possible to Recommend an 'Optimal' Postoperative Management After Hysteroscopic Metroplasty? A Retrospective Study With 52 Infertile Patients Showing a Septate Uterus

Nawroth F, Schmidt T, Freise C, et al (Univ of Cologne, Germany)
Acta Obstet Gynecol Scand 81:55-57, 2002   23–5

Introduction.—The recommendations for the postoperative management of hysteroscopic metroplasty in patients with septate uterus vary in the literature and have included postoperative estrogenization, the insertion of an intrauterine device (IUD), or a combination of both. The "optimal" postoperative management after hysteroscopic metroplasty was examined retrospectively in 52 infertile women with septate uterus.

Methods.—The median septal length was 3.0 cm (range, 2.0-7.0 cm). There were 3 patient groups: group 1 received a cyclical hormone replacement therapy (HRT) postoperatively plus an IUD; group 2 patients received HRT alone for 3 months; and group 3 patients received no postoperative therapy. There were 22, 13, and 17 patients, respectively, in groups 1, 2, and 3. Groups were similar in patient age, median follow-up, and median septum length.

Results.—During a median follow-up of 21 months, 30.9%, 53.8%, and 41.2% of group 1, 2, and 3 patients, respectively, became pregnant and had delivery rates at term of 53.3%, 64.4%, and 88.9%, respectively ($P = $ NS). Groups did not differ in remaining septa or adhesions.

Conclusion.—The use of postoperative HRT plus IUD insertion or HRT alone is not needed after hysteroscopic metroplasty.

▶ The desire to prevent postoperative adhesions after hysteroscopic surgery has prompted the use of both stents (such as various IUDs) and hormonal therapies. In this retrospective analysis of 3 postoperative management methods, pregnancy outcomes were similar in each group. Neither postoperative estrogens nor a combination of HRT plus an IUD conferred a benefit. Given the lack of consensus regarding adhesion prevention after hysteroscopic surgery, prospective trials are indicated.

R. D. Arias, MD

Uterus

Vasopressin as an Etiologic Factor for Infection in Gynecologic Surgery: A Randomized Double-Blind Placebo-Controlled Trial

Kammerer-Doak DN, Rogers RG, Maybach JJ, et al (Univ of New Mexico, Albuquerque)
Am J Obstet Gynecol 185:1344-1348, 2001   23–6

Background.—The possibility of an increased risk of infection associated with vasoconstrictive agents deters many gynecologic surgeons from using vasopressin during vaginal hysterectomy. The risk of pelvic infection with the use of vasopressin at the time of vaginal hysterectomy was assessed.

Methods and Findings.—One hundred seventeen patients undergoing vaginal hysterectomy were randomly assigned to pericervical injections of vasopressin or normal saline solution. The infection rates in the saline group and vasopressin group were 7.3% and 1.6%, respectively, a nonsignificant difference. The vasopressin recipients had significantly less estimated blood loss and change in hemoglobin and hematocrit levels. No significant between-group differences were seen in interval blood pressure measurements after vasopressin administration.

Conclusions.—The use of vasopressin during vaginal hysterectomy does not appear to increase the risk of pelvic infection. However, it does reduce operative blood loss. Blood pressure in this series was unaffected.

▶ Vasopressin can be a useful adjunct to vaginal hysterectomy. The dual benefits of unobscured tissue planes and decreased blood loss have traditionally been weighed against a fear of increased infection or delayed bleeding. This trial addresses these fears with a result that confirms the place of dilute vasopressin as a safe "chemical tourniquet" in pelvic surgery.

R. D. Arias, MD

Total Hysterectomy for a Nonprolapsed, Benign Uterus in Women Without Vaginal Deliveries
Chauveaud A, de Tayrac R, Gervaise A, et al (Antoine Béclère Hosp, Clamart, France)
J Reprod Med 47:4-8, 2002   23–7

Introduction.—All large-scale surveys addressing hysterectomy practice have reported that 60% to 80% of hysterectomies are performed via the abdominal approach. Although the vaginal route for hysterectomy is usually contraindicated in nulliparity, it is associated with less morbidity, shorter hospitalization, and faster convalescence. Changes in obstetric practice, along with an increased rate of cesarean section, are responsible for an increased number of women who have never had a vaginal delivery. The different surgical approaches of hysterectomy for a nonprolapsed, benign uterus was examined retrospectively in women who had never had vaginal deliveries.

Methods.—Of 660 patients with nonprolapsed, benign uteri who underwent hysterectomy between August 1991 and June 2000, 148 (22%) had never had a vaginal delivery; 104 (70%) were nulliparous and 44 (30%) had undergone at least 1 cesarean section. The vaginal route was the preferred route for the 148 hysterectomies. The vaginal route was used for 77 patients (52%), 56 (38%) underwent laparotomies, and 15 (10%) had laparoscopically assisted vaginal hysterectomies (groups 1, 2, and 3, respectively).

Results.—The mean uterine weight was 275 g, 1830 g, and 331 g, respectively, for groups 1, 2, and 3. Mean surgical time was 87 minutes, 96 minutes, and 112 minutes for groups 1, 2, and 3, respectively. There was 1 serious injury (sigmoid injury) in the vaginal route group. The mean hospital stay was 4, 7.1, and 4.3 days, respectively, in groups 1, 2, and 3.

Conclusion.—Vaginal hysterectomy for a nonprolapsed benign uterus is recommended for women who had not had vaginal deliveries and was feasible in 72% of the patients scheduled for total hysterectomy by the vaginal route. This cohort had a low complication rate.

▶ Lower parity, the generous use of cesarean section, and a decline in the number of gynecologists trained in vaginal surgery combine to reduce the proportion of hysterectomies performed via the vaginal route. Vaginal hysterectomy is associated with a shorter hospital stay and quicker recovery because of the avoidance of an abdominal incision. Wound complications are also reduced. The vaginal route should be considered the preferred route of hysterectomy in benign cases and should be rejected only after careful consideration of risk factors known to make it unfeasible. As indicated by these authors, neither nulliparity, cesarean section, nor lack of descensus should necessarily preclude this route of hysterectomy by experienced gynecologists.

R. D. Arias, MD

Hysterectomy Rates in the United States 1990-1997
Farquhar CM, Steiner CA (Agency for Healthcare Research and Quality, Rockville, Md)
Obstet Gynecol 99:229-234, 2002   23–8

Background.—Nearly one third of all women aged 60 years have undergone a hysterectomy, which is the most common nonpregnancy-related surgery performed in the United States. Laparoscopically assisted vaginal hysterectomy was developed to allow a shorter hospital stay, reduce complications, lower hospital costs for the patient, and better surgical outcomes, all of which have been achieved, yet the frequency with which this approach is used is believed to be low. Vaginal hysterectomy has similar low rates, although it is accompanied by fewer postoperative infections, shorter hospital stays, and faster recovery times. The rates and types of hysterectomy performed between 1990 and 1997 in the United States were evaluated, along with various other data.

Methods.—National discharge data were obtained from the nationwide Inpatient Sample of the Healthcare Cost and Utilization Project for 1990 through 1997. International Classification of Diseases, 9th Revision, Clinical Modification procedure codes were used to classify the women having hysterectomy. Rate, type of hysterectomy, patient age, length of stay in the hospital, total hospital charges, and diagnostic categories were documented in a descriptive statistical analysis.

Results.—The rates for hysterectomy in 1990 and 1997 were 5.5 per 1000 women and 5.6 per 1000 women, respectively. Abdominal hysterectomy was the most common procedure performed, accounting for 63% of the hysterectomies done in 1997, whereas laparoscopic procedures accounted for

9.9% of them and vaginal hysterectomy was done in 23% of cases. The frequency of laparoscopic hysterectomy increased more than 30-fold over the period assessed. In 2% of hysterectomies, a subtotal procedure was performed; its frequency tripled over the 8 years of the study.

The shortest length of stay was found with laparoscopic hysterectomy (down from 3 days in 1990 to 2 days in 1997), whereas the lowest median total hospital charges were noted in women having a vaginal hysterectomy in all of the years covered. From 1990 to 1997, the total hospital charges for laparoscopic hysterectomy nearly doubled. Forty percent or more of the abdominal and subtotal hysterectomies were performed for fibroids. When the primary diagnosis was fibroids, endometriosis, cancer, or inflammatory pelvic disease, two thirds of the women had an abdominal hysterectomy. Vaginal hysterectomy was performed most frequently when the primary diagnosis was uterovaginal prolapse.

Conclusion.—The most common indication for hysterectomy is uterine fibroids and the most common approach is abdominal. No effect on the rates of hysterectomy was produced by the development of alternative techniques for controlling abnormal uterine bleeding. Laparoscopic procedures remain limited in number.

▶ The introduction of nonsurgical and nonextirpative treatments for excessive uterine bleeding have, thus far, failed to diminish enthusiasm for hysterectomy. Although the majority of hysterectomies performed for benign indications could be approached by the vaginal route, most women still receive an abdominal incision. The use of laparoscopy appears to have converted a minority of abdominal procedures to laparoscopically assisted vaginal hysterectomy. Hopefully, laparoscopy has not been gratuitously added to procedures better suited to the direct vaginal approach.

R. D. Arias, MD

Transplantation of the Human Uterus
Fageeh W, Raffa H, Jabbad H, et al (King Fahad Hosp, Jeddah, Saudi Arabia)
Int J Gynaecol Obstet 76:245-251, 2002   23–9

Introduction.—The greatest difficulty in uterine transplantation is the vascular anastomosis between the uterine vessels of the donor and the recipient. Reported is a case of human uterine transplantation.

> *Case Report.*—Woman, 26, lost her uterus 6 years earlier as a result of postpartum hemorrhage. She underwent uterine transplantation on April 6, 2000. The donor was a 46-year-old woman with multiloculated ovarian cysts who underwent hysterectomy modified to preserve tissue and vascular integrity. The donor uterus was attached in the orthotopic position to the recipient's vaginal vault. Additional fixation was achieved by shortening the uterosacral ligament. The uterine arteries and veins were extended by using reversed

segments of the great saphenous vein and then were attached to the external iliac arteries and veins, respectively. Immunosuppression was maintained by means of oral cyclosporine A (4 mg/kg body weight), azathioprine (1 mg/kg body weight), and prednisolone (0.2 mg/kg body weight). Allograft rejection was assessed by Echo-Doppler examination, MRI, and measurement of the CD4/CD8 ratio in peripheral blood by fluorescence-activated cell sorter. The patient experienced an episode of acute rejection, which was treated and controlled on the ninth day with antithrombocytic globulin. The transplanted uterus responded well to combined estrogen-progesterone therapy, with endometrial proliferation up to 18 mm. The patient had 2 episodes of withdrawal bleeding when hormonal therapy was discontinued. She experienced acute vascular thrombosis 99 days after transplantation and underwent hysterectomy. Macroscopic and microscopic histopathologic examination showed acute thrombosis in the vessels of the uterine body, with resulting infarction. Both fallopian tubes remained viable with no signs of rejection.

Conclusion.—The acute vascular occlusion seemed to be the result of inadequate uterine structure support, which probably led to tension, torsion, or kinking of the connected vascular uterine grafts.

▶ This article describes a procedure that breaches so many basic tenets of the humane and ethical practice of medicine that one is tempted to believe that it is a hoax. Far from a milestone in the treatment of infertile women, this case report would more accurately be described as an extreme example of disregard for a woman's value as an intrinsically worthwhile individual. The value of her reproductive potential was placed ahead of her life and well-being. Unfortunately, the editorial commenting on this article does not confront any of these ethical questions.[1] To rationally consider the transplant of the human uterus would first require that the donor suffer little additional risk associated with her hysterectomy. This is, after all, not a life-preserving procedure. On the contrary, however, the donor, who would have otherwise been a candidate for a simple hysterectomy, was subjected to a significantly more morbid and technically more challenging procedure that increased the risk of bleeding, ureteral injury, and prolonged recovery. In fact, ureteral injury did occur. Given the elective nature of the procedure, a cadaveric donor would have been far more ethical, although even then efforts would more appropriately be turned to the removal of organs necessary for life or sight before harvest of the uterus. When heart, liver, or lungs fail, transplant surgery and a lifetime of immunosuppression become a reasonable consideration. This case begins with a healthy woman and subjects her (and the donor) to risks associated with surgery and then compounds the recipient's risk with powerful immunosuppressive drugs. Should implantation have occurred in the interim before rejection of this questionably perfused organ, could anything resembling normal development have been expected? How much loss of function in the previously healthy organs would have been tolerated before extirpation would have been offered? This procedure stood little, if any, chance of restoring reproductive function. A few episodes of vaginal bleeding seem small reward for the expenses (physical, emotional, and financial) incurred in this experiment.

R. D. Arias, MD

Reference

1. Keith LG, Priore GD: Uterine transplantation in humans: A new frontier. *Int J Gynaecol Obstet* 76:243, 2002.

Vagina

Histologic Examination of "Fascia" Used in Colporrhaphy
Farrell SA, Dempsey T, Geldenhuys L (Dalhousie Univ, Halifax, NS, Canada)
Obstet Gynecol 98:794-798, 2001   23–10

Background.—Many gynecologic surgeons believe that identifying and using "fascia" is essential for achieving effective anterior and posterior colporrhaphy. A histologic examination of tissue identified as fascia and used during colporrhaphy was reported.

Methods.—Sixty samples obtained from 5 women undergoing primary anterior and posterior colporrhaphy were analyzed. Biopsies were obtained from 3 surgically distinct vaginal tissue types: the wall, the fascia, and the areolar tissue. Histologic examination included staining with hematoxylin-eosin, Masson trichrome for collagen, Movat for elastin, and immunoperoxidase stain for actin in smooth muscle. Histologic diagnoses were compared with surgical diagnoses.

Findings.—The specimens from 2 women were disqualified. Histologic diagnoses for vaginal wall were mucosa and underlying connective tissue; for fascia, moderately dense connective tissue with smooth muscle; and for areolar tissue, loose connective tissue. The histologic appearance of the fascia could not be distinguished from the deeper aspects of the vaginal wall. This tissue consisted of the same proportions of smooth muscle, elastin, and collagen. When histologic appearance was used as the gold standard, the accuracy of surgical diagnosis of vaginal wall was 100%; of fascia, 58%; and of areolar tissue, 67%.

Conclusions.—This analysis shows that the surgical "fascia" used during colporrhaphy is composed of moderately dense connective tissue with smooth muscle similar to the deep aspects of the vaginal wall. It is the same in both the anterior and posterior compartments. The fascia appears to be an artifact of the surgical dissection used to separate the vaginal wall from the underlying organs.

▶ The connective tissue that separates the vaginal epithelium from the bladder anteriorly, and the rectum posteriorly, was evaluated histologically in this study. Histologic examination revealed the anterior connective tissue to be identical to the posterior layer. Furthermore, this layer was indistinguishable from the tissue that remained adherent to the vaginal epithelium. It would appear, therefore, that the tissue used in vaginal colporrhaphy is an artifact of the dissection that separates the vagina from adjacent organs.

R. D. Arias, MD

Anterior Colporrhaphy: A Randomized Trial of Three Surgical Techniques
Weber AM, Walters MD, Piedmonte MR, et al (Cleveland Clinic Found, Ohio)
Am J Obstet Gynecol 185:1299-1306, 2001   23–11

Background.—The treatment of anterior vaginal prolapse is one of the most challenging aspects of pelvic reconstructive surgery. The standard treatment has been anterior colporrhaphy, but there are few prospective studies in the literature to document its success or failure. Anterior vaginal prolapse may recur after standard anterior colporrhaphy in up to 40% of patients. This high recurrence rate has spurred the use of synthetic materials such as absorbable or permanent synthetic mesh, and uncontrolled studies of this technique have yielded cure rates of 93% to 100%. However, in as many as one quarter of patients, the permanent mesh may erode through the vagina. Previously, there have been no controlled studies examining outcomes after anterior vaginal prolapse repair with absorbable synthetic mesh. Outcomes after anterior colporrhaphy with the use of 3 different surgical techniques were compared.

Methods.—The study group comprised 109 women with anterior vaginal prolapse. These patients were randomly assigned to undergo anterior repair by standard technique, standard technique with the addition of polyglactin 910, or ultralateral anterior colporrhaphy. The patients underwent physical examination staging of prolapse with the use of the International Continence Society system before and after surgery. Symptoms were assessed by questionnaire and visual analogue scales. Cure was defined as satisfactory (stage I) or optimal (stage 0) outcome at points Aa (midline anterior vagina 3 cm proximal to the external urethral meatus) and Ba (the most dependent position of the anterior vagina).

Results.—Eighty-three of 109 patients returned for follow-up. The mean age of the patients was 64.7 ± 11.1 years. At a median follow-up of 23.3 months, 10 of 33 patients (30%) in the standard colporrhaphy group had satisfactory or optimal anatomic results, compared with 11 of 26 patients (42%) with standard colporrhaphy plus mesh and with 11 of 24 patients (46%) with ultralateral anterior colporrhaphy. There was a significant improvement in the severity of symptoms related to prolapse. Twenty-three of 24 patients (96%) no longer required manual pressure to void after surgery.

Conclusions.—Similar anatomic cure rates and symptom resolution for anterior vaginal prolapse repair were obtained from the 3 surgical techniques. The cure rate was not improved with the addition of polyglactin 910 mesh compared with standard anterior colporrhaphy.

▶ Although the patient population evaluated in this randomized trial was diverse in terms of preoperative findings and complaints, the authors did a good job of evaluating a single aspect of their prolapse while varying the technique used to correct it. Women randomized to standard midline colporrhaphy, colporrhaphy with polyglactin mesh, and ultralateral anterior colporrhaphy all enjoyed a similar reduction in symptoms and objective evidence of anatomic improvement. One might reasonably conclude that when performed in the context of other indicated procedures, either standard or ultralateral colporrhaphy are acceptable techniques for reducing anterior vaginal prolapse. The addition of mesh appears superfluous, since outcomes were not improved by its contribution to the repair.

R. D. Arias, MD

Vaginal Creation for Müllerian Agenesis
Roberts CP, Haber MJ, Rock JA (Emory Univ, Atlanta, Ga)
Am J Obstet Gynecol 185:1349-1353, 2001   23–12

Introduction.—Most patients with vaginal agenesis have primary amenorrhea and the vagina is likely to be absent or hypoplastic. After observing that the need for surgery and its possible complications could be eliminated because coitus alone could create an adequate vagina in some patients, techniques for vaginal dilation were evaluated. The effectiveness of passive vaginal dilation and McIndoe vaginoplasty was examined in the creation of a neovagina in patients with müllerian agenesis.

Methods.—Fifty-one females with müllerian agenesis were treated between November 18, 1983, and June 6, 1998, and were followed up through August 1, 2000. Patients were given careful instructions for the correct use of Lucite vaginal dilators of gradual sizes that they were to use to create a vaginal space by increasing alternately the length and width until satisfactory vaginal creation was accomplished (Ingram method for vaginal dilation). Patients who refused a trial of vaginal dilation or were not able to create a functional vaginal space with dilation underwent a modified McIndoe vaginoplasty.

Results.—Four patients were lost to follow-up, and 10 refused vaginal dilation and went on to a successful modified McIndoe vaginoplasty. For the remaining 37 patients, 91.9% anatomic and functional success was achieved with the Ingram method for vaginal dilation. Passive dilation was not possible in 8.1% of the patients who underwent a modified McIndoe vaginoplasty; all neovaginal creations were successful. All patients who underwent the McIndoe vaginoplasty procedure were compliant with use of the postoperative vaginal form. No patients experienced loss of vaginal space through contractions or loss of skin graft. Of the patients for whom the dilation approach failed, 1 discontinued the trial as a result of bleeding and discomfort. Of the 3 unsuccessfully treated patients, 1 had undergone a previous hymenotomy. Six patients for whom dilation was successful (17.6%) also had undergone a previous hymenotomy. The mean overall follow-up was 111.1 months (25-188 months). The mean follow-up for patients for whom dilation failed or who refused dilation was significantly shorter (mean, 64.5 months and 65.3 months, respectively; $P < .005$). The mean time to successful dilation was 11.8 months (range, 3-33 months). There was no significant difference in dilation time for patients who failed to achieve anatomic or functional success (20.5 months; range, 8-33 months).

Conclusion.—Passive dilation with the Ingram method is capable of creating a sufficient vaginal canal in patients with vaginal agenesis, both functionally and anatomically, even in those with a previous hymenotomy and resultant scar formation. The modified McIndoe procedure was an excellent option in patients for whom conservative dilation approaches failed and who refused to attempt any dilation. It appears that patients may now be trending toward immediate surgical correction versus diligent use of dilation techniques to create a vaginal space.

▶ The concept of tissue expansion for reconstruction is well described by our colleagues in plastic surgery. Typically, this tissue expansion is initiated by an operative procedure and only unusually is it patient controlled. The authors of this study present a simple patient-controlled technique for vaginal creation or dilation for those with müllerian agenesis. More than 90% of the patients who attempted vaginal creation and dilation with the Ingram technique were successful. The advantages of this technique are not only that it is patient controlled and avoids a surgical procedure, but it also allows for some preservation of modesty and multitasking by the patient. This certainly appears to be the best first step in vaginal reconstruction for these patients before one resorts to more elaborate interventions.[1]

D. S. Miller, MD

Reference

1. Parsons JK, Gearhart SL, Gearhart JP: Vaginal reconstruction utilizing sigmoid colon: Complications and long-term results. *J Pediatr Surg* 37:629, 2002.

Complications

Management of Ureteric Injuries During Gynecological Operations: 10 Years Experience

Sakellariou P, Protopapas AG, Voulgaris Z, et al ("Alexandra" Maternity Hosp, Athens, Greece; Univ of Athens, Greece)
Eur J Obstet Gynecol Reprod Biol 101:179-184, 2002   23–13

Background.—The anatomy of the ureter places it in a position where it can be injured during various types of gynecologic surgery, yet the incidence of such injury is low, usually between 0.1% and 1.5%. Successful, complication-free gynecologic surgery depends on being aware of the potential for ureteric injury, plus recognizing injury before closure. The cases of ureteric injuries caused by various gynecologic surgeries occurring over 10 years were reviewed.

Methods.—Among the 76 patients, 29 injuries were detected intraoperatively and subjected to suturing, removal of ligatures, end-to-end anastomosis, and ureter reimplantation, as needed. Of the 47 cases detected postoperatively, all patients who had obstruction had ureteric catheterization. When this failed, ureterolysis and reimplantation were performed. Surgical evacuation and anastomoses were used for 2 patients who had urinomas.

Results.—Whether unilateral or bilateral injury occurred, when it was detected intraoperatively, management techniques restored patency. Adverse consequences included increased time to performance of surgery and prolonged time in the hospital. No significant increases were noted in postoperative morbidity, and the urinary tract was patent and functioning. With some injuries that were recognized later and required a secondary procedure, infection was found, requiring anti-inflammatory agents and antibiotics. One patient had a urine leak and required a pig-tail catheter. Fourteen percent of the reimplantations had transient ipsilateral distention of the urinary outflow tract; all of these patients had a ureteric stent removed on the twelfth day after surgery. Of 16 ureters with ureteric ligation in which catheterization was used, 4 had significant ureteric distention that required a pigtail ureteric catheter. After a minimum of 2 years of follow-up, long-term morbidity was minimal and relapses absent. Kidney function was maintained regardless of when the ureteric injury was diagnosed.

Conclusion.—Immediate recognition of ureteric damage can prevent prolonged postoperative morbidity and long-term adverse outcomes, whereas unrecognized injuries can go on to produce serious problems postoperatively and require more extensive interventions.

▶ Expert pelvic surgery requires not only a thorough understanding of the course of the ureter and normal variants but also an awareness of those pathologies that predispose to a distorted ureteric course. While prevention of injury is always preferable, the ability to assess ureteral patency when damage is suspected should also be within the scope of the gynecologic surgeon.

The importance of primary intraoperative intervention is illustrated by the findings in this review of 76 patients who suffered a variety of ureteric injuries during gynecological surgery. Intraoperative repairs were associated with few complications and little additional morbidity. Women whose injuries were discovered postoperatively fared much less well. Unfortunately, only the minority of ureteric injuries (27%) were discovered at the time of the initial surgery.

R. D. Arias, MD

Transfusion Rate Associated With Hysterectomy for Benign Disease
Otton GR, Mandapati S, Streatfeild KA, et al (John Hunter Hosp, New South Wales, Australia)
Aust N Z J Obstet Gynaecol 41:439-442, 2001   23–14

Background.—The rate of transfusion required perioperatively is an indirect indication of hemorrhage occurring during hysterectomy. This indicator is used as a quality assurance mark and reflects the standard of care. Patients often undergo a group and save (G and S) preoperatively because of the hemorrhage risk, which incurs extra cost and stress for the patient. The transfusion rate for hysterectomies done at a tertiary care hospital was assessed to determine which patients are likely to require transfusion and whether routine G and S procedures are necessary.

Methods.—The medical records of 532 women having vaginal hysterectomies and 688 having abdominal procedures were reviewed retrospectively. Patient data were collected, as well as individual G and S and transfusion records.

Results.—Two women having vaginal hysterectomy had intraoperative transfusions; 135 women having vaginal hysterectomies had no preoperative G and S. Fifteen women having abdominal hysterectomy received transfusions, with 12 done postoperatively and 3 intraoperatively. No preoperative G and S was performed in 98 women having the abdominal approach. Of the 3 women transfused intraoperatively, 2 had fibroids and 1 had pelvic adhesions. Thus, transfusion rates were 0.38% for the vaginal approach and 2.18% for the abdominal approach. The combined overall rate was 1.4%.

Conclusions.—Overall, under 2% of women undergoing hysterectomy required transfusions perioperatively. Based on these findings, there appears to be no need to perform preoperative G and S routinely on most hysterectomy patients.

▶ Less than 2% of patients undergoing hysterectomy for benign disease were transfused perioperatively in this study of 1220 cases. Hysterectomies evaluated in this series included only those cases approached by the vaginal or abdominal route. Laparoscopically assisted techniques were excluded. Only 2 of 532 women scheduled for a vaginal procedure received blood. This is an especially reassuring observation given that these procedures were performed in a training program under the supervision of several attending physicians. Women undergoing hysterectomy (especially vaginal hysterectomy) appear to be at low risk for requiring perioperative transfusion.

R. D. Arias, MD

Other

Korean Hand Acupressure Reduces Postoperative Nausea and Vomiting After Gynecological Laparoscopic Surgery

Boehler M, Mitterschiffthaler G, Schlager A (Univ of Innsbruck, Austria)
Anesth Analg 94:872-875, 2002   23–15

Introduction.—Without prophylactic antiemetics, gynecologic patients undergoing laparoscopic surgery frequently experience postoperative nausea and vomiting (PONV). Several trials have reported that stimulation of the Chinese acupuncture point P6 is as effective as antiemetic prophylaxis. The Korean hand acupressure point K-K9, whose antiemetic effect has been reported in several trials, is located on the middle phalanx of the fourth finger of each hand. The antiemetic effect of prophylactic acupressure, using the Korean hand acupuncture point K-K9, was assessed in women undergoing gynecologic laparoscopic surgery in a double-blind, randomized, placebo-controlled investigation.

Methods.—Eighty women scheduled for minor gynecologic laparoscopic surgery were randomly assigned to either acupressure performed on both hands on the Korean hand acupressure point K-K9 (using a special acupressure seed [2 mm in diameter] fixed on K-K9 with opaque adhesive tape) or to a placebo group (using acupressure seeds that were taped to sham points, points not defined in Korean hand acupressure [ulnar sides of both fifth fingers]). The seeds were placed ½ hour before surgery and remained in place for a minimum of 24 hours. Oral premedication with diazepam 0.15 mg/kg was administered 1 hour before the expected start of anesthesia. The incidence of PONV was recorded up to 24 hours after the start of anesthesia.

Results.—In the acupressure group, the incidence of nausea and vomiting was significantly less (40% vs 22.5%) than in the placebo group (70% and 50%) ($P = .006$ and $P = .007$, respectively). No patients complained of PONV 8 hours after surgery. Eight and 15 women in the acupressure and placebo groups, respectively, required tropisetron as antiemetic rescue therapy.

Conclusion.—The Korean hand acupressure point K-K9 was effective in decreasing PONV in women who had undergone minor gynecologic laparoscopic surgery.

▶ The use of acupressure would appear to provide an effective method of decreasing PONV. This is especially important in outpatient surgery where a delay in discharge results in patient transfer to an inpatient setting. The utility of this modality, however, is limited by a lack of availability of practitioners trained in its use. Given the importance of outpatient surgery in gynecology, perhaps there is a place for acupressure training in Ob-Gyn residency training.

R. D. Arias, MD

Effects of a Laboratory-Based Skills Curriculum on Laparoscopic Proficiency: A Randomized Trial

Coleman RL, Muller CY (Univ of Texas, Dallas)
Am J Obstet Gynecol 186:836-842, 2002   23–16

Background.—It is difficult to quantify objective measures of surgical performance. In addition to excellent motor control, good operative skills also require knowledge, judgment, and experience. Studies have found that surgical skill correlated not with speed and precision but with the ability of the resident to use landmarks to create a mental 3-dimensional space, to interpret sensory cues based on previous experience, and to distinguish essential from nonessential details. In an animal-based assessment model, construct validity was demonstrated among junior and senior residents by observing their performance of laparoscopic and open abdominal procedures. In a follow-up study in which inanimate tools were used, the findings suggested that this type of assessment can be accomplished in a more cost-efficient manner. More recently, 1 study suggested that intensive laboratory-based endoscopic video training can enhance skill performance of general surgical residents who perform laparoscopic cholecystectomy. The effect and validity of an intensive laboratory-based laparoscopic skills training curriculum on the operative proficiency of obstetrics and gynecology residents were determined.

Methods.—In a prospective, randomized, block-design trial of postgraduate year 3 and year 4 residents, a study schedule was set up as follows. The first week included an orientation to study objectives, administration of a laparoscopic experience questionnaire, timed video laparoscopic drills, and performance of a video-recorded laparoscopic partial salpingectomy. After week 1, the residents were randomly assigned to a skills group and a control group. During weeks 2 and 3, the residents in the skills group repeated the laparoscopic drills 30 minutes daily for 10 days, and the control group had no formal practice sessions. The week 1 evaluation was repeated in week 4. Operative proficiency was quantified by using the Global Skills Assessment Tool through blinded, independent scoring of videotapes.

Results.—At week 1, there were no significant differences between the skills and control groups in previous laparoscopic experience, timed video skills, or resident operative proficiency. Both groups significantly improved their timed drill test scores at week 4. There was a greater percent reduction in time from baseline in the skills group versus the control group (51% vs 18%). Both groups also improved their laparoscopic performance. However, only the skills group showed significant intracohort improvement from baseline.

Conclusions.—A core curriculum including intensive video laparoscopic skills training among postgraduate year 3 and 4 residents can improve not only technical but also operative performance.

▶ Surgery is one of those peculiar endeavors where the apprentice is turned loose on the patient with only a minimal skill set and familiarity with the instrumentation. Airline pilots probably spend much more time in trainers than do surgical trainees. Military and police recruits spend hours assembling and disassembling their weapons before they are ever allowed to load or fire them. Often our residents learn how to assemble a cystoscope, proctoscope, or a laparoscope with the patient under anesthesia. Now, with the increasing variety of laparoscopic and urogynecologic procedures, declining surgical case volumes in many residency programs, and looming resident work hour restrictions, many programs are recognizing the importance of developing efficient instructional guidelines to teach trainees. This is particularly evident in the ever-expanding realm of endoscopic surgery. Several residency programs have met this challenge by incorporating, to varying degrees, training modules patterned after the training set developed by the Council on Resident Education in Obstetrics and Gynecology.[1] This article demonstrates the validity of a similarly structured curriculum on third and fourth year residents in a prospective, randomized design. The unique end point in this trial was clear documentation that laboratory-based skill enhancement translated into surgical performance gains as assessed by the Global Surgical Assessment Tool. It remains to be seen whether such models can also be used to impart surgical judgment and precision.

D. S. Miller, MD

Reference

1. Goff BA, Nielsen PE, Lentz GM, et al: Surgical skills assessment: A blinded examination of obstetrics and gynecology residents. *Am J Obstet Gynecol* 186:613, 2002.

24 BRCA

Risk-Reducing Salpingo-Oophorectomy in Women With a *BRCA1* or *BRCA2* Mutation
Kauff ND, Satagopan JM, Robson ME, et al (Mem Sloan-Kettering Cancer Ctr, New York)
N Engl J Med 346:1609-1615, 2002   24–1

Introduction.—Risk-reducing salpingo-oophorectomy is an option for carriers of *BRCA1* and *BRCA2* mutations who have completed childbearing. Data are limited concerning the efficacy of this approach. The effect of risk-reducing salpingo-oophorectomy was prospectively compared with surveillance for ovarian cancer for incidence of subsequent breast cancer and *BRCA*-related gynecologic cancers in women with BRCA mutations.

Methods.—All women assessed between June 1, 1995, and May 30, 2001, for possible pathogenic *BRCA1* or *BRCA2* mutations during genetic counseling were offered enrollment in a prospective follow-up investigation. A total of 177 women from 153 families were advised to undergo surveillance for ovarian cancer with annual or twice yearly gynecologic examinations, twice yearly transvaginal ultrasonographic examinations, and twice yearly determinations of serum CA-125 concentrations. A total of 170 women 35 years of age or older who had not undergone bilateral oophorectomy chose to undergo either surveillance for ovarian cancer or risk-reducing salpingo-oophorectomy. Follow-up included an annual questionnaire, telephone contact, and reviews of medical records. The time to cancer was compared in both groups by Kaplan-Meier analysis and a Cox proportional-hazards model.

Results.—During a median follow-up of 24.2 months, breast cancer was diagnosed in 3 of 98 women who chose risk-reducing salpingo-oophorectomy. Among the 72 women who chose surveillance, breast cancer was diagnosed in 8, ovarian cancer in 4, and peritoneal cancer in 1. The time to breast cancer or BRCA-related gynecologic cancer was longer in the salpingo-oophorectomy versus the surveillance group, with a hazard ratio for subsequent breast cancer or BRCA-related gynecologic cancer of 0.25 (95% CI, 0.08-0.74).

Conclusion.—Salpingo-oophorectomy in carriers of *BRCA* mutations can reduce the risk of breast cancer and *BRCA*-related gynecologic cancer.

▶ The *BRCA1* and *BRCA 2* genes encode proteins involved in the cellular response to DNA damage. Women with mutation of these genes are at increased risk for development of breast and/or ovarian cancer. These 2 studies (Abstracts 24–1 and 24–2) provide further evidence that prophylactic oophorectomy can significantly decrease but not eliminate the risk of developing not only ovarian or peritoneal carcinoma but breast cancer as well. No survival advantage was reported. It will be important to determine whether this maneuver merely exchanges 1 cause of death for another or whether it is life saving, given the concern that some have for the use of hormone replacement therapy in this group of patients. It was also discouraging to note that in the group of patients who underwent increased surveillance most of the ovarian cancers were not found until they were of advanced stage in a proportion similar to that seen in an unscreened population.

D. S. Miller, MD

Prophylactic Oophorectomy in Carriers of *BRCA1* or *BRCA2* Mutations
Rebbeck TR, for the Prevention and Observation of Surgical End Points Study Group (Univ of Pennsylvania, Philadelphia; et al)
N Engl J Med 346:1616-1622, 2002   24–2

Introduction.—Prophylactic oophorectomy has been shown to diminish the risk of breast cancer by about 50% in women who are carriers of *BRCA1* mutations and those who are genetically uncharacterized. Women with *BRCA1* and *BRCA2* mutations were examined to determine whether oophorectomy decreases the risk of cancers of the coelomic epithelium and breast.

Methods.—Five hundred fifty-one women with disease-related germ-line *BRCA1* or *BRCA2* mutations were identified from several registries and evaluated for the occurrence of ovarian and breast cancer. The incidence of ovarian cancer was determined in 259 women who had undergone bilateral prophylactic oophorectomy and in 292 matched controls who had not had the surgery. In a subgroup of 241 women with no history of breast cancer or prophylactic mastectomy, the incidence of breast cancer was ascertained in 99 who had undergone bilateral prophylactic oophorectomy and in 142 matched controls. Postoperative follow-up was a minimum of 8 years for both groups.

Results.—Six women who underwent prophylactic oophorectomy (2.3%) were given a diagnosis of stage 1 ovarian cancer at the time of the procedure. In 2 women (0.8%), ovarian cancer was diagnosed at a mean follow-up of 8.8 years. Excluding the 6 women whose cancer was diagnosed at the time of surgery, prophylactic oophorectomy significantly diminished the risk of coelomic epithelium cancer (hazard ratio, 0.04; 95% CI, 0.01-0.16). Twenty-one (21.2%) of the 99 women who underwent bilateral prophylactic oophorectomy and were evaluated to ascertain the risk of breast cancer developed breast cancer compared with 60 (42.3%) in the control group (hazard ratio, 0.47; 95% CI, 0.29-0.77).

Conclusion.—Bilateral prophylactic oophorectomy diminishes the risk of coelomic bilateral cancer and breast cancer in females with *BRCA1* and *BRCA2* mutations. Surveillance does not decrease the proportion of ovarian cancers diagnosed in late stages or have an impact on mortality rate, which is estimated at 80% at 5 years for stage III disease.

Germline BRCA1–2 Mutations in Non-Ashkenazi Families With Double Primary Breast and Ovarian Cancer

Schorge JO, Mahoney NM, Miller DS, et al (Univ of Texas, Dallas)
Gynecol Oncol 83:383-387, 2001   24–3

Background.—Among Ashkenazi women who have double primary tumors in the breast and ovary, germline Jewish founder mutations in the BRCA1 and BRCA2 genes are prevalent, but those Ashkenazi women in whom only ovarian cancer develops also often have these mutations and they are also found among non-Ashkenazi women. BRCA1-2 mutations occur twice as often in families where breast cancer is prevalent when there is an individual who has a second non-breast–type primary cancer. The frequency and type of BRCA1-2 mutations in non-Ashkenazi families who have a member with double primary breast and ovarian cancer were explored.

Methods.—From 1992 through 2000, the University of Texas Southwestern Familial Cancer Registry enrolled women at increased risk for cancer based on their family history, with blood samples from persons who chose to have genetic testing done sent for complete DNA sequencing of the BRCA1 and BRCA2 genes. Clinical data were obtained particularly from individuals with breast and ovarian cancer.

Results.—Of the 900 families that enrolled, 62 had non-Ashkenazi ancestry and contained at least 1 member with breast plus ovarian cancer; genetic testing was performed in 21 of these families. Eleven had germline BRCA1 mutations and 2 had mutations of BRCA2, with 8 families testing negative. Six of 7 women who had double primary disease had a BRCA1-2 mutation. BRCA1 mutations were found 5 times as often as BRCA2 mutations. The median age at diagnosis for 60 women with double primary disease (55 families) was 46 years for breast cancer and 50 years for ovarian cancer, with 57% having a breast cancer diagnosis preceding ovarian cancer, 17% having both diagnosed within a year, and 26% having ovarian cancer diagnosed before breast cancer. In 17 families, at least 1 member had bilateral breast cancer.

Conclusion.—Sixty-two percent of the non-Ashkenazi families with double primary disease had a BRCA1-2 mutation, with 86% of women who had both breast and ovarian cancer and chose to undergo testing having a mutation found. These data indicate that non-Ashkenazi families with double primary disease run a risk similar to that of Ashkenazi families for having this mutation. These individuals often have the diagnosis of breast cancer made before that for ovarian cancer, so the diagnosis of breast cancer should trigger a search of the family history and referral for women at risk for these mutations.

▶ Ashkenazi women, in whom double primary breast and ovarian cancer develops, have a high prevalence (greater than 50%) of the 3 Jewish BRCA1-2 founder mutations. The authors of this study sought to determine whether non-Ashkenazis have similar predisposing germline mutations. Sixty-two such families with at least 1 member having double primary disease were identified via an institutional hereditary cancer registry. Twenty-one families underwent genetic testing; 41 did not. Thirteen (62%) of 21 had at least 1 member test positive for a germline BRCA1-2 mutation; only 1 was a Jewish founder mutation. Of 7 non-Ashkenazi women who themselves had double primary disease, 6 (86%) tested positive for a BRCA1-2 mutation. Thus, non-Ashkenazi women in whom both breast and ovarian cancer develop have a high prevalence (greater than 50%) of germline BRCA1-2 mutations. However, comprehensive sequencing is important since these mutations may occur throughout both genes.

R. D. Arias, MD

25 Ovarian Cancer

Risk Factors & Markers

Low-Dose Oral Contraceptives: Protective Effect on Ovarian Cancer Risk
Royar J, Becher H, Chang-Claude J (Deutsches Krebsforschungszentrum, Heidelberg, Germany; Univ of Heidelberg, Germany)
Int J Cancer 95:370-374, 2001   25–1

Background.—In the last decade, clinicians have preferred to prescribe low-dose oral contraceptive (OC) formulations, which contain 35 µg or less ethinyl estradiol. However, little is known about their relation to ovarian cancer risk. The effects of low-dose OC on the risk of ovarian cancer were determined in a population-based case-control study.

Methods.—Two hundred eighty-two patients, aged 20 to 75 years at diagnosis of incident primary invasive ovarian cancer or borderline tumor between 1993 and 1996, comprised the case group. The control group consisted of 533 control subjects matched individually to each case by age and study area.

Findings.—Ever using any type of OC significantly decreased ovarian cancer risk by 52%. The risk reduction was 7% per year of use. This reduction was more evident in first-use women younger than 25 years. The decrease in risk for ovarian cancer was marked for use of low-dose OC, with odds ratios of 0.86 per year of using OC containing less than 35 µg ethinyl estradiol, 0.91 per year of using OC containing 35 to 49 µg, and 0.95 per year of using OC containing 50 µg or more.

Conclusions.—Low-dose OCs confer marked protection against the development of ovarian cancer. These findings are consistent with previous observations of the strong protective effect of OCs on ovarian cancer risk.

► The reduction in ovarian cancer risk associated with oral contraceptive use has been well demonstrated for pills containing higher doses of estrogen and progestin. In this population-based case-control study, lower-dose estrogen formulations were even more strongly protective than higher-dose pills. A stronger protective effect was also seen when women initiated OC use before the age of 25 years. This protection persisted for at least 20 years after discontinuation. It appears that newer formulations also reduce ovarian cancer risk.

R. D. Arias, MD

Prostasin, a Potential Serum Marker for Ovarian Cancer: Identification Through Microarray Technology

Mok SC, Chao J, Skates S, et al (Harvard Med School, Boston; Med Univ of South Carolina, Charleston; Dana-Farber Cancer Inst, Boston; et al)
J Natl Cancer Inst 93:1458-1464, 2001   25–2

Objective.—Ovarian cancer is the fifth leading cause of death in US women, and only 28% of women with distant disease survive for 5 years. Because the 5-year survival rate for women with confined disease is 90%, it is important to identify markers for the disease. Microarray technology allows identification of differentially expressed genes. Novel molecular markers for ovarian cancer were identified and the clinical value of 1 (prostasin) was prospectively assessed.

Methods.—RNA was isolated from cultures of normal human surface epithelial cells and from fresh biological specimens collected from 3 women having surgery for primary ovarian cancer. Complementary DNA was hybridized in a microarray system, amplified, and subjected to reverse transcription–polymerase chain reaction. Prostasin, a serine protease, was identified by immunohistochemical localization and measured by enzyme-linked immunosorbent assay. Serum prostasin was determined in 64 case patients and in 137 control women for whom CA 125 levels had been determined.

Results.—Adjusted prostasin levels were significantly increased in epithelial cells and stroma in women with ovarian cancer, compared with control women (13.7 µg/mL in 64 case patients vs 7.5 µg/mL in control women). Prostasin levels were highest in women with stage II disease. Prostasin levels were lower in mucinous-type ovarian tumors than in ovarian tumors of other types. In control women, archived specimens had lower prostasin levels than did current specimens. In 16 women with preoperative and postoperative specimens of their nonmucinous tumors, 14 had lower prostasin levels after surgery. Postoperative prostasin levels for the group were significantly lower than preoperative levels.

Conclusion.—Microarray technology is a powerful tool for identifying markers of ovarian cancer. Prostasin may be a clinically significant ovarian cancer marker.

▶ Prostasin is a secretory protein present in the prostate that is overexpressed in epithelial ovarian tumors. It was identified using microarray complementary DNA technology. Its function and biological plausibility in relationship to ovarian cancer are not yet clear. However, given our lack of sensitive and specific screening tests for ovarian cancer, this and other markers should receive further scrutiny. Microarray complementary DNA technology will be an important technique in studying the molecular carcinogenesis of ovarian and other cancers.

D. S. Miller, MD

Osteopontin as a Potential Diagnostic Biomarker for Ovarian Cancer
Kim J-H, Skates SJ, Uede T, et al (Catholic Univ of Korea, Kyong-Ki-Do; Harvard Med School, Boston; Dana Farber Cancer Inst, Boston; et al)
JAMA 287:1671-1679, 2002   25–3

Background.—Of the 25,000 women given a diagnosis of ovarian cancer each year, 15,000 die secondary to the malignancy, reflecting the fact that most diagnoses are made when the disease is in stages III or IV (survival under 30%) rather than stage I (survival 95%). Detecting the disease at an earlier stage would greatly improve survival, and tumor markers are being sought to enable that detection. Using high-throughput complementary DNA (cDNA) microarray techniques, potential serum markers have been detected. Specific to ovarian cancer, a spot with an ovarian cancer/healthy human ovarian surface epithelial (HOSE) ratio of 184 was identified, corresponding to the protein osteopontin. Validation studies were conducted for this upregulated gene to verify its clinical usefulness.

Methods.—Samples were taken from 144 patients being evaluated for a pelvic mass, in addition to ovarian cancer and healthy human ovarian surface epithelial cell lines and cultures and archival paraffin-embedded ovarian tissue. Healthy controls consisted of plasma samples from 107 women chosen from an epidemiologic study of ovarian cancer. Being sought were the relative messenger RNA expression in cancer cells versus fresh ovarian tissue (expressed as $2^{-\Delta\Delta ct}$), the production of osteopontin in the various tissues, and the amount of osteopontin found in the plasma of patients versus controls.

Results.—High levels of osteopontin expression occurred in 10 of the ovarian cancer cell lines and in the 27 ovarian cancer tissues when compared with 2 samples of healthy ovarian surface epithelium. No significant differences in the expression of osteopontin were noted among the tumors of various subtypes. Healthy ovarian epithelium and stroma showed no osteopontin immunoreactivity, with the highest degree of positive staining found in cancer tissues in the cellular membrane and cytoplasm, extracellular matrix component, or psammoma bodies. A statistically significant difference in immunostaining scores from the various tissue sections was found among the diagnostic groups and the histologic groups, with the mucinous cases having the highest expression. The various stages and grades of cancer cells showed no significant differences in osteopontin immunoreactivity.

Combining the plasma samples from healthy controls, those with benign disease, those with nonovarian gynecologic cancers, and those with ovarian cancers, the mean osteopontin level was 230.9 ng/mL. This was broken down to 147.1 ng/mL for healthy tissues, 254.4 ng/mL for those with benign disease, 260.9 ng/mL for those with other gynecologic cancers, and 486.5 ng/mL for those with ovarian cancer. The specificity was 80% (cutoff value, 252 ng/mL), the sensitivity for detecting early-stage ovarian cancer was 80%, and the sensitivity for detecting late-stage ovarian cancer was 85%.

Conclusion.—The osteopontin levels in plasma were significantly higher for women with ovarian cancer than for any of the other groups assessed.

Thus, osteopontin holds promise for application as a tumor marker indicating the presence of ovarian cancer.

▶ Potential biomarkers for several cancers have been identified using recently developed high-throughput cDNA microarray technology. The authors of this study identified an RNA "spot" that was dramatically overproduced in ovarian cancer compared to normal ovarian tissue. This putative tumor marker (osteopontin) also had plasma levels that were significantly higher in ovarian cancer patients than healthy controls, patients with benign ovarian disease, and patients with other gynecologic cancers. In the near future, osteopontin could be included in a screening panel of putative biomarkers to obtain sensitivity and specificity estimates for the early detection of ovarian cancer. This investigation has demonstrated the potential value of cDNA microarray analysis in identifying overexpressed genes in ovarian cancer and its clinically meaningful link to a protein measurable in plasma.

D. S. Miller, MD

Use of Proteomic Patterns in Serum to Identify Ovarian Cancer
Petricoin EF III, Ardekani AM, Hitt BA, et al (Food and Drug Administration, Bethesda, Md; NIH, Bethesda, Md; Correlogic Systems Inc, Bethesda, Md; et al)
Lancet 359:572-577, 2002   25–4

Background.—New technologies to detect early-stage ovarian cancer are needed. Pathologic changes in an organ may be reflected in proteomic patterns in serum. Thus, a bioinformatics tool was developed and used to identify proteomic patterns in serum distinguishing neoplastic from nonneoplastic disease in the ovary.

Methods.—Serum samples were obtained from 50 patients with ovarian cancer and 50 healthy women. Mass spectroscopy, involving a surface-enhanced laser desorption and ionization, was used to produce proteomic spectra. A preliminary set of spectra derived from serum analysis was examined with an iterative searching algorithm that identified a proteomic pattern that completely discriminated cancer from noncancer. The pattern identified was then used to classify an independent set of masked serum samples from 50 women with ovarian cancer and 66 women without malignancy.

Findings.—In the preliminary set of samples, the algorithm identified a cluster pattern that completely discriminated between cancer and nonmalignancy. This pattern correctly identified all 50 ovarian cancer cases in the masked set, including 18 cases of stage I disease. Sixty-three of the 66 cases of nonmalignant disease were identified as nonmalignancy. The sensitivity and specificity were 100% and 95%, respectively, and the positive predictive value was 94%. The positive predictive value for CA125, measured in the same masked set, was only 34%.

Conclusions.—A prospective population-based assessment of proteomic pattern technology is a feasible screening tool for all stages of ovarian cancer in high-risk and general populations. The production of the mass spectra requires a small serum sample, which could be acquired by fingerprick. Results are available in less than 30 minutes.

▶ I am often asked by patients about a blood test that would determine whether they have cancer. Previously I have told them that no such test exists. However, the future may now be here. Using a supercomputer, the authors were able to teach it to differentiate between the serum proteome pattern of patients with ovarian cancer versus those without. Previous studies have been hampered by lack of computer power.[1] What these small peptides are and the genes that encode them have not yet been determined. Nonetheless, the patterns can be accurately discriminated. Because the device required for this costs $150,000, it remains to be seen whether this technology can be adopted in a high throughput fashion that would lend itself to mass screening.

D. S. Miller, MD

Reference

1. Lawson S, Latter G, Miller DS, et al: Quantitative protein changes in metastatic versus primary epithelial ovarian carcinoma. *Gynecol Oncol* 41:22-27, 1991.

Surgery

Survival Effect of Maximal Cytoreductive Surgery for Advanced Ovarian Carcinoma During the Platinum Era: A Meta-analysis

Bristow RE, Tomacruz RS, Armstrong DK, et al (Johns Hopkins Med Institutions, Baltimore, Md)
J Clin Oncol 20:1248-1259, 2002   25–5

Background.—Approximately 14,000 women in the United States receive a diagnosis of advanced epithelial ovarian carcinoma each year. Standard therapy for these patients consists of primary surgical cytoreduction followed by platinum-based chemotherapy. The positive effect of platinum-based chemotherapy on the survival of these patients is widely accepted, but the relative effect of aggressive surgical intervention on long-term outcome has been difficult to quantify. Proponents of aggressive surgery in patients with advanced ovarian carcinoma point out that a large body of retrospective data consistently demonstrates that prognosis and survival are strongly correlated with the amount of postoperative residual disease. However, critics of this approach argue that the survival advantage associated with minimal residual disease results more from the inherent biologic predisposition of the tumor than from the predisposition and skill of the surgeon. The relative effect of percent maximal cytoreductive surgery and other prognostic variables on survival among cohorts of patients with advanced-stage ovarian carcinoma treated with platinum-based chemotherapy was evaluated.

Methods.—For this meta-analysis, 81 cohorts of patients with stage III or IV ovarian carcinoma were identified from articles in MEDLINE for the years 1989 through 1998, for a total of 6885 patients. Linear regression models with weighted correlation calculations were used to assess the effects on log median survival time of the proportion of each cohort undergoing maximal cytoreduction, dose-intensity of the platinum maximal cytoreduction, dose-intensity of the platinum compound, the proportion of patients with stage IV disease, the median age, and the year of publication.

Results.—A statistically significant positive correlation was noted between the percent maximal cytoreduction and the log median survival time. This correlation was significant after controlling for all other variables. Every 10% increase in maximal cytoreduction was associated with a 5.5% increase in median survival time. Estimation of actuarial survival showed that cohorts with a maximal cytoreduction of 25% or less had a mean weighted median survival time of 22.7 months, whereas cohorts with more than 75% maximal cytoreduction had a mean weighted median survival time of 33.9 months. This difference represents an increase of 50%. There was no statistically significant relationship between platinum dose-intensity and log median survival time.

Conclusions.—During the platinum era, one of the most powerful determinants of cohort survival for patients with stage III or IV carcinoma was maximal cytoreduction. Currently, the best method for improving overall survival may be the consistent referral of patients with apparent advanced ovarian cancer to expert centers for primary surgery.

▶ It is the opinion of most gynecologic oncologists supported by case series data as well as their own clinical experience that aggressive surgical debulking of ovarian cancer at the time of initial surgery contributes substantially to the outcome of ovarian cancer patients. However, a few of our other oncologic colleagues remain skeptical as the concept of tumor debulking is usually an unsatisfactory approach for most other cancer types where a significant role of surgery is usually only seen when all the cancer is removed rather than most of it. It is highly unlikely that a randomized controlled trial will be accomplished to settle this issue. This quite thorough meta-analysis adds weight to the preponderance of evidence supporting cytoreduction. Unfortunately only 20% to 30% of patients with advanced ovarian cancer are seen by surgeons experienced and prepared to do aggressive surgical debulking.[1]

D. S. Miller, MD

Reference

1. Eisenkop SM, Spirtos NM, Montag TW, et al: The impact of subspecialty training on the management of advanced ovarian cancer. *Gynecol Oncol* 47:203, 1992.

Bowel Resection at the Time of Primary Cytoreduction for Epithelial Ovarian Cancer

Gillette-Cloven N, Burger RA, Monk BJ, et al (Univ of California Irvine, Orange; City of Hope Natl Med Ctr, Duarte, Calif)
J Am Coll Surg 193:626-632, 2001   25–6

Introduction.—Bowel resection at the time of primary surgery for advanced ovarian cancer is performed to achieve optimum resection and manage intestinal obstruction. Morbidity and survival associated with bowel resection at the time of primary cytoreductive surgery for advanced epithelial ovarian cancer were examined in 105 patients whose surgeries were performed between 1983 and 1995.

Methods.—The median patient age was 65 years (range, 34-84 years). There were 76 and 24 stage III and IV cancers, respectively. For 92% of patients, the primary indication for bowel resection was tumor debulking. For less than 5% of patients, bowel injury or abscess were indications for intestinal resection.

Results.—Seventy patients underwent segmental resection of the colon only and 22 had resections that included both the large and small bowels. Forty-five percent of patients required a stoma. Of these, one third were eventually reversed, resulting in 71% of patients with an intact gastrointestinal system. Of 105 patients, 33 (31%) were optimally cytoreduced to less than 1 cm residual disease.

Ten patients had major complications directly associated with bowel resection, including 4 with bowel fistulas, 5 with early postoperative bowel obstruction, and 1 with stomal hernia. Other morbidities included 18 patients with ileus for more than 10 days, 17 with cardiac complications, 8 with pneumonia, 5 with sepsis, and 4 with thromboembolism. Six patients died and 5 needed reexploration within 30 days of surgery. Postoperative morbidity was more common among patients with preoperative bowel obstruction and suboptimal residual disease.

Only 1 of 16 patients with bowel obstruction was optimally debulked ($P = .01$). Multivariate analysis showed that optimal debulking ($P = .009$) and platinum chemotherapy ($P = .00006$) were independently correlated with improved survival. Survival was not influenced by age, International Federation of Gynecologia Oncologists stage, American Society of Anesthesiologists class, or paclitaxel chemotherapy.

Conclusion.—Optimal resection to less than 1 cm residual disease at the time of primary cytoreduction for ovarian cancer resulted in improved survival. A median survival of 35 months for optimally debulked patients was similar to that of earlier series of optimally debulked patients. Patients with preoperative bowel obstruction and suboptimal residual disease were more likely to have serious morbidity.

▶ This article adds observational evidence that intestinal resection is often helpful in achieving optimal tumor cytoreduction, and that optimal reduction can result in a survival advantage. But what is the appropriate role for bowel resection for the patient in whom optimal cytoreduction cannot be accomplished? Since most major complications and all perioperative deaths occurred in the suboptimally debulked group of bowel resection patients, there does not seem to be any compelling reason, except for bowel obstruction, to perform bowel resection as part of primary ovarian cancer surgery unless that resection will contribute toward an eventual optimal debulking.

D. S. Miller, MD

Chemotherapy

Phase II Trial of Oral Altretamine for Consolidation of Clinical Complete Remission in Women With Stage III Epithelial Ovarian Cancer: A Southwest Oncology Group Trial (SWOG-9326)
Rothenberg ML, Liu PY, Wilczynski S, et al (Vanderbilt Univ, Nashville, Tenn; Southwest Oncology Group Statistical Ctr, Seattle; City of Hope Med Ctr, Duarte, Calif; et al)
Gynecol Oncol 82:317-322, 2001   25–7

Objective.—The aim of this study was to evaluate the 2-year survival rate in a group of women in complete clinical remission (cCR) from Stage III ovarian cancer following front-line therapy who were then treated with a 6-month course of altretamine.

Methods.—Patients were documented to be in cCR by physical examination, computed tomography or magnetic resonance imaging scan, and serum CA-125. Treatment consisted of altretamine (Hexalen)® 260 mg/m²/day po divided into four doses taken after meals and at bedtime for 14 of 28 days for six cycles. Based on previous experience in the Southwest Oncology Group (SWOG), the treatment would be considered promising if the 2-year survival rate was ≥65% as measured from study registration.

Results.—From 9/1/93 and 7/1/97, 112 patients were registered and 97 were fully evaluable. The majority of patients had optimally debulked (≤1 cm: 63%), high-grade (Grade 3: 82%) tumors. The 2-year survival rate in this study was 75% (95% CI: 66-84%). For those patients with optimal disease, the 2-year survival rate was 82% (95% CI: 72-92%) and for those with suboptimal disease it was 64% (95% CI: 48-79%). Four patients (4%) experienced Grade 4 and 21 patients (22%) experienced Grade 3 toxicities consisting primarily of nausea/vomiting, neutropenia, fatigue, anxiety, and paresthesias.

Conclusions.—The 2-year survival rate in this study warrants further evaluation of consolidation therapy for women in clinical complete remission following front-line chemotherapy for Stage III ovarian cancer. Caution is advised in the interpretation of these data, however, because of the nonrandomized nature of the trial and the unknown contribution of front-line use of paclitaxel to the durability of clinical complete response.

▶ Most patients with advanced ovarian cancer will respond to platinum-based chemotherapy. Many of these responses will be complete, yet most of these patients will suffer a relapse of their cancer and die of it. Modification of treatment regimens by increasing the number of treatment cycles beyond 6 or increasing drug dose intensity has not resulted in a significant improvement in outcomes. The use of consolidation therapy to sustain a complete response has been seen in other malignancies, especially breast cancer. The 2-year survival rates seen in this study exceeded that attained in this group of patients on previous Southwest Oncology Group (SWOG) trials.

A subsequent study has been done by SWOG and the Gynecologic Oncology Group comparing 3 versus 12 months of paclitaxel. It has recently been presented that there was a significant (7-month) progression-free survival advantage for the 12-cycle paclitaxel arm.[1] The obvious next step is to compare altretamine and paclitaxel in this group of patients.

D. S. Miller, MD

Reference

1. Markman M, Liu PY, Wilczynski S, et al: Phase 3 randomized trial of 12 versus 3 months of single-agent paclitaxel in patients with advanced ovarian cancer who attained a clinically defined complete response to platinum/paclitaxel-based chemotherapy. *Gynecol Oncol* 84:479, 2002.

Recurrent Epithelial Ovarian Carcinoma: A Randomized Phase III Study of Pegylated Liposomal Doxorubicin Versus Topotecan
Gordon AN, Fleagle JT, Guthrie D, et al (Texas Oncology, Professional Assoc, Dallas; Rocky Mountain Cancer Ctr, Boulder, Colo; Hosp General de Asturias, Oviedo, Spain; et al)
J Clin Oncol 19:3312-3322, 2001   25–8

Background.—Often, ovarian carcinoma is not diagnosed until it becomes symptomatic, in stages III and IV. Patients then have a drastically reduced rate of survival and often have recurrence, even after complete response to surgery and first-line chemotherapy. Patients with recurrent disease are classified as either platinum-sensitive or platinum-resistant, with those who are platinum-sensitive having a stronger likelihood of responding to subsequent chemotherapy. Agents used at this point include pegylated liposomal doxorubicin (PLD) and topotecan. The efficacy and safety of these 2 agents were compared.

Methods.—In this phase III study, 474 patients were randomly assigned to receive either 50 mg/m^2 of PLD as a 1-hour infusion every 4 weeks (239 patients) or 1.5 mg/m^2/day of topotecan for 5 consecutive days every 3 weeks (235 patients). All of the participants had measurable, assessable disease; they were subclassified according to platinum sensitivity and the presence or absence of bulky disease.

Results.—While not reaching statistical significance, the progression-free survival was more favorable for PLD than for topotecan. The difference in response rates between the 2 groups was insignificant, as was overall survival. For PLD, the time to death was 60 weeks and for topotecan it was 56 weeks. No difference in outcome was associated with the presence of bulky disease, but platinum-sensitive patients had a higher objective response than platinum-resistant patients, regardless of the agent they received. For platinum-resistant patients, the progression-free survival and overall survival favored topotecan. PLD was significantly more effective in the platinum-sensitive group compared with topotecan, with a significant difference in overall survival of 108 weeks for PLD and only 71.1 weeks for topotecan. Most patients in the topotecan group (90.2%) suffered hematologic toxicity, with most of these cases severe and related to dosage modification, growth factor, or blood product use. PLD toxicities were considered to be mild to moderate.

Conclusion.—PLD and topotecan were shown to be equally efficacious for recurrent ovarian carcinoma. Subgroup differences were noted, showing PLD was more effective in platinum-sensitive patients and topotecan of greater efficacy among patients who were platinum-resistant. Safety factors were comparable between the 2 agents.

▶ Most patients with advanced ovarian cancer treated by aggressive debulking surgery followed by platin and taxane-based chemotherapy will respond to that treatment.Unfortunately, most of those patients will suffer relapse of that cancer. Thus, the question of what is the best salvage therapy is an important one. While the response rates were similar, there was an advantage for PLD in terms of toxicity, progression-free interval, and survival. Since most of the "platinum sensitive" patients were probably retreated with a platin when they progressed on study, PLD more than topotecan appears to increase the "platinum-free interval."[1] The role of both of these agents in first-line therapy is currently being evaluated in a large, randomized trial—Gynecologic Oncology Group No. 182.

D. S. Miller, MD

Reference

1. Bookman MA: Extending the platinum-free interval in recurrent ovarian cancer: The role of topotecan in second-line chemotherapy. *Oncologist* 4:87, 1999.

Results of Reinduction Therapy With Paclitaxel and Carboplatin in Recurrent Epithelial Ovarian Cancer
Gronlund B, Høgdall C, Hansen HH, et al (Univ of Copenhagen)
Gynecol Oncol 83:128-134, 2001   25–9

Introduction.—Epithelial ovarian cancer is the most deadly malignant disease of the female genital tract. Most patients with advanced disease will relapse and die of chemoresistant disease, even in the presence of high sensitivity to chemotherapy. There are few data concerning the issue of retreatment therapy with paclitaxel and carboplatin in relapsing patients who were previously treated with paclitaxel and a platinum analogue. The treatment results and toxicity of a re-treatment regimen of paclitaxel and carboplatin were assessed in patients with ovarian cancer relapse.

Methods.—A retrospective review was conducted of 241 consecutive patients with primary epithelial ovarian cancer who received paclitaxel and a platinum analogue as a first-line treatment. Relapse treatment of platinum-sensitive patients included paclitaxel 175 mg/m^2 over 3 hours followed by carboplatin at an area under the concentration-time curve of 5, repeated every 3 weeks.

Results.—Forty-three patients with relapse received paclitaxel and carboplatin at a median progression-free interval from completion of first-line chemotherapy of 15.8 months (range, 6.0-41.7 months). For patients with evaluable disease, the overall response rate was 84% (95% CI, 68.0-93.8%). Progression-free survival from start of relapse treatment was a median of 9.7 months (range, 1.4-26.9 months); overall survival from start of relapse treatment was 13.1 months (range, 4.5-35.5 months). The independent prognostic factors for progression-free survival after first relapse were determined by multivariate Cox analysis and included response to relapse treatment ($P = .002$; hazard ratio, 13.9) and time to first recurrence ($P = .016$; hazard ratio, 0.167). The planned treatment was accomplished by 9.3% of the cohort. Thirty percent of the patients experienced grade 1-2 peripheral neuropathy. The paclitaxel dose was attenuated because of a grade 4 neutrocytopenia in 1 patient.

Conclusion.—Retreatment with paclitaxel and carboplatin in patients with platinum-sensitive epithelial ovarian cancer relapse resulted in a high response rate and encouraging progression-free survival and overall survival rates. This treatment strategy is generally well tolerated, and the toxicity is manageable.

▶ When ovarian cancer recurs after treatment with first-line platin and taxane chemotherapy, it has become the practice of many oncologists to retreat the patient with 1 or more of the agents the patient had previously received. This practice has evolved with limited data to support it.[1] The reader should note that although the response rates in this study and that by Rose were quite high, the progression-free interval was only modestly better and the survival rate was inferior to that seen in the liposomal doxorubicin versus topotecan trial.[2] The obvious conclusion from this is that reinduction therapy does not address the platin- and taxane-resistant cells, which can be treated only by a new agent that could be incorporated into the reinduction regimen or follow shortly thereafter.

D. S. Miller, MD

References

1. Rose PG, Fusco N, Fluellen L, et al: Second-line therapy with paclitaxel and carboplatin for recurrent disease following first-line therapy with paclitaxel and platinum in ovarian or peritoneal carcinoma. *J Clin Oncol* 16:1494, 1998.
2. Gordon AN, Fleagle JT, Guthrie D, et al: Recurrent epithelial ovarian carcinoma: A randomized phase III study of pegylated liposomal doxorubicin versus topotecan. *J Clin Oncol* 19:3312, 2001.

Randomized Controlled Trial of Single-Agent Paclitaxel Versus Cyclophosphamide, Doxorubicin, and Cisplatin in Patients With Recurrent Ovarian Cancer Who Responded to First-Line Platinum-Based Regimens
Cantù MG, Buda A, Parma G, et al (Università degli Studi di Milano-Bicocca, Monza, Italy; Istituto di Ricerche Farmacologiche "Mario Negri," Italy; European Inst of Oncology, Milan, Italy)
J Clin Oncol 20:1232-1237, 2002   25–10

Background.—Ovarian cancer is the fifth leading cause of death from cancer among European women and is the leading cause of death among women with gynecologic malignancies. Often it is diagnosed in the advanced phase (stage III or IV), and patients in these stages have a generally poor prognosis, despite activity by chemotherapy agents. As many as 80% of patients achieve an objective response with platinum-containing regimens, but 40% of patients relapse or have disease progression within 12 months. This percentage decreases to 20% after 12 months have passed since the end of first-line chemotherapy. These patients can be rechallenged with the same agent, but there is no consensus second-line treatment. Secondary responses to chemotherapeutic agents by patients with previous tumor regression in response to the same or similar drugs have been described in a number of malignancies other than ovarian cancer, including Hodgkin disease and small-cell lung cancer. Paclitaxel is active against recurring and platinum-resistant ovarian cancer and is well tolerated by most patients. The activity, efficacy, and tolerability of single-agent paclitaxel and a platinum-containing regimen were assessed in previously treated patients with recurrent ovarian cancer.

Methods.—Patients who experienced complete remission with platinum-based regimens and whose disease recurred after a progression-free interval of more than 12 months were studied. Patients received paclitaxel, 175 mg/m^2 intravenously over 3 hours, or a combination of cyclophosphamide 500 mg/m^2, doxorubicin 50 mg/m^2, and cisplatin 50 mg/m^2 (CAP) intravenously.

Results.—A total of 97 consecutive patients were enrolled from June 1992 to May 1995. The paclitaxel group comprised 50 patients, and the CAP group included 47 patients. The median number of cycles for each arm was 6. Toxicities included grade 3/4 leukopenia (4% for paclitaxel vs 34% for CAP), grade 3/4 neutropenia (13% vs 36%), grade 1/2 myalgia (19% vs 4%), allergic reactions (15% vs 2%), and grade 2/3 nausea and vomiting (17% vs 51%). Among the paclitaxel group, complete responses were achieved in 17% of patients, whereas 30% of patients receiving CAP achieved complete responses. Partial responses were obtained in 28% of paclitaxel patients and 25% of CAP patients. At a median follow-up of 49 months, the median progression-free intervals were 9 months for paclitaxel and 15.7 months for CAP. The median overall survival time was 25.8 months for paclitaxel and 34.7 months for CAP.

Conclusions.—In previously treated patients with recurrent ovarian cancer, rechallenge with either single-agent paclitaxel or platinum-based chemotherapy is effective. However, the findings suggest that single-agent pacli-taxel may not be as active as platinum-based chemotherapy in these patients.

▶ Since most patients with advanced ovarian cancer will respond to platinum-based chemotherapy and most of these cancers will then recur, the issue of what is the best second-line therapy is pertinent. Though the study is under-powered, it does appear that there was an advantage for retreatment of "platinum-sensitive" patients with platinum. It does not give us any informa-tion as to whether extending the platinum-free interval by using a nonplatinum agent is of any advantage to the patient. The whole concept of "platinum sen-sitivity" is misleading. If a patient's cancer was truly "platinum sensitive," the cancer would not recur. Those are the truly "platinum sensitive" patients. The patients we usually call "platinum sensitive" are, in fact, patients who proba-bly have few platinum-resistant cells. When the platinum chemotherapy is stopped, the platinum resistant cells regrow. Since they are no longer being suppressed by platinum, they no longer maintain the metabolic mechanisms of platinum resistance. However, laboratory studies as well as clinical experi-ence show that many of these cells retain in their genetic makeup the capabil-ity to reexpress platinum resistance. Thus, although many patients will re-spond to retreatment and those responses may be durable, all of them eventually fail. The issue really is what to do about these platinum-resistant cells. Clearly, further studies should be devoted to some sort of consolidation therapy after platinum response in an effort to eliminate all the cancer cells.[1]

D. S. Miller, MD

Reference

1. Rothenberg ML, Liu PY, Wilczynski S, et al: Phase II trial of oral altretamine for consolidation of clinical complete remission in women with stage III epithelial ovarian cancer: A Southwest Oncology Group Trial (SWOG-9326). *Gynecol On-col* 82:317, 2001.

In Vivo **Molecular Chemotherapy and Noninvasive Imaging With an Infectivity-Enhanced Adenovirus**
Hemminki A, Zinn KR, Liu B, et al (Univ of Alabama, Birmingham)
J Natl Cancer Inst 94:741-749, 2002   25–11

Background.—Although adenovirus-based gene therapy is a promising approach to cancer treatment, many primary cells lack the requisite coxsackie-adenovirus receptor (CAR), which limits the efficacy of gene ther-apy in vivo. Recent developments include a modified adenovirus that does not depend on CAR expression for infectivity. Noninvasive imaging was used to investigate the in vivo antitumor efficacy of gene therapy using this adenovirus in an animal model of ovarian cancer.

Methods.—Using highly aggressive SKOV3.ip1 cells, subcutaneous or peritoneal human xenograft ovarian cancers were established in immune-deficient mice. Adenoviral constructs were infected every day for 3 days intratumorally or intraperitoneally. Control mice were injected with a CAR-dependent adenoviral vector that included a luciferase marker gene. A somastatin analog was used for in vivo imaging of RGDTKSSTR injected into subcutaneous tumors. CAR-independent RGDTKSSTR and CAR-dependent AdTKSSTR express herpes simplex virus thymidine kinase (TK) for molecular chemotherapy and the human somastatin receptor subtype 2 (SSTR) for noninvasive nuclear imaging.

Findings.—Tumor-related RGDTKSSTR was detected 15 days after the vector was introduced. In the intraperitoneal model, mice treated with RGDTKSSTR had a longer survival rate than those treated with AdTKSSTR.

Conclusions.—The adenoviral vector RGDTKSSTR has antitumor efficacy against ovarian cancer in vivo in animal models. The virus, which can be imaged noninvasively, may be useful in the treatment of ovarian cancer.

▶ As more of the molecular genetics of carcinogenesis, progression, metastasis, and death are identified, potential targets may be found for gene therapy. Unfortunately, technical difficulties have hampered scientists from simply deleting oncogenes or repairing or replacing defective tumor suppressor genes in cancers.[1] The main challenge has been selecting the appropriate vector that can deliver the therapeutic gene to the cancer cells. This is usually accomplished with a virus such as the adenovirus used in this study, which was specially modified to facilitate its entry into cancer cells. The other challenge has been selecting the appropriate gene because it is often not sufficient simply to affect one step involved in the multistep process of carcinogenesis.[2] In this study a suicide gene was inserted that made the cancer cells susceptible to another drug. The authors have addressed many of these challenges in this study and present encouraging work.[3] However, much remains to be done before gene therapy becomes a standard part of cancer therapy.

D. S. Miller, MD

References

1. von Gruenigen VE, O'Boyle JD, Coleman RL, et al: Efficacy of intraperitoneal adenovirus-mediated p53 gene therapy in ovarian cancer. *Int J Gynecol Cancer* 9:365-372, 1999.
2. Muller CY, Coleman RL, Rogers P, et al: Phase I intraperitoneal adenoviral p53 gene transfer in ovarian cancer. 37th Annual Meeting of the American Society of Clinical Oncology, San Francisco, May 12-15, 2001.
3. Russell W: Adenovirus gene therapy for ovarian cancer (editorial). *J Natl Cancer Inst* 94:706, 2002.

Survivorship

"What Doesn't Kill You Makes You Stronger": An Ovarian Cancer Survivor Survey

Stewart DE, Wong F, Duff S, et al (Univ of Toronto; *CONVERSATIONS!* The Internatl Newsletter for Those Fighting Ovarian Cancer)
Gynecol Oncol 83:537-542, 2001   25–12

Background.—Advances in treatment have enabled more women to survive ovarian cancer with no recurrence for 2 years or more. A survey was conducted to investigate the physical health and quality of life of women surviving ovarian cancer with no known active disease and receiving no treatment.

Methods.—Two hundred women in Canada and the United States responded to a survey. This represented a response rate of 67.5%. The mean age was 55.3 years. Ovarian cancer diagnosis had been established a mean 7.2 years earlier. Seventy-three percent of the respondents had children.

Findings.—Eighty-nine percent of the women considered their health to be good or excellent. However, 53.5% had current pain or discomfort. Compared with the general population, they reported better mental health and equivalent energy levels. Fifty-seven percent reported that their sex lives had been adversely affected by cancer and its treatment. However, their overall sense of loss about sexual functioning appeared to be moderate to low. Women younger than 55 years reported a greater sense of loss related to sexual function and fertility. Younger age and being in a stable relationship were the only 2 reliable predictors of the effects of cancer on sexuality. Women receiving radiation therapy had more frequent or severe sexual symptoms. Most women said that their experience with cancer had changed their views on life and relationships in an overwhelmingly positive way.

Conclusions.—Despite the presence of some symptoms, most survivors of ovarian cancer appear to enjoy good physical, psychological, social, and spiritual health. Specific concerns about the impact of the disease and its treatment on sexuality should be addressed in patient education. The current findings may be useful when counseling newly diagnosed women.

▶ One of the things I have most enjoyed about gynecologic oncology are the patients. Many of them have clarity of vision and a sense of purpose to life that I have presumed comes from figuratively looking down the barrel of a gun and living to tell about it. The title of this article is a platitude that I frequently use in response to the complaints of some about irksome tasks they must do or a heavy burden they must bear. It is not something I have heretofore said to patients. But, as the authors of this study show, it appears quite applicable. Despite the fact that as a consequence of their disease and/or its treatment, most have become menopausal, have ongoing pain or discomfort, have a decrease in their sexual functioning and memory, most of the patients reported that having ovarian cancer and undergoing treatment had changed their views on life in an overwhelmingly positive way, especially with respect to their relationships with family, friends, and others and their role performance as mother, partner, working woman, or caregiver.

D. S. Miller, MD

Communication About Sexual Problems and Sexual Concerns in Ovarian Cancer: Qualitative Study
Stead ML, Fallowfield L, Brown JM, et al (Northern and Yorkshire Clinical Trials and Reserarch Unit, Leeds, England; Univ of Sussex, Brighton, England; St James's Univ Hosp, Leeds, England)
BMJ 323:836-837, 2001   25–13

Objective.—Although treatment of gynecologic cancers affects sexual activity, communication about these consequences is poor. A qualitative study of the psychosexual impact of ovarian cancer and the level of communication between women and health care professionals was explored.

Methods.—Fifteen women, aged 42 to 71 years, with ovarian cancer, who were identified as sexually active or inactive because of their disease, participated in a detailed interview regarding their current sexual behavior and response, their satisfaction with their sex life, and the importance of sex. Semistructured interviews were conducted with 43 clinicians and nurses concerning their attitudes and communications regarding the sexual impact of ovarian cancer treatment on their patients.

Results.—Although patients felt that the medical staff should have discussed psychosexual issues with them and provided written information, no patient received written information and only 2 patients discussed the topic briefly. Women felt that they needed reassurance about a variety of psychosexual issues and permission to discuss concerns. All but 1 clinician felt that the staff should talk about psychosexual issues, but only 4 clinicians and 5 nurses did so, and few were aware of the functional problems that can arise.

Conclusion.—There is a lack of awareness among medical staff of the psychosexual problems facing women with ovarian cancer. Oral and written communication with patients about psychosexual functioning after treatment for ovarian cancer is inadequate.

▶ This study plainly shows that while our media may be focused heavily on sex and many are thinking about it, sexual problems are not being dealt with. Patients with ovarian cancer would like to talk to their health care providers about their sexual problems, but don't. Health care providers think that they should talk about patients' sexual problems, but don't. The sexual problems of these patients are not complex and can usually be solved, if they are addressed.

D. S. Miller, MD

26 Uterine Malignancies

Localized Endometrial Cancer

Simultaneously Detected Endometrial and Ovarian Carcinomas—A Prospective Clinicopathologic Study of 74 Cases: A Gynecologic Oncology Group Study
Zaino R, Whitney C, Brady MF, et al (Pennsylvania State Univ, Hershey; Thomas Jefferson Univ, Philadelphia; Roswell Park Cancer Inst, Buffalo, NY; et al)
Gynecol Oncol 83:355-362, 2001   26–1

Background.—About 10% of women with ovarian carcinoma have carcinomas coexisting in the endometrium and ovary. Often it is unclear whether this finding represents synchronous primary tumors or metastasis from endometrium to ovary or from ovary to endometrium. Thus, staging, therapy, and expected outcome in these patients are uncertain. Findings of the Gynecologic Oncology Group's study of patients with simultaneously detected adenocarcinomas in the endometrium and ovary with disease grossly confined to the pelvis were reported. The possible correlation among discrete tumor subsets, natural history, and survival was investigated.

Methods.—From 1985 to 1991, a total of 85 patients were prospectively enrolled. Of these patients, 74 were eligible for participation. All the patients were treated first with total abdominal hysterectomy, bilateral salpingo-oophorectomy, and staging laparotomy. Radiation therapy and chemotherapy were performed at the discretion of the treating physician and the patient. Differences in tumor behavior were identified by analysis of 15 pathologic variables.

Results.—Among the 74 patients, 23 (31%) had microscopic spread of tumor in the pelvis or abdomen. Sixty-four patients (86%) had endometrioid carcinomas in both the endometrium and the ovary, and endometriosis was found in the ovary of 23 patients (31%). Concordance between the histologic grade of the tumor in the ovary and the uterus occurred in 51 patients (69%). The probability of recurrence at 5 years after staging surgery is estimated to be 15.1%. Two groups of patients with different probabilities of recurrence within 5 years were identified by the presence of metastasis. The 5-year probability of recurrence was 10% for patients with tumors confined to the uterus and ovary, compared with 27.1% for patients with metastasis. The histologic grades of ovarian and uterine tumors also differentiated groups of patients with different probabilities of recurrence at 5 years. Patients with no more than grade 1 disease at either site had a 5-year probability of recurrence of 8%, whereas those with a higher grade in either the endometrium or the ovary had a 5-year probability of recurrence of 22.4% at either site. The overall probability of survival at 5 years is estimated at 85.9%; the estimated survival at 10 years is 80.3%.

Conclusions.—Women with simultaneously detected carcinomas in the uterus and ovary, with gross disease confined to the pelvis, have a surprisingly good prognosis. This is particularly true when the disease is microscopically limited to the uterus and ovary or has a low histologic grade.

▶ It would be expected that an adenocarcinoma found both in the endometrium and the ovary would represent the metastasis of one from the other. This study and others have shown that in most cases, these appear to be concomitant separate primary tumors. Interestingly, molecular studies have not confirmed this. Fortunately, the outcome for most of these patients is good, and the mortality rate of having 2 cancers does not appear to be additive. Unfortunately, the most interesting questions are not answered by this study. The fact that 2 cancers arise at roughly the same time usually confined to their organ of origin certainly implies a common molecular genetic pathway that should be identifiable. It also implies a germ line as opposed to a somatic cell mutation. Otherwise you would expect the occurrence of this to be quite rare. Therefore, are these patients at high risk for subsequent malignancies of some other type? We have devoted much attention to families of patients who develop the same tumor type, but what are the genetics of the patient who develops multiple tumors, and is there something to be learned there?

D. S. Miller, MD

Reference

1. Lin WM, Forgacs E, Warshal DP, et al: Loss of heterozygosity and mutational analysis of the PTEN/MMAC1 gene in synchronous endometrial and ovarian carcinoma. *Clin Cancer Res* 4:2577, 1998.

Conservative Management of Stage I Endometrial Carcinoma After Surgical Staging
Straughn JM Jr, Huh WK, Kelly FJ, et al (Univ of Alabama, Birmingham)
Gynecol Oncol 84:194-200, 2002   26–2

Background.—More than three fourths of women diagnosed as having endometrial cancer have early-stage disease. The outcomes of patients with stage I endometrial carcinoma managed without adjuvant radiation after comprehensive surgical staging were reported.

Methods.—A review of the charts of patients diagnosed as having endometrial adenocarcinoma from 1993 to 1998 identified 864 women who had primary surgery. A total of 670 of these women had comprehensive surgical staging with total hysterectomy, bilateral salpingo-oophorectomy, pelvic or para-aortic lymphadenectomy, and peritoneal cytology. Fifty-seven patients with high-risk histologic subtypes were excluded, leaving 613 patients for the final analysis.

Findings.—Ninety-nine percent of patients with stage IB disease did not receive adjuvant radiation. In this group, the recurrence rate was 5%. Nine of the 15 recurrences were in the pelvis or vagina. All 9 were salvaged with whole pelvic radiation and brachytherapy. Of the 77 patients with stage 1C disease, 69% received no adjuvant treatment. In this group, the recurrence rate was 8%. Two of the 4 recurrences were in the vagina. Salvage was successful in 3 of the 4 patients, 2 with whole pelvic radiation and brachytherapy and 1 with surgery and chemotherapy. Among all patients with stage I disease, 5-year disease-free survival rate was 93%. Overall 5-year survival rate was 98%.

Conclusions.—The risk of recurrence in surgically staged patients with endometrial carcinoma limited to the uterine corpus is small. Most of these recurrences can be salvaged with radiation therapy. Conservative management of stage I endometrial carcinoma is effective.

▶ Most patients with endometrial cancer will do quite fine with the removal of the uterus, fallopian tubes, and ovaries. However, a small but significant percentage of them will have occult metastases that doom them to recurrence. Because of this, thorough surgical staging usually involving pelvic and periaortic lymph node sampling as well as peritoneal cytology with or without omentectomy has been advocated by my gynecologic oncology colleagues and incorporated into the International Federation of Gynecology and Obstetrics staging system. The justification has been that surgical staging will identify those patients with occult advanced disease who might be treated by radiation therapy as well as correctly identify those patients who do not have disease spread beyond the uterus who should not require radiation therapy. Yet many patients still receive postoperative radiation therapy. The published results of the PORTEC study show minimal, if any, survival advantage for patients who have not been surgically staged.[1] Likewise, the presented but not yet published results of the Gynecologic Oncology Group trial, #99, show no survival advantage for adjuvant radiation in patients who are surgically staged.[2] The study presented here is the authors' retrospective experience of putting gynecologic oncology surgical staging philosophy into action in that the vast majority of their surgically staged patients did not receive radiation therapy. They did very well. The few patients who did receive radiation, for reasons not well described, did not do significantly better stage for stage. Encouragingly, most of the patients who had recurrence after surgical staging alone were successfully treated with radiation therapy. Clearly too many patients with endometrial cancer, whether they are surgically staged or not, receive radiation therapy. Unfortunately, we have yet to identify clearly who, if anyone, might benefit. Some should given the small but real risk of recurrence.

D. S. Miller, MD

References

1. Creutzberg CL, van Putten WL, Koper P, et al: Surgery and post-operative radio-therapy versus surgery alone for patients with stage 1 endometrial carcinoma: Multicentre randomized trial. *Lancet* 355:1404-1411, 2000.
2. Roberts JA, Brunetto VL, Keys HM, et al: A phase III randomized study of surgery vs surgery plus adjunctive radiation therapy in intermediate-risk endometrial adenocarcinoma. *Gynecol Oncol* 68:135, 1998.

The Morbidity of Treatment for Patients With Stage I Endometrial Cancer: Results From a Randomized Trial
Creutzberg CL, for the PORTEC Study Group (Univ Hosp Rotterdam, The Netherlands; et al)
Int J Radiat Oncol Biol Phys 51:1246-1255, 2001   26–3

Background.—The most common gynecologic cancer is endometrial carcinoma. A recent prospective multicenter randomized study was performed to determine the role of postoperative pelvic radiation therapy (RT) in patients with stage I endometrial carcinoma. The treatment complications associated with surgery plus RT were compared with those associated with surgery alone.

Methods.—Patients had endometrial cancer limited to the uterine corpus, grade 1 or 2 with more than 50% myometrial invasion or grade 2 or 3 with less than 50% myometrial invasion. Surgical treatment consisted of abdominal hysterectomy and oophorectomy without lymphadectomy. Postoperatively, patients were randomly assigned to pelvic RT, 46 Gy, or to no further treatment. Seven hundred fifteen patients were randomly assigned. The median follow-up was 60 months.

Results.—Six hundred ninety-one patients were evaluable. The 5-year actuarial rates of late complications, grades 1 to 4, were 26% in the group receiving RT and 4% in those receiving no RT. Most complications were grade 1, the 5-year rates being 17% in the RT group and 4% in the control group. All severe complications, grades 3 and 4, occurred in the RT group, with a rate of 3%. Most complications affected the gastrointestinal tract. After some years, half the patients had symptom resolution. Grades 1 and 2 genitourinary complications occurred in 8% of RT recipients and in 4% of non-recipients. Bone complications occurred in 1% of patients undergoing RT. Two percent of patients quit RT because of acute treatment-related symptoms. The risk of late RT complications was increased in patients with acute morbidity. A lower risk of late complications correlated with the 4-field box technique.

Conclusions.—Pelvic RT increases treatment-related morbidity in patients with stage I endometrial cancer. Severe complications occurred in 3% of treated patients. More than 20% had mild symptoms. Because pelvic RT in stage I endometrial carcinoma significantly decreased locoregional recurrence rate without significantly improving survival, its use in the adjuvant setting should be carefully considered, with judicious patient selection.

▶ Many patients receive RT after surgical treatment of endometrial cancer, but few benefit from it.[1] The authors provide us with some numbers that will be helpful in counseling patients. Their previous study showed that pelvic radiation decreased 5-year local recurrence from 14% to 4% but had no effect on overall survival.[2] Seventy-nine percent of the patients in the observation arm who had recurrence were salvaged with RT. Thus, 79% of the 14% of surgery-only patients who had recurrence is 11% of the total, leaving a recurrence-free benefit of only 3%, but no survival benefit. Interestingly, 3% was also the proportion of patients in the radiation arm who had severe complications. We still await the final results of Gynecologic Oncology Group Study #99, which can give us some of this information in patients who are surgically staged.

D. S. Miller, MD

References

1. Straughn JM, Huh WK, Kelly FJ, et al: Conservative management of stage I endometrial carcinoma after surgical staging. *Gynecol Oncol* 84:194-200, 2002.
2. Creutzberg CL, van Putten WL, Koper P, et al: Surgery and post-operative radiotherapy versus surgery alone for patients with stage 1 endometrial carcinoma: Multicentre randomized trial. *Lancet* 355:1404-1411, 2000.

Chemotherapy

Phase II Trial of the Pegylated Liposomal Doxorubicin in Previously Treated Metastatic Endometrial Cancer: A Gynecologic Oncology Group Study

Muggia FM, Blessing JA, Sorosky J, et al (New York Univ; Roswell Park Cancer Inst, Buffalo, NY; Univ of Iowa, Iowa City; et al)
J Clin Oncol 20:2360-2364, 2002   26–4

Background.—Patients with endometrial cancer sometimes have advanced disease and distant metastases on initial diagnosis. The success of treatment is limited in these cases, with cytotoxic agents being one of the more recent therapy additions. The Gynecologic Oncology Group (GOG) has found doxorubicin to be more useful in endometrial cancer when combined with cisplatin than when used alone. The effectiveness of another cytotoxic agent, paclitaxel, also has been compared with that of doxorubicin. A significantly different pharmacologic profile and spectrum of toxicity are linked to pegylated liposomal doxorubicin (PLD) when compared with doxorubicin itself. PLD was investigated to see whether it has antitumor activity in patients with persistent or recurrent endometrial carcinoma who have failed previous treatment. The nature of PLD and its toxicity also were assessed.

Methods.—The 42 patients ranged in age from 40 to 79 (median, 62.5); all had recurrent or persistent measurable endometrial carcinoma and had failed 1 previous treatment. Intravenous PLD was given over a 1-hour period in a dose of 50 mg/m^2 every 4 weeks. When toxic reactions occurred, the dose was adjusted accordingly.

Results.—Patients received 1 to 14 courses of PLD; 4 of them (9.5%) achieved a partial response that lasted from 1.1 to 5.4 months. Three of the responding patients had received doxorubicin previously; the fourth had been treated with nondoxorubicin combination chemotherapy. The 95% CI for the true response rate ranged from 2.7% to 22.6%. The disease remained stable over at least 2 cycles in 29% of the patients, and median survival overall was 8.2 months. Brain metastases developed in 4 patients and vertebral metastases in 4 patients, with 2 of these exhibiting neurologic complications. Five patients received additional chemotherapy, and 1 who received paclitaxel achieved stable disease. Adverse effects were generally mild and usually involved the hematologic, pulmonary, neurologic, and dermatologic systems, with rare severe gastrointestinal effects. Six patients required that the doses be reduced, 7 discontinued use because of side effects, and 2 ceased participation for no clear reason.

Conclusions.—Only limited success was achieved in these patients using PLD. Its usefulness also should be assessed among patients who have not undergone previous treatment and in anthracycline-naive patients. The toxicity attending its use was minimal.

▶ Doxorubicin along with cisplatin and paclitaxel are active against advanced or recurrent endometrial cancer. Recently, doxorubicin has been repackaged in a pegylated liposome, which alters its toxicity with a decrease in cardiac and myelotoxicity but an increase in cutaneous reactions. It was expected that its activity against various tumors would be similar. Thus, the GOG tested it against endometrial cancer in patients who had previously failed other chemotherapy. Many of these patients had previously received unpegylated doxorubicin. The PLD was reasonably well tolerated and demonstrated moderate activity. This should allow its substitution for doxorubicin in combination therapy for endometrial cancer.

D. S. Miller, MD

Paclitaxel in the Treatment of Carcinosarcoma of the Uterus: A Gynecologic Oncology Group Study
Curtin JP, Blessing JA, Soper JT, et al (Cornell Univ, New York; Roswell Park Canc Inst, Buffalo, NY; Duke Univ, Durham, NC; et al)
Gynecol Oncol 83:268-270, 2001   26–5

Introduction.—Carcinosarcoma (mixed mesodermal tumor) of the uterus is characterized by a high rate of advanced stage at diagnosis and high recurrence rates after local therapy. Paclitaxel is reported to have a relatively high rate of response to tumors with demonstrated resistance to previous chemotherapy. A phase II trial of paclitaxel was performed by the Gynecologic Oncology Group (GOG) in 53 patients with persistent or recurrent carcinosarcoma of the uterus in whom other treatments had failed.

Methods.—After receiving a pretreatment regimen designed to abrogate allergic reactions to paclitaxel, 53 patients with histologic verification of carcinoma and measurable disease in whom appropriate local therapy had failed received 170 mg/m² paclitaxel (135 mg/m² in patients who received prior irradiation) intravenously every 3 weeks.

Results.—Of 53 patients who entered the trial between September 1994 and January 1997, 44 were evaluable for response. Median patient age was 65 years (range, 38-79 years). Twenty-six and 18 patients, respectively, had heterologous mixed mesodermal tumors and homologous tumors. Patients received a median of 3 courses (range, 1-18 courses). Fifteen patients had undergone previous radiation treatment, and in 33 prior chemotherapy had failed. Of 8 patients (18.2%) with a response to paclitaxel, 4 had a complete response and 4 had a partial response. The most frequent toxic effect was neutropenia.

Conclusion.—There was a moderate 18% total response rate to paclitaxel in patients with persistent or recurrent carcinosarcoma of the uterus in whom other treatments had failed.

▶ Carcinosarcoma, also known as malignant mixed mesodermal tumor (MMMT), is the most common uterine sarcoma, which accounts for only 2% to 3% of uterine malignancies. Unlike uterine carcinomas, carcinosarcomas are often already metastatic at the time of surgery or usually recur. Thus, the issue of salvage chemotherapy is pertinent. The active drugs identified by the GOG include adriamycin, ifosfamide, and cisplatin. To this modest list we can now add paclitaxel. Accordingly, paclitaxel has now been incorporated into the experimental arm of an ongoing phase III trial by the GOG study #161 comparing ifosfamide with or without paclitaxel in patients with advanced or recurrent carcinosarcoma.

D. S. Miller, MD

27 Cervical Cancer

Risk Factors

Advancing Age and Cervical Cancer Screening and Prognosis
Sawaya GF, Sung H-Y, Kearney KA, et al (Univ of California, San Francisco; Kaiser Permanente Med Care Program, Oakland, Calif; Kaiser Permanente Med Care Program, Sacramento, Calif; et al)
J Am Geriatr Soc 49:1499-1504, 2001   27–1

Background.—Half of all invasive cervical cancer (ICC) cases in the United States occur in women who have never had a cervical smear. Case series have reported that never-screened women tend to be elderly. The relation of advancing age and screening behavior with prognosis in patients with ICC was investigated.

Methods.—The case series included long-term members of a prepaid health plan. The medical records of 455 women were reviewed for age, stage at diagnosis, tumor histology, and results of and reasons for previous cervical smears.

Findings.—Compared with younger women, those in older age groups were less likely to have had screening within the 3 years preceding diagnosis of ICC. Noncompliance with follow-up of abnormal findings was uncommon and unassociated with age. The proportions of ICC that were interval cancers (ICC diagnosed within 3 years of a negative screening smear) were highest in women younger than 30 years. Multivariate analyses adjusting for stage at diagnosis demonstrated that women aged 60 and older were not more likely to die of ICC within 3 years of diagnosis than were women younger than 60 years.

Conclusions.—Although older women were more likely than younger women to die of ICC within 3 years of diagnosis, this appears to be because of their higher likelihood of having advanced stage disease at diagnosis. There is no evidence that older women with cervical cancer are more likely to be diagnosed with an interval cancer than were younger women.

▶ In the United States and other developed countries, most cervical cancers occur in women who have never or infrequently been screened. Women who have never been screened are more likely to be older. Younger women usually undergo screening as part of prenatal or contraceptive care. However, when these services are no longer required by the patient, particularly if she is without third-party coverage, she may not seek or receive Pap smear screening. This study showed that older women were less likely to have been screened recently and were more likely to have advanced cervical cancer. Although there is little advantage to annual Pap smears in postmenopausal patients who have previously been well screened, this study and others have clearly shown that a significant number of elderly and aged women have not been well screened and would benefit from a Pap smear.

D. S. Miller, MD

Male Circumcision, Penile Human Papillomavirus Infection, and Cervical Cancer in Female Partners

Castellsagué X, for the International Agency for Research on Cancer Multicenter Cervical Cancer Study Group (Institut Català d'Oncologia, Barcelona; et al)
N Engl J Med 346:1105-1112, 2002   27–2

Introduction.—During the past 15 years, the International Agency for Research on Cancer has performed several large case-control investigations of cervical cancer in various countries. Data were used from these investigations to evaluate the effect of male circumcision on the risk of genital human papillomavirus (HPV) infection in males themselves and the risk of cervical cancer in their female sexual partners.

Methods.—Data were used from 1913 couples from 5 countries enrolled in 1 of the 7 case-control investigations of cervical cancer in situ and cervical cancer. The status of circumcision was self-reported. Accuracy of data were verified by physical examination at 3 trial sites. The presence or absence of penile HPV DNA was examined by a polymerase chain reaction assay in 1520 males and yielded a valid result in 1139 males (74.9%).

Results.—Penile HPV was identified in 166 of 847 uncircumcised males (19.6%) and in 16 of 292 circumcised males (5.5%). After adjusting for age at first intercourse, lifetime number of sexual partners, and other potential confounders, circumcised males were less likely than uncircumcised males to have HPV infection (odds ratio [OR], 0.37; 95% CI, 0.16-0.85). Monogamous females whose male partners had 6 or more sexual partners and were circumcised were at lower risk of cervical cancer than were females whose partners were uncircumcised (adjusted OR, 0.42; 95% CI, 0.23-0.79). Findings were similar in the subgroup of males in whom circumcision was verified by medical examination.

Conclusion.—Male circumcision is correlated with a decreased risk of penile HPV infection. In males with a history of multiple sexual partners, circumcision decreased the risk of cervical cancer in their current female sexual partners.

▶ Since antiquity, circumcision of the newborn baby boy has been a part of the religious traditions of several cultures. For decades our pediatric colleagues have been telling us that there is no medical benefit to circumcising.

This study shows that perhaps our ancestors were wiser than we thought. Although there may be minimal advantage to the male, the risk of penile HPV infection was less and circumcision reduced the risk of cervical cancer in the female partners of promiscuous men. Based merely on the evidence from this study, it is probably premature to change our public health policy in regards to infant circumcision. However, I am reminded of the admonition "those who fail to remember history are doomed to repeat it."

D. S. Miller, MD

Effect of Oral Contraceptives on Risk of Cervical Cancer in Women With Human Papillomavirus Infection: The IARC Multicentric Case-Control Study
Moreno V, for the International Agency for Research On Cancer (IARC) Multicentric Cervical Cancer Study Group (L'Hospitalet de Llobregat, Barcelona; et al)
Lancet 359:1085-1092, 2002   27–3

Background.—Research has shown that oral contraceptive (OC) use appears to increase the risk of cervical cancer. However, the effect of human papillomavirus (HPV), the main cause of cervical cancer, has not been considered. The effects of OC use on cervical cancer risk in women testing positive for HPV DNA were investigated.

Methods.—Data from 8 case-control studies of patients with histologically confirmed invasive cervical carcinoma and from 2 of patients with carcinoma in situ were analyzed. Personal interviews were conducted to obtain information on OC use.

Findings.—Ninety-four percent of 1561 patients with invasive cervical carcinoma, 72% of 292 patients with carcinoma in situ, and 13% of 1916 control subjects were HPV positive. Compared with women who never used OCs, women who had used OCs for less than 5 years did not have an increased cervical cancer risk (odds ratio, 0.73). The odds ratios for OC use of 5 to 9 years and for 10 or more years were 2.82 and 4.03, respectively. These risks did not vary by length of time since first or last use.

Conclusions.—Long-term OC use may be a cofactor that increases cervical carcinoma risk as much as 4-fold in women testing positive for cervical HPV DNA. Efforts should be made to include long-term OC users in cervical screening programs.

▶ This study is another in a recent series that reports to show a relationship between OCs and cervical carcinogenesis. In this report, that association was only seen in HPV-positive patients. But there was no correlation between OCs and HPV positivity. While some confounding factors were controlled, this study does not appear to use appropriate controls, since it is not known whether the non-OC control group were using barrier methods or were not sexually active. Both factors would play a role in the persistence or reinfection with HPV that appears to be required for progression to cervical cancer.

D. S. Miller, MD

Surgery

Laparoscopic Retroperitoneal Lymphadenectomy Followed by Immediate Laparotomy in Women With Cervical Cancer: A Gynecologic Oncology Group Study

Schlaerth JB, Spirtos NM, Carson LF, et al (Women's Cancer Ctr at Pasadena, Calif; Women's Cancer Ctr of Northern California, Palo Alto; Univ of Minnesota, Minneapolis; et al)

Gynecol Oncol 85:81-88, 2002   27–4

Background.—Therapeutic pelvic lymphadenectomy and sampling of pelvic and aortic lymph nodes can reportedly be done by laparoscopy. Whether retroperitoneal lymphadenectomies done by laparoscopy are comparable to those done by laparotomy was investigated.

Methods.—Forty women with stage IA, IB, or IIA cancer of the cervix were studied. Laparoscopy was performed and lymph node removal was attempted immediately before radical abdominal hysterectomy, pelvic lymphadenectomy, and aortic lymph node sampling. The adequacy of lymph node removal was determined by surgeon opinion during laparoscopy, photographic records reviewed by 2 independent observers, inspection of the surgical site at laparotomy, and lymph node count.

Findings.—By all 4 methods of evaluation, bilateral laparoscopic aortic lymph node sampling was judged to be adequate in all patients. Six laparoscopic pelvic lymphadenectomies were judged to be incomplete at laparotomy, 3 of which were also considered incomplete by the independent reviewers. The mean number of right pelvic nodes and left pelvic nodes removed was 16.6 and 15.5, respectively. A mean 6.2 right aortic nodes and 5.9 left aortic nodes were removed.

Conclusions.—These findings suggest that laparoscopic bilateral aortic lymph node sampling is feasible and safe. The adequacy of laparoscopic therapeutic bilateral pelvic lymphadenectomy was problematic but can probably be corrected.

▶ With the wholesale headlong rush to laparoscopy in the 1990s, many reports emerged of various open abdominal procedures that could be accomplished laparoscopically. Fortunately, in some quarters, cooler heads and objective minds prevailed and sought to evaluate this emerging technology trend scientifically. The Gynecologic Oncology Group has taken the lead in applying science to laparoscopy. This group, the study's authors, and most especially the study patients should be saluted for embarking on a protocol that had little advantage to the individual patient. However, the important information was obtained and showed that laparoscopic lymphadenectomy was feasible and potentially comparable to that accomplished by laparotomy.

D. S. Miller, MD

Lymphatic Mapping and Sentinel Node Identification in Patients With Cervix Cancer Undergoing Radical Hysterectomy and Pelvic Lymphadenectomy

Levenback C, Coleman RL, Burke TW, et al (Univ of Texas, Houston; Univ of Texas, Dallas)
J Clin Oncol 20:688-693, 2002   27–5

Background.—Although patients with the most favorable cervical cancer stage, stage IB_1, have positive nodes in about 15% of cases, 80% must undergo lymphadenectomy with its associated adverse events for no benefit. In addition, because the cervix is a midline structure with complex lymphatic drainage, an extensive pelvic dissection is required to ensure that all the lymph nodes are included. Clinical findings do not indicate which nodes are positive. In addition, if nodal status can be determined accurately, node-positive patients can begin chemoradiation and avoid radical pelvic surgery. The feasibility of applying sentinel node identification and lymphatic mapping techniques in patients with invasive cervical cancer was explored. Preoperative lymphoscintigraphy and intraoperative lymphatic mapping were augmented with both blue dye and radiocolloid.

Methods.—Two institutions identified 39 patients (age range, 27 to 70 years; median, 40 years) who had preoperative lymphoscintigraphy and intraoperative lymphatic mapping with blue dye and a handheld gamma probe. Four patients had metastatic disease identified on frozen section analysis of the sentinel node, and avoided radical hysterectomy.

Results.—On the preoperative lymphoscintigrams, 85% of patients had at least 1 sentinel node identified, and 55% had bilateral sentinel nodes localized. The 6 patients for whom a sentinel node could not be identified preoperatively had bilateral hot nodes at operation. At least 1 sentinel node was identified intraoperatively in all 39 patients, and all had a hot sentinel node in the pelvis or para-aortic area on gamma probing. Eighty-seven percent of patients had pelvic or para-aortic sentinel nodes bilaterally or unilaterally. Eighty percent of the sentinel nodes were found in 3 areas: obturator, parametrial, and iliac below the bifurcation of the common iliac artery, with the most common sites being the interiliac and obturator basins. Nine percent of nodes were in the para-aortic area. Eight patients had metastatic disease. Twenty-five positive nodes were removed, 21 of which were sentinel and 4 nonsentinel. One patient had false-negative sentinel nodes. While 4 sentinel nodes had been identified preoperatively, all were hot and blue intraoperatively. Sensitivity was 87.5% and negative predictive value was 97% for the sentinel node.

Conclusions.—The method used identified sentinel nodes in all the patients studied. Preoperative lymphoscintigraphy and intraoperative lymphatic mapping could be used successfully in patients who are scheduled to undergo radical hysterectomy.

▶ Lymphatic mapping and sentinel node evaluation in gynecologic sites has principally been evaluated in patients with carcinoma of the vulva. This

2-center clinical trial of lymphatic mapping of the cervix was conducted to evaluate its potential in cervical cancer. By design, candidates for radical hysterectomy are infrequently found with metastatic lymphatic disease, and no one nodal basin in the pelvis is immune to direct lymphatic drainage. The ambiguity of cervical tumor location in the cervix and its primary draining site was demonstrated in this study which included involvement of the para-aortic nodal basins. Directed molecular evaluation of these nodes by cytokeratin copy count has been suggested as a risk factor of recurrence in otherwise-histologically negative nodes.[1] However, it remains to be seen if the technique can be fine-tuned enough to be generally applicable and if the hypothesis of the sentinel node applies to this tumor site.

D. S. Miller, MD

Reference

1. Van Trappen PO, Gyselman VG, Lowe DG, et al: Molecular quantification and mapping of lymph-node micrometastases in cervical cancer. *Lancet* 357:15-20, 2001.

Effect of Hemodilution on Tissue Perfusion and Blood Coagulation During Radical Hysterectomy

Santoso JT, Hannigan EV, Levine L, et al (Univ of Texas, Galveston)
Gynecol Oncol 82:252-256, 2001   27–6

Introduction.—Radical hysterectomy often necessitates blood transfusion after surgery. Acute normovolemic hemodilution is more cost-effective than intraoperative blood salvage. The safety of hemodilution has not been well examined in patients who undergo radical hysterectomy. The measurement of gastric mucosal pH (pHi) is a sensitive method for detecting hypoperfusion and has been used to identify subclinical shock. The safety of hemodilution on global and splanchnic perfusion and blood coagulation during radical hysterectomy was examined in 16 patients with cervical carcinoma.

Methods.—During surgery, a pulmonary artery catheter and a gastric tonometry catheter were placed. Measurements were taken of global perfusion indices, splanchnic perfusion index, and coagulation tests. Blood was removed before skin incision to obtain a hemoglobin measurement of 8 to 9 g/dL. Measurements were repeated after hemodilution, at completion of surgery, and after retransfusion of blood.

Results.—The mean amount of blood removed was 1 L. Mean blood loss was 0.8 L. Hemodiluted preoperative hemoglobin value was 8.7 g/dL. All of the global perfusion indices, except for arterial pH and oxygen consumption, diminished after hemodilution and recovered with blood retransfusion ($P \le .004$). Splanchnic perfusion and coagulation tests did not vary ($P \le .1$). One patient experienced pulmonary edema.

Conclusion.—Hemodilution during radical hysterectomy in this select cohort did not seem to compromise tissue perfusion or coagulation.

▶ Acute normovolemic hemodilution is a technique that has been applied in other surgical disciplines for patients expected to have significant intraoperative blood loss. It involves removal of red blood cells from the patient in the operating room, before the anticipated blood loss, and then replacement of that blood volume with crystalloid or colloid solutions. After the procedure during which hemodiluted blood loss occurs, the previously removed red cells are then reinfused into the patient. It has been shown in other operations to decrease the requirement for intraoperative and postoperative transfusions. The authors in this study show that hemodilution is technically feasible and that vital organ perfusion does not appear to be compromised as measured by several sophisticated technologies. Because there was not a control group, the authors were not able to determine whether the transfusion rate was decreased or whether the postoperative course was improved. Nonetheless, this technique should be considered in patients undergoing other high-blood-loss procedures in gynecology, such as ovarian cancer tumor debulking and pelvic exenteration.

D. S. Miller, MD

Radiation Therapy

Neoadjuvant Chemotherapy and Radical Surgery Versus Exclusive Radiotherapy in Locally Advanced Squamous Cell Cervical Cancer: Results From the Italian Multicenter Randomized Study

Benedetti-Panici P, Greggi S, Colombo A, et al (Campus Bio-Medico Free Univ, Rome; Catholic Univ, Rome; Regina Elena Inst, Rome; et al)
J Clin Oncol 20:179-188, 2001   27–7

Background.—The long-term outlook for women with locally advanced cervical cancer is grim, and survival among these women has changed little during the past 2 decades. The overall 5-year survival rate among these women is approximately 40% when conventional treatments are used. Neoadjuvant chemotherapy (NACT) followed by radical surgery (RS) has emerged as a possible alternative to conventional radiation therapy in locally advanced cervical carcinoma. The results of a phase 3 trial initiated in 1990 to evaluate the feasibility of this technique in terms of survival and treatment-related mortality were reported.

Methods.—Patients were eligible for this study if they had International Federation of Gynecology and Obstetrics stages IB2 to III squamous cell cervical cancer. Eligible patients received cisplatin-based NACT followed by RS (type III to V radical hysterectomy plus systematic pelvic lymphadenectomy) (arm A) or external-beam radiation therapy (45-50 Gy) followed by brachyradiotherapy (20-30 Gy) (arm B).

Results.—A total of 210 patients were eligible for arm A (NACT plus RS), and 199 patients were eligible for arm B (radiation therapy). Treatment was administered according to protocol in 76% of patients in arm A and 72% of patients in arm B. Adjuvant treatment was administered in 48 patients (29%) who underwent surgery. Both treatments were well tolerated, and there were no treatment-related deaths in either arm. Overall, severe morbidity affected 32% of patients in the chemosurgery arm and 28% of patients in the radiotherapy arm. A 27% severe additional toxicity was considered for the NACT group. The 5-year overall survival and progression-free survival rates were 58.9% and 55.4%, respectively, for arm A (chemosurgery) and 44.5% and 41.3%, respectively, for arm B (radiotherapy). Treatment significantly affected overall survival and progression-free survival.

Conclusions.—A survival benefit appears to be associated with the use of NACT plus RS compared with conventional radiotherapy, but this benefit was found to be significant only for the patients with stages IB2 to IIB2 cervical cancer.

▶ The concept of using chemotherapy to shrink an advanced cervical cancer to a point where surgery can be applied is an appealing one for the gynecologic surgeon, as it is also for patients who often prefer having the cancer removed. This study showed that there was a small but significant progression-free and survival advantage to patients who received preoperative NACT. Limitations to this study temper one's enthusiasm for the approach. First, many of the patients who received NACT followed by RS then also received radiation therapy. Second, the patients randomized to radiation therapy received that modality alone and not the contemporary standard of care, which is radiation with concomitant chemotherapy. The main advantage for the NACT was seen in the stage IB2 and IIB patients, but not in stage III patients. Since the likelihood of lymph node metastasis, as well as distant spread, is higher in patients with stage III tumors than in those with stage I or II, the advantage seen in lower-stage patients was probably because those patients likely had locally advanced but node-negative tumors. Also, since several different chemotherapeutic regimens were used, one cannot determine which was the best and which should be selected for further trials. Nonetheless we await the results of the Gynecologic Oncology Group's study #141 to further evaluate this interesting approach.

D. S. Miller, MD

Phase III Trial Comparing Radical Radiotherapy With and Without Cisplatin Chemotherapy in Patients With Advanced Squamous Cell Cancer of the Cervix

Pearcey R, Brundage M, Drouin P, et al (Univ of Alberta, Edmonton, Canada; Univ of Calgary, Alta, Canada; Queen's Univ, Kingston, Ont, Canada; et al)
J Clin Oncol 20:966-972, 2002   27–8

Background.—Invasive cervical cancer has traditionally been treated by surgery or radiotherapy or, in some patients, by a combination of both. Radiotherapy is the primary modality of treatment for more locally advanced disease with spread beyond the uterus. For these patients, cure rates decrease with advancing stage and tumor bulk. One major reason for treatment failure in many patients is the inability to achieve control over the primary cancer and first-echelon lymph node metastases. The local control rate can be increased by increasing the dose of radiotherapy, but this strategy also increases the complication rate. It was hypothesized that cisplatin administered concurrently with standard radiotherapy would improve pelvic control and survival in patients with advanced squamous cell cancer of the cervix.

Methods.—The study group included 259 patients with International Federation of Gynecology and Obstetrics stage IB to IVA squamous cell cervical cancer with central disease of 5 cm or greater, or histologically confirmed pelvic lymph node involvement. These patients were randomly assigned to receive either radiotherapy plus weekly cisplatin chemotherapy (40 mg/m^2) or the same radiotherapy protocol without chemotherapy.

Results.—The median follow-up was 82 months, and 253 patients were available for follow-up. There was no significant difference in progression-free survival, and no significant difference in 3- and 5-year survival rates was found. The hazard ratio for survival was 1.10.

Conclusions.—Pelvic control or survival was not improved by the addition of concurrent weekly cisplatin chemotherapy in a dose of 40 mg/m^2 to radical radiotherapy. However, the balance of evidence favors the use of combined-modality treatment for the type of patient included in this trial. Optimal results are obtained by careful attention to radiotherapy details.

▶ Based on the results of 5 large clinical trials, the United States National Cancer Institute issued a clinical alert in 1999 advising that strong consideration should be given to incorporating concurrent cisplatin-based chemotherapy with radiation therapy for the treatment of cervical cancer.[1] Those recommendations have been adopted by many cancer centers and have been incorporated into the control arms of subsequent cooperative group trials. The results of this study do not appear to support previous findings. As pointed out in the excellent editorial by Rose and Bundy,[2] there were factors at play that may account for these seeming irreconcilable differences. The patients in this study did not undergo surgical staging of their para-aortic lymph nodes as did the patients in most of the positive studies. Thus, it is not known how many patients had positive para-aortic nodes that were outside the treatment field. In addition, as seen in Figure 1 from the editorial, the confidence interval for this study overlaps those of the 5 previous trials as well as the pooled data from those 5 trials. The difference could merely be caused by statistical variation. Thus, it remains the consensus of most that cisplatin-based chemoradiation should be the standard of care for those patients who are not surgical candidates. A recent meta-analysis confirms this conclusion.[3]

D. S. Miller, MD

References

1. National Cancer Institute: *Clinical Announcement: Concurrent Chemoradiation for Cervical Cancer.* Washington DC, United States Department of Public Health, February 1999.
2. Rose PG, Bundy BN: Chemoradiation for locally advanced cervical cancer: Does it help? (editorial) *J Clin Oncol* 20:891-893, 2002.

3. Green JA, Kirwan JM, Tierney JF, et al: Survival and recurrence after concomitant chemotherapy and radiotherapy for cancer of the uterine cervix: A systematic review and meta-analysis. *Lancet* 358:781, 2001.

Long-term Follow-up of RTOG 92-10: Cervical Cancer With Positive Para-Aortic Lymph Nodes

Grigsby PW, Heydon K, Mutch DG, et al (Washington Univ, St Louis; Radiation Therapy Oncology Group, Philadelphia; Univ of Alabama, Birmingham; et al)
Int J Radiat Oncol Biol Phys 51:982-987, 2001   27–9

Background.—When positive para-aortic lymph nodes accompany carcinoma of the cervix, survival is poor: only 30% at 5 years. Treatment consists of hyperfractionated radiotherapy to increase the pelvic and para-aortic radiation dose and chemotherapy to increase the sensitivity of tumor cells in these areas to the irradiation and to provide a cytotoxic agent for micrometastatic disease beyond the irradiation portals. The late toxicity and efficacy of using twice-daily external irradiation to the pelvic and lumbar para-aortic areas using brachytherapy and concurrent chemotherapy was evaluated for these carcinomas of the cervix.

Methods.—The patients chosen had clinical stages I to IV carcinoma of the cervix with documented metastases to the para-aortic lymph nodes; they ranged in age from 29 to 72 (median, 47). All 30 patients were given twice-daily radiation doses of 1.2 Gy to the designated areas at 4- to 6-hour intervals 5 days each week. The whole pelvis thus had a total external radiation dose of 24 to 48 Gy, with a 12- to 36-Gy parametrial boost, and 48 Gy to the lumbar para-aortic area, with a total dose of 54 to 58 Gy to positive para-aortic lymph nodes. The minimum total dose was 85 Gy to point A. Either 3 or 4 cycles of chemotherapy were given on days 1, 22, and 43 (cisplatin 75 mg/m^2 and 5-fluorouracil 1000 mg/m^2/24 hours for 4 consecutive days).

Results.—Only 7 patients were alive when data were assessed; these were followed for a median of 57 months. Twenty patients died of cervical cancer and 1 patient died of a myocardial infarction secondary to chemotherapy. The degree of acute toxicity associated with chemotherapy was grade 1 in 3% of patients, grade 2 in 17%, grade 3 in 47%, and grade 4 in 30%. With respect to radiotherapy, toxicity was grade 1 in 10% of patients, grade 2 in 33%, grade 3 in 27%, and grade 4 in 13%. Of the 15 nonhematologic grade 4 toxic reactions, all were related to the bowel. Late complications ranked as grade 1 in 10% of patients, grade 2 in 17%, grade 3 in 7%, and grade 4 in 17%; 1 patient had a grade 5 toxicity during therapy but not late. At 36 months, the cumulative incidence of toxicities of at least grade 3 was 34%. At 1 year, the local regional control was 40%. This increased to 50% at years 2 and 3. At 1 year, the probability of disease failure was 46%, increasing to 60% at year 2 and 63% at year 3.

Conclusions.—The acute and late toxicity rates associated with the regimen of twice-daily external irradiation to the pelvis and para-aortic area with brachytherapy and concurrent cisplatin and 5-fluorouracil were unacceptably high. Far too many patients were unable to complete the course, and survival rates were not improved over the use of standard fractionation irradiation without chemotherapy.

▶ As is the case with many cancers, metastasis of cervical cancer to the para-aortic lymph nodes indicates possible systemic carcinomatosis and portends a grave prognosis. The original intent of this study was to evaluate effectiveness of twice-daily radiation therapy. That treatment schedule was not more effective than traditional once-daily radiation. The important clinical point to be gained from this article is that a significant minority of patients with para-aortic nodal metastasis from their cervix cancer can be salvaged with aggressive treatment.

D. S. Miller, MD

28 Vulvar Cancer

Intraoperative Lymphatic Mapping and Sentinel Node Identification With Blue Dye in Patients With Vulvar Cancer
Levenback C, Coleman RL, Burke TW, et al (Univ of Texas, Houston; Univ of Texas, Dallas)
Gynecol Oncol 83:276-281, 2001   28–1

Background.—One method of reducing the morbidity associated with radical vulvectomy and bilateral inguinal femoral lymphadenectomy for cancer of the vulva uses sentinel node identification. The 8 to 10 superficial inguinal lymph nodes have been designated sentinel nodes, with the understanding that if these are negative for metastatic disease, the femoral nodes also are negative in all cases. This obviates the need for femoral lymphadenectomy. The strategy was begun in 1993. The data reported update and expand the information concerning the effectiveness of intraoperative lymphatic mapping with blue dye in patients with vulvar cancer.

Methods.—From 1993 to 1999, 52 patients undergoing primary surgical treatment for vulvar cancer (age range, 18 to 92 years; median, 58 years) were enrolled. Of these women, 87% had T1 or T2 lesions and 92% had nonsuspicious lymph nodes palpated. Each had isosulfan blue dye injected intradermally at the edge of the primary tumor nearest the adjacent groin. When the tumor was within 2 cm of the midline, bilateral dye injections and groin dissections were carried out.

Results.—In 88% of the patients, at least 1 sentinel node was identified, consisting of 22 patients with lateral tumors and 24 with midline tumors. Of the 76 groins examined, 57 (75%) had successful identification of the sentinel node. Type of previous biopsy, location of primary tumor, and extent of clinical experience with the procedure influenced the ability to identify sentinel nodes, with failures linked to incisional or excisional biopsy (44%) versus punch biopsy (16%); to midline versus lateral tumors; and to the first 2 years of the study (16% of patients and 36% of groin dissections) versus the remaining years (7% of patients and 15% of groin dissections). Of the 556 nodes removed, 83 were designated as sentinel nodes. Twenty-one percent of patients had lymph node metastases, with most (10 of the 11 patients) being unilateral. In 10 of the 12 groins dissected, a positive sentinel node was found. No false-negative sentinel nodes were detected. Of the cases examined since 1995, the sentinel lymph node was successfully identified in 16 of

16 patients and 25 of 25 groin dissections involving T1 or T2 primary vulvar tumors of squamous cell histology with clinically nonsuspicious nodes.

Conclusions.—Overall, lymphatic mapping with blue dye done by experienced physicians identifies the sentinel node in 95% of the selected group of patients with vulvar cancer. Mapping accuracy can be compromised by prior surgery, prior excisional biopsy, and infection. Patients whose tumors are limited to the vulva, who have no grossly positive groin nodes or infection, and who have had a punch biopsy to confirm diagnosis constitute the ideal population for this procedure.

▶ Intraoperative lymphatic mapping and sentinel node identification, first developed for penile cancer and subsequently expanded to melanoma and breast cancer, continues to be evaluated in several solid tumors. The hope of less-radical nodal extirpation, specifically directed nodal evaluation, and reduced postoperative complications has driven this charge. It is no surprise then that work continues in patients with cancer of the vulva. The authors have supplemented their clinical experience in this current report, detailing by subset analysis cohorts in which successful localization might be augmented. In addition, they demonstrate that in experienced hands, their blue dye-only technique can achieve rates of success rivaling that seen with the combined technique (lymphoscintigraphy and blue dye). The infrequency of this tumor, though, places special challenges on widespread adaptation of the technique, which must follow validation as is being investigated in a group-wide prospective trial within the Gynecologic Oncology Group.

D. S. Miller, MD

Bleomycin, Methotrexate, and CCNU in Locally Advanced or Recurrent, Inoperable, Squamous-Cell Carcinoma of the Vulva: An EORTC Gynaecological Cancer Cooperative Group Study
Wagenaar HC, Colombo N, Vergote I, et al (Leiden Univ, The Netherlands; EORTC Data Ctr, Brussels, Belgium; European Inst of Oncology, Milan, Italy; et al)
Gynecol Oncol 81:348-354, 2001   28–2

Background.—Squamous cell carcinoma of the vulva is relatively rare, accounting for 4% to 8% of all gynecologic cancers. Although most cases are detected at an early stage, many are not caught until an advanced stage. The effects of a modified combination chemotherapy consisting of bleomycin, methotrexate, and CCNU were investigated in patients with locally advanced, squamous cell carcinoma of the vulva not amenable to resection by standard radical vulvectomy or recurrent disease after incomplete resection.

Methods.—Twenty-five eligible patients, aged 39 to 82 years, were enrolled in the phase II trial. Treatment consisted of 5 mg bleomycin given intramuscularly on days 1 to 5; 40 mg of oral CCNU on days 5 to 7; and 15 mg of oral methotrexate on days 1 and 4 during the first week. Between weeks 2 and 6, patients were given bleomycin, 5 mg intramuscularly, on days 1 and 4, and methotrexate, 15 mg orally, on day 1. This 6-week cycle was repeated every 49 days.

Findings.—Treatment resulted in 2 complete and 12 partial responses for a response rate of 56%. Major hematologic side effects and mild signs of bleomycin-related pulmonary toxicity occurred. Three patients were still alive at a median of 8 months. Eighteen patients died from malignancy, and 2 died from toxicity. The remaining 2 died from intercurrent disease and unknown causes, respectively. Median progression-free survival was 4.8 months. Median survival was 7.8 months. Survival at 1 year was 32%.

Conclusions.—The BMC regimen had therapeutic activity in locoregionally advanced or recurrent squamous cell carcinoma of the vulva. The overall response rate after neoadjuvant chemotherapy was 56%. This treatment regimen may have a role in the palliative care of advanced or recurrent vulvar cancer.

▶ There is little literature on the treatment of recurrent or advanced vulvar cancer with chemotherapy. That literature consists of several case reports and a few case series. Until recently, the problem has not been addressed by our cooperative groups. These unfortunate patients are typically offered platinum-based regimens that had reported activity in cervical cancer with the assumption that activity may also be seen in vulvar cancer. As seen in this paper, that practice may not be serving our patients well in that their 3-drug combination consists of drugs not typically used in North America for the treatment of cervical cancer. The 56% response rate is notable, but unfortunately we have little to compare it to. Clearly the Gynecologic Oncology Group should consider developing a phase II program in vulvar cancer.

D. S. Miller, MD

29 Surgical Oncology

Ureteroileoneocystostomy: The Use of an Ileal Segment for Ureteral Substitution in Gynecologic Oncology

Manolitsas TP, Copeland LJ, Cohn DE, et al (Ohio State Univ, Columbus)
Gynecol Oncol 84:110-114, 2002   29–1

Background.—As a result of various circumstances, the distal two thirds of the ureter may be extensively damaged and require reimplantation of the ureter into the bladder, or ureteroneocystostomy. The ureter also may be reanastamosed or anastamosed to the contralateral ureter; percutaneous nephrostomy may be a short-term solution. In ureteroileoneocystostomy (UINC), a segment of the ileum is interposed between the bladder and the distal ureter to bridge the gap caused by resection of the ureter. This technique is safe and effective but not used frequently.

Methods.—All 8 patients (average age, 56 years) underwent 12 UINC procedures at the Ohio State University Medical Center's James Cancer Hospital from 1988 to 2000. Their medical records were reviewed retrospectively.

Results.—Epithelial ovarian cancer was the principal diagnosis in 6 cases, low-grade endometrial stromal sarcoma in 1 case, and vaginal squamous cell carcinoma in 1 case. Bilateral UINC was performed in 1 patient in a single procedure. Unilateral UINC was done in 7 patients, 2 of whom required repeat or revision procedures and 1 a contralateral UINC. It was performed as part of reductive surgery for the primary tumor in 2 cases, and at subsequent laparotomy in 10 cases. Ureteric obstruction occurred after tumor recurrence in 8 of the laparoscopic cases. Two cases had obstruction without tumor recurrence; 1 was caused by radiation fibrosis and 1 by postsurgical fibrosis. One patient died from non-UINC–related aspiration pneumonia. Pelvic abscess and ureteric obstruction on the right side required temporary percutaneous nephrostomy and drainage that produced resolution of the obstruction in 1 patient. One fibrosis-related obstruction required revision of the ureteroileal anastamosis, and 1 tumor recurrence–related obstruction required repeat UINC. Cystitis developed in 3 patients, but no ascending infections were seen. Mean follow-up was 34 months (range, 38 days to 77 months), and 3 additional patients died. Of the 4 living patients, 3 have no evidence of disease and 1 has recurrent ovarian cancer that is being treated. Thus, 82% of patients had successful long-term integrity of renal drainage with the first UINC procedure and 100% at repeat or revision procedures.

Conclusions.—Overall, the UINC procedure proved to be safe and effective treatment for achieving lower ureteric resection.

▶ Occasionally, it is necessary to remove the terminal portion of the ureter to achieve an optimal tumor resection in gynecologic oncology. A typical approach to restore urinary tract integrity is usually a bladder advancement procedure such as a psoas hitch or Boari flap to accomplish ureteroneocystostomy. This approach may not be practical because of bladder immobility from tumor involvement, partial bladder resection, or the relatively inflexible radiated bladder. In some circumstances, anastomosis of a segment of intestine between the distal ureteral remnant and the bladder, ureteroileoneocystostomy, a procedure used by our urologic colleagues on occasion, may provide the best reconstruction. This appropriately small series shows that this procedure can be feasible and helpful in well selected patients. Another obvious indication for ureteroileoneocystostomy is for reconstruction of ureteral stricture due to radiation-induced retroperitoneal fibrosis.

D. S. Miller, MD

Surgical Blood Loss in Abdominal Hysterectomy
Santoso JT, Dinh TA, Omar S, et al (Univ of Texas, Galveston)
Gynecol Oncol 82:364-366, 2001   29–2

Background.—Estimating surgical blood loss is important because it can affect the patient's condition both intraoperatively and postoperatively, yet the methods used most often are felt to be inaccurate. More accurate ways are time consuming, impractical, and/or expensive. Generally, surgeons estimate blood loss from the volume of blood in the suction container and the amount of blood lost in surgical laparotomy pads. The assessment using volume in the suction container increases in inaccuracy because red cell concentration grows more diluted as time passes. In a group of patients undergoing abdominal hysterectomy, the red cell concentration in the suction container was evaluated as a function of the duration and type of hysterectomy performed.

Methods.—The 72 patients completing the study had either simple or radical hysterectomy with pelvic and periaortic lymphadenectomy. In each case, the suction tubing system was heparinized to prevent clotting and the vacuum pressure was reduced to minimize red cell lysis. The hematocrit was determined immediately after surgery and compared with the hematocrit of the patient's venous blood and of the suction container blood.

Results.—Simple hysterectomy was performed in 54 patients and type III radical hysterectomy in 18 patients; the 2 groups did not differ significantly with respect to age or preoperative hematocrit. None of the patients received blood or albumin transfusions intraoperatively. All patients had a lower hematocrit in the suction container than in venous blood. Patients having radical hysterectomy lost more blood and their surgery lasted longer than those who had the simple hysterectomy, as would be expected. The longer the surgery, the more the suction container hematocrit fell, suggesting that fluid other than blood was diluting the blood in the container.

Conclusions.—The hematocrit in the suction container blood was consistently lower than in the patient's venous sample. The hematocrit discrepancy between the suction container and the patient's venous sample was found to be closely correlated with the performance of radical surgery, lymphadenectomy, and duration of surgery. Thus, the current method of estimating red cell loss during surgery is more inaccurate because of the dilution that takes place. A comprehensive measurement, such as photometric or radioisotopic determination of blood volume and red cells preoperatively, intraoperatively, and postoperatively, would provide a more-accurate determination.

▶ This study adds a new layer of complexity to the already-challenging art of estimating blood loss during surgery. It would appear that a progressive hemodilution is observed in the blood suctioned from the surgical field. This decline in hematocrit is greater than that seen in the patient's venous sample. The authors postulate that the excess fluid is lymphatic in origin since they controlled for the effect of irrigation. This effect appears to be more pronounced in longer cases and those involving retroperitoneal dissection.

R. D. Arias, MD

Pneumatic Compression Versus Low Molecular Weight Heparin in Gynecologic Oncology Surgery: A Randomized Trial

Maxwell GL, Synan I, Dodge R, et al (Duke Univ, Durham, NC)
Obstet Gynecol 98:989-995, 2001   29–3

Introduction.—There are nearly 260,000 cases of clinically diagnosed deep vein thrombosis (DVT) and 100,000 deaths caused by pulmonary embolism annually. Thromboembolism occurs in 14% of patients undergoing gynecologic surgery for benign indications and 38% of those undergoing gynecologic oncology surgery. Pulmonary embolism is an important cause of postoperative death in higher-risk patients with uterine and cervical carcinoma. The unfractionated heparin regimen is correlated with a significantly increased transfusion requirement, compared with pneumatic calf compression.

Low molecular weight (LMW) heparin has more anti-Xa and less anti-thrombin activity, producing less effect on partial thromboplastin time. The efficacy and treatment-related complications of LMW heparin and external pneumatic compression were examined in the prevention of venous thromboembolism after major gynecologic oncology surgery in 211 patients aged more than 40 years.

Methods.—Patients were randomly assigned to perioperative thromboembolism prophylaxis with either LMW heparin or external pneumatic compression (105 and 106 patients, respectively). Data were gathered regarding demographics and clinical outcome. All patients underwent bilateral Doppler US of the lower extremities on postoperative day 3 to 5 to determine the presence of occult DVT. Bleeding complications were determined using operative estimated blood loss and number of transfusions needed intraoperatively and postoperatively. A follow-up interview at 30 days after surgery was performed determine whether DVT or PE developed in any patients after hospital discharge.

Results.—Two patients who received LMW heparin and 1 who received external pneumatic compression were given a diagnosis of DVT. LMW heparin was discontinued postoperatively in 3 patients because of intraoperative hemorrhage. The frequency of bleeding complications was similar in both groups.

Conclusion.—LMW heparin and external pneumatic compression are similarly effective in the postoperative prophylaxis of thromboembolism. The use of LMW heparin is not correlated with an increased risk of bleeding complications when compared with external pneumatic compression. Both modalities are efficacious in this high-risk group of patients.

▶ Although very rare, pulmonary embolism is the most common cause of perioperative death following presumed "routine" obstetric or gynecologic surgical procedures. The vast majority of these emboli arise from pelvic and lower extremity DVT, which can be prevented with a number of interventions. Studies have identified patients at high risk: smokers and those with obesity or cancer. Unfortunately, many of these patients are not afforded the benefit of a prophylactic maneuver. This study confirms evidence seen in other surgical sites that therapeutic maneuvers directed at just one aspect of Virchow's triad of stasis, hypercoagulability, and endothelial injury can minimize the patient's risk of this most unfortunate complication.

D. S. Miller, MD

30 Quality of Life

Preventing Anxiety and Depression in Gynaecological Cancer: A Randomised Controlled Trial
Petersen RW, Quinlivan JA (Univ of Melbourne, Australia)
Br J Obstet Gynaecol 109:386-394, 2002   30–1

Background.—Immediately after receiving a diagnosis of gynecologic cancer, from 47% to 70% of women experience psychological symptoms that qualify as moderate to severe depression or anxiety. If these symptoms are not addressed, the woman suffers not only immediate morbidity but also the potential for adverse effects on disease progression and even survival. Interventions were designed to address this problem, and their efficacy was assessed.

Methods.—All patients responded to baseline questionnaires, specifically the Hospital Anxiety and Depression Scale (HADS) and the General Health Questionnaire-28 (GHQ-28). Twenty-six patients served as control subjects, and 27 received the intervention, which consisted of a 1-hour relaxation and counseling session conducted by a senior medical practitioner involved in the patient's care. This intervention was instituted within 24 hours of hospital discharge and included emotional support and care as well as information. Follow-up questionnaires were completed at 6 weeks. The scores on the HADS were compared.

Results.—Fifty patients completed the protocol; both groups reported high levels of social support, and no demographic or disease-related factors differed significantly between them. The baseline HADS and GHQ-28 scores were similar. Tumor site was found to be a significant predictor of the baseline score. At 6 weeks, the intervention group had significantly lower HADS and GHQ-28 scores than the control group. The total HADS score was significantly reduced from baseline. On regression analysis, only the intervention and baseline HADS score showed a significant relationship with outcome. Thus, the intervention produced a significant reduction in total HADS score. A high baseline HADS score was significantly related to patients' tendency to improve over time. Secondarily, the intervention was associated with reductions in anxiety, mild to moderate depression subscale score, total GHQ-28 scores, and 3 of the GHQ-28's 4 subscales (anxiety, somatization, and personality development). Seventy-nine percent of patients felt that the intervention was a positive experience, 14% were neutral, and 7% were negative. Fifty-seven percent would have preferred that the treating doctor conduct the intervention rather than another health professional. Patients appreciated the opportunity to talk with a doctor, felt that the intervention made them feel important, appreciated the effort to make them feel relaxed and comfortable before the intervention, valued the provision of specific information about the disease and care options, and felt motivated to succeed. On the negative side, 1 patient felt the intervention was too short and 1 considered the bed in the counseling room too hard.

Conclusions.—Significant reductions were found in various psychological symptoms in response to the 1-hour relaxation and information session carried out by a treating doctor. These reductions were evident at 6 weeks' follow-up and included all the psychological subscales measured except severe depression. When patients had a high baseline HADS score, they tended to improve over the period of follow-up, but the intervention was in addition to that effect. Patients reported high levels of appreciation, particularly for the time spent with their doctor.

▶ Obviously, the postoperative period for the gynecologic cancer patient can be anxiety provoking if not frightening, as she worries about prognosis and what further interventions might be required. The authors found that an intervention consisting of relaxation and counseling performed by senior doctors reduced psychological symptoms in these patients. Whether the positive outcome resulted from the relaxation techniques or the counseling was not identified. However, I would speculate that similar results could be achieved by having a senior member of the team hold the patient's hand, listen carefully, and speak kindly. I am reminded of a quote from Hippocrates that is framed and hangs on the wall in my office that says, "For some patients though conscious that their condition is perilous, recover their health simply through their contentment with the goodness of the physician."

D. S. Miller, MD

Effect of Soy Phytoestrogens on Hot Flashes in Postmenopausal Women With Breast Cancer: A Randomized, Controlled Clinical Trial
Van Patten CL, Olivotto IA, Chambers GK, et al (British Columbia Cancer Agency; Vancouver Cancer Centre, BC, Canada; Vancouver Hosp and Health Sciences Centre, BC, Canada; et al)
J Clin Oncol 20:1449-1455, 2002
30–2

Background.—Women who have been treated for breast cancer may experience vasomotor symptoms including hot flashes and night sweats. The symptoms may be caused by chemotherapy or worsened by tamoxifen or the abrupt withdrawal of hormone replacement therapy. Soy beverages have been suggested as treatment for such symptoms. The efficacy and acceptability of a soy beverage for treating hot flashes were assessed in symptomatic postmenopausal women who had received treatment for breast cancer.

Methods.—The 123 women assessed had received treatment for early-stage breast cancer and now suffered moderate hot flashes. Fifty-nine received the soy beverage, which contained 90 mg of isoflavones, and 64 women received a placebo rice beverage. The participants had been stratified for their use of tamoxifen. A daily menopause diary was kept for 4 weeks at baseline and 12 weeks while drinking the beverages (500 mL a day). Data included the number and severity of hot flashes experienced each day.

Results.—Both groups noted significant reductions in the number of hot flashes that occurred during the day, at night, and over 24 hours as well as in the hot flash scores from the study's onset until its last 4 weeks. Women taking soy had a 30% reduction in the 24-hour hot flash score; those taking placebo had a 40% reduction. More frequent and more severe gastrointestinal side effects occurred with the soy beverage, leading more women to drop out. Weight gain occurred equally in the 2 groups; 1 woman taking placebo and 4 taking soy had vaginal spotting. Women in both groups perceived a decline in the number and severity of hot flashes both during the day and at night. The soy beverage was given overall acceptability ratings of 1.9 and 2.0 by the soy and placebo groups, respectively, out of a possible 5; 1 was the highest rating.

Conclusion.—There was no support for the use of a soy beverage to treat hot flashes. The decline in the number and severity of hot flashes did not differ significantly between the 2 groups, but the placebo group tended to experience a better effect. In addition, the gastrointestinal symptoms that resulted with the soy beverage led some women to discontinue its use. While some of the results may be attributable to the effects of the anticancer therapy these women received, insufficient data are available to justify the use of a soy beverage or phytoestrogens as a viable alternative for the treatment of hot flashes.

▶ The profound placebo response associated with alternative therapies for vasomotor symptoms has contributed to their widespread popularity. Soy products, in particular, are sold for this purpose. In no subset of the menopausal population are vasomotor symptoms more vexing than in cancer survivors. These women have often received therapies for cancer which have contributed either directly or indirectly to premature climacteric. They are then denied the most effective therapy because of their cancer. This randomized clinical trial compared a soy beverage with a beverage containing a rice base. The women studied had been previously treated for primary breast cancer. This and other studies have failed to show a therapeutic effect for currently available soy preparations for vasomotor symptoms. Soy was actually less effective than placebo at reducing vasomotor symptoms (though this difference did not achieve statistical significance). Adverse effects (mostly gastrointestinal) were higher in the soy users compared to the rice beverage users.

R. D. Arias, MD

31 Breast Disease

Cost-Effectiveness of Raloxifene and Hormone Replacement Therapy in Postmenopausal Women: Impact of Breast Cancer Risk
Armstrong K, Chen T-M, Albert D, et al (Univ of Pennsylvania, Philadelphia)
Obstet Gynecol 98:996-1003, 2001   31–1

Background.—Deciding whether to initiate hormone replacement therapy (HRT) or raloxifene after menopause can be difficult. The life expectancy and the cost-effectiveness of HRT and raloxifene therapy for healthy 50-year-old postmenopausal women were analyzed.

Methods and Findings.—A cost-effectiveness analysis was performed using a Markov model. Both HRT and raloxifene therapy increased life expectancy. In addition, both were cost effective compared with no therapy. For women with an average risk for breast cancer and coronary heart disease, lifetime HRT increased quality-adjusted life expectancy more and cost

TABLE 1.—Disease Incidence and Mortality

		Sensitivity Analysis Range	Source(s) (References)
Coronary heart disease			
Incidence	0.32 lifetime	0.30-0.90	11, 12
Mortality	0.1-0.3 first y	0.05-0.4	14, 15
	0.01-0.04 subsequent y	0.005-0.02	
Hip fracture			
Incidence	0.14 lifetime	0.10-0.40	25
Mortality	0.17 first y	0.08-0.35	26
Vertebral fracture			
Incidence	0.18 lifetime	0.04-0.20	27
Mortality			
Breast cancer			
Incidence	0.10 lifetime	0.05-0.50	28
Mortality	0.025 first y	0.01-0.05	28
	0.032 subsequent y	0.01-0.05	
Endometrial cancer			
Incidence	0.026 lifetime	0.01-0.05	28
Mortality	0.15 first y	0.05-0.3	28
Thromboembolism			
Incidence	0.00072 annually	0.0003-0.002	4
Mortality	0.016 first y	0.008-0.03	29

TABLE 2.—Effect of Interventions on Disease Incidence

	Relative Risk	Sensitivity Analysis Range	Source(s) (References)
HRT			
Coronary heart disease	0.56	0.3-1.0	1
Hip fracture	0.53	0.3-1.0	2
Vertebral fracture	0.53	0.3-1.0	2
Breast cancer	1.35	1.0-2.0	3
Endometrial cancer	1.00	1.0-6.0	30
Thromboembolism	2.10	1.0-7.8	29
Raloxifene			
Coronary heart disease	0.87	0.5-1.0	5, 6
Hip fracture	0.93	0.5-1.0	5
Vertebral fracture	0.67	0.5-1.0	7
Breast cancer	0.24	0.1-1.0	4
Endometrial cancer	1.00	1.0-6.0	4
Thromboembolism	3.10	1.0-6.2	4

Abbreviation: HRT, Hormone replacement therapy.
(Reprinted with permission from The American College of Obstetricians and Gynecologists courtesy of Armstrong K, Chen T-M, Albert D, et al: Cost-effectiveness of raloxifene and hormone replacement therapy in postmenopausal women: Impact of breast cancer risk.*Obstet Gynecol* 98:996-1003, 2001.)

less than lifetime raloxifene treatment. However, raloxifene was more cost effective than HRT for women with an average coronary risk and a lifetime breast cancer risk of 15% or greater or who received postmenopausal therapy for 10 years or less. In addition, raloxifene was more cost effective when HRT decreased the coronary heart disease risk by less than 20% (Tables 1 and 2).

Conclusion.—Long-term HRT appears to be the most cost-effective treatment for women with an average risk of breast cancer and coronary heart disease. However, raloxifene is more cost effective for women with an average coronary risk and with 1 or more major risk factors for breast cancer.

▶ Epidemiologic studies comparing therapies for similar indications are important. However, such studies can be fraught with pitfalls due to selective assumptions and the published sources that form the "data" for the analysis. Furthermore, clinicians must remain vigilant in appraising such studies as the conclusions are usually from a population-based public health point of view, which is often in contrast to an individual patient's situation and desires. In addition, HRT has been scrutinized and researched for more than 50 years, whereas recently available therapies have just begun to receive critical investigation. Detailed analysis of quality-of-life issues and application of this analysis in terms of absolute risk would be of keen clinical interest.

In a related comparison, a digitalized mammography study revealed raloxifene therapy to have no influence on mammographic density in postmenopausal women who had previously had a hysterectomy,[1] whereas multiple reports have shown that a definite percentage of similar women will have increased mammographic density on estrogen replacement therapy (ERT).

However, this ERT-associated mammographic density subsides to pretreatment levels within weeks of stopping ERT.

W. H. Hindle, MD

References

1. Freedman M, San Martin J, O'Gorman J, et al: Digitized mammography: A clinical trial of postmenopausal women randomly assigned to receive raloxifene, estrogen or placebo. *J Natl Cancer Inst* 93:51-56, 2001.

SUGGESTED READING

Olsson H, Bladstrom A, Ingvar C, et al: A population-based cohort study of HRT use and breast cancer in southern Sweden. *Brit J Cancer* 85:674-677, 2001.

▶ This Swedish study has impressive numbers (29,508 women, aged 25-65). "Among about 3,663 ever users of HRT, there was no increase in overall tumor incidence (SIR = 0.98, 95% CI 0.86-1.12) but a significant excess of breast cancer (SIR = 1.35, 95% CI 1.09-1.64) compared with never users (SIR = 1.07, 95% CI 0.96-1.19)." There was increasing incidence of breast cancer with increasing duration of HRT use (SIR 1.92, 95% CI 1.32-2.70 for 48-120 months of use). Beyond 5 years after stopping HRT, there was no increased risk. There was no significant interaction with previous use of oral contraception or family history of breast cancer. These findings are similar to other published reports showing low levels of increased risk of breast cancer associated with current and recent HRT use. Though mathematically correct, the data should not alter clinical management.

O'Meara et al[1] reviewed data on 2755 women with breast cancer of which 174 used HRT after treatment. The breast cancer risks of recurrence and mortality were lower in the HRT treated women compared to those who did not use HRT. This adds to the clinically reassuring data concerning HRT treatment of women after diagnosis and treatment for breast cancer.

Manier et al[2] reported on a population-based prospective cohort study of 5,865 postmenopausal women followed for an average of 9.9 years. Twenty percent were current users of HRT. One hundred forty-one incident breast cancer cases were identified with a relative risk of 1.72 (95% CI 1.17-2.52) for HRT users: "Among HRT users, there was over-representation of tumours that, with regard to stage, type and grade, are associated with a favourable prognosis."

Zera et al[3] studied breast biopsies of women who had taken estrogen and/or progesterone within 3 months of biopsy with women who had not taken any hormones. Exogenous hormone use was significantly higher for women with atypical hyperplasia compared to women with non-proliferative fibrocystic changes. The authors conclude that this data supports that a continuum exists for undefined subsets of women from normal epithelium to hyperplasia and ultimately to carcinoma for some, and that exogenous hormone use influences progression along this continuum.

William H. Hindle, MD

References

1. O'Meara ES, Rossing MA, Daling JR, et al: Hormone replacement therapy after a diagnosis of breast cancer in relation to recurrence and mortality. *J Natl Cancer Inst* 93:754-762, 2001.

2. Manier J, Malina J, Berglund G, et al: Increased incidence of small and well-differentiated breast tumors in post-menopausal women following hormone-replacement therapy. *Int J Cancer* 92:919-922, 2001.
3. Zera RT, Danielson D, Van Camp JM, et al: Atypical hyperplasia, proliferative fibrocystic change, and exogenous hormone use. *Surgery* 30:732-737, 2001.

Five Versus More Than Five Years of Tamoxifen for Lymph Node-Negative Breast Cancer: Updated Findings From the National Surgical Adjuvant Breast and Bowel Project B-14 Randomized Trial
Fisher B, Dignam J, Bryant J, et al (Univ of Pittsburgh, Pa; Allegheny Gen Hosp, Pittsburgh, Pa)
J Natl Cancer Inst 93:684-690, 2001   31–2

Background.—The value of tamoxifen for patients with estrogen receptor–positive breast tumors and negative axillary lymph nodes was assessed in 4127 women by the National Surgical Adjuvant Breast and Bowel Project B-14 trial in 1982. This showed a significant improvement in disease-free survival (DFS) through 5 years of follow-up with the use of tamoxifen. However, these women were then redistributed randomly to receive tamoxifen or placebo and no advantage from tamoxifen was found through 4 years of follow-up. How long to continue tamoxifen therapy continues to be in question, so the B-14 study was updated.

Methods.—A total of 1172 patients completed 5 years of taking tamoxifen and were disease free. These women were then randomly reassigned, with 579 receiving tamoxifen and 593 given placebo. Measures included survival, DFS, and relapse-free survival (RFS).

Results.—Women who received placebo had a DFS of 82% through 7 years after being randomly reassigned, whereas those taking tamoxifen had a DFS of 78% (Fig 1). The placebo group's RFS was 94% and survival was 94%; the tamoxifen group's RFS was 92% and survival was 91%. Neither

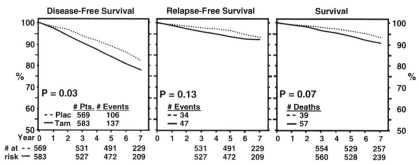

FIGURE 1.—Disease-free survival, relapse-free survival, and survival through 7 years of follow-up of all patients who were randomly reassigned after 5 years of tamoxifen to receive either placebo (*Plac*) or prolonged tamoxifen (*Tam*) therapy. All P values were 2-sided. (Courtesy of Fisher B, Dignam J, Bryant J, et al: Five versus more than five years of tamoxifen for lymph node-negative breast cancer: Updated findings from the National Surgical Adjuvant Breast and Bowel Project B-14 Randomized Trial. *J Natl Cancer Inst* 93:684-690, 2001. By permission of Oxford University Press.)

TABLE 3.—Sites and Rates of First Events

Site	Placebo (n = 569) No. of Events	%	Rate*	Tamoxifen (n = 583) No. of Events	%	Rate*	Rate Ratio	Placebo Versus Tamoxifen 95% Confidence Interval	P†
All breast cancer re-currences	34	6.0	8.9	47	8.1	12.5	1.4	0.9 to 2.2	.13
Local-regional‡	17	3.0	4.4	21	3.6	5.6	1.3	0.6 to 2.6	
Distant	17	3.0	4.4	26	4.5	6.9	1.6	0.8 to 3.1	
Second primary can-cer	54	9.5	14.1	63	10.8	16.7	1.2	0.8 to 1.7	
Contralateral breast	20	3.5	5.2	17	2.9	4.5	0.9	0.4 to 1.7	
Endometrial	6	1.1	1.6	12	2.1	3.2	2.0	0.7 to 6.6	
Other	28	4.9	7.3	34	5.8	9.0	1.2	0.7 to 2.1	
Death, no evidence of disease	18	3.2	4.7	27	4.6	7.2	1.5	0.8 to 2.9	
All events	106	18.6	27.6	137	23.5	36.3	1.3	1.0 to 1.7	.03
Alive, event free	463	81.4	—	446	76.5	—			

*Average annual rate per 1000 patients.
†Two-sided P from log-rank test.
‡Includes ipsilateral breast tumor recurrence in patients treated with lumpectomy.
(Courtesy of Fisher B, Dignam J, Bryant J, et al: Five versus more than five years of tamoxifen for lymph node-negative breast cancer: Updated findings from the National Surgical Adjuvant Breast and Bowel Project B-14 Randomized Trial. *J Natl Cancer Inst* 93:684-690, 2001. By permission of Oxford University Press.)

age nor tumor size appeared to influence the outcome. The rate of breast cancer or other events was higher in the tamoxifen women than in the placebo group, although the difference did not reach statistical significance (Table 3). Rates of occurrence of contralateral breast cancer did not differ between the 2 groups. Endometrial cancer occurred in 1.1% of the placebo group and 2.1% of the tamoxifen group. Women in the tamoxifen group suffered more second primary cancers as first events (Table 4) and more deaths (Table 5) than those receiving placebo.

TABLE 4.—Number of Second Primary Cancers as First Events

Site*	Placebo	Tamoxifen
Colon/rectum	7†	5
Liver	0	0
Other gastrointestinal organs	4	3
Lung and bronchus	4	6
Soft tissue	2	2
Skin (melanoma)	3	3
Endometrium	6	12
Urinary system	1	3
Lymphatic system (non-Hodgkin's lymphoma)	0	2
Other	8	9
Unknown	0	1
Total	35†	46

*Contralateral breast cancers were excluded.
†Includes 1 ineligible patient.
(Courtesy of Fisher B, Dignam J, Bryant J, et al: Five versus more than five years of tamoxifen for lymph node-negative breast cancer: Updated findings from the National Surgical Adjuvant Breast and Bowel Project B-14 Randomized Trial. *J Natl Cancer Inst* 93:684-690, 2001. By permission of Oxford University Press.)

TABLE 5.—Causes of Death as First Events

Cause of Death	Placebo	Tamoxifen
Septicemia	2	2
Ischemic heart disease	2	6
Other heart disease	1	0
Cerebrovascular disease	1*	4
Diseases of the respiratory system	1	1
Diseases of the liver, gallbladder, and pancrease	1	2
Diseases of the genitourinary system	2	1
Miscellaneous	6	6
Unknown	3	5
Total	19*	27

*Includes 1 ineligible patient.
(Courtesy of Fisher B, Dignam J, Bryant J, et al: Five versus more than five years of tamoxifen for lymph node-negative breast cancer: Updated findings from the National Surgical Adjuvant Breast and Bowel Project B-14 Randomized Trial. *J Natl Cancer Inst* 93:684-690, 2001. By permission of Oxford University Press.)

Conclusion.—The findings noted in the original B-14 trial were upheld, with no benefit accruing to women with estrogen receptor–positive tumors and negative axillary lymph nodes who continue tamoxifen therapy for more than 5 years. Both the overall number of events and the number of deaths were higher among those taking tamoxifen than those receiving placebo.

▶ With 4 years of follow-up after re-randomization to placebo or continuing tamoxifen therapy, no additional benefit from tamoxifen could be demonstrated after the initial 5 years of therapy. This lack of benefit for continued therapy after 5 years was observed for disease-free survival, relapse-free survival, and overall survival. In fact, "a slight advantage" was observed in the placebo group, compared to those continuing tamoxifen, for estrogen receptor–positive axillary lymph node–negative breast cancers. The mechanism for this seemingly paradoxical result is unknown. However, the current generally accepted clinical recommendation for this particular subset of breast cancer patients is to give tamoxifen therapy for 5 years and no more.

The Scottish adjuvant tamoxifen trial (initially, n = 1323 patients), with a median follow-up of 15 years, reported similar findings with no advantage of tamoxifen therapy beyond 5 years of treatment.[1] Furthermore, the benefits of the initial 5 years of tamoxifen therapy "persisted" even after a 15-year follow-up suggesting that the breast cancer was eradicated "permanently," at least for some women in the study.

W. H. Hindle, MD

Reference

1. Stewart HJ, Prescott RJ, Forrest APM: Scottish adjuvant tamoxifen trial: A randomized study updated to 15 years. *J Natl Cancer Inst* 93:456-462, 2001.

Institutional Validation of Breast Cancer Treatment Guidelines

Minter RM, Spengler KK, Topping DP, et al (Univ of Florida, Gainesville)
J Surg Res 100:106-109, 2001   31–3

Background.—Although many groups have created clinical practice guidelines for the management of breast cancer, most guidelines have not yet been validated. Therefore, whether compliance with the National Comprehensive Cancer Network (NCCN) guidelines would have an effect on survival, quality of life (QOL), or hospital costs of women with breast cancer was examined.

Methods.—The medical records of 129 women with stages I to III invasive breast carcinoma treated in 1991 and 1992 were reviewed. None of the subjects had carcinoma in situ, inflammatory cancer, or comorbid conditions that would affect treatment. Five-year survival, QOL, and hospital costs were assessed according to whether the patient had been treated per the NCCN guidelines (Fig 1). Five-year survival was calculated by Kaplan-Meier analysis. QOL was determined on the basis of 12 parameters, each rated according to a 5-point Likert-type scale, and scores were averaged to produce a cumulative QOL score. Hospital costs included emergency department, inpatient, and outpatient charges.

Results.—The 36 patients who had been treated according to the NCCN guidelines (NCCN+ group) did not differ significantly from the 93 patients who had not been treated according to these guidelines (NCCN− group) in age (mean, 53.7 vs 55.7 years), race (86% vs 94% white), or tumor characteristics. Five-year survival was higher in the NCCN+ group than in the NCCN− group (87.6% vs 83.3%), but this difference was not statistically significant. Given the small sample size, however, the study was of insufficient power to detect a significant between-group difference in survival rate. The cumulative QOL score also did not differ significantly between the NCCN+ and NCCN− groups (4.18 vs 4.24). However, hospital costs in the NCCN+ group were almost one third lower ($20,300 vs $59,700), and the difference between groups was significant. The higher costs in the NCCN− group were related to higher laboratory, pharmacy, and operating room charges.

Conclusion.—Compliance with the NCCN guidelines can significantly reduce treatment costs for stages I to III breast cancer without adversely affecting survival rate or quality of life.

▶ Authoritative breast cancer treatment guidelines are clinically important, not only for those who are directly involved in the treatment but for primary health care providers and others who work with and counsel breast cancer patients. The specific treatment plan information is useful to both potential patients and their physicians even though following the guidelines does not seem to influence to quality of life or survival of the patients involved, as documented in this analysis. The estimated cost figures are fascinating with a range from $22,100 for those following the guidelines to $84,900 for those treated outside the guidelines.

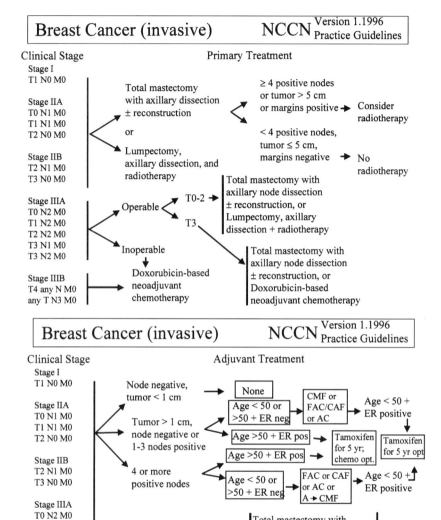

FIGURE 1.—NCCN guidelines for the primary and adjuvant treatment of invasive breast cancer, version 1.1996. (Courtesy of Minter RM, Spengler KK, Topping DP, et al: Institutional validation of breast cancer treatment guidelines. *J Surg Res* 100:106-109, 2001.)

Several associated articles relate to breast cancer treatment and outcome. Hoover et al[1] compared the methods of detecting recurrences and found that tests prompted by symptoms and/or physical findings identified most of the recurrences versus routine screening tests. Velanovic et al[2] used the National Comprehensive Cancer Network Breast Cancer Practice Guidelines as a standard and compared breast cancer treatment for women less than 65 years of age with those older than 65.[3] In the older age group, the omitted treatments were: 11.4%, no tumor extirpation; 39.1%, no axillary dissection; 47.7%, no radiation therapy; and 18.2%, no chemotherapy. The causes of the omissions in the older age group were 40.9% prohibitive associated medical conditions, 13.6% favorable primary tumor pathology, 31.8% patient refusal, and 13.6% unexplained. In general, upon detailed review, the older aged patients did not receive standard care for specific documented reasons. Grogan et al[4] calculated 10-year actuarial cause-specific survival tables based on tumor size and histologic grade for 1200 women with node-negative breast cancers of less than 30mm diameter in the Swedish Two-Count Trial database. The subsets were women aged less than 50 years and women aged 50 years or older. The tables give absolute 10-year survival benefits, which is accurate information for clinicians to utilize in counseling their patients. Given et al[5] reviewed Medicare claim files of 205 women aged 65 and older who were treated for breast cancer and found that within a 6-week interval, 54% of the women treated by breast conserving surgery (BCS) underwent a second surgery. Subsequently, only a successful first BCS was less expensive than a mastectomy ($4,955 vs $9,049 USD).

W. H. Hindle MD

References

1. Hoover S, Fodera T, Peters G, et al: Breast cancer recurrences—a comparison of detection methods. [Abstract] *Breast J* 7:370, 2001.
2. Carlson RW, Edge SB, McCormick B: Update: NCCN Breast Cancer Practice Guidelines. Rockledge, PA: National Comprehensive Cancer Network, Inc., 1999.
3. Velanovich V, Gabel M, Walker EM, et al: Causes for undertreatment of elderly breast cancer patients: Tailoring treatments to individual patients. *J Am Coll Surg* 194:8-13, 2002.
4. Grogan M, Tabar L, Chua B, et al: Estimating the benefits of adjuvant systemic therapy for women with early breast cancer. *Br J Surg* 88:1513-1518, 2001.
5. Given C, Bradley C, Luca A, et al: Observation interval for evaluating the cost of surgical interventions for older women with a new diagnosis of breast cancer. *Med Care* 39:1146-1157, 2001.

SUGGESTED READING

Allweis TM, Boisvert ME, Otero SE, et al: Immediate reconstruction after mastectomy for breast cancer does not prolong the time to starting adjuvant chemotherapy. *Am J Surg* 183:218-221, 2002.

▶ This retrospective analysis (n = 49) compared patients who had mastectomy, immediate reconstruction and then chemotherapy to 308 similar patients without reconstruction. Overall the reconstructed women were younger (46 vs 55 years of age, P < .001), had more advanced disease, and had shorter time to chemotherapy (41 vs 53 days, P = 0.039). The latter is surprising. The type of reconstruction did not affect the time to chemotherapy.

Lin et al[1] at the University of Virginia Health Sciences Center, Charlottesville, Va, reviewed the presurgical risk factors for complications of breast reconstruction (123 reconstructions in 98 patients). The statistically significant risk factors were: (1) increasing obesity, defined by body mass index, 2) an active or recent (<5 year) history of cigarette smoking, and 3) a history of previous radiation exposure. A nomogram based on ordinal regression analysis was developed to calculate a patient's presurgical risk. Such risk analysis should be useful to referring physicians, their patients, and plastic surgeons.

Jansen et al[2] the Tulane University Plastic Surgery Service, New Orleans, La, described 2 cases of "traumatic injury to the breast bud while the body was under increased physical stress." Both were gymnasts who sustained premenarchal injuries that resulted in subsequent breast asymmetry "severe enough to prevent them from leading a normal life." Modified breast reconstruction is a surgical option in such cases.

William H. Hindle, MD

References

1. Lin KY, Johns FR, Gibson J, et al: An outcome study of breast reconstruction: Presurgical identification of risk factors for complications. *Ann Surg Oncol* 8:586-591, 2001.
2. Jansen DA, Stoetzel RS, Leveque JE: Premenarchal athletic injury to the breast bud as the cause of asymmetry: Prevention and treatment. *Breast J* 8:108-111, 2002.

Bruera E, Willey JS, Palmer JL, et al: Treatment decisions for breast carcinoma: Patient preferences and physician perceptions. *Cancer* 94:2076-2080, 2002.

▶ This prospective study from the M. D. Anderson Cancer Center, Houston, Texas, has small numbers (n = 57) but vital information about active shared decisions for breast cancer treatment that was preferred by 89% (51/57) of the breast cancer patients. "The agreement between patients and physicians with regard to decision-making preference occurred in only 24 cases (42%)." The covariates of age, education, and income were not statistically significant. The authors conclude: "Enhanced agreement between patient preferences and physician expectations most likely will improve communication and patient satisfaction with the treatment decision-making process."

Keating et al[1] surveyed 1081 women with diagnosed early stage breast cancer and found that 64% desired a collaborative role in decision-making "but only 33% reported actually having such a role when they discussed treatments with their surgeons." The women whose actual role matched their desired role in decision-making were 83.5% "very satisfied" with their treatment choice.

Te Boekhorst et al[2] from Nijmegen, The Netherlands, did a retrospective review of 250 patients with recurrent breast cancer. When detected, 63% were symptomatic and 37% were not. The recurrent breast cancer was local in 45% (45/100) of the asymptomatic patients and in 14% (23/170) of the symptomatic patients. "There was no significant difference in the disease-free survival between the two groups." Furthermore, "when locoregional and distant recurrences were analysed separately, no significant differences were found between both groups in overall survival after primary treatment or in survival after detection of recurrence." The authors questioned the value of the current follow-up management of breast cancer.

The International Consensus Conference on image-detected breast cancer discusses screening mammography, pathologic processing, prognostic issues, sentinel lymph node biopsy, percutaneous biopsy, breast conserving therapy, partial breast irradiation, quality of life issues, and tamoxifen therapy.[3] The conference concluded: "Wider implementation of currently available techniques will improve patient selection, reduce recurrence rates, mortality, and morbidity of therapy, improve cosmetic results and decrease overall cost."

Pijnappel et al[4] reviewed 749 non-palpable breast lesions treated in multiple routine daily practices. A primary surgery approach was the initial procedure in 42% of the lesions which "were more frequently not visible on ultrasound (62%) and mainly consisted of microcalcifications only (56%)." However, the authors state: "In 45%, this primary surgical approach could have been avoided." In conclusion, the authors stressed "the importance of protocols in order to standardise diagnostic procedures and prevent unnecessary surgery."

William H. Hindle, MD

References

1. Keating NL, Guadagnoli E, Landrum MB, et al: Treatment decision making in early-stage breast cancer: Should surgeons match patient's desired level of involvement? *J Clin Oncol* 20:1473-1479, 2002.
2. te Boekhorst DS, Peer NG, van der Sluis RF, et al: Periodic follow-up after breast cancer and the effect on survival. *Eur J Surg* 167:490-496, 2001.
3. International Breast Cancer Consensus Conference: Image-detected breast cancer: State of the art diagnosis and treatment. *J Am Col Surg* 193:297-302, 2001.
4. Pijnappel RM, Peeters PHM, van den Donk M, et al: Diagnostic strategies in non-palpable breast lesions. *Eur J Cancer* 38:550-555, 2002.

Benedict S, Cole DJ, Baron L, et al: Factors influencing choice between mastectomy and lumpectomy for women in the Carolinas. *J Surg Oncol* 76:6-12, 2001.

▶ This study based on mailed questionnaires of women in North and South Carolina, USA, who were treated for breast cancer during 1995-1998 confirmed the low rate of breast conserving surgery (BCS) in this area. In fact, the rate of BCS actually dropped from 23% in 1995 to 18% overall (1995-1998). This contrasts sharply with other areas in the USA which have reported rates as high as 63% BCS.[1] USA national figures (1995) reveal that 45.8% of the women diagnosed with breast cancer were stage I and of these, 58% were treated by partial mastectomy (lumpectomy). In this current survey, the major reasons given for choosing mastectomy were: (1) perceived better cure rate, (2) "quickly getting rid of all cancer cells," and (3) avoiding irradiation.

The sources of information for the mastectomy group in addition to their physicians were (in order of descending frequency): (1) friends, (2) American Cancer Society, (3) relatives, (4) the media, (5) nurses and (6) the Internet. Thus, this wide spectrum of sources of patient information needs to be educated about the data supporting BCS as the preferred method of treatment for Stage I and II breast cancer.

William H. Hindle, MD

Reference

1. Stanton A, Estes M, Estes N, et al: Treatment decision making and adjustment to breast cancer: A longitudinal study. *J Consult Clin Psycho* 66:313-322, 1998.

510 / Obstetrics, Gynecology, and Women's Health

2. Bland K, Menck H, Scott-Conner C, et al: The national cancer data base 10-year survey of breast carcinoma treatment at hospitals in the United States. *Cancer* 83:1262-1273, 1998.

Surgical Management of High-Risk Patients
Rhei E, Nixon AJ, Iglehart JD (Brigham and Women's Hosp, Boston; Elliot Hosp, Manchester, NH; Wentworth-Douglass Hosp, Dover, NH)
Breast Dis 12:3-12, 2001   31–4

Background.—The state of knowledge about genes that predispose to breast cancer is reviewed, with an emphasis on how this knowledge may alter treatment approaches.

Hereditary genes that cause breast cancer.—To date, 5 hereditary breast and ovarian cancer genes have been identified (Table 1); BRCA1 and BRCA2 are the most common and are the focus of this report. All of these genes are located on autosomal chromosomes, and thus men and women each have a 50% likelihood of inheriting a mutation from a parent who is a carrier. The penetrance of the mutation (ie, the likelihood that a mutation carrier will actually develop the disease), however, is higher in women and in certain ethnic or geographic populations, such as Ashkenazi Jews. The risk of Ashkenazi Jewish women with the BRCA1 mutation of developing breast cancer by the age of 70 years is estimated at 50% to 60%; the corresponding risk for BRCA2 carriers is 30% to 60%. Having 1 or more close relatives with breast cancer is also a risk factor. The risk of non-Ashkenazi Jewish women with a family history of breast cancer of developing breast cancer by age 70 years is 70% to 80%. Nonetheless, not all BRCA1/BRCA2 carriers will develop breast cancer, nor are most cases of breast cancer associated with mutations in these 2 genes. Among 206 families with breast cancer (but not ovarian cancer), even in those families with 5 or more women who developed breast cancer before the age of 50 years, about half of the cases were attributable to BRCA1/BRCA2 mutations (Table 2). Thus, identifying which patients should be referred for genetic counseling is important (Table 3).

Treatment of BRCA1/BRCA2 carriers.—Women with BRCA1/BRCA2 mutations should perform monthly breast self-examinations and undergo annual or semiannual clinical breast examinations. Mammography should

TABLE 1.—Hereditary Breast Cancer Genes and the Syndromes They Cause

Hereditary Genes That Cause Breast Cancer	Syndrome	Population Frequency Estimate (%)
p53	Li-Fraumeni Syndrome	<<1%
CHK2	Atypical Li-Fraumeni	<<1% (individual reports)
PTEN	Cowden's Disease	<<1% (too small to estimate)
BRCA1	Familial Breast & Ovarian Cancer	0.1-0.2% (general population) 1% in certain populations
BRCA2	Familial Breast & Ovarian Cancer	0.08-0.1% (general population) 1% in certain populations

(Courtesy of Rhei E, Nixon AJ, Iglehart JD: Surgical management of high-risk patients. *Breast Dis* 12:3-12, 2001.)

TABLE 2.—BRCA1 and BRCA2 Mutations in Breast Cancer Families

Number of Female Breast Cancers < 50	Number of Families Studied	Number Attributable to BRCA1	Number Attributable to BRCA2	Number Attributable to either (%)
2	84	3	12	17.8
3	67	6	8	20.9
4	34	6	7	38.2
>4	21	4	8	57.1

Based on 206 breast cancer-only families from Duke University and the Imperial Cancer Research Fund in London, England.
(Courtesy of Rhei E, Nixon AJ, Iglehart JD: Surgical management of high-risk patients. *Breast Dis* 12:3-12, 2001.)

be performed annually beginning between ages 25 and 35. Prophylactic mastectomy can dramatically reduce the incidence of breast cancer in women with an inherited predisposition, but patients must be carefully evaluated and educated before and after the procedure to minimize adverse physical and psychological effects. Chemoprevention may be another option, but whether antiestrogen therapy or estrogen withdrawal via oophorectomy will have the same beneficial effects in BRCA1/BRCA2 carriers as in the general population is unknown at present. For patients who develop BRCA1/BRCA2-associated breast cancer, breast-conserving therapy may be an option for those with early disease. Studies addressing treatment outcomes after breast-conserving therapy in women with an inherited susceptibility to breast cancer are sparse but indicate that relapse-free and overall survival are similar in these patients and in patients with sporadic breast cancer. The risk of contralateral breast cancer, however, is much higher (15% to 40%) in patients with BRCA1/BRCA2-associated breast cancer, and this higher risk should be considered in the decision-making process. Whether women with hereditary breast cancer should undergo radiation therapy remains controversial, because some evidence suggests that radiation therapy actually increases the risk of tumor formation in these patients.

► The excitement surrounding the initial identification of the BRCA1 and BRCA2 genes has been muted by the limitations of the application of this information to clinical practice, as only a small percentage eg (5%) of invasive breast cancers are associated with the more than 100 breast cancer related mutations currently identified on these genes. The mechanisms of the biolog-

TABLE 3.—Criteria for Referral to Genetic Counseling

1. Family with > 1 breast cancers < age 50 and ≥ 1 ovarian cancer diagnosed at any age
2. Family with > 3 breast cancers diagnosed before age 50

3. Two sisters diagnosed before age 50 with	2 breast cancers or 2 ovarian cancers or 1 breast and 1 ovarian cancer

Modified from American Society of Clinical Oncology criteria defining families with >10% likelihood of harboring BRCA1 mutation.
(Courtesy of Rhei E, Nixon AJ, Iglehart JD: Surgical management of high-risk patients. *Breast Dis* 12:3-12, 2001.)

ic actions of these mutations in the "cause" of cancer is as yet unknown. Identification of other breast cancer related genes and elucidation of the microbiologic actions of the individual mutations urgently awaits further research and discovery. Tables 1 through 3 give current sound guidance for clinicians in counseling their patients. A trained and experienced medical genetics counselor in a multidisciplinary setting should do further detailed counseling. However, clear and concise patient information is available in such soft cover books[1] such as authored by Dr Pat Kelly, one of the pioneers in medical genetic counseling, particularly about breast cancer.

W. H. Hindle, MD

Reference

1. Kelly PT: Assess your true risk of breast cancer. New York, Henry Holt and Company, 2000.

SUGGESTED READING

Hultman CS, Bostwick J III: Breast reconstruction following mastectomy: Review of indications, methods, and outcomes. *Breast Disease* 12:113-130, 2001.

▶ Ob-Gyns need to be aware of the opportunities for breast reconstruction for breast cancer patients. This overview and summary of the authors' experience with ample illustrations and references offer a good basis for discussions with patients. Since the introduction in 1982 of the TRAM (transverse rectus abdominis myocutaneous) flap,[1] immediate reconstruction, which does not compromise oncologic management, has become increasingly popular. Skin-sparing mastectomy (1996)[2] (except in smokers, diabetics and women who have had chest irradiation) allows superior cosmetic results and has not been shown to alter recurrence or survival rates. Nipple-areolar reconstruction is usually performed about 3 months after the initial reconstruction. The authors prefer a "nipple sharing procedure."[3] Other "aesthetic refinements" often include (1) suction-assisted lipectomy of the donor sites, (2) revisions of redundant skin, (3) dermal-fat grafts for scar depressions, and (4) multiple Z-plasties in lines of scar tension. In 1996, the authors instituted breast reconstruction "Clinical Pathways" at their institutions with goals to improve patient education, standardize physician practice patterns, streamline nursing care, decrease complications, and improve resource utilization. With the Clinical Pathways program, the use of immediate TRAM reconstruction increased from 61% to 70%, the flap loss rate decreased from 7.4% to 1.4%, seroma formation decreased from 14.9% to 5.4%, pulmonary complications decreased from 4% to 1%, and fat necrosis remained at 25%.

William H. Hindle, MD

References

1. Hartrampf CR, Scheflan M, Black PW: Breast reconstruction with a transverse abdominal island flap. *Plast Reconstr Surg* 69:216-224, 1982.
2. Singletary SE: Skin-sparing mastectomy with immediate breast reconstruction: The M.D. Anderson Center expereince. *Ann Surg Oncol* 3:411-416, 1996.
3. Jones G, Bostwick J: Nipple-areolar reconstruction. *Operative Tech Plast Reconstr Surg* 1:35-38, 1994.

Smith BL: Complications of breast surgery. *Breast Dis* 12:95-101, 2001.

▶ Noting that "complications rates are no higher when breast procedures are performed on an outpatient or short-stay basis," Smith et all present a clinical overview of (1) wound infection, (2) hematoma, (3) seroma, (4) flap necrosis, (5) Mondor's diseases, (6) injuries to adjacent structures, (7) missed lesions on breast biopsy, (8) complications of sentinel node biopsy, (9) effects of isosulfan blue in node mapping, (10) lymphedema, (11) chronic breast edema and cellulitis, (12) pain syndromes and (13) mobility problems. This summary from the Massachusetts General Hospital, Boston, Mass, briefly reviews the current literature relevant to each of the above with ample references (54 in all). Except for lymphedema, morbidity from current surgical procedures is low.

Gajdos et al[1] at the Robert H Lurie Comprehensive Cancer Center, Northwestern University, Chicago, Ill, reviewed a clinical experience (1978-1998) of 206 women aged 70 years and older and compared the risk factors, presentation, pathology, treatment, and outcomes to 920 younger patients. The cancers of the older group were more often visible on mammography (usually a mass), had better differentiated cancers, which were more likely ER negative and PR positive, and were treated with fewer mastectomies, fewer axillary node dissections, less irradiation, and less chemotherapy compared to the younger patients. Tamoxifen was given to 57% of the older group and 36% of the younger group. The mean follow-up was 63 months. "Elderly patients' rates of local and distant recurrence were comparable to those of younger patients after both mastectomy and breast conservation." Even though 57% (98/180) of the older group received "under treatment by conventional criteria, the rates of local recurrence and distant metastasis are not increased in comparison with conventionally treated elderly patients."

Schnaper & Hughes[2] provide a clinical overview of breast cancer patients older than age 70 and note that approximately 31.6% of breast cancers in women occur in this older age group. The authors cite ongoing research sugesting ". . .that tamoxifen alone is effective in preventing breast tumor recurrence and eventual mastectomy, then radiotherapy can potentially be omitted without increasing risk to the patient."

William H. Hindle, MD

References

1. Gajdos C, Tartter PI, Bleiweiss IJ, et al: The consequence of undertreating breast cancer in the elderly. *J Am Coll Surg* 192:698-707, 2001.
2. Schnaper LA, Hughes KS: Special considerations when treating breast cancer in the elderly. *Breast Dis* 12:83-93, 2001.

Chemoprevention for High-Risk Women: Tamoxifen and Beyond
Fabian CJ, Kimler BF (Univ of Kansas, Kansas City)
Breast J 7:311-320, 2001   31–5

Background.—Among the 75% of women with a diagnosis of breast cancer who survive, some long-term morbidity from local or systemic treatment is probable. Thus, prevention must focus on reducing morbidity related to treatment as well as mortality. Changes termed intraepithelial neoplasia oc-

Intraepithelial Neoplasia in the Breast

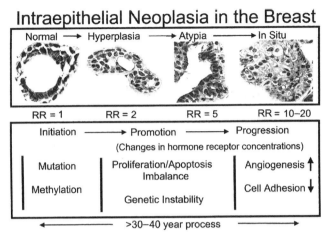

FIGURE 1.—Pathway for the development of intraepithelial neoplasia in the breast. The stepwise progression that is discernible morphologically is associated with processes of initiation, promotion, and progression. The various biological processes may occur over a 30- to 40-year span before reaching the in situ stage and subsequently progressing to invasive breast cancer. *Abbreviation: RR,* Relative risk. (Courtesy of Fabian CJ, Kimler BF: Chemoprevention for high-risk women: Tamoxifen and beyond. *Breast J* 7(5):311-320, 2001. Reprinted by permission of Blackwell Science, Inc.)

cur over decades before breast cancer is found and reflect an increased cancer risk (Fig 1). Chemopreventive efforts are directed at blocking or reversing precancerous progression and diminishing the incidence or delaying the appearance of invasive cancer.

Chemopreventive Agent.—Tamoxifen can selectively regulate estrogen receptors (ERs) by binding to them and blocking the transcription process they direct (Fig 2). As the only drug fulfilling the criteria for breast chemoprevention, it is used for premenopausal and postmenopausal women aged 35 years or older whose 5-year predicted probability of breast cancer devel-

Tamoxifen Inhibits ER-Directed Transcription

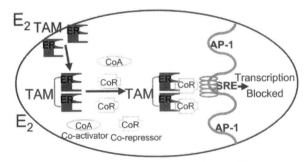

FIGURE 2.—Schematic of the pathway through which tamoxifen can inhibit transcription that is mediated via the estrogen receptor (*ER*). Tamoxifen competitively binds with the ER, displacing estrogen. The resultant complex preferentially binds co-repressors rather than coactivators, which promote transcription. With only co-repressors bound to the receptor, the steroid response element does not function and transcription is blocked. (Courtesy of Fabian CJ, Kimler BF: Chemoprevention for high-risk women: Tamoxifen and beyond. *Breast J* 7(5):311-320, 2001. Reprinted by permission of Blackwell Science, Inc.)

The Gail Risk Model
for Development of Breast Cancer

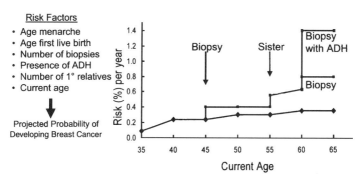

FIGURE 3.—Representation of the risk for development of breast cancer according to the Gail model. For example, a woman with menarche at age 14 and no first live birth before age 30, but no other risk factors, would experience a gradual increase in risk per year with increasing age. A biopsy at age 45 would result in an increased calculated risk, as would a sister with a diagnosis of breast cancer when the woman is 55. Finally, a second biopsy at age 60 would increase risk again, and if the biopsy showed evidence of atypical hyperplasia, would be an additional increase in risk. (Courtesy of Fabian CJ, Kimler BF: Chemoprevention for high-risk women: Tamoxifen and beyond. *Breast J* 7(5):311-320, 2001. Reprinted by permission of Blackwell Science, Inc.)

opment at least equals that of a typical 60-year-old woman. The National Surgical Adjuvant Breast Project (NSABP) found that 5 years of tamoxifen reduced breast cancer incidence in high-risk women by about 50%, yet side effects such as hot flashes, menstrual abnormalities, and bone loss in premenopausal women, plus uterine cancer, deep venous thrombosis, pulmo-

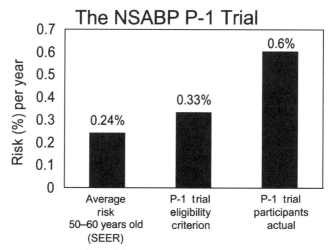

FIGURE 4.—Comparison of risk of development of breast cancer for the average 50- to 60-year-old woman, the criterion for entry into the National Surgical Adjuvant Breast Project (*NSABP*) P-1 trial, and the actual mean value for all participants in the P-1 trial. (Courtesy of Fabian CJ, Kimler BF: Chemoprevention for high-risk women: Tamoxifen and beyond. *Breast J* 7(5):311-320, 2001. Reprinted by permission of Blackwell Science, Inc.)

Pathways to Breast IEN

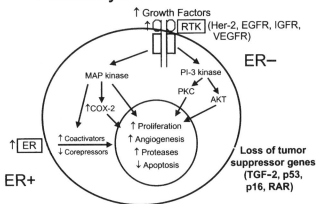

FIGURE 5.—Pathways to breast intraepithelial neoplasia (*IEN*). An estrogen receptor (*ER*)-dependent pathway functions through the ER to promote transcription. An ER-independent pathway is initiated by various growth factors and is mediated via kinase cascades. For both pathways, the simultaneous loss of tumor suppressor gene function may exacerbate the preneoplastic processes of increased proliferation, decreased apoptosis, increased angiogenesis, and increased protease activity. (Courtesy of Fabian CJ, Kimler BF: Chemoprevention for high-risk women: Tamoxifen and beyond. *Breast J* 7(5):311-320, 2001. Reprinted by permission of Blackwell Science, Inc.)

nary embolism, and stroke in women over age 50 years make its use unwise for all high-risk women. Women with ER-positive invasive breast cancer or ductal carcinoma in situ who take tamoxifen reduce their risk of development of contralateral breast cancer by 40% to 50% and are excellent candidates for this therapy. Tamoxifen appears a good choice for women aged 35 years or older meeting NSABP P-1 eligibility criteria (5-year Gail predicted probability of 1.7% or greater) (Fig 3), but participants in this trial had a high average Gail risk (Fig 4). Women with a prior ductal carcinoma in situ, ER-positive invasive cancer, or a *BRCA1* or *BRCA2* germline mutation and no history of thromboembolic events or precancerous uterine biopsy are also good candidates.

Biomarkers.—Biomarkers indicate a drug's potential as a chemoprevention agent. Of the biomarkers investigated thus far, breast intraepithelial neoplasia is most closely allied with the underlying neoplastic process (Fig 5). While tamoxifen has been linked to reduced mammographic breast density volume and serum insulin-like growth factor–1, indicating a favorable clinical response, these findings are not validated.

Conclusion.—Currently, only tamoxifen is approved for breast cancer risk reduction, and it carries an increased risk for serious side effects, especially for women over age 50 years. Tamoxifen reduces the incidence of ER-positive cancers by 67% but does not reduce the risk for ER-negative cancers. Those who benefit most from its use have the highest short-term risk of breast cancer and the lowest risk of thromboembolic events and uterine cancer, especially those who have had a biopsy of atypical hyperplasia, lobular or ductal carcinoma in situ, or ER-positive invasive breast cancer. Other women who may benefit are white women aged 35 to 49 years whose 5-year Gail risk is 1.7% or greater and women aged 50 years or older whose 5-year Gail risk is 2.5% or greater for those without a uterus and 5.0% or greater for those with a uterus. Tamoxifen should not be used for women who have had deep venous thrombosis or uterine precancerous conditions.

▶ This clinically oriented overview with 117 references summarizes the current status of chemoprevention of breast cancer. The accompanying 5 figures clearly illustrate the current knowledge of the development and pathways of breast intraepithelial neoplasia, the action of tamoxifen, and the application of the Gail risk model. Research continues in the search of predictable and consistent risk and response biomarkers. Molecular abnormalities observed in intraepithelial neoplasia, breast density volume, and serum markers (for example, insulin-like growth factor–1) are under study. Other chemotherapeutic agents, such as raloxifene, are undergoing clinical trials with the goal of avoiding the tamoxifen side effects of hot flashes, menstrual abnormalities, and—particularly in postmenopausal women—uterine cancer and thromboembolic phenomena.

The authors conclude, "Those individuals likely to derive greatest benefits are women with a prior biopsy of atypical hyperplasia, lobular or ductal carcinoma in situ, or ER-positive invasive breast cancer." They note further, "Tamoxifen does not reduce the incidence of ER-negative cancers and only reduces the incidence of ER-positive cancers by 67%."

Of related interest, Port et al reported a low level of acceptance (less than 5% in this study) of chemoprevention with tamoxifen by women who met the criteria for entry into the NASABP P-1 clinical trial.[1] Most of the women declined treatment due to fear of the known side effects of tamoxifen. Educational sessions did not increase the level of acceptance. The work of Cameron et al indicates the multifactorial and complex actions of tamoxifen that result in altered apoptotic:mitotic ratios with shift of the balance between apoptosis and mitosis, compared to untreated cancer growth, being directly dependent only on the mitotic rate.[2]

W. H. Hindle, MD

References

1. Port ER, Montgomery LL, Heerdt AS, et al: Patient reluctance toward tamoxifen use for breast cancer primary prevention. *Ann Surg Oncol* 8:580-585, 2001.
2. Cameron DA, Ritchie AA, Miller WR: The relative importance of proliferation and cell death in breast cancer growth and response to tamoxifen. *Eur J Cancer* 37:1545-1553, 2001.

SUGGESTED READING

Cole BF, Gelber RD, Gelber S, et al: Polychemotherapy for early breast cancer: An overview of the randomised clinical trials with quality-adjusted survival analysis. *Lancet* 358:277-286, 2001.

▶ This overview analysis of 47 randomized breast cancer trials (n = 18,000) summarizes the chemotherapy benefits within 10 years' follow-up. Women less than 50 years of age "gained an average of 10.3 months of relapse-free survival and 5.4

months of overall survival." The quality-adjusted benefit ranged from −0.6 to 10.3 months. Women aged 50 to 69 years gained "6.8 months of relapse free survival and 2.9 months of overall survival." Statistically, all these benefits were close to or at P = 0.0001. The quality-adjusted benefit ranged from −3.1 to 6.8 months. Similar analysis needs to be done for tamoxifen therapy in both age groups.

William H. Hindle, MD

Kuerer HM, Singletary SE: Integration of neoadjuvant chemotherapy and surgery in the treatment of patients with breast carcinoma. *Breast Dis* 12:69-81, 2001.
▶ This clinically oriented overview points out that neoadjuvant chemotherapy has been documented to (1) increase the resectability of primary breast cancers, (2) facilitate more women having breast conserving surgery by "down staging" the cancer, and (3) has no survival disadvantage compared to standard adjuvant chemotherapy. Neoadjuvant chemotherapy has become the preferred initial treatment for locally advanced and inflammatory breast carcinomas. The authors state that, "The clinical and pathologic response of the primary breast tumor to neoadjuvant chemotherapy appears to be a surrogate maker for the response of occult micrometastases and therefore patient outcome."

Johnson et al[1] reviewed the assessment of margins in maximizing local control by breast conserving surgery. Touch prep cytology and intraoperative ultrasound are effective intraoperative methods of evaluating "clear" surgical margins.[2] MRI, where the technology is available, is effective in the preoperative assessment of the potential success of breast conserving surgery and "in assessing the completeness of initial breast cancer surgery in the referred patient."[3]

William H. Hindle, MD

References

1. Johnson AT, Henry-Tillman R, Klimberg VS: Breast conserving surgery: Optimizing local control in the breast with assessment of margins. *Breast Dis* 12:35-41, 2001.
2. Klimber VS, Harms S, Korourian S: Assessing margin status. *Surg Oncol* 8:77-84, 1999.
3. Harms SE: Technical report of the International Working Group on Breast MRI. *J Magn Reson Imaging* 10:978-1015, 1999.

Bonneterre J, Buzdar A, Nabhlotz J-MA, et al: Anastrozole is superior to tamoxifen as first-line therapy in hormone receptor positive advanced breast cancer. *Cancer* 92:2247-2258, 2001.
▶ These 2 randomized, double-blind trials (n = 1021 postmenopausal women) compared tamoxifen 20 mg daily with anastrozole (a selective nonsteroidal aromatase inhibitor) 1 mg daily. The end points were (1) time to progression, (2) objective response, and (3) tolerability. The mean duration of follow-up was 18.2 months. Comparatively, somewhat increased benefits were noted in the anastrozole arm of the trials. Anastrozole therapy led to less thromboembolic events and vagina bleeding compared to tamoxifen. However, long-term clinical trials will be required to assess the occurrence of uterine abnormalities and the effects on osteoporosis and cardiovascular disease. For now, anastrozole appears to be at least an alternate first or second line therapy for advanced breast cancer.

William H. Hindle, MD

Bartlelink H, Horiot JC, Poortmans P, et al: Recurrence rates after treatment of breast cancer with standard radiotherapy with or without additional radiation. *N Engl J Med* 345:1378-1387, 2001.

▶ This report of the European Organization for Research and Treatment of Cancer Radiotherapy and Breast Cancer Groups covers 5318 stage I or II breast cancer patients. About half of the patients received 16 Gy to the tumor bed in addition to the standard 50 Gy to the entire breast. With a mean duration follow-up of 5.1 years, the additional tumor bed irradiation decreased the local recurrence rate from 7.3% to 4.3%. The largest benefit was noted in the group of women 40 years of age or younger. Only age and additional irradiation significantly affected the local recurrence rates. Survival free of distant metastases, overall survival, and cause of death were similar in both the groups treated with and without additional irradiation. It is of particular clinical interest that re-excision was necessary in 24% of the patients in order to obtain clear surgical margins. This adverse effect of breast conserving surgery (re-excision) needs further attention, awareness, and clinical investigation.

William H. Hindle, MD

Breast Carcinoma in Women Age 25 Years or Less
Kothari AS, Beechey-Newman N, D'Arrigo C, et al (Guy's Hosp, London; St James' Univ, Leeds, England)
Cancer 94:606-614, 2002   31–6

Background.—Breast cancer occurs in few women younger than age 35, although young age at diagnosis has been variously found to be an independent risk factor and to carry a poor prognostic outlook. The effects of age on the prognosis for breast cancer was explored, comparing women age 25 to 35 with those age 36 to 65 in terms of long-term survival, presentation and extent of disease at diagnosis, and aspects of tumor pathology.

Methods.—The 15 participants (median age, 24 years) were selected from women who received care at Guy's Hospital's Breast Unit and consisted of 2 age groups (younger than age 25 and age 25 to 35) whose tumor characteristics and survival were gleaned from their medical charts. When it was possible and appropriate, the women from the 2 groups were individually matched for tumor size and histologic grade. The term *young* was used to refer to women age 26 to 35 and the term *very young* referred to those under age 25 (Fig 1). Comparisons were made with women age 36 to 65 who were received the diagnosis of breast cancer and who were in the same unit over the same period.

Results.—Symptoms were present for 1 to 104 weeks (median, 4 weeks), and delay to diagnosis after the first visit ranged from 3 to 350 days (median, 14 days). Twelve patients (80%) had a distinct palpable mass at the time of diagnosis; 3 had focal nodularity of the breast on palpation only. Of those with palpable lumps, 58% had T1 lesions, 24% had T2 lesions, and 17% had T3 lesions. No statistical differences in tumor size were found between the young and very young women (Table 1). None of these women had mammograms taken. Two patients (13%) had DCIS (1 high grade and 1 low

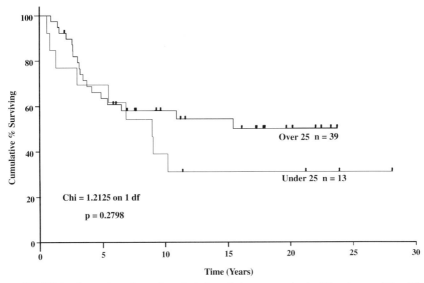

FIGURE 1.—Comparison of overall survival of matched very young (under 25) and young (26 to 35) patients with invasive disease. (Courtesy of Kothari AS, Beechey-Newman N, D'Arrigo C, et al: Breast carcinoma in women age 25 years or less. *Cancer* 94:606-614, 2002. Copyright 2001 American Cancer Society. Reprinted by permission of Wiley-Liss, Inc, a subsidiary of John Wiley & Sons, Inc.)

grade) and 13 (87%) had invasive ductal carcinoma. In 4 patients (31%), the lesions were moderately differentiated and in 9 (69%) they were poorly differentiated invasive tumors. In 4 patients (33%) who had axillary clearance had nodal involvement. No statistical differences in preponderance of Grade II tumors, frequency of estrogen receptor positive status, C-erb B2 overexpression, or proportion of node-positive cases were noted between the young and very young groups. In comparison to the age 36-to-65–years group, the combined young and very young group had a higher proportion of Grade III carcinomas and a lower proportion of estrogen receptor positive

TABLE 1.—Comparative Clinicopathologic Features of All Patients ≤35 Years of Age Compared to Older Age Groups Seen In the Guy's Breast Unit Between 1970 and 1995

Feature/Age	≤ 35 yr	P Value ≤ 35 v. 36-65 yr (1 df)	36-45 yr	46-55 yr	56-65 yr	P Value 36-45, 46-55, 56-65 yr (2 df)	P Value Between All Decades (4 df)
n	13	118	514	904	867		
Mean tumor size (cm)	2.51	0.2162	2.56	2.64	2.83	0.005 (sig.)	0.011 (sig.)
Proportion of Grade III	63%	9×10^{-12} (sig.)	39%	32%	30%	0.005 (sig.)	1.3×10^{-11} (sig.)
Proportion expressing ER	63%	1.8×10^{-4} (sig.)	61%	68%	75%	7.3×10^{-6} (sig.)	4×10^{-7} (sig.)
Proportion with positive axillary nodes	54%	0.6208	54%	52%	48%	0.0518	0.072
50% survival (years)	10.3	0.0003 (sig.)	18.69	17.93	16.6	0.613	0.007 (sig.)

Abbreviations: Yr, Years; *ER,* estrogen receptor.
(Courtesy of Kothari AS, Beechey-Newman N, D'Arrigo C, et al: Breast carcinoma in women age 25 years or less. *Cancer* 94:606-614, 2002. Copyright 2001 American Cancer Society. Reprinted by permission of Wiley-Liss, Inc, a subsidiary of John Wiley & Sons, Inc.)

TABLE 5.—Clinicopathologic Features of Patients Aged ≤25 Years Who Relapsed

Tumor Size (mm)	Symptom Duration (Weeks)	Tumor Grade	Nodal Status	Primary Treatment	Adjuvant Treatment	ER/PgR	C-erb B-2	Relapse Site
10	4	2	Negative	MRM	CT	Neg/Neg	Pos	SCF
10	3	3	Negative	BCT	None	Neg/Neg	Neg	Lung
30	2	3	Negative	MRM	None	Neg/Neg	Neg	SCF
40	4	2	Negative	BCT	None	Pos/Neg	Neg	Local
10	8	3	Positive	BCT	None	Pos/Pos	Neg	SCF
20	3	2	Positive	MRM	CT	Pos/Pos	Neg	Bone
40	6	2	Positive	MRM	None	Pos/Pos	Neg	SCF +Bone
60	26	3	Positive	MRM	CT	Pos/Neg	Neg	Bone

Abbreviations: PR, Progesterone receptor; *ER,* estrogen receptor; *BCT,* breast conservation therapy; *CT,* chemotherapy; *MRM,* modified radical mastectomy; *SCF,* supraclavicular fossa.

(Courtesy of Kothari AS, Beechey-Newman N, D'Arrigo C, et al: Breast carcinoma in women age 25 years or less. *Cancer* 94:606-614, 2002. Copyright 2001 American Cancer Society. Reprinted by permission of Wiley-Liss, Inc, a subsidiary of John Wiley & Sons, Inc.)

tumors. Of the women with invasive carcinoma, 8 patients had mastectomy, 4 were offered breast conservation therapy, and 1 had primary chemotherapy, followed by radiotherapy. Of the DCIS cases, 1 had wide excision only and 1 had simple mastectomy without axillary surgery. Median duration to relapse was 24 months, and the 8 patients who had relapse died of their disease (Table 5). The survival of young women did not differ significantly from that of very young women (Fig 2), but when combined, the survival of wom-

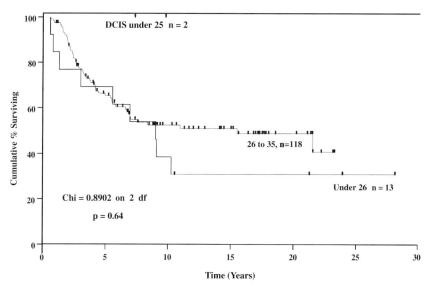

FIGURE 2.—Overall survival of all patients aged 25 or less compared to those aged 26 to 35 years. (Courtesy of Kothari AS, Beechey-Newman N, D'Arrigo C, et al: Breast carcinoma in women age 25 years or less. *Cancer* 94:606-614, 2002. Copyright 2001 American Cancer Society. Reprinted by permission of Wiley-Liss, Inc, a subsidiary of John Wiley & Sons, Inc.)

en younger than 35 was significantly worse than that for women age 36 to 65.

Conclusions.—Among women younger than age 35 who have breast cancer, the prognosis differs little between those younger than 25 and those older than 25. However, all women younger than 35 have a significantly worse prognosis than those who are older than 35. This high mortality rate can be addressed with careful selection of both local treatment and adjuvant systemic therapy.

▶ It took 25 years (1970-1995) at the Guy's Hospital Breast Unit, London, UK, to accumulate 15 cases of breast cancer in women aged 25 years or younger and of these, 2 were ductal carcinoma in situ. More so than in some other reports (all with small numbers), the cases in this series were similar in cancer characteristics to groups of older women. However, 69% (9/13) developed recurrences and died of their cancers. The seemingly worse prognosis in this young age group appeared to be related to higher grade and estrogen receptor negative cancers, even though two thirds of the patients were node negative. However, any such conclusions are tentative due to the small numbers (n = 13) and, not surprisingly, no differences in tumor characteristics reached statistical significance.

W. H. Hindle, MD

SUGGESTED READING

Skinner KA, Silberman H, Sposto R, et al: Palpable breast cancers are inherently different from nonpalpable breast cancers. *Ann Surg Oncol* 8:705-710, 2001.

▶ Intuitively, it would seem that there is some inherent difference between palpable and nonpalpable T1 breast cancers. This study of 1263 T1 breast cancers (1981-2000) found that palpability correlated with higher S-phase, lymphovascular invasion, mitotic grade, nodal positivity, nuclear grade, pathologic tumor size, and worse breast cancer specific survival, but had less extensive intraductal component, multicentricity, and multifocality. Only the differences of nodal positivity and less multifocality were statistically significant. However, no changes in treatment were recommended. The authors estimated that even with 100% annual mammography compliance and 100% accurate mammographic interpretation, "13% of breast cancers would still be detected only when they became palpable. . ." Thus, clinical breast examination remains an essential component of annual screening for breast cancer.

Moore et al[1] reported a prospective study of intraoperative ultrasound for the assessment of surgical margins for invasive carcinoma. The radial margin was most commonly the location of the "nearest" (or cut, ie positive). These reported results are encouraging and add to those published by Smith et al.[2] Clear surgical margins continue to be a vexing and major problem, particularly for breast conserving surgery.

William H. Hindle, MD

References

1. Moore MM, Whitney LA, Cerilli L, et al: Intraoperative ultrasound is associated with clear lumpectomy margins for palpable infiltrating ductal breast cancer. *Ann Surg* 233:761-768, 2001.
2. Smith LF, Rubio IT, Henry-Tillman R, et al: Intraoperative ultrasound-guided breast biopsy. *Am J Surg* 180:419-423, 2000.

Familial Breast Cancer: Collaborative Reanalysis of Individual Data From 52 Epidemiological Studies Including 58 209 Women With Breast Cancer and 101 986 Women Without the Disease
Beral V, for the Collaborative Group on Hormonal Factors in Breast Cancer (Radcliffe Infirmary, Oxford, England; et al)
Lancet 358:1389-1399, 2001   31–7

Introduction.—Women with a family history of breast cancer are at increased risk for the disease, yet no trials have been large enough to characterize reliably how, over a women's life, the risk of breast cancer is affected by particular patterns of disease in first-degree relatives. The relevance of the pattern of breast cancer in first-degree female relatives to a woman's risk of breast cancer at various ages was examined.

Methods.—Individual data on breast cancer in first-degree relatives of 58,209 women with breast cancer and 101,986 controls were collected, examined, and analyzed. Risk ratios for breast cancer were determined by conditional logistic regression stratified by trial, age, menopause status, number of sisters, parity, and age when the first child was born. Breast cancer and mortality rates for particular family histories were determined by applying age-specific risk ratios to breast cancer rates usual for more-developed countries.

Results.—A total of 7496 (12.9%) women with breast cancer and 7438 (7.3%) control subjects reported having 1 or more first-degree relatives with a history of breast cancer; 12% of women with breast cancer had 1 affected relative; 1% had 2 or more (Fig 2). Risk ratios for breast cancer rose with increasing numbers of affected first-degree relatives, compared with women with no affected relatives. The ratios were 1.80 (99% CI 1.69-1.91); 2.93 (CI, 2.36-3.64), and 3.90 (CI, 2.03-7.49), respectively, for 1, 2, and 3 or more affected first-degree relatives ($P < .0001$ each). The risk ratios were highest for younger ages. For women of a given age, the risk ratios were greater the younger the relative was when the diagnosis was made. Findings did not differ notably between women reporting an affected mother (1904) or sister (6386).

Other factors, including childbearing history, did not significantly impact the risk ratios linked to a family history of breast cancer. For women from more-developed countries with 0, 1, or 2 affected first-degree relatives, the estimated cumulative incidences of breast cancer up to age 50 years were 1.7%, 3.7%, and 8.0%, respectively (Fig 4). Corresponding figures for the incidence up to age 80 years were 7.8%, 13.3%, and 21.1%, respectively.

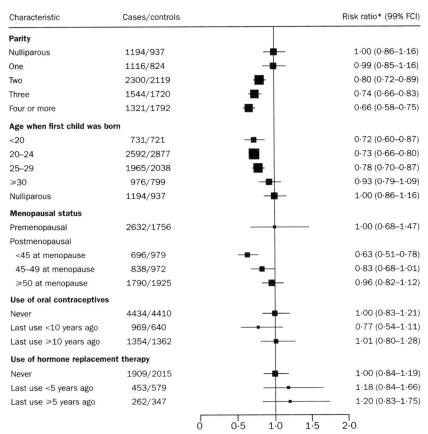

Characteristic	Cases/controls	Risk ratio* (99% FCI)
Parity		
Nulliparous	1194/937	1·00 (0·86–1·16)
One	1116/824	0·99 (0·85–1·16)
Two	2300/2119	0·80 (0·72–0·89)
Three	1544/1720	0·74 (0·66–0·83)
Four or more	1321/1792	0·66 (0·58–0·75)
Age when first child was born		
<20	731/721	0·72 (0·60–0·87)
20–24	2592/2877	0·73 (0·66–0·80)
25–29	1965/2038	0·78 (0·70–0·87)
≥30	976/799	0·93 (0·79–1·09)
Nulliparous	1194/937	1·00 (0·86–1·16)
Menopausal status		
Premenopausal	2632/1756	1·00 (0·68–1·47)
Postmenopausal		
<45 at menopause	696/979	0·63 (0·51–0·78)
45–49 at menopause	838/972	0·83 (0·68–1·01)
≥50 at menopause	1790/1925	0·96 (0·82–1·12)
Use of oral contraceptives		
Never	4434/4410	1·00 (0·83–1·21)
Last use <10 years ago	969/640	0·77 (0·54–1·11)
Last use ≥10 years ago	1354/1362	1·01 (0·80–1·28)
Use of hormone replacement therapy		
Never	1909/2015	1·00 (0·84–1·19)
Last use <5 years ago	453/579	1·18 (0·84–1·66)
Last use ≥5 years ago	262/347	1·20 (0·83–1·75)

FIGURE 2.—Risk ratios for breast cancer according to various factors among women who had 1 or more first degree relatives with a history of breast cancer. Risk ratios calculated as floating absolute risks. Stratified by study, age at diagnosis, number of sisters, and where appropriate parity, age at first birth, and menopausal status. (Courtesy of Beral V, for the Collaborative Group on Hormonal Factors in Breast Cancer: Familial breast cancer: Collaborative reanalysis of individual data from 52 epidemiological studies including 58 209 women with breast cancer and 101 986 women without the disease. *Lancet* 358:1389-1399, 2001. Reprinted with permission from Elsevier Science.)

For estimates for death from breast cancer up to age 80, rates were 2.3%, 4.2%, and 7.6%, respectively. The age when the relative was given a diagnosis had a moderate influence on these estimates.

Conclusion.—Eight of 9 women in whom breast cancer develops do not have an affected mother, sister, or daughter. Women who have first-degree relatives with a history of breast cancer are at increased risk for the disease. Most will never have breast cancer and most who do will be over age 50 years when the diagnosis is made. In countries where breast cancer is common, the lifetime excess incidence of breast cancer is 5.5% for women with 1 affected first-degree relative and 13.3% for those with 2 first-degree relatives.

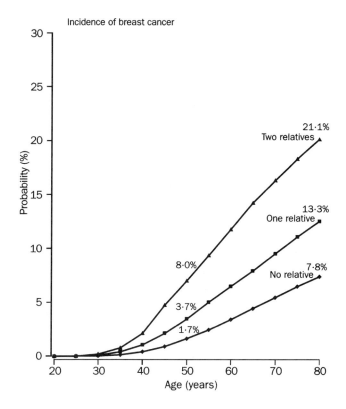

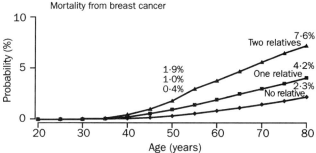

FIGURE 4.—Probability (percentage) that women in more-developed countries who are free from breast cancer at age 20 will have the disease (**top**) or die from it (**bottom**) by various ages, according to the number of affected relatives. (Courtesy of Beral V, for the Collaborative Group on Hormonal Factors in Breast Cancer: Familial breast cancer: Collaborative reanalysis of individual data from 52 epidemiological studies including 58 209 women with breast cancer and 101 986 women without the disease. *Lancet* 358:1389-1399, 2001. Reprinted with permission from Elsevier Science.)

▶ With these impressive numbers, the statistical power of this re-analysis is clinically meaningful. As seen in Figure 2, women reporting a first-degree relative with diagnosed breast cancer showed decreased risk ratios with (1) parity of 2 or more, (2) age when first child was born 29 years or less, and (3) onset of menopause at age 45 or less. Reported use of oral contraceptives and use of hormone replacement therapy did not significantly alter the risk ratio of women with first-degree relatives with breast cancer.

Furthermore, the potential risk factors of race, education, height, body mass index, parity (overall), age at first birth (overall), use of oral contraceptives in previous 10 years, use of hormone replacement therapy in previous 5 years, alcohol use, smoking, age at menarche, and age at menopause (overall) did not significantly alter the base risk of breast cancer for women with first-degree relatives diagnosed with breast cancer. Importantly, the authors conclude: (1) ". . .there was no strong evidence of an interaction between the effects of family history and the other factors, in terms of relative risk of breast cancer" and (2) [there is] ". . . little evidence to suggest an adverse interaction between use of such hormonal therapies and having first-degree relatives with a history of breast cancer with respect to the relative risk of developing the disease."

W. H. Hindle, MD

Sanderson M, Shu XO, Dai Q, et al: Abortion history and breast cancer risk: Results from the Shanghai Breast Cancer Study. *Int J Cancer* 92:899-905, 2001.
▶ Numerous epidemiologic studies have documented that lack of impact of spontaneous abortions upon the risk of breast cancer. This population-based case-control breast cancer study of women aged 25 to 64 years, with impressive numbers of patient interviews, found "no relation between ever having had an induced abortion and breast cancer (odds ratio [OR] = 0.9, 95% confidence interval [CI] 0.7-1.2)." Increased risk was not demonstrated for either pre- or postmenopausal breast cancer for women who had had 3 or more induced abortions. Thus, neither spontaneous nor induced abortions appear to have any impact on the incidence of breast cancer.

William H. Hindle, MD

Breast Cancer Risks: Some Clinically Useful Approaches
Kelly PT (Saint Francis Mem Hosp, Berkeley, Calif)
Curr Womens Health Rep 2:128-133, 2002   31–8

Background.—The way risk information regarding breast cancer is presented promotes confusion and can be misunderstood. The average woman's breast cancer risk, prognosis after a diagnosis of breast cancer, breast cancer risks accompanying hormone replacement therapy (HRT), use of tamoxifen as a preventive agent, risks linked to BRCA mutations, and how genetic testing is used were evaluated and expressed in clinically significant but comprehensible terms.

Cancer Risk, Prognosis, and HRT.—At any age, the magnitude of the risk of breast cancer depends on the number of years being discussed. Average risk from age 20 to 50 years is 2%, from age 50 to 70 years it is 6%, and from age 70 to 80 years it is 3% (Fig 1). Risks for past years no longer apply. Prognosis can be expressed in absolute terms, such as reporting a better than 90% survival to 20 years, or as comparisons, for example, between women receiv-

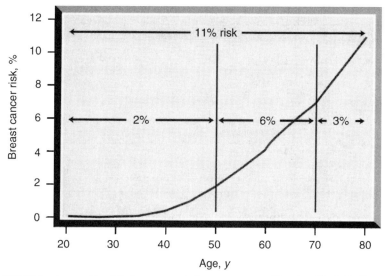

FIGURE 1.—Age-specific risk for breast cancer in the average woman. (Data from Ries LAG, Eisner MP, Kosary CL, et al: *SEER Cancer Statistics Review, 1973-1996*. Bethesda, Md, National Cancer Institute, 1999.) (Courtesy of Kelly PT: Breast cancer risks: Some clinically useful approaches. *Curr Womens Health Rep* 2:128-133, 2002.)

ing tamoxifen and those who did not (Table 1). The absolute format of conveying survival, involving number of women studied and number of years of follow-up, may offer a more meaningful expression of prognosis.

Dealing with the risk-to-benefit dilemma presented by HRT, if the relative risk or odds ratio is 3.0 or more, the difference in risk results from the agent being studied rather than undetected differences or methodologic problems. Duration of use must also enter into the equation, as illustrated by the relationship between the risks of current and past users (Table 2). HRT users who are concerned that they run a higher risk of death from coronary heart disease should be made aware of the Nurses' Health Study (Table 3). The growth of cancer cells showed no increased rapidity with HRT.

Tamoxifen, BRCA, and Genetic Testing.—The 49% reduction in breast cancer risk with the use of tamoxifen reflects only the number of breast can-

TABLE 1.—Proportional Mortality Reduction and Absolute Breast Cancer Survival Differences Following Adjuvant Tamoxifen Treatments

Group*	Overall Proportional Mortality Reduction, %	10-Year Absolute Difference, %
Node negative	25	6
Node positive	28	11

Note: Data indicate 5 years of use. Data from Early Breast Cancer Trialists' Collaborative Group: Tamoxifen for early breast cancer: An overview of the randomised trials. *Lancet* 351:1451-1467, 1998.

*No significant difference in tamoxifen effects in node-positive and node-negative disease.

(Courtesy of Kelly PT: Breast cancer risks: Some clinically useful approaches. *Curr Womens Health Rep* 2:128-133, 2002.)

TABLE 2.—Mammography Use and Breast Cancer Risk in
Current and Past Hormone Replacement Therapy Patients

Use of HRT For ≥ 10 Years	Mammography Use in Past Year, %	Breast Cancer Risk to ≥ 10 Years
Never	49	1.0 (ref.)
Past	50	1.5*
Current	64	1

Note: Data from Colditz GA, Hankinson SE, Hunter DJ, et al: The use of estrogens and progestins and the risk of breast cancer in postmenopausal women. *N Engl J Med* 332:1589-1593, 1995 and Colditz GA, Stampfer MJ, Willett WC, et al: Prospective study of estrogen replacement therapy and risk of breast cancer in postmenopausal women. *JAMA* 64:2648-2653, 2990.
*Significant.
Abbreviation: HRT, Hormone replacement therapy. (Courtesy of Kelly PT: Breast cancer risks: Some clinically useful approaches. *Curr Womens Health Rep* 2:128-133, 2002.)

cers, not the total number of women included or the time period over which these women were studied. Cumulative rate per 100 women would be more instructive (Table 4). The presence of mutations of either the BRCA1 or the BRCA2 gene indicates that the woman has a higher risk of cancer but not that cancer will occur.

The population in which genetic studies are carried out must be evaluated; for example, the BRCA mutations data are based on specially selected families who have large numbers of cancers diagnosed at very young ages and on all known mutations—not an average family. Usually, genetic testing is most informative after a mutation that increases the risk of cancer is found in a family. Cost, likelihood of finding a mutation, and effect of test results on future medical care or quality of life are important considerations in deciding to undergo genetic testing.

Conclusion.—Risk considerations must be expressed in terms of a specific time frame, as an absolute risk rather than in a comparison, and in light of the limitations attending current understanding.

▶ In spite of a plethora of epidemiologic studies of potential breast cancer risk factors, few clinicians, and even fewer patients, actually understand relative

TABLE 3.—Current Use of Hormone Replacement
Therapy and Risk of Death

Cause	Deaths, *n*	Risk*
All	2051	0.6†
Coronary heart disease	289	0.5†
Stroke	91	0.7
All cancer	1103	0.7†
Breast cancer	246	0.8

Note: Data from Grodstein F, Stampfer MJ, Colditz GA, et al: Postmenopausal hormone therapy and mortality. *N Engl J Med* 336:1769-1775, 1997.
*Compared with patients who never used hormone replacement therapy.
†Significant.
(Courtesy of Kelly PT: Breast cancer risks: Some clinically useful approaches. *Curr Womens Health Rep* 2:128-133, 2002.)

TABLE 4.—Tamoxifen Use in Women Without Breast Cancer Diagnosis
and Breast Cancer Rates at 5.75 Years

Numbers and Rates	No Tamoxifen	Tamoxifen For 5 Years
Women, *n*	6599	6576
Breast cancers, *n*	175	89
Average annual rate/100 women	0.6	0.3
Cumulative rate (to 5.75 years)/100 women	3.8	2

Note: Data from Fisher B, Constantino IP, Wickerham DL, et al: Tamoxifen for prevention of breast cancer: Report of the National Surgical Adjuvant Breast and Bowel Project P-1 Study. *J Natl Cancer Inst* 90:1371-1388, 1998.

(Courtesy of Kelly PT: Breast cancer risks: Some clinically useful approach., *Curr Womens Health Rep* 2:128-133, 2002.)

risk, odds ratios and, proportional risk reductions. Percentage figures can be grossly misleading, particularly if the incidence and/or number of cases is small, eg, less than 100. Furthermore, the patient's age and the time frame of the calculation are critical to the clinical utility of the mathematical results. Most women desperately want to know exactly their own individual risk of having breast cancer. Unfortunately, no currently available data or methodology yields the precise, accurate answer for an individual patient.

The available data are mathematic evaluations of raw data from groups of patients, usually with similar demographic characteristics. Furthermore, the specific criteria and methods of patient selection and the details of obtaining, reporting, and processing the data are essential information for the evaluation of the results. All these factors tend to make the typical medical "sound bite" on the evening news almost scientifically meaningless.

All women's health care providers should read this cogent and readily understood article by Dr. Kelly. A detailed soft cover book for patients is available and is helpful reading for clinicians who wish to counsel their patients appropriately.[1]

Examples of reports with conflicting results in case-controlled studies of physical activity and breast cancer risk are the articles of Lee et al[2] and Breslow et al.[3] The former concludes, ". . .no significant trends were observed in any age group," and "These data do not support a role of physical activity in preventing breast cancer." And the latter states, "High recreational physical activity over the long-term may reduce breast cancer risk in women >50 years of age; in this sample, it did so regardless of weight history."

Selection bias, confounding factors, or other multifactorial variables must be at play in these contrary results. The detailed reading of the published methodology does not yield an explanation. What are patients to think and how should they be counseled?

W. H. Hindle, MD

References

1. Kelly PT: *Assess Your True Risk of Breast Cancer.* New York, Henry Holt & Co, 2000.
2. Lee I-M, Cook NR, Rexrode KM, et al: Lifetime physical activity and risk of breast cancer. *Br J Cancer* 85:962-965, 2001.

3. Breslow RA, Ballard-Barbash R, Munoz K, et al: Long-term recreational physical activity and breast cancer in the National Health and Nutrition Examination Survey I epidemiologic follow-up study. *Cancer Epidemiol Biomarkers Prev* 10:805-808, 2001.

SUGGESTED READING

Morris KT, Johnson N, Krasikov N, et al: Genetic counseling impacts decision for prophylactic surgery for patients perceived to be at high risk for breast cancer. *Am J Surg* 181:431-433, 2001.

▶ It is now widely accepted that breast cancer is a multifactorial multigene disorder. The mystery of the occurrence and progression of breast cancer and the various modes of prevention and inhibition/destruction of breast cancer are just beginning to be understood. Genetics plays a fundamental role in all aspects of the biology and natural history of breast cancer. Genetic counseling and risk assessment are becoming essential to the management of women perceived to be at "high risk" and those diagnosed with breast cancer.

This report from the Oregon Health Sciences University, Portland, Oregon, followed 60 women (of which 47% [28/60] actually had "high risk" by calculation) who were considering prophylactic mastectomy or oophorectomy. Thirty-one (37%) considered themselves to be at "high risk." Testing was recommended for 23 of the 31. Of the 10 women who were actually tested, 5 were positive. Seven had proceeded with prophylactic surgery based solely on their risk assessment. Three women with negative tests decided to proceed with surgery anyway. One woman with a positive test declined surgery. "After counseling, prophylactic surgery was performed in just over half [58%] of the initial candidates."

Khabele and Runowicz[1] provide a balanced clinical overview of screening, counseling, and testing for breast and ovarian cancer. The accompanying algorithms, table, and guidelines of the American Society of Clinical Oncology, which "state that testing should be offered to patients with a risk greater than 10% only if a test is interpretable and only if it will affect further medical management,"[2] should assist clinicians and patients in interpretation of technically detailed but often inconclusive genetic data.

William H. Hindle, MD

References

1. Khabele D, Runowicz CD. Genetic counseling, testing and screening for breast and ovarian cancer: practical and social considerations. *Curr Womens Health Rep* 2:163-169, 2002.
2. Statement of the American Society of Clinical Oncology: Genetic testing for cancer susceptibility, adopted February 30, 1996. *J Clin Oncol* 14:1730-1736, 1996.

Understanding Mathematical Models for Breast Cancer Risk Assessment and Counseling
Euhus DM (Univ of Texas, Dallas)
Breast J 7:224-232, 2001   31–9

Background.—Although chemoprevention and prophylactic surgery effectively reduce breast cancer incidence, these approaches are associated with certain risks. Accurate assessment of individualized breast cancer risk is

TABLE 1.—Breast Cancer Risk Factors

Risk Factor	Index Value	Comparison Value	RR	Reference
Reproductive factors				
Total parity	Uniparous	≥5	0.69	30
Early age at menopause	50	≤39	0.71	31
Late age at menarche	13	≥16	0.76	30
Early age at menarche	13	≤11	1.20	14
Late age at menopause	50	≥54	1.31	31
Age at first live birth	20	≥35	1.32	32
Benign breast disease				
Atypical hyperplasia (AH)	No PD	Yes AH	4.3	5
Lobular carcinoma in situ (LCIS)	No PD	Yes LCIS	6.9	9
Family history				
First-degree relative (FDR)	No FDR	Yes FDR	2.4	33

Abbreviations: RR, Relative risk; *PD*, proliferative disease.
(Courtesy of Euhus DM: Understanding mathematical models for breast cancer risk assessment and counseling. *Breast J* 7(4):224-232, 2001. Reprinted by permission of Blackwell Science, Inc.)

essential in the risk-benefit analysis done before either strategy is implemented. In the past decade, several mathematical models have been developed for estimating individual breast cancer risk. These models were discussed.

Discussion.—The most generally accepted model is the Gail model. However, this model does not include family history information regarding second-degree relatives or personal history of lobular neoplasia. In addition, it treats premenopausal and postmenopausal breast cancer as though they are the same. Although the Claus model accounts for family history, it does not assign any special relevance to histories of bilateral breast cancer

TABLE 3.—Relative Strengths and Weaknesses of the Models

Model	Relative Strengths	Relative Weaknesses

Gail	Nonfamily history risk factors
	  Reproductive factors
	  Breast biopsies
	  Atypical hyperplasia
	Caucasian and African American
	Independent validation
		Limited family history information
		  No age at breast cancer diagnosis
		  No second-degree relatives
		Does not account for lobular neoplasia

Claus	Family history information
	  Age at breast cancer diagnosis
	  Pattern of affected relatives
	Likely to recognize non-BRCA familial clusters
		Neglects nonfamily history factors
		Caucasian only
		No independent validation

BRCAPRO	Family history information
	  Age at breast cancer diagnosis
	  Age at ovarian cancer diagnosis
	  Bilateral breast cancer
	  Pattern of affected relatives
	  Unaffected relatives
	Independent validation (partial)
		Neglects nonfamily history factors
		Caucasian only
		Likely to miss non-BRCA familial clusters

(Courtesy of Euhus DM: Understanding mathematical models for breast cancer risk assessment and counseling. *Breast J* 7(4):224-232, 2001. Reprinted by permission of Blackwell Science, Inc.)

TABLE 4.—Selecting the Model Best Able to Account for the Clinical Information

Clinical Scenario	Gail	Claus	BRCAPRO
A 45-year-old woman with benign breast disease whose mother was diagnosed with breast cancer at age 58	√		
A 45-year-old woman with menarche at age 13, first live birth at age 20, and a family history of breast cancer in a maternal aunt at age 57 and a maternal grandmother at age 62		√	√
A 45-year-old woman whose mother developed bilateral breast cancer at ages 39 and 42, and a maternal aunt developed ovarian cancer at age 54			√

(Courtesy of Euhus DM: Understanding mathematical models for breast cancer risk assessment and counseling. *Breast J* 7(4):224-232, 2001. Reprinted by permission of Blackwell Science, Inc.)

or ovarian cancer. It also neglects nonfamily history information included in the Gail model. The BRCAPRO is a Bayesian family history model that determines individual breast cancer probabilities based on the probability that a family carries a mutation in one of the BRCA genes. This model accounts for family history more thoroughly than the other models do but neglects nonfamily history risk factors included in the Gail model. Thus, it may not appreciate familial clustering unassociated with BRCA gene mutation (Tables 1, 3, and 4).

Conclusion.—Clinicians wishing to perform intervention counseling need a thorough understanding of the principles of risk analysis and the mathematical models available. This article describes the basic components of risk analysis, how these models work, and the strengths and weaknesses of each.

▶ Ideally, a computerized mathematical model could accurately estimate breast cancer risk. However, breast cancer is a multifactorial heterogonic disease that is unique to each woman's circumstances, and breast cancer treatment is unique to the specific health care resources available to the individual patient and her informed decisions about that treatment. A basic pitfall of risk models is the reliance on various published data on relative risk in studies that were designed for specific purposes, none of which was to form the basis of mathematical models.

Unfortunately, few published epidemiologic studies of risk factors validate associated causality with (1) review of several studies with similar results, (2) relative risk or odds ratios of 3-fold or greater to rule out methodological biases, and (3) statistical significance. Furthermore, what is critically important is the actual (absolute) risk. In addition, anyone using multiple risk factors must remember that the factors are not additive, much less multiplicative. An easy to read and understand, clear, concise soft cover book on true breast cancer risk written for women by Kelly[1] offers a straightforward review of the subject which could be invaluable for clinicians to read and use as a foundation for discussion with their patients.

W. H. Hindle, MD

Reference

1. Kelly PT: *Assess Your True Risk of Breast Cancer.* New York, Henry Holt & Co, 2000.

SUGGESTED READING

Euhus DM, Leitch AM, Huth JF, et al: Limitations of the Gail model in the specialized breast cancer risk assessment clinic. *Breast J* 8:23-27, 2002.

▶ Though the Gail model is mathematically correct and based on extensive Breast Cancer Detection Demonstration Project data, its potential application to clinical practice is neither clear nor agreed upon. Potential confounding factors for the Gail model are (1) family history of breast cancer in 2nd degree relatives, (2) family history of breast cancer before the age of 50, (3) family history of bilateral breast cancer, (4) family history of ovarian cancer, and (5) personal history of lobular neoplasia. This study of 213 women attending a specialized breast cancer risk assessment clinic utilized the Gail, Claus, and BRCAPRO models and Boding tables to calculate breast cancer risk and found that the risk level assigned was increased in 13% of the cases. The authors concluded that the Gail model by itself was an appropriate risk assessment tool. However, the use of the Gail (or any other model or tables) in general clinical practice continues to be debated.

William H. Hindle, MD

Brinkmann E, Morrow M: The surgeon's role in breast cancer chemoprevention. *Breast Dis* 12:103-112, 2001.

▶ This clinical overview is applicable to Ob-Gyns and evaluates the risk factors for breast cancer and the current prevention options. The relative risk (RR) at RR <2 are (1) early menarche, (2) late menarche, (3) nulliparity, (4) proliferative benign breast disease, (5) obesity, (6) alcohol use and (7) hormone replacement therapy. Factors at RR 2 to 4 are (1) age greater than 35 at first birth, (2) lst degree relative with breast cancer, (3) radiation exposure, and (4) prior breast cancer. Factors at RR >4 are (1) gene mutation, (2) lobular carcinoma in situ, (3) ductal carcinoma in situ, and (4) atypical hyperplasia. In 1995, a survey reported[1] that women visiting a high risk clinic estimated their own risk at levels 10 times higher than their actual risk as calculated by the Gail model,[2] which is the generally accepted (with some known limitations) model for calculating relative risk of breast cancer.

A summary of the NSABP P-1 trial[3] reveals "a 49% risk reduction in the development of invasive breast cancer and a 50% risk reduction in the development of noninvasive breast cancer" with 5 years of tamoxifen therapy. However, in postmenopausal women, an increased risk of endometrial carcinoma and thrombotic vascular events was noted. "The absolute increase in endometrial cancer was from 0.91 cases per 1,000 women in the placebo group to 2.3 per 1,000 in the tamoxifen group."

Dunn and Ford of the National Cancer Institute (Bethesda, Md) provide a clinical overview of the NSABP Breast Cancer Prevention Trial (BCPT) P-1[3] and the Study of Tamoxifen and Raloxifene (STAR) NSABP P-2 clinical trials with 122 references. The STAR trial, based on the observations of the beneficial effects of raloxifene upon the incidence of breast cancer in the MORE trial,[4] is designed to evaluate the effects of tamoxifen 20mg per day or raloxifene 60 mg per day for 5 years given to postmenopausal women with increased risk of breast cancer by the Gail model[2] criteria. The STAR trial is ongoing, and the results are not yet reported.

Cummings et al[5] reported the "baseline serum estradiol concentrations levels measured by a central laboratory using a sensitive assay" from the MORE trial. The assay is not commercially available. However, the results indicate that a subset of women with elevated estradiol levels can be identified and are the women who benefit most from raloxifene therapy to decrease the incidence of breast cancer. Women with "undetectable" levels were found to have no such benefit. If confirmed by similar studies and made commercially available, such testing would be a useful tool in selecting women for raloxifene breast cancer prevention.

Rockhill et al[6] point out that the Gail model 1 estimates probability of both invasive and in situ breast carcinoma whereas the Gail model 2 predicts the incidence of only invasive breast carcinoma. Using data from the Nurses Health Study (n = 82,109) and Gail model 2, this study calculated the Observed and Expected cases (O/E ratio). "Good fit" was found in predicting the number of breast cancer cases in specific age and risk factor strata. "However, its capability to discriminate risk in any given individual was only modest. These findings have important implications at the individual level, given that 96.7% of invasive cancer cases developed in women in age and risk strata that would not be expected to benefit from chemoprophylactic tamoxifen."

William H. Hindle, MD

References

1. Stefanek M, Helzsourer KJ, Wilcox PM, et al: Prediction of satisfaction with bilateral prophylactic mastectomy. *Prev Med* 24:412-419, 1995.
2. Gail MH, Brinton LA, Byar DP, et al: Projecting individual probabilities of developing breast cancer for white females who are being examined annually. *J Natl Cancer Inst* 81:1879-1886, 1989.
3. Fisher B, Costantino JP, Wickerham DL, et al: Tamoxifen for prevention of breast cancer: Report of the National Surgical Adjuvant Breast and Bowel Project P-1 study. *J Natl Cancer Inst* 90:1371-1388, 1998.
4. Dunn BK, Ford LG: From adjuvant therapy to breast cancer prevention: BCPT and STAR. *Breast J* 7:144-157, 2001.
5. Cummings SR, Eckert S, Krueger KA, et al: The effect of raloxifene on risk of breast cancer in postmenopausal women: Results from the MORE randomized trial. *JAMA* 281:2189-2197, 1999.
6. Rockhill B, Spiegelman D, Byrne C, et al: Validation of the Gail et al model of breast cancer risk prediction and implications for chemoprevention. *J Natl Cancer Inst* 93:358-366, 2001.

Herrington DM, Klein KP: Effects of SERMs on important indicators of cardiovascular health: Lipoproteins, hemostatic factors, and endothelial function. *Womens Health Iss* 11:95-102, 2001.

▶ As new SERMs are developed and applied to clinical practice it is essential that the major multifaceted effects on various proteins, factors, and functions are known. This article from the Wake Forest University School of Medicine, Winston-Salem, NC, reviews (and summarizes in clear tables) the literature on tamoxifen, raloxifene, and droloxifene and cardiovascular risk factors. In general, these SERMs all lower LDL, have no effect on HDL or triglyceride levels, and lower fibrinogen and Lp(a). In addition there is evidence of favorable effects on endothelial function. The Raloxifene Use for The Heart (RUTH) clinical trial (10,000 women with or at risk of coronary heart disease treated with 60 mg raloxifene or placebo) should eventually shed some light on the effects on the known cardiovascular risk factors.

Marttunen et al[1] reported on 167 postmenopausal women with stage II-III breast cancer, treated with tamoxifen 20 mg per day (n = 84) and toremifene 40 mg per day (n = 83). The mean follow-up was 2.3 years. Prior to therapy, 35% of the women had vasomotor symptoms, and this increased to 57.21% on tamoxifen and 62.7% on toremifene. The mean endometrial thickness increased from 3.9 mm to 6.8 mm after 6 months of therapy. One patient on toremifene developed endometrial cancer. The endometrium was somewhat more often proliferative and the increased number of polyps somewhat more common in the tamoxifen group compared to the women on toremifene. The authors concluded that close endometrial surveillance was not mandatory—at least during the first 3 years of therapy.

Bergman et al[2] performed a nationwide (The Netherlands) case-control study on the risk and progression of endometrial cancer after tamoxifen use for breast cancer (n = 309 in the study group and 860 controls). The relative risk for endometrial cancer on tamoxifen increased from 2.0 for 2 to 5 years to 6.9 for at least 5 years of therapy compared to non-users. The endometrial cancer was stage III or IV in 17.4% in the tamoxifen group (after more than 2 years) versus 5.4% in the non-users. The endometrial cancer in the tamoxifen group was ER negative in 60.8% compared to 26.2% in the non-users. "3-year endometrial cancer specific survival was significantly worse for long-term tamoxifen users than for non-users (76% for >5 years, 85% for 2-5 years vs 94% for non-users P = 0.02)."

In a semi-structured telephone interview of 25 women on tamoxifen, Arnold et al[3] found "a pattern of ambivalence in attributing symptoms to the drug." "Of all the symptomatic changes noted, the women only attributed 51% to tamoxifen." Flushes, fatigue and depression were the most commonly reported symptoms. Though frequently voiced by the women, the symptoms appear to be under reported as treatment-specific side effects.

William H. Hindle, MD

References

1. Marttunen MB, Cacciatore B, Hietanen S, et al: Prospective study of gynecological effects of two antioestrogens tamoxifen and toremifene in postmenopausal women. *Brit J Cancer* 84:897-902, 2001.
2. Bergman L, Beelen MLR, Gallee MPW, et al: Risk and prognosis of endometrial cancer after tamoxifen for breast cancer. *Lancet* 356:881-887, 2000.
3. Arnold BJ, Cumming CE, Lees AW, et al: Tamoxifen in breast cancer: Symptom reporting. *Breast J* 7:97-100, 2001.

Horn-Ross PL, John EM, Lee M, et al: Phytoestrogen consumption and breast cancer risk in a multiethnic population: The Bay Area Breast Cancer Study. *Am J Epidemiol* 154:434-441, 2001.

▶ This study of 1326 women diagnosed with breast cancer and 1657 control subjects used a questionnaire evaluating their intake of 7 phytoestrogen compounds in 4 ethnic groups. The average intake was "equivalent to less than one serving of tofu per week." "Phytoestrogen intake was not associated with breast cancer risk (odds ratio = 1.0). Pre- and postmenopausal women and all the various ethnic groups had similar results.

Several additional articles relate to soy, nutrition, and body mass. Dai et al[1] in a population-based case-controlled Shanghai, China, study of 1459 breast cancer cases and 1556 age-matched controls concluded: "No clear monotonic dose-response relation was found between soyfood intake and breast cancer risk among regular soy eaters, but nevertheless the results suggest that regular soy-food consumption may reduce the risk of breast cancer, particularly for those positive of ER and PR; the effect may be modified by body mass index."

Shu et al[2] reported a population-based age-matched case-controlled Shanghai, China, study of 1459 breast cancer cases and 1556 controls. The information covered soy food intake by young people [female] aged 13 to 15 years. The author's detailed analysis concluded ". . .that high soy intake during adolescence may reduce the risk of breast cancer in later life."

Van Patten et al[3] from Vancouver, British Columbia, Canada, reported on postmenopausal breast cancer patients with hot flashes who were given soy beverage (n = 50) or placebo (n = 64). "Both groups had significant reduction in hot flashes." However, "The soy beverage did not alleviate hot flashes in women with breast cancer any more than did a placebo."

Byrne et al analyzed[4] data from the Nurses Health Study of 44,697 postmeno-pausal women without benign breast disease (BBD) and "found no increase in the rate of breast cancer with greater intake of dietary fat and fat subtypes among postmenopausal women without a history of BBD."

Ciu et al[5] at the University of Maryland, Baltimore, reported 966 newly di-agnosed breast cancer cases. "Women who were obese (body mass index [BMI] >27.3) were more likely to be at an advanced stage at diagnosis compared with women with a BMI of <27.3." Apparently, obesity interferes with early diagnosis of breast cancer.

William H. Hindle, MD

References

1. Dai Q, Shu X-O, Potter JD, et al: Population-based case-control study of soyfood intake and breast cancer risk in Shanghai. *Brit J Cancer* 85:372-378, 2001.
2. Shu XO, Jin F, Dai Q, et al: Soyfood intake during adolescence and subsequent risk of breast cancer among Chinese women. *Cancer Epidemiol Biomarkers Prev* 10:483-488, 2001.
3. Van Patten CL, Olivotto IA, Chambers GK, et al: Effect of soy phytoestrogens on hot flashes in postmenopausal women with breast cancer: a randomized, controlled clinical trial. *J Clin Oncol* 20:1449-1455, 2002.
4. Byrne C, Rockett H, Homes MD. Dietary fat, fat subtypes, and breast cancer risk: lack of an association among postmenopausal women with no history of benign breast disease. *Cancer Epidemiol Biomarks Prev* 11:261-265, 2002.
5. Cui Y, Whiteman MK, Flaws JA, et al: Body mass and stage of breast cancer at diagnosis. *Int J Cancer* 98:279-283, 2002.

Extent of Ductal Carcinoma *In Situ* Within and Surrounding Invasive Primary Breast Carcinoma

Crombie N, Rampaul RS, Pinder SE, et al (City Hosp NHS Trust, Nottingham, England)
Br J Surg 88:1324-1329, 2001   31–10

Background.—Ductal carcinoma in situ (DCIS), possibly the main precursor lesion for invasive breast cancer, in its pure form accounts for about 5% of palpable breast lumps and more than 20% of cases seen on mammography. The pathologic and morphological characteristics of DCIS in and surrounding invasive ductal carcinoma were reported.

Methods.—One hundred seven patients with primary, operable invasive breast tumors and associated DCIS were included in the study. Treatment consisted of simple or subcutaneous mastectomy or wide local excision plus radiotherapy. Patients with pure DCIS and insufficient tumor available for analysis were excluded. In the remaining 91 patients, the most representative hematoxylin and eosin–stained sections were selected and examined. The entire section was assessed, and the cell under each point of the graticule was categorized as normal, DCIS surrounded by normal tissue, invasive tu-

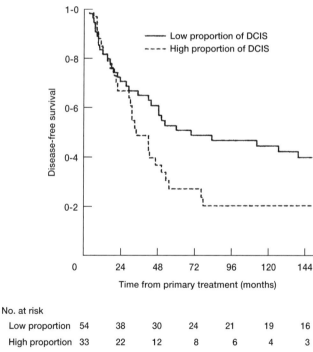

FIGURE 1.—Disease-free interval for patients with tumors showing low and high proportions of ductal carcinoma in situ (*DCIS*) ($\chi^2 = 3.86$; $P = .048$). (Courtesy of Crombie N, Rampaul RS, Pinder SE, et al: Extent of ductal carcinoma in situ within and surrounding invasive primary breast carcinoma. *Br J Surg* 88:1324-1329, 2001. Reprinted by permission of Blackwell Science, Inc.)

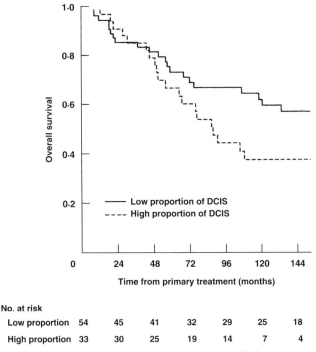

FIGURE 2.—Overall survival for patients with tumors showing low and high proportions of ductal carcinoma in situ (*DCIS*) ($\chi^2 = 2.88$; $P = .089$). (Courtesy of Crombie N, Rampaul RS, Pinder SE, et al: Extent of ductal carcinoma in situ within and surrounding invasive primary breast carcinoma. *Br J Surg* 88:1324-1329, 2001. Reprinted by permission of Blackwell Science, Inc.)

mor, or DCIS surrounded by invasive malignancy. Volume ratios of DCIS in the normal and invasive tissue were then determined.

Findings.—The DCIS volume in invasive tumor did not correlate with outcomes. However, the volume in adjacent normal tissue was related to local recurrence, disease-free interval, occurrence of distant metastases, death, and disease-free survival (Figs 1 and 2). Volume ratios of DCIS in normal and invasive tumors were unassociated with known prognostic factors such as lymph node stage, grade, tumor size, vascular invasion, and patient age.

Conclusion.—The extent of DCIS associated with invasive cancer had a significant prognostic effect, especially in local tumor recurrence. This effect is limited to DCIS volume in tissue surrounding the invasive lesion, not in the intratumoral component.

▶ The quest to understand the natural history and biological behavior of DCIS became urgent with the advent of effective mammography and its resultant detection of a multitude of nonpalpable malignancies. Numerous studies have evaluated the prognostic factors of axillary lymph node involvement, nuclear grade, patient age, presence of necrosis, and tumor size. The size of the area of DCIS involvement appears to be the most important factor. This study from the United Kingdom utilized a volume ratio of DCIS within and without invasive cancer and found associations with disease-free interval, disease-free survival, local recurrence, occurrence of distant metastases, and death. Unfortunately, the procedure requires careful histologic evaluation of the surgical pathologic specimen in order to calculate the volume ratio of DCIS. Hopefully, a reliable tumor marker or surrogate will be identified that gives similar prognostic information.

Lymph node mapping such as advocated by Cox[1] is an essential step in gaining knowledge about DCIS. The mapping identified a 13% incidence of cancer cells in the sentinel lymph nodes of women with DCIS. What is the significance of these cells? Further research and follow-up of clinical outcomes should yield the answer.

Hieken[2] analyzed factor VIII–related antigen, p53, and vascular endothelial growth factor in pure DCIS specimens and found correlation between mutant p53 expression and ipsilateral recurrence which suggests biological aggressiveness, possibly by promoting angiogenesis. When strong correlation of molecular markers with colonial outcomes occurs, specific treatments at the molecular level might then be developed. This is an exciting field of breast cancer research.

W. H. Hindle, MD

References

1. Cox CE, Nguyen K, Gray RJ, et al: Importance of lymphatic mapping in ductal carcinoma in situ (DCIS): Why map DCIS? *Am Surg* 67:513-521, 2001.
2. Hieken TJ, Farolan M, D'Alessandro S, et al: Predicting the biologic behavior of ductal carcinoma in situ: An analysis of molecular markers. *Surgery* 130:593-601, 2001.

SUGGESTED READING

King TA, Farr GH Jr, Cederbom GJ, et al: A mass on breast imaging predicts co-existing invasive carcinoma in patients with a core biopsy diagnosis of ductal carcinoma in situ. *Am Surg* 67:907-912, 2001.

▶ This report from the Ochsner Clinic, New Orleans, La, evaluated the 148 (4.9%) of the 2995 imaging-guided core-needle breast biopsies (July1993-May 2000), which demonstrated ductal carcinoma in situ (DCIS). Pathologic review eliminated 8 cases. Invasive carcinoma was diagnosed in 140 (26%) of the complete excision specimens, which showed DCIS by core-needle biopsy. When comedo-type necrosis, nuclear grade, periductal fibrosis, periductal inflammation, and presence of a mass were analyzed histologically, only the presence of a mass was a significant predictor of invasive carcinoma (P = 0.04). Subsequently, it became institutional policy to perform sentinel lymph node mapping and excision biopsy as the initial surgical procedures for patients with a core-needle biopsy diagnosis of DCIS and the presence of a mass.

DCIS-related clear clinically oriented overviews by Winchester[1] on DCIS and by Edwards and Mahoney[2] on image-guided needle biopsy merit reading by Ob-Gyns and other health care providers for women. Winchester notes "that the mortality of DCIS is virtually equivalent in all studies" and that the problem is local recurrence, half of which recur as invasive carcinoma. Irradiation decreases the recurrent rate by about half (50%). However, there is increasing evidence that clear surgical margins (10mm) produce an even lower local recurrence rate, approximately 3%. Edwards and Mahoney state that "Over one million breast

540 / Obstetrics, Gynecology, and Women's Health

biopsies are performed each year in the U.S., with approximately 80% confirming benign pathology." After review of all the available image-guided needle breast biopsy techniques, the authors conclude that ultrasound guided vacuum-assisted core needle biopsy is the procedure of choice.

Stallard et al[3] in a study of 220 DCIS patients in Glasgow, UK, found that only "mammographic nipple to lesion distance of <40mm and high/intermediate nuclear grade" correlated with increased likelihood of recurrence. Of clinical interest is that 70% (153/220) had breast conserving surgery and 30% (67/220) had a mastectomy. Of the 97 (44%, 97/220) adjuvant therapy patients, 56% (54/97) had only tamoxifen, 23% (22/97) had only irradiation, and 22% (21/97) had both tamoxifen and irradiation.

William H. Hindle, MD

References

1. Winchester DJ: Ductal carcinoma in situ. Breast Dis 12:23-33, 2001.
2. Edwards MJ, Mahoney MC: Image-guided needle breast biopsy. Breast Dis 12:13-21, 2001.
3. Stallard S, Hole DA, Purushotham AD, et al: Ductal carcinoma in situ of the breast—among factors predicting for recurrence, distance from the nipple is important. Eur J Surg Oncol 27:373-377, 2001.

Histopathology of Fibroadenoma of the Breast
Kuijper A, Mommers ECM, van der Wall E, et al (Free Univ, Amsterdam)
Am J Clin Pathol 115:736-742, 2001   31–11

Background.—Fibroadenoma of the breast is generally considered benign but it may be associated with a higher risk of subsequent breast carcinoma. Diagnosed most often in the second and third decades of life, it is not an infrequent finding. It is composed of epithelial and stromal components. The histologic features occurring in these components and in adjacent areas were inventoried in 396 cases.

Methods.—The 396 fibroadenomas were found in 358 patients (Table 1) who ranged in age from 12 to 81 years (mean age, 33.4 years). The size of the

TABLE 1.—Revised Diagnosis of 426 Cases
Originally Diagnosed as Fibroadenoma

Diagnosis	No. (%) of Cases
Fibroadenoma	396 (93.0)
Sclerosing lobular hyperplasia	5 (1.2)
Phyllodes tumor	5 (1.2)
Hamartoma	4 (0.9)
Tubular adenoma	3 (0.7)
Pseudoangiomatous stromal hyperplasia	6 (1.4)
Adenomyoepithelioma	1 (0.2)
Normal tissue	6 (1.4)

(Courtesy of Kuijper A, Mommers ECM, van der Wall E, et al: Histopathology of fibroadenoma of the breast. Am J Clin Pathol 115:736-742, 2001. Copyright 2001 by the American Society of Clinical Pathologists. Reprinted with permission.)

tumors was 0.1 to 22 cm, and 28 patients (7.8%) had multiple tumors. All samples were assessed histopathologically for proliferative epithelial changes, fibrocystic epithelial changes, stromal changes, and various other modifications.

Results.—Pericanalicular fibroadenomas were noted in 60.2% of cases; 20.8% were classified as intracanalicular and 19.0% were of mixed histologic types (Table 2). The most common finding was hyperplasia of various degrees; this occurred in 43.9% of the cases, with 32.3% being hyperplasia of a more than mild degree. The complexity of the fibroadenoma was significantly related to the presence of hyperplasia within the fibroadenoma. While no invasive carcinoma was found, 3 patients had lobular carcinoma in situ and 5 had ductal carcinoma in situ. These patients' mean age was 51.7 years, which is significantly older than the mean age of those without this lesion. Apocrine metaplasia was the most common complex feature, occurring in 28.0% of cases.

Overall, 40.4% of the fibroadenomas were complex, and 18.4% had more than 1 complex feature, with 2.5% having more than 2. Older patients were more likely to have complex fibroadenomas. Complexity showed no link to the presence of hyperplasia in surrounding tissues. In 317 cases, enough adjacent breast tissue was present to be evaluated (Table 3). Some form of hyperplasia was found in adjacent tissue in 13.9% of cases, most

TABLE 2.—Frequency of Histopathologic Changes in
396 Cases of Fibroadenoma

Lesion	No. (%) of Cases
Proliferative epithelial changes	
Mild ductal hyperplasia	46 (11.6)
Moderate ductal hyperplasia	106 (26.8)
Florid ductal hyperplasia	21 (5.3)
Atypical ductal hyperplasia	1 (0.3)
Atypical lobular hyperplasia	0 (0.0)
Lobular carcinoma in situ	3 (0.8)
Ductal carcinoma in situ	5 (1.3)
Invasive carcinoma	0 (0.0)
Fibrocystic epithelial changes	
Apocrine metaplasia	111 (28.0)
Cysts	20 (5.1)
Sclerosing adenosis	49 (12.4)
Calcifications	15 (3.8)
Microglandular adenosis	1 (0.3)
Papilloma	7 (1.8)
Pseudolactational changes	2 (0.5)
Squamous metaplasia	1 (0.3)
Stromal changes	
Pseudoangiomatous changes	15 (3.8)
Smooth muscle	11 (2.8)
Other	
Foci of tubular adenoma	2 (0.5)
Focal phyllodes tumor	3 (0.8)

(Courtesy of Kuijper A, Mommers ECM, van der Wall E, et al: Histopathology of fibroadenoma of the breast. *Am J Clin Pathol* 115:736-742, 2001. Copyright 2001 by the American Society of Clinical Pathologists. Reprinted with permission.)

TABLE 3.—Frequency of Histopathologic Changes in the Adjacent
Parenchyma of 317 Cases of Fibroadenoma

Lesion	No. (%) of Cases
Proliferative epithelial changes	
Mild ductal hyperplasia	16 (5.1)
Moderate ductal hyperplasia	22 (6.9)
Florid ductal hyperplasia	3 (0.9)
Atypical ductal hyperplasia	2 (0.6)
Atypical lobular hyperplasia	2 (0.6)
Lobular carcinoma in situ	1 (0.3)
Ductal carcinoma in situ	6 (1.9)
Invasive carcinoma	3 (0.9)
Fibrocystic epithelial changes	
Apocrine metaplasia	75 (23.7)
Cysts	8 (2.5)
Sclerosing adenosis	46 (14.5)
Calcifications	11 (3.5)
Microglandular adenosis	6 (1.9)
Papilloma	1 (0.3)
Pseudolactational changes	4 (1.3)
Squamous metaplasia	0 (0.0)
Stromal changes	
Pseudoangiomatous changes	0 (0.0)
Smooth muscle	0 (0.0)
Other	
Foci of tubular adenoma	0 (0.0)
Focal phyllodes tumor	0 (0.0)

(Courtesy of Kuijper A, Mommers ECM, van der Wall E, et al: Histopathology of fibroadenoma of the breast. *Am J Clin Pathol* 115:736-742, 2001. Copyright 2001 by the American Society of Clinical Pathologists. Reprinted with permission.)

often in older patients (mean age, 45.5 years). Adjacent tissues showed lobular carcinoma in situ in 1 patient and ductal carcinoma in situ in 6. Three cases showed invasive carcinoma in the surrounding parenchyma of the fibroadenoma but not involving the fibroadenoma itself. Apocrine metaplasia was also the most common fibrocystic epithelial change noted in adjacent tissues, found in 23.7% of cases.

Conclusion.—A variety of histologic changes accompany the finding of fibroadenoma. A long list of benign lesions mimic fibroadenoma, making diagnosis difficult and the differentiation important in some cases. Hyperplasia was a common finding, both in the fibroadenoma and in the surrounding tissues, as was apocrine metaplasia. Most often, it is in older patients (over age 35 years) that factors leading to elevated risk are found.

▶ Although fibroadenomas are the most common benign tumors of the breast, we await the findings of molecular biology and genetic research to achieve a clear understanding of the origin, variants, and natural history of fibroadenomas. Dupont was helpful in differentiating the "simple fibroadenomas" (by far the most common type) from "complex fibroadenomas."[1] The latter are associated with various histologic changes within and neighboring the fibroadenoma and appear to be associated with a low level of increased risk of eventual invasive carcinoma—usually elsewhere in the breast, and not within the fibroadenoma. Invasive carcinoma arising within a fibroadenoma is exceptionally rare and should be diagnosed and treated in the same manner as invasive carcinoma arising elsewhere in the breast.

This study from the Free University Hospital, Amsterdam, the Netherlands demonstrated the prevalence and wide variety of histologic changes within and adjacent to breast fibroadenomas. Hyperplasia (of varying degrees) was commonly noted within the fibroadenomas. Complex histologic features were present in 40%, mostly in older patients (mean age, 35.4 years). The risk-related changes in or adjacent to the fibroadenomas occurred mostly in women 35 years of age or older. Thus, conservative management of a definitively diagnosed fibroadenoma appears to be a rational option for women less than 35 years of age, if the patient so desires. When there is doubt about the histologic implications of the triple test, a tissue core-needle biopsy (often with US guidance) should be performed to establish a definite histologic diagnosis.

In a related report, p53 gene mutations and microsatellite alterations were studied in fibroadenomas. The authors concluded, ". . .fibroadenoma does not constitute a significant increase in the relative risk of later contracting breast cancer."[2]

W. H. Hindle, MD

References

1. Dupont WD, Page DL, Parl FF, et al: Long-term risk of breast cancer in women with fibroadenoma. *N Engl J Med* 331:10-15, 1994.
2. Franco N, Picard S-F, Mege F, et al: Absence of genetic abnormalities in fibroadenomas of the breast determined at p53 gene mutations and microsatellite alterations. *Cancer Res* 61:7955-7958, 2001.

Evaluation and Management of the Woman With an Abnormal Ductal Lavage

Morrow M, Vogel V, Ljung B-M, et al (Northwestern Univ, Chicago; Univ of Pittsburgh, Pa; Univ of California, San Francisco; et al)
J Am Coll Surg 194:648-656, 2002   31–12

Background.—Prophylactic tamoxifen and prophylactic mastectomy can reduce the risk of breast cancer in high-risk women, but only if we develop methods for reliably identifying these women. Ductal lavage appears to be such a method, and its use in risk assessment is described.

How ductal lavage works.—Ductal lavage is a minimally invasive method that collects large quantities of epithelial cells from the breast ductal system. In brief, the nipple is aspirated to identify fluid-containing ducts, which are then lavaged with about 10 mL of saline solution. The samples are prepared and stained according to standard cytologic techniques, and results are categorized as benign, mild atypia, marked atypia, malignant, or inadequate cellular material for diagnosis. Cytologic atypia appears to have the same implications for breast cancer risk as histologic atypia. However, until more

TABLE 1.—Risk Factors for Breast Cancer

Risk Factor	Comparison Category	Risk Category	Relative Risk	Prevalence (%)
Age at menarche	16 years	Younger than 12 years	1.3	16
Age when first child born alive	Before 20 years	Nulliparous or older than 30 years	1.9	21
Benign breast disease	No biopsy or fine-needle aspiration	Any benign disease	1.5	15
		Proliferative disease	2.0	4
		Atypical hyperplasia	4.0	1
Family history of breast cancer	No first-degree relative affected	Mother affected	1.7	8
		Two first-degree relatives affected	5.0	4
Estrogen replacement therapy	Never used	Current use, between ages 50 to 59 years	1.5	18

(Courtesy of Morrow M, Vogel V, Ljung B-M, et al: Evaluation and management of the woman with an abnormal ductal lavage. *J Am Coll Surg* 194: 648-656, 2002. Reprinted with permission from the Journal of the American College of Surgeons.)

data are available, ductal lavage should be considered not as a diagnostic tool but as an adjunct in risk assessment in carefully selected women.

Patient selection.—Ductal lavage should be integrated into a comprehensive assessment approach that also includes known factors that increase the risk of breast cancer, such as age, gynecologic history, history of benign breast disease, family history of breast cancer, and estrogen replacement therapy (Table 1). In models that included these risks, the presence of atypical hyperplasia approximately doubled an individual's risk of developing breast cancer. At present, ductal lavage seems to be most appropriate for high-risk women who are facing decisions about initiation of early mammographic screenings, beginning tamoxifen prophylaxis, using hormone replacement therapy, or undergoing prophylactic mastectomy. In these women, ductal lavage results can enhance the value of a comprehensive risk assessment program (Fig 1).

▶ This is an up-to-date clinical summary of the status of ductal lavage beginning with a review of risk factors for breast cancer. Rapidly advancing technology has produced ductal endoscopy tools and ductal lavage systems, which are now commercially available. However, it is essential that multi-institutional clinical trials be carefully carried out to establish the indications for and the specificity/sensitivity of detecting malignancy of these ductal tools and systems. Even theoretically, it seems highly unlikely that ductal evaluation of any kind will have any potential for screening.

Ductograms (Galactograms) have been utilized for the evaluation of nipple discharge for more than 20 years,[1] though the technique receives limited attention in the USA. When an intraductal lesion is identified, the approximate location can be ascertained which assists in the surgical excision of the lesion. All intraductal lesions should be excised, as there are no reliable imaging criteria to definitively differentiate benign from malignant lesions.

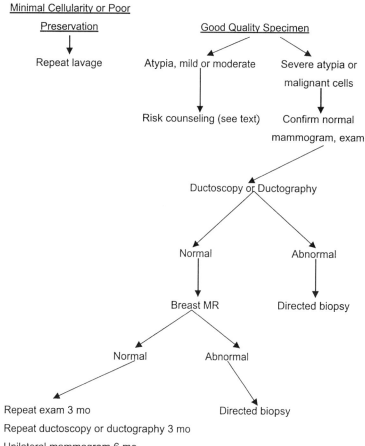

Minimal Cellularity or Poor
Preservation

Repeat lavage

Good Quality Specimen

Atypia, mild or moderate

Severe atypia or
malignant cells

Risk counseling (see text)

Confirm normal
mammogram, exam

Ductoscopy or Ductography

Normal

Abnormal

Breast MR

Directed biopsy

Normal

Abnormal

Repeat exam 3 mo

Repeat ductoscopy or ductography 3 mo

Unilateral mammogram 6 mo

Consider tamoxifen

Directed biopsy

FIGURE 1.—Algorithm for evaluation of the woman with an atypical or malignant ductal lavage. The workup is determined by the quality of the specimen and the severity of the cytologic changes. (Courtesy of Morrow M, Vogel V, Ljung B-M, et al. Evaluation and management of the woman with an abnormal ductal lavage. *J Am Coll Surg* 194: 648-656, 2002. Reprinted with permission from the Journal of the American College of Surgeons.)

Lawler[2] reported on 175 ductal flush cytology specimens of which 92 had follow-up surgical data. More than 75% of the specimens were reported as atypical. Only 3 of the 20 cancers had malignant cytology, and 2 were reported as negative. Thus, in this series, the ductal flush cytology had low sensitivity (3/20) and 10% (2/20) false-negatives. Certainly much more evaluation needs to be done in research settings before the clinical practice application of these ductal techniques can occur.

W. H. Hindle, MD

References

1. Tabar L, Dean PB, Pentek Z: Galactography: The diagnostic procedure of choice for nipple discharge. *Radiology* 149:31-38, 1983.
2. Lawler MJ, Levin E, Newton A, et al: Can the cytological evaluation of nipple aspirate fluid predict the diagnosis of breast carcinoma? [Abstract] *Breast J* 7:371, 2001.

SUGGESTED READING

Schwarz RJ, Shrestha R: Needle aspiration of breast abscesses. *Am J Surg* 182:117-119, 2001.

▶ This prospective study from Kathmandu, Nepal, of 33 breast abscesses (83% [25/30] of the 30 patients were lactating) achieved an overall cure rate of 82% with needle aspiration (18-guage needle with a 10-mL syringe) of the abscesses. All received oral cloxacillin 500 mg four times a day and were outpatients. Ultrasound was not used. Nine patients (30%) required multiple aspirations. Six patients (20%) ultimately required incision and drainage. The initial volume of aspirated pus was less (4.0 mL vs 21.5 mL, P = 0.002) and the presentation was earlier (5.0 days versus 8.5 days, P = 0.006) for the successfully aspirated patients compared to those requiring incision and drainage. Since 1988, Dixon[1,2] has recommended this technique for both lactating and non-lactating women. At the Breast Diagnostic Center, Women's and Children's Hospital, Los Angeles, Calif, the technique has been modified by the use of local anesthesia and ultrasound for confirmation of a liquid center (abscess), visualization and direction of the aspiration, and ascertaining complete drainage, with similar results. However, patients requiring eventual incision and drainage usually had 100 cc or more of pus upon initial aspiration.

Foxman[3] followed 946 breast-feeding women for three months postpartum and found that "9.5% reported provider-diagnosed lactation mastitis at least once during the 12-week period" of which 64% were diagnosed via the telephone. History of mastitis with a previous child, cracks and nipple sores in the same week as the mastitis, using an antifungal nipple cream, and using a manual breast pump strongly predicted mastitis (OR = 4.0-3.3). Protective effect was seen for women breast-feeding less than 10 times a day (OR = 0.4). Mastitis was not associated with the duration of breast-feeding.

William H. Hindle, MD

References

1. Dixon JM: Repeated aspiration of breast abscesses in lactating women. *BMJ* 297:1517-1518, 1988.
2. Dixon JM: Outpatient treatment of non-lactating breast abscesses. *Br J Surg* 79:56-57, 1992.
3. Foxman B, D'Arcy H, Gillespie B, et al: Lactation Mastitis: Occurrence and Medical Management among 946 breastfeeding women in the United States. *Am J Epidemiol* 155:103-114, 2002.

Usefulness of the Triple Test Score for Palpable Breast Masses

Morris KT, Pommier RF, Morris A, et al (Oregon Health Sciences Univ, Portland)
Arch Surg 136:1008-1013, 2001   31–13

Background.—The "triple test" in the evaluation of palpable breast masses includes physical examination, mammography, and fine-needle aspiration (FNA) in women 40 years and older. The triple test score (TTS) was hypothesized to be useful and accurate in assessing palpable breast masses.

Methods.—Four hundred seventy-nine women with 484 palpable breast lesions were examined between 1991 and 2000. Physical examination, mammography, and FNA were scored as 1, 2, or 3 for benign lesions, lesions suggestive of malignancy, or malignant lesions, respectively. The TTS is the sum of these scores. Results from subsequent histopathologic analysis or follow-up were correlated with the TTS.

Findings.—On clinical follow-up, all lesions with a TTS of 4 or less were benign, including 8 lesions for which the FNA results were considered suggestive of malignancy. Fifty-one of the 60 lesions that underwent biopsy were normal breast tissue, 4 showed fibrocystic changes, 1 was a papilloma, and 4 were atypical hyperplasia. All lesions with a TTS of 6 or greater were confirmed to be malignant on biopsy. The specificity of a TTS of 4 or less was 100%, and the sensitivity of a TTS of 6 or more was 100%. Thirty-nine lesions had scores of 5. Forty-nine percent of these proved to be malignant, and 51% proved to be benign.

Conclusions.—The TTS reliably guides the assessment and treatment of palpable breast masses. In the current series, masses with scores of 3 or 4 were always benign, and masses with scores of 6 or greater were malignant. Confirmatory biopsy is needed only for the masses with a TTS of 5, which occurred in 8% of this series.

▶ The authors represent a multidisciplinary breast clinic at the Oregon Health Sciences University, Portland. The triple test "initially described in 1975"[1] was utilized in their clinic for the evaluation of palpable masses in women aged 40 or older. In 1995, they published their results and noted a substantial reduction in the number of open surgical biopsies in their instituion.[2] In response to the occurrence of 40% non-concordant triple test, a triple test score (TTS) was developed which further allowed the reduction in open surgical biopsies.[3] This current report covers 484 palpable breast masses evaluated by their TTS. The results are impressive. However, "the cytopathologists are present to perform all FNAs." Though this undoubtedly limits non-diagnostic FNAs and poor quality cellular material on the slides, many (probably most, in the editor's experience) breast clinics do not have this idea personnel situation. What about the vast majority of women with palpable breast lumps who are seen by solo practitioners or in small (or even large) medical groups without such ideal personnel on site? Hindle et al[4] have suggested modification of the FNA technique, which potentially makes FNA applicable in most medical office and clinic circumstances.

An example of the continuing cutting edge FNA research is the work of Mountford et al[5] with magnetic resonance spectroscopy of FNA aspirates predicting malignancy, lymph node involvement, and vascular invasion with overall accuracies of 93% to 95%.

W. H. Hindle, MD

References

1. Johanses C: A clinical study with special reference to diagnostic procedures. *Acta Clin Scand* 451:1-70, 1975.
2. Vetto JT, Pommier PF, Schmidt WA, et al: Use of the "triple test" for palpable breast lesion yields high diagnostic accuracy and cost savings. *Am J Surg* 169:519-522, 1995.
3. Morris A, Pommier RF, Schmidt WA: Accurate evaluation of palpable breast masses by the triple test score. *Arch Surg* 133:930-934, 1998.
4. Hindle WH, Arias RD, Felix JC, et al: Breast cancer: Adaptation of fine needle aspiration to office practice. *Clinical Obstet Gynecol* 45(3):761-766, 2002.
5. Mountford CF, Somorjai RL, Malycha P, et al: Diagnosis and prognosis of breast cancer by magnetic resonance spectroscopy of fine-needle aspirates analysed using a statistical classification strategy. *Brit J Surg* 88:1234-1240, 2001.

Critical Clinicopathologic Analysis of 23 Cases of Fine-Needle Breast Sampling Initially Recorded as False-Positive: The 44-Year Experience of the Institut Curie
Klijanienko J, Zajdela A, Lussier C, et al (Institut Curie, Paris)
Cancer 93:132-139, 2001   31–14

Background.—A major limitation of fine-needle sampling (FNS) is finding false-positive cytologic diagnoses, which affect surgical management decisions, the pathologist/surgeon relationship, the psychologic aspects of accepting the presence of a malignant disease, and medicolegal considerations. Because these false-positive findings are rare, a large number of cases must be reviewed to produce enough to assess their causes. The experience of the Institut Curie, a French anticancer facility that sees about 1700 new cases of breast cancer each year, was assessed retrospectively over 44 years to determine why false-positive diagnoses occur.

Methods.—FNS was used to assess 9334 benign breast lesions preoperatively. Twenty-three cases were identified as false-positive results (0.25% of cases), and these were reviewed retrospectively.

Results.—In 16 cases (70%), the tumors were distant from the nipple and in 7 they were located centrally (30%). One was T0, 18 were T1, and 4 were T2; all patients were N0M0. Radiologically, 9 were judged to be benign, 7 were suspicious or indeterminate, and 6 were malignant. On follow-up mammograms done 3 to 15 months postoperatively, all patients showed an absence of radiologic abnormalities. Retrospectively, the cytologic diagnoses were benign in 12 cases, suspicious in 7 cases, and malignant in 4 cases (Table 1). On multidisciplinary clinicopathologic analysis, 20 of the preoperative FNSs were determined to be false-positive and 3

TABLE 1.—Clinicopathologic Characteristics of the Patients

Patient No.	Age (yrs)	Site/Radiology	TNM	Cytology Review	Histology Material	Histology Review	DNA Index	Clinical Course (mos)	Follow-up (mos)
1	71	Distant benign	T2N0	Benign	Lumpectomy	Phyllodes tumor	—	Colon carcinoma (73)	DOD (75)
2	60	Central benign	T2N0	Suspicious	Lumpectomy	Fibroadenoma	—	No evidence of disease	DDF (62)
3	49	Central benign	T1N0	Benign	Drill biopsy	Fibroadenoma	—	Ipsilateral breast cancer (93)	ADF (266)
4	35	Distant malignant	T1N0	Benign	Lumpectomy + LN	Fibroadenoma	—	No evidence of disease	ADF (218)
5	62	Central indeterminate	T1N0	Benign	Lumpectomy	Duct ectasia	—	No evidence of disease	ADF (16)
6	50	Distal benign	T1N0	Suspicious	Lumpectomy	Phyllodes tumor	—	No evidence of disease	ADF (15)
7	72	Distant malignant	T1N0	Suspicious	Lumpectomy	Fibrocystic changes	—	No evidence of disease	ADF (132)
8	65	Distal suspicious	T1N0	Suspicious*	Mumpectomy	Inflammation	—	Radiotherapy	ADF (30)
9	42	Central malignant	T1N0	Benign	Lumpectomy + LN	Radial scar	—	No evidence of disease	ADF (160)
10	55	Distant suspicious	T1N0	Benign	Lumpectomy + LN	Duct ectasia	—	No evidence of disease	ADF (42)
11	51	Distant not done	T1N0	Suspicious	Lumpectomy + LN	Fibroadenoma	—	No evidence of disease	ADF (129)
12	67	Central suspicious	T2N0	Benign	Mastectomy + LN	Fibroadenoma	1.0	Controlateral breast cancer (4)	LWD (4)
13	56	Distant benign	T1N0	Suspicious	Lumpectomy	AIH	1.0	No evidence of disease	ADF (58)
14	44	Distant malignant	T2N0	Benign	Lumpectomy	Sclerosing adenosis	1.0	Cancer of ovary (52)	ADF (59)
15	52	Distant benign	T1N0	Benign	Lumpectomy	Fibroadenoma	—	No evidence of disease	ADF (43)
16	30	Distant benign	T1N0	Benign	Lumpectomy + LN	Fibroadenoma	1.0	Ipsilateral breast cancer (20)	ADF (39)
17	77	Distant benign	T0N0	Suspicious†	Lumpectomy	Fibrocystic changes	—	No evidence of disease	ADF (4)
18	48	Distant benign	T1N0	Malignant	Lumpectomy	AIH	—	No evidence of disease	ADF (200)
19	66	Central indeterminate	T1N0	Benign	Lumpectomy + LN	Duct ectasia	1.76	No evidence of disease	ADF (120)
20	42	Distant suspicious	T1N0	Benign	Drill biopsy	Sclerosing adenosis	1.50	No evidence of disease	ADF (29)
21	52	Central suspicious	T1N0	Malignant	Lumpectomy	Fibrocystic changes	—	Local recurrence + metastases (12)	DOD (26)
22	47	Distant malignant	T1N0	Malignant	Lumpectomy	AIH	1.30	Lymph nodes metastases (70)	ADF (127)
23	63	Distant malignant	T1N0	Malignant	Lumpectomy	AIH	—	Local recurrence (25)	ADF (82)

*Diagnosed initially as lymphoma.
†Diagnosed initially as mucinous carcinoma.
Abbreviations: DOD, Dead of disease; *DF*, disease free; *ADF*, alive disease-free; *LN*, axillary lymph node dissection; *LWD*, lost with disease; *AIH*, atypical intraductal hyperplasia.
(Courtesy of Klijanienko J, Zajdela A, Lussier C, et al: Critical clinicopathologic analysis of 23 cases of fine-needle breast sampling initially recorded as false-positive: The 44-year experience of the Institut Curie. *Cancer* 93(2):132–139, 2001. ©2001, American Cancer Society. Reprinted by permission of Wiley-Liss, Inc, a subsidiary of John Wiley & Sons, Inc.)

were true-positive based on the finding of local or metastatic progression on short-term follow-up.

Conclusion.—In these cases, the false-positive rate resulted from overdiagnosis of cytologic benign patterns and the presence of atypical morphological criteria. The cytopathologist's level of experience was the most important technical factor involved, along with the number of cytopathologists in the laboratory, the quality of the smears, and the number of smears evaluated by a cytopathologist per day. Morphologically, false-positive diagnoses were more likely with certain types of breast tumors, including fibrocystic change, papillomatosis, sclerosing adenosis, dystrophic cysts with apocrine cells, tubular adenosis, gynecomastia, pregnancy-related epithelial modifications, fat necrosis, granulomas, and organizing hematomas. If all tumors found to be benign radiologically but showing suspicious or positive FNS results were further assessed in an intraoperative frozen section examination, surgical overtreatment might be reduced.

▶ This detailed and illustrated report from the Department of Tumor Biology, Institut Curie, Paris covers a 44 year experience of 245,116 cytology reports of which 25,156 were breast diagnostic FNSs on previously untreated breast tumors with histologic correlations. Histologically, 15,822 were malignant and 9,334 were benign. Upon review, 23 (0.25%) were considered to be false-positive. However, 3 of the "false-positives" (malignant by FNS but benign by histology) subsequently developed local (recurrent) malignancy and/or metastasis. Thus, 20 (0.21%) were true false-positive FNS. This gives a false-positive ratio of 1:467 FNS. The ratio for false-negative histology was 1:3111. In addition, 6 of the FNS false-positives were radiologically malignant, that is, the failed triple test (FNS, breast imaging and clinical examination) ratio was 1:1556. The authors conclude by recommending that positive/suspicious FNSs with benign radiologic findings should be subjected to intraoperative frozen section examination before definitive surgery.

The authors state, "collective analysis shows that among experienced cytopathologists, the false-positive rate varies between 0% and 0.86% with an average rate of 0.17%" which "is comparable to the false-positive rate reported on frozen sections." Unfortunately, when dealing with biological/pathologic processes, no diagnostic test is perfect.

A related study from the Breast Care Centre, Waikato Hospital, Hamilton, New Zealand demonstrated improvement of FNA results by the "near patient" (the authors term for immediately available reporting by an on-site cytopathologist) FNA diagnosis by an experienced cytopathologist.[1] Definite reports increased from 82.4% to 91.9%; discrete breast lump FNA specificity increased from 76.5% to 89.1%; and the unsatisfactory rate decreased from 19.6% to 9.4%. These findings are consistent with other similar reports of the near ideal situation of having an experienced cytopathologist performing and evaluating the FNAs on site in the breast clinic. However, in the fragmented health care system of the USA, this is rarely the logistical situation.

W. H. Hindle, MD

Reference

1. Hamil J, Campbell ID, Mayall F, et al: Improved breast cytology results with near patient FNA diagnosis. *Acta Cytol* 46:19-24, 2002.

A Comparison of Aspiration Cytology and Core Needle Biopsy in the Evaluation of Breast Lesions

Westenend PJ, Sever AR, Beekman-de Volder HJC, et al (Albert Schweitzer Hosp, Dordrecht, The Netherlands)
Cancer 93:146-150, 2001

31–15

Background.—Differences among reported trials in patient selection, setting, biopsy techniques, and the incidence of disease in a population make it difficult to compare the accuracy of fine-needle aspiration cytology (FNAC) with that of core needle biopsy (CNB) for the prediagnostic evaluation of breast lesions. Direct comparisons between these 2 techniques were made possible by having the same operator perform FNAC and CNB of the same breast lesion in the same session.

Methods.—Between 1994 and 1997, both US-guided FNAC and CNB were performed by the same operator on 286 breast lesions during the same session. Symptomatic lesions and lesions detected by screening were included, but cysts and microcalcifications without a soft tissue mass were excluded from analyses. Both FNAC and CNB results were graded into 5 categories and were compared with excisional biopsy (if performed) or with the most recent mammographic findings.

Results.—The sensitivity and positive predictive value of FNAC and CNB were similar, as was the rate of inadequate samples (Tables 1 and 2). However, specificity was significantly higher with CNB than with FNAC, and CNB had significantly higher positive predictive values for suspicious lesions

TABLE 1.—Diagnostic Accuracy of Fine-Needle Aspiration Cytology

Parameter	This Study (95% CI)	Acceptable Values (%)[8]
Absolute sensitivity	72 (67-78)	> 60
Complete sensitivity	92 (89-95)	> 80
Specificity (biopsy cases only)	58 (53-64)	
Specificity (full)	82 (78-87)	> 60
Ppv malignant	100 (100-100)	> 95
Ppv suspicious	78 (73-83)	
Ppv atypia	18 (13-22)	
False-negative rate	6 (3-8)	< 5
False-positive rate	0 (0-0)	< 1
Inadequate rate	7 (4-10)	< 25
Inadequate rate from cancers	2 (1-4)	
Suspicious rate	13 (9-17)	< 20

Abbreviation: Ppv, Positive predictive value.
Note: Please see article in original journal of publication for references.
(Courtesy of Westenend PJ, Sever AR, Beekman-de Volder HJC, et al. A comparison of aspiration cytology and core needle biopsy in the evaluation of breast lesions. *Cancer* 93(2):146-150. Copyright 2001 American Cancer Society. Reprinted by permission of Wiley-Liss, Inc., a subsidary of John Wiley & Sons, Inc.)

TABLE 2.—Diagnostic Accuracy of Core Needle Biopsy

Parameter	CNB (95% CI)	Compared With FNAC (P Value)
Absolute sensitivity	75 (70-80)	NS
Complete sensitivity	88 (84-91)	NS
Specificity (biopsy cases only)	78 (73-83)	< 0.05
Specificity (full)	90 (87-94)	< 0.05
Ppv malignant	99 (97-100)	NS
Ppv suspicious	100 (100-100)	< 0.05
Ppv atypia	80 (75-85)	< 0.05
False-negative rate	9 (6-12)	NS
False-positive rate	1 (0-2)	NS
Inadequate rate	7 (4-10)	NS
Inadequate rate from cancers	3 (1-6)	NS
Suspicious rate	5 (2-7)	< 0.05

Abbreviations: CNB, Core needle biopsy; *FNAC*, fine-needle aspiration cytology; *NS*, not significant; *Ppv*, positive predictive value.
(Courtesy of Westenend PJ, Sever AR, Beekman-de Volder HJC, et al. A comparison of aspiration cytology and core needle biopsy in the evaluation of breast lesions. Cancer 93(2):146-150, 2001. Copyright 2001 American Cancer Society. Reprinted by permission of Wiley-Liss, Inc., a subsidiary of John Wiley & Sons, Inc.)

and for lesions with atypia. The rate of suspicious lesions was also significantly lower with CNB. Combining FNAC and CNB findings significantly improved absolute sensitivity (88% combined vs 72% for FNAC and 75% for CNB) and the rate of inadequate specimens for cancer (0% combined vs 2% for FNAC and 3% for CNB). However, combining the results of both techniques also significantly decreased the positive predictive value of atypia (7% combined vs 18% for FNAC and 80% for CNB).

Conclusion.—This direct comparison reveals that, for most parameters, FNAC and CNB are equally accurate in the prediagnostic evaluation of breast lesions. CNB, however, does have significantly higher specificity and a significantly lower suspicious rate; the latter finding reflects the difficulty in interpreting some FNAC specimens. Combining the results of FNAC and BNC improved absolute sensitivity without adversely affecting specificity and improved the inadequate rate for cancers.

▶ This smaller (n = 286) study from The Netherlands obtained similar results as the Shannon study (Abstract 31–16). Tissue core-needle biopsies were found to have higher specificity and lower suspicious rates than fine-needle aspirations (FNA), though combining both biopsy techniques resulted in increased absolute sensitivity without affecting specificity and decreased inadequacy rates.

Clarke et al[1] at the royal Gwent Hospital, Newport, UK, reported on the triple assessment (clinical examination, mammography, and FNA) [triple test] for 52 symptomatic breast lumps. Motivated by numerous inconclusive cytology reports, automated tissue core-needle biopsy was added to the triple assessment. During the study period the sensitivity of FNA was 60% while the sensitivity of tissue core-needle biopsy was 96%. Subsequent to this study, the authors concluded that tissue core-needle biopsy "should replace fine needle aspiration cytology in the assessment of symptomatic breast lumps."

W. H. Hindle, MD

Chapter 31–Breast Disease / **553**

Reference

1. Clarke D, Sudhakaran N, Gateley CA. Replace fine needle aspiration cytology with automated core biopsy in the triple assessment of breast cancer. *Ann Royal Coll Surg Engl* 83:110-112, 2001.

Conversion to Core Biopsy in Preoperative Diagnosis of Breast Lesions: Is It Justified by Results?

Shannon J, Douglas-Jones AG, Dallimore NS (Univ of Wales, Cardiff; Lland-ough Hosp, Penarth, UK)
J Clin Pathol 54:762-765, 2001
31–16

Background.—Increasingly, core biopsy (CB) is replacing the use of fine-needle aspiration cytology (FNAC) in the preoperative diagnosis of patients with symptomatic or screening-detected breast lesions. But is CB more accurate than FNAC in the preoperative diagnosis of breast cancer? The accuracy of CB for patients with screened and symptomatic breast lesions was compared with that of FNAC in a single center's experience.

Methods.—Tissue samples were obtained from 1768 consecutive patients with symptomatic breast lesions or lesions detected by screening. At the institution involved, CB began to become more common than FNAC in 1998 (Fig 1). Thus, quality-assessment parameters were determined and compared for 4 groups of patients: 561 patients with screening-detected lesions who underwent FNAC from October 1996 through September 1998, 473 patients with symptomatic breast lesions who underwent FNAC from October 1996 through September 1998, 385 patients with screening-detected lesions who underwent CB from January 1998 through October 1999, and 349 patients with symptomatic breast lesions who underwent CB from January 1998 through October 1999. Both FNAC and CB results were graded into 5 categories (C1-C5, B1-B5) according to National Health Service Breast Screening Programme guidelines, and were confirmed with excisional biopsy (if performed).

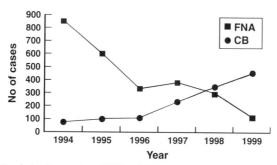

FIGURE 1.—Graph showing number of FNA and CB investigations performed in screening practice by year. (Courtesy of Shannon J, Douglas-Jones AG, Dallimore NS: Conversion to core biopsy in preoperative diagnosis of breast lesions: Is it justified by results? *Clin Pathol* 54:762-765, 2001. With permission from the BMJ Publishing Group.)

TABLE 3.—Performance Parameters for the 4 Groups of Patients

	Symptomatic		Screening	
Number of patients	473	349	561	385
Predominant type of investigation	FNAC	Core	FNAC	Core
	%	%	%	%
Absolute sensitivity	70.4	98.5	59	89
Complete sensitivity	88.8	99.5	78.9	93.1
Specificity (biopsy)	38.5	65	19.7	20
Specificity (full)	47.6	85.5	46.4	52.7
PPV: C5/B5	100	99.5	98.8	99.5
PPV: C4/B4	84	—	84.6	66.7
PPV: C3/B3	8	40	32	16.7
False negatives	0	0	1.5	0.9
False positives	0	0.5	0.7	0.5
Inadequate	34.7	4.6	32.4	21.3
Inadequate for cancer	11.2	0.5	19.6	6
Suspicious rate	12.7	2.3	13.7	4.7

Abbreviations: FNAC, Fine-needle aspiration cytology; PPV, positive predictive value.
(Courtesy of Shannon J, Douglas-Jones AG, Dallimore NS: Conversion to core biopsy in preoperative diagnosis of breast lesions: Is it justified by results? *Clin Pathol* 54:762-765, 2001. With permission from the BMJ Publishing Group.)

Results.—In both symptomatic and screened patients, CB had much higher absolute sensitivity and complete sensitivity than FNAC (Table 3). The inadequate specimen rate and the suspicious rate were also lower with CB in both types of patients. In screened patients, the overall premalignant diagnosis rate (C5 or B5 ratings) increased from 86% with FNAC to 90% with CB. In patients with symptomatic lesions, typing of tumor was attempted in 141 (86.7%) of those undergoing CB and was accurate in 132 cases (93.6%). Grading of invasive carcinomas was attempted in 111 cases (63.5%). The provisional grade provided by CB was subsequently confirmed histologically to be correct in 6 of 8 grade 1 cases(75%), in 42 of 60 grade 2 cases(70%), and in 37 of 43 grade 3 cases(86%).

Conclusion.—Converting from FNAC to CB for the preoperative diagnosis of symptomatic and screened breast lesions suspected of being cancerous improved specificity and reduced the rates of inadequate specimens or suspicious findings. CB accurately identified the grade and type of tumor in most cases. Furthermore, CB specimens can be examined immunohistochemically to determine estrogen receptor status. The conversion from FNAC to CB in the preoperative diagnosis of suspected breast cancer seems justified and has implications for FNAC quality assessment.

▶ Though the concept originated in the USA in 1930[1] and was proven effective and popularized by the Swedish in 1967[2] with documentation of the efficiency, accuracy, convenience and cost effectiveness in 1968[3] and 1970[4] and subsequently confirmed by multiple international studies, fine-needle aspiration (FNA) of palpable breast masses has not obtained wide-spread clinical practice application in the USA (except in a limited number of breast centers and rare medical practices). New technically modified tissue core-needle biopsies appear to be filling the same indications with almost the same advantages of FNA. Perhaps tissue core-needle biopsies will be offered to patients throughout the USA in individual medical offices and clinics fulfilling the original promise of near immediate on-site initial visit definitive diagnosis of palpable breast masses no matter what type of medical setting the patient visits.

This impressive study from the University of Wales College of Medicine, Cardiff, UK, of 1768 tissue core-needle biopsies confirmed by resection histology reports increased specificity and reduced inadequate and suspicious rates. Is this the office/clinic diagnostic wave of the future? Perhaps appropriate specialty and primary care residency training programs should include training and experience in tissue core-needle biopsy technique.

W. H. Hindle MD

References

1. Martin HE, Ellis EB: Biopsy by needle puncture and aspiration. *Ann Surg* 92:169-181, 1930.
2. Zajicek J, Franzen S, Jakobsson P, et al: Aspiration biopsy of mammary tumors in diagnosis and research—a critical review of 2,200 cases. *Acta Cytol* 11:169-175, 1967.
3. Franzen S, Zajicek J: Aspiration biopsy in diagnosis of palpable lesions of the breast: critical review of 3,479 consecutive biopsies. *Acta Radiol Ther Phys Biol* 7:241-262, 1968.
4. Zajiceck J, Caspersson T, Jakobsson P, et al: Cytologic diagnosis of mammary tumors from aspiration biopsy smears: Comparison of cytologic and histologic findings in 2,111 lesions and diagnostic use of cytophotometry. *Acta Cytol* 14:270-276, 1970.

SUGGESTED READING

Morrow M, Venta L, Stinson T, et al: Prospective comparison of stereotactic core biopsy and surgical excision as diagnostic procedures for breast cancer patients. *Ann Surg* 233:537-541, 2001.

▶ Granting that the choice of open surgical biopsy or image-guided tissue core-needle biopsy was based on the preferences of the radiologist, patient, and referring physician (surgeon), which indicates potential selection bias as there were no strict criteria of each assessment and preference, 1852 nonpalpable mammographically detected abnormalities were biopsied. Open surgical biopsy was performed in 545 and core-needle biopsies in 1307. The lesions were mass (50%), calcifications (43%), and architectural distortion (7%). The corresponding malignancy percentages were mass (23.7%), calcifications (19.4%), and architectural distortion (28.3%). The diagnostic open surgical biopsy was also the definitive surgery in 33% of the 142 cancer patients who were diagnosed by that technique. However, the percentage requiring re-excision to complete their breast conserving surgery is not stated. As regards the issue of understaging invasive cancer by tissue core-needle biopsy, such understaging occurred in 14%. However, the rate of understaging was 7% for the surgical biopsies, so it could be said that the "net rate" for tissue core-needle biopsies was also 7% understaging. Furthermore, the mammographic prediction of "pure" ductal carcinoma in situ (without invasive) remains problematic, particularly when tissue core-needle biopsy is the initial diagnostic technique.

William H. Hindle, MD

Percutaneous Imaging-Guided Core Breast Biopsy: 5 Years' Experience in a Community Hospital

Margolin FR, Leung JWT, Jacobs RP, et al (California Pacific Med Ctr, San Francisco; Harvard Med School, Boston)

AJR 177:559-564, 2001   31–17

Background.—Percutaneous imaging-guided core biopsy of breast lesions has been touted as accurate and cost-effective in the literature, which comes largely from academic centers. The experience of 1 community hospital breast center over 5 years, including follow-up for benign lesions, was reported.

Methods.—The prospectively collected results from 1994 to 1998 included 1333 lesions in 1183 patients (Table 1). Ninety-four percent of these were in Breast Imaging Reporting and Data System (BI-RADS) assessment category 4; those who were in category 5 were referred for surgery. For 506 lesions, stereotactic guidance was used for the core biopsy; for 827 solid masses, sonography guided the core biopsy, which usually used a 16-gauge needle.

Results.—For 1027 biopsies, a BI-RADS assessment category was available (Table 2). Of 506 lesions detected with stereotactically guided core biopsy, 344 were microcalcified clusters and 162 were noncalcified (Table 3). Of the 59 cancers thus diagnosed, 18 were invasive and 41 ductal carcinomas in situ, for a positive yield of 12%. None of the lesions detected stereotactically were palpable. Of 827 lesions detected with sonographically guided core biopsy, 88 cancers were found; 80 were invasive and 8 ductal carcinoma in situ, for a positive yield of 11%. Six hundred ninety-eight masses had palpa-

TABLE 1.—Five-Year Summary of Mammograms, Management
Recommendations, and Interventions

Procedures/Recommendations	No. of Patients
Mammograms performed*	180,818
Management recommendation	
6-month follow-up visit	3,877
Biopsy	3,138
Imaging-guided core	790
Surgical procedure	1,336
Both options offered	1,012
Procedures performed	2,958
Stereo guided core biopsy†	506
Sono guided core biopsy‡	827
Sono guided FNA§	63
Surgical biopsy	1,562
Cancers diagnosed	705

Note: Period summarized in table is January 1, 1994, to December 31, 1998.
*Mammograms = 72% screening, 7% call-back rate.
†Stereotactically guided core biopsy.
‡Sonographically guided core biopsy.
§Sonographically guided fine-needle aspiration.
(Courtesy of Margolin FR, Leung JWT, Jacobs RP, et al: Percutaneous imaging-guided core breast biopsy: 5 years' experience in a community hospital. *AJR* 177:559-564, 2001. Reprinted with permission from the American Journal of Roentgenology.)

TABLE 2.—Breast Imaging Reporting and Data System (BI-RADS) Assessment and Malignant Core Biopsy Results in 1027 Lesions

	BI-RADS 3		BI-RADS 4		BI-RADS 5	
Procedure	No. of Lesions	No. (%) Lesions Found Malignant	No. of Lesions	No. (%) Lesions Found Malignant	No. of Lesions	No. (%) Lesions Found Malignant
Stereotactically guided	16	1 (6)	299	39 (13)	6	5 (83)
Sonographically guided	18	0 (0)	668	61 (9)	20	19 (95)
Total	34	1 (3)	967	100 (10)	26	24 (92)

Note: BI-RADS assessment category was not reported for 306 lesions.
(Courtesy of Margolin FR, Leung JWT, Jacobs RP, et al: Percutaneous imaging-guided core breast biopsy: 5 years' experience in a community hospital. *AJR* 177:559-564, 2001. Reprinted with permission from the American Journal of Roentgenology.)

bility recorded, of which 514 were palpable (Table 4). All patients who had malignant core biopsy results were referred for surgical excision, during which the results were confirmed in all cases (100% positive predictive value). None of the patients had serious complications, although 2 required oral antibiotics for cellulitis that developed at the entrance site of the 14-gauge stereotactic biopsy needle. Atypical ductal hyperplasia was found in 24 patients, 18 of whom had stereotactic core biopsies for calcifications and 6 of whom had sonographically guided biopsies of solid masses. Twenty-two of these patients had surgery to excise the biopsied area, with cancer found in 12 patients (55%) at surgery. Of 962 patients with benign core biopsy results, follow-up mammograms were tracked for 15 to 75 months, with no cancer found in the area biopsied in any case.

Conclusions.—The use of imaging-guided core biopsies allowed the differentiation between benign and malignant tumors and was an accurate, cost-effective alternative to surgical biopsy. The community hospital site was a plus for the patients and did not diminish the method's effectiveness.

TABLE 3.—Stereotactic Core Biopsy Results for 506 Lesions

Core Biopsy Diagnosis	Mass*	Calcification	Asymmetric Density†	Total No.
Benign lesions				
Fibroadenomas	46	89	2	137
Other types of benign lesions	77	195	19	291
Malignant lesions				
Ductal carcinomas in situ	5	35	1	41
Invasive cancers	8	6	4	18
Atypical hyperplasias	0	10‡	0	19
Total overall	136	344	26	506

*Includes masses with calcification.
†Includes 3 cases of architectural distortion.
‡Includes 18 cases of atypical ductal hyperplasia and 1 case of atypical lobular hyperplasia.
(Courtesy of Margolin FR, Leung JWT, Jacobs RP, et al: Percutaneous imaging-guided core breast biopsy: 5 years' experience in a community hospital. *AJR* 177:559-564, 2001. Reprinted with permission from the American Journal of Roentgenology.)

TABLE 4.—Sonographically Guided Core Biopsy Results for 827 Solid Masses

Core Biopsy Diagnosis	Palpable Mass (n = 515)	Nonpalpable Mass (n = 184)	Palpability Not Recorded (n = 128)	Total No.
Benign lesions				
Fibroadenomas	317	109	81	507
Other benign lesions	125	57	42	224
Malignant lesions				
Ductal carcinomas in situ	2	3	3	8
Invasive cancers	65	14	1	80
Atypical hyperplasias*	6	1†	1†	8
Total overall	515	184	128	827

*Includes 6 cases of atypical ductal hyperplasia and 2 cases of atypical lobular hyperplasia.
†Atypical lobular hyperplasia.
(Courtesy of Margolin FR, Leung JWT, Jacobs RP, et al: Percutaneous imaging-guided core breast biopsy: 5 years' experience in a community hospital. *AJR* 177:559-564, 2001. Reprinted with permission from the American Journal of Roentgenology.)

▶ This study from the California Pacific Medical Center, San Francisco, demonstrates the practical clinical application of breast imaging/biopsy techniques initially described in research/academic centers. This documented "testing in the field" is essential before the widespread application of new techniques. In this report of 1333 lesions, 94% of which were BI-RADS category 4 upon breast imaging, demonstrates 7% were diagnosed as invasive carcinoma and 4% in situ carcinoma. (Ed: The latter require surgical excision to rule out a focus of invasive carcinoma.) There were no false-positives in the series. Of particular interest, 55% (12/22) of the core biopsies revealing atypical ductal hyperplasia had associated carcinoma upon subsequent surgery.

Parker et al[1] used a handheld sonographically guided directional vacuum-assisted breast biopsy techniques to remove 124 breast masses 1.5 cm or less in greatest dimension. Even though the biopsies were continued, "until no sonographic evidence of the lesion remained," subsequent surgery revealed: "Only one infiltrating ductal carcinoma was entirely removed histologically at Mammatome biopsy." Citing numerous advantages, the authors recommend this biopsy technique "for all sonographically guided biopsies of breast masses smaller than 1.5 cm."

Becker et al[2] (London, Ontario, Canada) described the effective use of an add-on stereotactic unit for core biopsies of indeterminate microcalcifications and compared this equipment with digital and conventional stereotactic guidance systems. Retrospective reviewed revealed that 94.4% (219/232) of the targeted lesions were successfully sampled. The target lesions were missed in 7.4% (9/121) using conventional radiography and in 3.5% (4/111) of the digital imaging. Further advantages of less cost and space and greater accuracy are cited for an add-on unit using digital imaging.

W. H. Hindle, MD

References

1. Parker SH, Klaus AJ, McWey PJ, et al. Sonographically guided directional vacuum-assisted breast biopsy using a handheld device. *AJR* 177:405-408, 2001.

2. Becker L, Taves D, McCurdy L, et al. Stereotactic core biopsy of breast microcalcifications: comparison of film versus digital mammography, both using an add-on unit. *AJR* 177:1451-1457, 2001.

SUGGESTED READING

Liberman L, Cody HS III: Percutaneous biopsy and sentinel lymphadenectomy: Minimally invasive diagnosis and treatment of nonpalpable breast cancer. *AJR Am J Roentgenol* 177:887-891, 2001.

▶ This retrospective review from the Memorial Sloan-Kettering Cancer Center, in New York, NY, covers 200 consecutive nonpalpable breast cancers diagnosed by percutaneous imaging guided core biopsy treated with surgery and sentinel lymph node mapping utilizing intradermal injection radioisotope and intraparenchymal injection of blue dye. The technical success rate (identification of sentinel nodes at surgery) was 100% (200). The sentinel node was cancer free in 79% (158). In 2% (3), the sentinel node was negative but other suspicious nodes were positive. Axillary node dissection revealed cancer in non-sentinel nodes in 23% (7/31). "A single surgical procedure was performed for 164 (82%) of the 200 carcinomas; the breast was preserved in 191 (96%) of the 200 carcinomas."

William H. Hindle, MD

Llatjos M, Castella E, Fraile M, et al: Intraoperative assessment of sentinel lymph nodes in patients with breast carcinoma: Accuracy of imprint cytology compared with definitive histologic workup. *Cancer* 96:150-156, 2002.

▶ This report from Barcelona, Spain, is on 77 patients who underwent successful sentinel lymph node biopsy. Intraoperative imprint smears were made from all cut surfaces on the node, which had been freshly sectioned at 2 mm intervals. The sensitivity was 67.7%, specificity 100%, accuracy 86.8% and negative predictive value 81.8% with this technique. Eight of the 10 false-negative cases were discovered only with cytokeratin immunostained sections. The authors conclude: "Imprint cytology examination of MGG [May-Grunwald-Giemsa] smears appears to be a reliable technique for the intraoperative assessment of SNs [sentinel nodes] in patients with breast carcinoma."

Ollila et al[1] provide a clinical overview, with 65 references, on the clinical significance of micrometastases in axially lymph nodes for women with invasive breast cancer and the conundrum produced upon the use of immunohistochemical staining for keratin cells. Even a single cell can be identified with cytokeratin stains, but are the cells viable, capable of sustained growth, and able to metastasize? It does appear that such cells, which cannot be seen on hematoxylin-eosin (H&E) stain do not impact the patient's survival. Extracapsular extension is another perplexing variable of sentinel node metastasis. The authors conclude: "For the medical oncologist, SN [sentinel node] metastases visible by H&E should be considered prognostically relevant, and the patient treated for node-positive breast cancer."

Sachdev et al[2] reviewed a prospective database of 212 breast cancer patients who had sentinel node biopsy followed by complete axillary node dissection. "Tumor size greater than 2 cm, lymphatic invasion of the primary tumor, macrometastases in the sentinel node, and use of radioisotope all positively correlated independently with metastasis in the nonsentinel lymph nodes. . ."

Ahlgren et al[3] in Uppsala, Sweden, evaluated 5-node axillary biopsy compared to traditional level I-II axial lymph node dissection. In all patients the sensitivity of the five-node biopsy was 97.3%, the negative predictive value 98.5%, and the negative likelihood ratio .027. The results were essentially the same for the screening detected patients (n = 204) and the clinically detected patients (n = 197).

Mincey et al[4] at the Mayo Clinic, Jackson, Fla and Rochester, Minn, reported on the role of axillary node dissection in patients with T1a and T1b breast cancer (n = 163). "Node positivity was 0% for T1a and 11.3% for T1b tumors (P = 0.03)." As the tumor size increased, the risk of lymph node positivity became significantly higher (P = 0.002). A higher risk of lymph node involvement was indicated by a higher tumor grade (P = 0.02). The authors' conclude: "T1a tumors have minimal risk of nodal positivity and may not require subsequent axillary lymph node dissection in the future."

William H. Hindle, MD

References

1. Ollila DW, Carey LA, Sartor CI: Clinical significance of micrometastatic disease in the era of sentinel node. *Breast Dis* 12:57-67, 2001.
2. Sachdev U, Murphy K, Derzie A, et al: Predictors of nonsentinel node metastasis in breast cancer patients. *Am J Surg* 183:213-317, 2002.
3. Ahlgren J, Holmberg L, Bergh J, et al: Five-node biopsy of the axilla: An alternative to axillary dissection of levels I-II in operable breast cancer. *Eur J Surg Oncol* 28:97-102, 2002.
4. Mincey BA, Bummer T, Atkinson EJ, et al: Role of axillary node dissection in patients with T1a and T1b breast cancer. *Arch Surg* 136:779-782, 2001.

Wong SL, Edwards MJ, Chao C, et al: Sentinel lymph node biopsy for breast cancer: Impact of the number of sentinel nodes removed on the false-negative rate. *J Am Coll Surg* 192:684-691, 2001.

▶ This multi-institutional study involved 148 surgeons and 1436 women with clinical stage T1-2, N0 breast cancer. Sentinel lymph nodes were detected in 90% (1287/1436) with an overall false negative rare of 8.3%. However, the false negative rate was 14.3% when only a single node was removed and 4.3% when multiple "sentinel" nodes were removed. All of the patients had level I and II axillary lymph node dissections. Generally, about a third of breast cancer patients, who are surgical candidates, have a single sentinel node. In the current study, if only a single sentinel node had been removed, the false negative rate would have been 28.8%. As with many other studies, the use of radioactive colloid combined with blue dye improved the detection of multiple sentinel nodes.

In related studies, McCarter et al[1] reported on 1561 successful sentinel lymph node biopsies without blue dye and radioisotope injection. Three or more "sentinel" nodes were identified in 15% (241/1561) of the biopsies. Of the 449 women with node-positive disease, 98% (440/449) had sentinel nodes identified within the first 3 sentinel node sites. In 8 patients, the first positive sentinel node was identified only after examining 4 to 8 sites. Thus 0.2% (3/1561) required more than 4 sentinel nodes to be removed before a positive node was identified.

McMasters[2] reported on 2206 patients (229 surgeons) with clinical stage T1-2 N0 breast cancer who had sentinel node biopsies followed by level I and II axillary lymph node dissections. The radioactive colloids injected were peritumoral (n = 1074), subdermal (n = 297) and dermal (n = 251). The corresponding sentinel node identification rates were 89.9%, 95.3%, and 98.0%. The false negative rates were 9.5%, 7.8%, and 6.5%. The authors state that "The sentinel lymph nodes were 5 to 7 times more radioactive after dermal injection than after peritumoral injection." The University of Louisville Breast Cancer Sentinel Lymph Node Study conducted this multicenter trial. Others have confirmed the increased isotope success of 97% with intradermal injection versus prior 78% for peritumoral injection.[3]

William H. Hindle, MD

References

1. McCarter MD, Yeung H., Fey J, et al: The breast cancer patient with multiple sentinel nodes: When to stop? *J Am Coll Surg* 192:692-697, 2001.
2. McMasters KM: Dermal injection of radioactive colloid is superior to peritumoral injection for breast cancer sentinel lymph node biopsy: Results of a multiinstitutional study. *Ann Surg* 233:676-687, 2001
3. Lineham DC, Hill ADK, Akhurst T, et al: Intradermal radiocolloid and intraparenchymal blue dye injection optimize sentinel node identification in breast cancer patients. *Ann Surg Oncol* 6:450-454, 1999.

Cox CE, Salud CJ, Cantor A, et al: Learning curves for breast cancer sentinel lymph node mapping based on surgical volume analysis. *J Am Coll Surg* 193:573-600, 2001.

▶ This study from the H. Lee Moffitt Cancer Center and Research Institute at the University of South Florida, Tampa, followed the surgical performance of 16 surgeons after a 2-day CME course in sentinel node biopsy technique. The combined radiocolloid and blue dye injections were utilized in the 2255 patients in the study. The learning curve showed that it took about 63 cases to reach a 5% failure rate and then plateaued after 75 cases. Subsequently, "Surgeons performing more than six SLN biopsies per month had a success rate of 97.81% ± 0.44%."

Harlow and Krag[1] provide a clinical overview of sentinel lymph node biopsy and reviewed the literature (1994-2001) of 3240 reported cases with a mean identification rate of 89%, an accuracy rate of 98%, and a mean false-negative rate of 6%. The authors' discussion of the implications of immunohistochemical (IHC) positive cells in the excised lymph nodes is of particular clinical interest. "Tumor cell aggregates that are greater than 1 mm in size may be more likely to represent a truly independent focus of monastic disease and may be a better indicator of the risk of similar lesions elsewhere in the body." Furthermore, the authors quote that Klauber-DeMore et al[2] ". . .reported a 12% incidence of IHC positive sentinel nodes in patients with "pure DCIS."

Schrenk et al[3] in Linz, Austria, compared 165 breast cancer patients with sentinel node (SN) biopsies to 195 patients with standard level I and II axillary lymph node dissections (ALND). Patient demographics and tumor characteristics were comparable between the 2 groups. However, they reported that "Micrometastases were more frequently found in the SN group when compared to the ALND group (six of 70 positive nodes) (P = 0.04)." The authors conclude: "SN biopsy may be as accurate as standard axillary lymph-node dissection for the evaluation of the axillary lymph-node status in breast cancer patients."

Roumen et al[4] in Veldhoven, The Netherlands, report on 100 patients with sentinel node-negative breast cancer with further axillary dissection. The median questionnaire follow-up was 24 months (range 16-40). "No patient developed lymphedema or needed physiotherapy after the operation." One woman developed axillary relapse (a = 14 months) after her initial diagnosis. "There were no other local recurrences."

William H. Hindle, MD

References

1. Harlow SP, Krag DN: Sentinel lymph node biopsy in breast cancer. *Breast Dis* 12:43-55, 2001.
2. Klauber-DeMore N, Tan LK, Liberman L, et al: Sentinel node biopsy: Is it indicated in patients with high-risk ductal carcinoma-in-situ and ductal carcinoma-in-situ with microinvasion? *Ann Surg Oncol* 7:636-642, 2000.
3. Schrenk P, Shamiyeh A, Wayand W: Sentinel lymph-node biopsy compared to axillary lymph-node dissection for axillary staging in breast cancer patients. *Eur J Surg Oncol* 27:378-382, 2001.
4. Roumen RMH, Kuijt GP, Liem IH, et al: Treatment of 100 patients with sentinel node-negative breast cancer without further axillary dissection. *Brit J Surg* 88:1639-1643, 2001.

Simmons RM: Review of sentinel lymph node credentialing: How many cases are enough? *J Am Coll Surg* 193:206-209, 2001.

▶ This review has pertinent value to Ob-Gyns and others involved in sentinel lymph node biopsies (SLNB). The advantages of sentinel node mapping/biopsy are (1) elimination of postoperative axillary drainage, (2) almost no lymphedema or neurovascular injury, and (3) less discomfort for the patient. The American College of Surgeons task force on SLNB has recommended "that the identification rate for SLNB be 85% or higher and that a false-negative rate be 5% or less." Summary of 5 published studies indicates that it takes more than 15 SLNB cease for a surgeon to achieve the recommended rates. Furthermore, it is often recommended that a surgeon perform as many as 50 SLND cases with verification by traditional axillary lymph node dissection (ALND) on the same patients before operating without the supervision of a "credentialed" SLNB surgeon.

Ahrendt et al[1] studied (n = 174) the influence of tumor location and other variables upon success of SLNB. The authors confirmed, as have many other similar reports, that the combined use of blue dye and radiocolloid is superior to either method alone. The combinations gave 93% mapping success in this series. Lower inner quadrant tumor location adversely affected the mapping success. Obesity and non-palpability adversely affected the success rate when the cancer was in the upper outer or upper inner quadrants.

Burak et al[2] at Ohio State University, Columbus, used quantitative arm measurements and return to "normal activity" to compare SLNB with ALND in their institution (n = 96) with mean follow-up of 15 months. Subjective arm measurements, arm numbness and arm complaints were less (P < 0.001) with the SLNB group. The SLNB group were 88% outpatients and 71% returned to normal activity in <4 days whereas the ALND group were 15% outpatients and 7% returned to normal activity in <4 days.

William H. Hindle, MD

References

1. Ahrendt GM, Laud P, Tjoe J, et al: Does breast tumor location influence success of sentinel lymph node biopsy? *J Am Coll Surg* 194:278-284, 2002.

2. Burak WE, Hollenbeck ST, Zervos EE, et al: Sentinel lymph node biopsy results in less postoperative morbidity compared with axillary lymph node dissection for breast cancer. *Am J Surg* 183:23-27, 2002.

Preventive Health Care, 2001 Update: Should Women Be Routinely Taught Breast Self-Examination to Screen for Breast Cancer?
Baxter N, and the Canadian Task Force on Preventive Health Care (Univ of Toronto, et al)
Can Med Assoc J 164:1837-1846, 2001   31–18

Background.—Even in highly screened populations, many breast tumors are detected by the women themselves. However, many are detected incidentally, not during a breast self-examination (BSE). The efficacy of BSE in breast cancer screening was investigated by a literature review, and recommendations for routine teaching of BSE to women in various age groups were provided.

Methods and Findings.—Research on the efficacy of BSE for reducing breast cancer mortality published from 1966 to October, 2000 was reviewed. To date, 2 large randomized, controlled trials; a quasi-randomized study; a large cohort study; and several case-control studies have shown no benefit associated with regular performance of BSE or BSE education when compared with no BSE (Table 1). Instruction in BSE appears to be associated with significant increases in physician visits for assessment of benign breast lesions and significantly greater rates of benign biopsy results.

Recommendations.—Routine BSE instruction should be omitted from the periodic health examination of women aged 40 to 69 years. Sufficient evidence for women in other age groups to make a recommendation is lacking (Table 3).

▶ This clear and precise analysis of the pertinent literature documents little evidence that teaching BSE alters breast cancer mortality. With 78 references and 3 concise summary tables, the author makes a strong case for questioning the actual health care value of what has become a "time honored" recommendation in the fight against breast cancer. Clinicians must now reflect on (1) the allocation of health care resources, (2) the potential for misleading patients as to the effectiveness of BSE, even under optimal circumstances, and (3) the "downside" of increased physician office visits and increased rates of benign breast biopsies. As expected, the American Cancer Society offers a rebuttal in support of their longtime recommendation of BSE.[1] In addition, the editorial accompanying the Baxter article suggests that there is insufficient evidence to support abandoning BSE.

W. H. Hindle, MD

Reference

1. News & Views (American Cancer Society): Breast self-exam is too valuable to discard. *CA Cancer J Clin* 51:268-270, 2001.

TABLE 1.—Summary of Randomized and Quasi-randomized Controlled Trials Evaluating the Effects of Breast Self-examination on Breast Cancer Outcomes

Trial	Participants	Follow-up/ Outcomes Measured	Results	Strengths/Potential Biases
Shanghai RCT of BSE training[27]	Women aged 31-64; residents of Shanghai and current or former employees of Shanghai Textile Industry Bureau (STIB). Randomly assigned at factory level to BSE training group ($n =$ 133 375) or control group ($n =$ 133 665)	Follow-up: 5 yr Outcomes: breast cancer mortality (from STIB tumour and death registry), and follow-up of breast cancer cases, tumour stages and no. of benign lesions detected	No difference between groups in breast cancer mortality or stage of breast cancer; higher rate of benign biopsy results in BSE group than in control group (1.1% v. 0.5%)	Randomized trial, high participation and compliance rates; no concurrent screening programs. Inadequate length of follow-up (further follow-up underway). Political changes in China may affect ability to complete the study
Russian/WHO RCT of BSE training[28-32]	Women aged 40-64; residents of Leningrad (St. Petersburg), randomly assigned at medical clinic level to BSE training group ($n =$ 57 712 at 9 yr) or control group ($n =$ 64 759 at 9 yr)	Follow-up: 9 yr Outcomes: breast cancer mortality among women diagnosed with breast cancer at oncology referral centre and medical clinic, tumour stages and rate of benign biopsy results	No difference between groups in breast cancer mortality or stage of breast cancer; higher rate of benign biopsy results in BSE group than in control group (at 5 yr; RR = 1.5, 95% CI 1.1-1.9)	Randomized trial, high participation rate; no concurrent screening. Decrease in compliance over time; inadequate power (further follow-up underway). Political changes in Russia may affect ability to complete the study
United Kingdom quasi-randomized controlled trial of breast cancer screening[33-34]	Women aged 40-49 from 8 geographic areas assigned to following groups by centre: Screening by CBE and mammography (2 centres) ($n =$ 45 607) BSE instruction (2 centres) ($n =$ 63 373) Control group (4 centres) ($n =$ 127 123)	Follow-up: mean 14.4 yr (98.2% of women traced) Outcome: breast cancer mortality (from tumour registry records), rate of benign biopsy results	No difference between groups in breast cancer mortality (RR = 0.99, 95% CI 0.87-1.12); no significant difference detected in secondary analysis by 5-yr age groups. Rate of benign biopsy results significantly higher in BSE group than in control group (0.91% v. 0.61%)	Differences across centres in demographics, rates of breast cancer, medical services, attendance at BSE instruction sessions (31% and 53% at 2 centres respectively) and breast cancer treatment patterns. No assessment of prevalent cancers, or BSE frequency or technique. Last years of follow-up overlapped with large national breast cancer screening study

Abbreviations: BSE, Breast self-examination; *RCT,* randomized, controlled trial; *WHO,* World Health Organization; *CBE,* clinical breast examination; *RR,* relative risk.

Note: Please see original journal article for references.

(Reprinted from Baxter N, and the Canadian Task Force on Preventive Health Care: Preventive Health Care, 2001 update: Should women be routinely taught breast self-examination to screen for breast cancer? *Can Med Assoc J* 164:1837-1846. Copyright 2001, Canadian Medical Association.)

TABLE 3.—Summary Table of Recommendations for the Routine Teaching of Breast Self-Examination to Women

Manoeuvre	Effectiveness	Levels of Evidence*	Recommendation*
Routine teaching of BSE to women aged 40-49 yr	Evidence of no benefit in terms of survival from breast cancer	RCTs (I),[27,31,32] non-randomized trial (II-1),[34] cohort study (II-3),[35] case–control studies (II-3)[36-38]	Because there is fair evidence of no benefit, and good evidence of harm, there is fair evidence to recommend that routine teaching of BSE be excluded from the periodic health examination of women aged 40-49 (grade D†)
	Evidence of increased no. of physician visits for breast problems and increased rate of benign biopsy results	RCTs (I),[27,31,32] non-randomized trials (II-1)[34]	
Routine teaching of BSE to women aged 50-69 yr	Evidence of no benefit in terms of survival from breast cancer	RCTs (I),[27,31,32]non-randomized trial (II-1),[34] cohort study (II-3)[35] case–control studies (II-3)[36-38]	Because there is fair evidence of no benefit, and good evidence of harm, there is fair evidence to recommend that routine teaching of BSE be excluded from the periodic health examination of women aged 50-69 (grade D†)
	Evidence of increased no. of physician visits for breast problems and increased rate of benign biopsy results	RCTs (I),[27,31,32] non-randomized trial (II-1)[34]	

Note: The lack of sufficient evidence to evaluate the effectiveness of the manoeuvre in women younger than 40 years and those 70 years and older precludes making recommendations for teaching breast self-examination (*BSE*) to women in these age groups. The following issues may be important to consider: For women younger than 40 years, there is little evidence for effectiveness specific to this group. Because the incidence of breast cancer is low in this age group, the risk of net harm from BSE and BSE instruction is even more likely. For women 70 years and older, although the incidence of breast cancer is high in this group, there is insufficient evidence to make a recommendation concerning BSE for women 70 years and older.

*Although the evidence indicates no benefit from routine instruction, some women will ask to be taught breast self-examination (*BSE*). The potential benefits and harms should be discussed with the woman, and if BSE is taught, care must be taken to ensure that she performs it in a proficient manner.

Note: Please see original journal article for references.

(Courtesy of Baxter N, and the Canadian Task Force on Preventive Health Care: Preventive Health Care, 2001 update: Should women be routinely taught breast self-examination to screen for breast cancer? *Can Med Assoc J* 164:1837-1846. Copyright 2001, Canadian Medical Association.)

Mammography-Related Anxiety: Effect of Preprocedural Patient Education

Mainiero MB, Schepps B, Clements NC, et al (Brown Univ, Providence, RI)
Womens Health Issues 11:110-115, 2001   31–19

Background.—Mammography can be considered uncomfortable, painful, or anxiety provoking, leading women to avoid participating in routine screenings. Efforts to minimize anxiety related to mammography include education about the procedure and providing a pleasant atmosphere at the time, but these have not been proven effective. How much anxiety is related

TABLE 1.—Anxiety Associated With Mammography

	Anxiety About Procedure n (%)	Anxiety About Results n %
None	218 (36)	75 (12)
Slight	108 (18)	102 (17)
Mild	78 (13)	69 (11)
Moderate	146 (24)	214 (35)
Severe	13 (2)	42 (7)
Extreme	44 (7)	107 (18)
Did not know	5 (1)	4 (1)
Frequency missing	1 (<1)	0

(Reprinted by permission of the Jacobs Institute of Women's Health from Mammography-related anxiety: Effect of preprocedural patient education by Mainiero MB, Schepps B, Clements NC, et al. *Womens Health Issues* Vol. No.11, pp. 110-115, copyright 2001.)

to the procedure itself and how much is attributable to fear of breast cancer has not been determined. Preprocedural education was offered to diminish procedure-related anxiety, whereas distraction was offered to lessen cancer-related anxiety.

Methods.—A survey concerning mammography and its expected results involved 613 women who were undergoing the procedure. For 424 patients, it was a screening examination and for 185, a diagnostic procedure. Before the procedure began, half of the women were shown an educational videotape and half viewed an entertaining movie. Preprocedural and postprocedural anxiety levels were measured by questionnaire.

Results.—Regardless of whether the examination was for screening or diagnosis, women expressed a greater degree of anxiety about the results of the mammogram than about the procedure itself (Table 1). Women being screened had lower levels of anxiety about the procedure and the results than those undergoing diagnosis (Table 2). Women under diagnosis expected and experienced more pain than those being screened. Patients with a higher degree of education had decreased odds of reporting moderate to high anxiety concerning the results of the mammogram. Patients who had greater anxiety experienced more pain than those who were less anxious.

TABLE 2.—Pain and Discomfort With Mammography

	Pain n (%)	Discomfort n (%)
None	168 (28)	46 (8)
Slight	167 (27)	201 (33)
Mild	114 (19)	143 (23)
Moderate	135 (22)	189 (31)
Severe	22 (4)	26 (4)
Extreme	6 (1)	8 (1)
Frequency missing	1 (<1)	0

(Reprinted by permission of the Jacobs Institute of Women's Health from Mammography-related anxiety: Effect of preprocedural patient education by Mainiero MB, Schepps B, Clements NC, et al. *Womens Health Issues* Vol. No.11, pp. 110-115, copyright 2001.)

More anxiety about the result than about the procedure was felt by women undergoing their first mammogram; these women also had higher levels of anxiety about both the procedure and the results than did women who had had previous mammograms. No differences were found in anxiety or pain between women viewing the educational versus the entertaining videotapes. The women who watched the educational videotape reported enjoying the program statistically significantly more than those watching the entertaining movie.

Conclusion.—Most mammography-related anxiety was caused by fear of the results rather than of the procedure itself. Women for whom the mammography is a screening procedure had less anxiety than those for whom it was diagnostic. Offering educational or entertaining distraction before the procedure had no impact on the degree of anxiety felt by the women.

▶ This report quantifies what most clinicians already were aware of, namely, that women have moderate anxiety about mammography based on their fear of breast cancer. The surprising finding was that viewing a preprocedural educational video had little impact on the frequency and levels of anxiety in this survey study. The patients' evaluation of pain upon mammography is of clinical interest (Table 2.).

Several mammography-related articles demonstrate the changing indications for and applications of breast imaging in clinical practice. Dennis et al report on 600 palpable breast lumps with no focal masses on sonograms and no abnormalities on mammograms with either biopsy or 2 years of follow-up.[1] The biopsy results were all benign and no carcinomas occurred in the areas of initial concern. Thus, under these particular circumstances, biopsy can be avoided. Ashkanani et al reported on a series of 695 breast-conserving cancer patients from Scotland.[2] The local recurrences were initially identified by physical examination in 52% and by mammography in 48%. Mammography identified or confirmed the recurrence in two thirds of the women. However, the false-positive rate was 2.3%. Focused US evaluation may have improved the imaging performance.

Rosen et al[3] reviewed 295 cases with initial short-term follow-up–interval mammography. Malignancy occurred in 51 cases of which 45% were microcalcifications, 24% a mass, 8% architectural distortion, and 24% developing densities. Results reported that "None fulfilled strict criteria for a probably benign lesion when reviewed in retrospect." Progression was mammographically demonstrated in 92% of the malignant lesions at the time of follow-up. Thus, the critical need for mammographers to follow the strict diagnostic imaging criteria for probably benign lesions is apparent.

W. H. Hindle, MD

References

1. Dennis MA, Parker SH, Klaus AJ, et al: Breast biopsy avoidance: The value of normal mammograms and normal sonograms in the setting of a palpable lump. *Radiology* 219:186-191, 2001.

2. Ashkanani F, Sarkar T, Needham G, et al: What is achieved by mammographic surveillance after breast conservation treatment for breast cancer? *Am J Surg* 182:207-210, 2001.
3. Rosen EL, Baker JA, Soo MS: Malignant lesions initially subjected to short-term mammographic follow-up. *Radiology* 223:221-228, 2002.

SUGGESTED READING

Olsen O, Gotzsche PC: Cochrane review on screening for breast cancer with mammography. *Lancet* 358:1340-1342, 2001.

▶ This highly controversial re-analysis of the prospective randomized, mostly population-based, clinical trials of screening mammography (1963-1980) received intense media attention and stirred instant heated public and professional debate. The major premise presented is "that breast cancer mortality is a misleading outcome measure" and that randomization was adequate in only 3 of the 7 clinical trials and that only 1 had reliable mortality data. This 2-page summary of a 46 page online Cochrane review (http://image.thelancet.com/lancet/extra/fullreport.pdf)[1] is subsequent documentation of their initial publication.[2] Both the initial and current manuscripts had accompanying editorial critiques and commentary.[3,4] Similarly both have been followed by thoughtful and detailed "rebuttals."[5,6] Unfortunately, none of the above mentioned articles lends itself to abstractions or brief summations and each requires careful detailed reading of the entire manuscript.

Clinically, it seems counterintuitive that screening mammography, the only currently available effective technique for the systematic detection of non-palpable breast cancers, does not diagnose cancers before metastasis has occurred. There is ample evidence that small non-metastatic breast cancers can truly be "cured" by primary therapy with resultant disease-free (breast cancer) survival.[7-12]

William H. Hindle, MD

References

1. Gotzsche PC, Olsen O: Is screening for breast cancer with mammography justifiable? *Lancet* 355:129-134, 2000
2. Olsen O, Gotzsche PC: Screening for breast cancer with mammography (Cochrane Review). In: The Cochrane Library, Issue 4, 2001. Oxford: Update Software. Cochrane Review: Cochrane Database Syst Rev 4:CD001877, 2001
3. de Koning HJ: Assessment of nationwide screening programs (editorial). *Lancet* 355:80-81, 2000.
4. Horton R: Screening mammography—an overview revisited (commentary). *Lancet* 358:1284-1285, 2001.
5. Smith R: Ongoing analysis of breast cancer screening trial data: two steps forward, one step back. *Breast Diseases: A Year Book Quarterly* 11:252-253, 2000
6. Duffy SH, Tabar L, Smith RA: The mammographic screening trials: Commentary on the recent work by Olsen and Gotzsche. *CA Cancer J Clinc* 52:68-71, 2002.
7. Tabar L, Dean PB, Kaufman CS, et al: A new era in the diagnosis of breast cancer. *Surg Oncol Clin N Am* 9:233-277, 2000
8. Tabar L, Chen H-H, Duffy SW, et al: A novel method for prediction of long-term outcome of women with T1a, T1b, and 10-14 mm invasive breast cancers: A prospective study. *Lancet* 355:429-433, 2000
9. Joensuu H, Pylkkanen L, Toikkanen S: Late mortality from pT1N0M0 breast carcinoma. *Cancer* 85:2183-2189, 1999.
10. Lopez MJ, Smart CR: Twenty-year follow-up of minimal breast cancer from the breast cancer detection demonstration project. *Surg Oncol Clin N Am* 6:393-401, 1997.

11. Arnesson LG, Smeds S, Fagerberg G: Recurrence-free survival in patients with small breast cancer. *Eur J Surg* 160:271-276, 1994

12. Rosen PP, Groshen S, Kinne DW: Survival and prognostic factors in node-negative breast cancer; results of long-term follow-up studies. *J Natl Cancer Inst Monogr* 11:159-162, 1992.

Kinsinger LS, Harris R: Breast cancer screening discussions for women in their forties. Breast Disease 13:21-31, 2001
▶ This comprehensive clinical overview focuses on shared decision making and is generally applicable to all age groups. The authors stress that "the decision must be individualized for each woman" and that "The choice ultimately belongs to the patient and the provider's role is to make sure the patient is well informed and has weighed the options against her own values." The essential elements of shared decision making for providers have been articulate by Braddock:[1] open mutual discussion with the patient of (1) the patient's role in decision making, (2) the clinical issues or nature of the decision, (3) the alternatives, (4) the pros (potential benefits) and cons (harms) of the alternatives, (5) the uncertainties associated with the decision, (6) the assessment of the patient's understanding, and (7) the exploration of the patient's preferences. The editor urges all Ob-Gyns and other health care providers for women to carefully read this article, to take to heart the message therein, and to apply the information and techniques to their practice. So doing will improve doctor-patient communication and yield greater patient satisfaction with the medical care rendered.

William H. Hindle, MD

Reference

1. Braddock CH III, Edwards K, Hasenberg NM, et al: Informed decision making in outpatient practice: Time to get back to basics. *JAMA* 282:2313-2320, 1999.

Tabar L, Vitak B, Ceh H-HT, et al: Beyond randomized controlled trails: Organized mammographic screening substantially reduces breast carcinoma mortality. *Cancer* 91:1724-1731, 2001.
▶ This study utilizes data from before, during, and after the Swedish Two-County Mammography Clinical Trial. Compared to the period "before" offering screening mammography, the latter 2 periods ("during" and "after") showed a 57% decreased incidence of breast cancer mortality (RR 0.43; 95% CI 0.34-0.55). During the "after" period (service mammography) the rate decreased 63% (RR 0.37; 95% CI 0.30-0.46). Over the entire 29 years of data collection, 6807 women (aged 20-69) were diagnosed with breast cancer and 1863 (27%) died of their disease. The authors concluded that "Service screening mammography reduced breast cancer specific mortality rates by 63% among women 40-69 years old who underwent screening and by 50% among all women in the age group regardless of whether they underwent screening." The Swedish Two-County Clinical Trial and follow-up data continue to be the strongest support for routine screening mammography.

William H. Hindle, MD

Geographical Distribution of Breast Cancers on the Mammogram: An Interval Cancer Database

Brown M, Eccles C, Wallis MG (Coventry and Warwickshire Hosp, England)
Br J Radiol 74:317-322, 2001   31–20

Background.—Auditing interval cancers is important in breast screening. Whether the position of interval cancers on the mammogram differs from those found on screening was investigated.

Methods.—Seven hundred seventy-three interval cancers and the first 200 screen-detected cancers were entered into a database that records pathologic and radiologic features, such as the position of the cancer on a stylized diagram. Reports showing the positions of all interval cancers by classification and reader were generated.

Findings.—On both views, the distribution of true interval cancers was significantly different from that of screen-detected cancers. The distribution of the false-negative and screen-detected cancers differed only on the oblique view. False-negative and true interval cancers had the same distribution on both craniocaudal and oblique views. These differences did not appear to be of use, however, when applied to individual readers.

Conclusion.—The database developed permits systematic recording of pathologic and radiologic information on breast cancers. The database can also record the geographic position of the cancer with minimal memory requirements. The current analysis demonstrated statistical differences in the distribution of false-negative and screen-detected cancers.

▶ Where in the breast do most cancers occur? Does the location pattern of interval cancers differ from the location pattern of cancers detected by screening? Are the patterns of false-negatives and false-positives different from the biological location distribution of actual cancers?

This intriguing analysis found some statistical differences but did not identify any practical use for the differences when applied to individual readers (mammographers). Perhaps further analysis of this continuing study will give some guidance for the increased detection of both screening and interval cancers. It is of interest that in 1975 similar location distributions were reported with 38% upper outer quadrant, 25% upper inner quadrant, 22% subareolar, 9% lower outer quadrant, and 6% lower inner quadrant.[1] These rounded percentages roughly equate to the amount of glandular tissue in each location.

W. H. Hindle, MD

Reference

    1. Hanley RS: Carcinoma of the breast. *Ann R Coll Surg Engl* 57:59-66, 1975.

SUGGESTED READING

Lundstrom E, Christow A, Kersemackers W, et al: Effects of tibolone and continuous combined hormone replacement therapy on mammographic breast density. *Am J Obstet Gynecol* 186:717-722, 2002.

▶ This prospective, randomized, double-blind placebo-controlled Scandinavian study (n = 166) showed mammographic density to be increased 46% to 50% with hormone replacement therapy (estradiol 2 mg/norethisterone acetate 1 mg po) 2% to 6% with tibolone (2.5 mg po) and 0% with placebo. The therapies were continuous for 6 months. Tibolone is reported to be effective for menopausal symptoms and converts to metabolites with estrogenic, progesterogenic and androgenic activities.[1] In addition, tibolone *acts to* inhibit sulfatase activity and therefore decrease local estradiol levels, stimulates apoptosis, and inhibits breast tissue proliferation.[2] Tibolone is not available in the USA.

Rutter et al[3] in a retrospective observational study (n = 5212), evaluated 2 screening mammograms (1996-1998) for changes in mammographic density and correlated the findings with hormone replacement therapy (HRT). The second mammogram showed increased density in 705 women of whom 28% (200/705) initiated HRT before the second mammogram and 12% (82/705) were not taking HRT. Of the 345 women whose mammographic density decreased, 13% (45/345) discontinued HRT and 65% (224/345) were not taking HRT.

Khalkhali et al[4] reported the accuracy of scintimammography (99mTc Sestamibi) on 580 women of whom 48% (276/580) had mammographically dense breasts and 228 had malignant lesions. No significant differences in sensitivity, specificity, positive predictive value, negative predictive value, or accuracy were found in comparing dense breasts to fatty breasts. Thus, mammographic density did not interfere with scintimammography evaluation.

Gram et al[5] reported on the effect on mammographic density of women discontinuing gonadotropin-releasing hormone agonist (GnRHA) and low-dose add-back estrogen-progestin therapy (n = 21). The treatment-induced reductions in mammographic density were found to have returned to baseline (pretreatment) levels. The authors speculate that the hormonal treatment regimen may be chemopreventive for breast cancer.

William H. Hindle, MD

References

1. Moore RA: Livial: A review of clinical studies. *Br J Obstet Gynecol* 106:1-21, 1999.
2. Rymer JM: The effects of tibolone. *Gynecol Endocrinol* 12:213-220, 1998.
3. Rutter CM, Mandelson MT, Laya MB, et al: Changes in breast density associated with initiation, discontinuation, and continuing use of hormone replacement therapy. *JAMA* 285:171-176, 2001.
4. Khalkhali I, Baum JK, Villanueva-Meyer J, et al: 99mTc Sestamibi breast imaging for the examination of patients with dense and fatty breast: multicenter study. *Radiology* 222:149-155, 2002.
5. Gram IT, Ursin G, Spicer DV, et al: Reversal of gonadotropin-releasing hormone agonist induced reductions in mammographic densities on stopping treatment. *Cancer Epidemiol Biomarks Prev* 10:1117-1120, 2001.

Defense of Breast Cancer Malpractice Claims

Zylstra S, D'Orsi CJ, Ricci BA, et al (Univ of Massachusetts, Worcester; Pro-Mutual, Boston)
Breast J 7:76-90, 2001   31–21

Background.—Breast cancer is the most frequently involved disease in legal claims filed for medical malpractice resulting from misdiagnosis. Legal and medical records of breast cancer cases were reviewed to identify practitioner risk management issues and to develop multidisciplinary algorithms for improving diagnosis.

Methods.—A total of 124 breast cancer misdiagnosis cases that closed in Massachusetts between January 1986 and November 1997 were reviewed. These cases involved 212 defendants and 176 plaintiffs, including 97 women's health practitioners (obstetrician-gynecologists, family medicine, internal medicine), 43 radiologists, 33 surgeons, and 3 pathologists. Demographic, medical, and legal data were extracted for each case, and multivariate stepwise logistic and linear regression analyses were used to determine the associations between clinical factors and case outcomes. Then these data were used in concert with National Comprehensive Cancer Network prac-

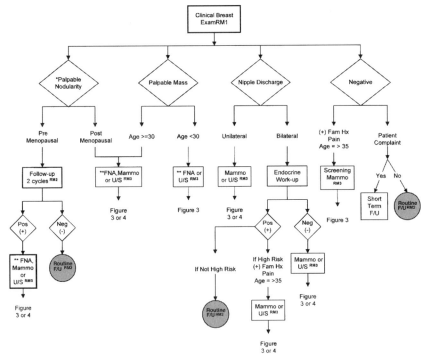

FIGURE 2.—Multidisciplinary clinical breast care algorithm: Clinical breast examination. (Courtesy of Zylstra S, D'Orsi CJ, Ricci BA, et al: Defense of breast cancer malpractice claims. *Breast J* 7:76-90, 2001. Reprinted by permission of Blackwell Science, Inc.)

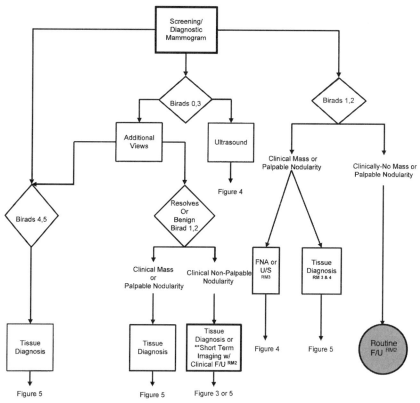

FIGURE 3.—Multidisciplinary clinical breast care algorithm: Mammography. (Courtesy of Zylstra S, D'Orsi CJ, Ricci BA, et al: Defense of breast cancer malpractice claims. *Breast J* 7:76-90, 2001. Reprinted by permission of Blackwell Science, Inc.)

tice guidelines to formulate multidisciplinary algorithms for breast cancer care.

Results.—Models based on cases involving women's health practitioners predicted that the probability of successful defense was significantly lower when record keeping was inadequate, when a patient's cancer had metastasized and she was still alive, and when the diagnosis was delayed by ≥12 months. Total indemnity (ie, payment to the plaintiff based on case outcome) for all plaintiffs was significantly greater when the disease had spread at the time of evaluation, when a patient's cancer had metastasized and she was still alive, and when the date of occurrence was closer to the present. Alternatively, overall indemnity was significantly lower in patients who underwent lymph node dissection, who had died, or who were alive without metastasis. Among women's health practitioners, indemnity was increased when the disease had spread at the time of the evaluation and when a mass without pain was noted at presentation. Indemnity was reduced for patients with a history of pregnancy, without symptoms at presentation, with pain at presentation with or without a mass, and when lymph node dissection was

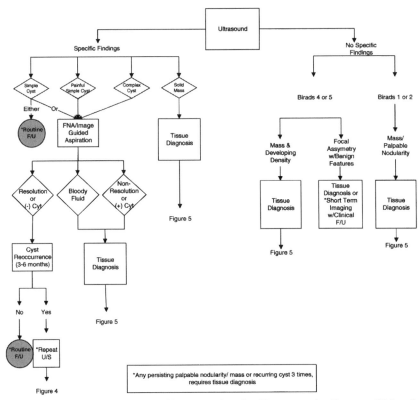

FIGURE 4.—Multidisciplinary clinical breast care algorithm: Ultrasonography. (Courtesy of Zylstra S, D'Orsi CJ, Ricci BA, et al: Defense of breast cancer malpractice claims. Breast J 7:76-90, 2001. Reprinted by permission of Blackwell Science, Inc.)

performed. These data were used to create multidisciplinary algorithms for clinical breast examination, mammography, ultrasonography, and tissue diagnosis (Figs 2 to 6). Multispecialty risk management issues associated with the largest indemnity payments included inadequate follow-up, referral, and communication.

Conclusion.—Incorporation of the management algorithms and risk management strategies described may reduce the risk of failure to diagnose cancer and the indemnity associated with such legal claims.

▶ Careful review of Figures 2 to 6 will provide clinicians with algorithms of appropriate evaluations of breast lesions, which should help them avoid the potential pitfalls that might lead to lawsuits. The algorithms are based on National Comprehensive Cancer Network practice guidelines. In this detailed analysis of 156 malpractice cases handled by ProMutual, Boston, Mass, Ob-Gyns made up 31% of the defendants. We are not immune, no matter the quality of care actually given. Inadequate record keeping weakens any defense case. Unfortunately, these cases usually come to trial or settlement, years af-

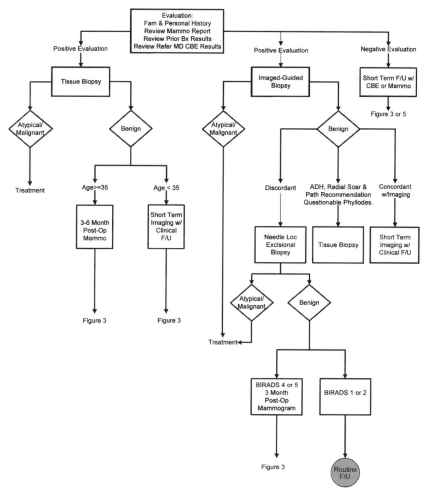

FIGURE 5.—Multidisciplinary clinical breast care algorithm: Tissue diagnosis. (Courtesy of Zylstra S, D'Orsi CJ, Ricci BA, et al: Defense of breast cancer malpractice claims. *Breast J* 7:76-90, 2001. Reprinted by permission of Blackwell Science, Inc.)

ter the actual events, so that plaintiff's attorneys can vigorously challenge non-documented recall. Furthermore, an apparent delay in diagnosis, that is, lacking documentation otherwise, of 12 months or more is difficult to defend.

Kern,[1] in a similar article, presents the current Physician Insurers Association of America data (1990, 1995) with detailed analysis and cites 47 cogent references. Of particular clinical interest are 2 risk-prevention profiles of the patient most likely to sustain a delayed diagnosis, listing 7 characteristics, and the physician most likely involved in the delayed diagnosis, listing 8 characteristics. All women's health care providers would do well to carefully read these profiles. Direct tissue sampling is suggested as the means to interrupt the cycle of error leading to delayed diagnosis. "In fact, immediate tissue sampling

Key to Breast Cancer Risk Prevention Algorithm:

Dark Black outlined box represent the top 10 areas where physicians deviated from the algorithm in our closed claims.

Clinical Breast Exam:

*Palpable Nodularity = Fibrocystic Changes (FCC = vague thickening, nodularity, fullness, cystic, lumpy, etc.)

**Any persistent palpable nodularity requires tissue diagnosis.

Pregnant patients who present with a breast complaint or abnormal CBE should have FNA or U/S. Lactating patients or patients who have recently given birth and present with a breast complaint or abnormal CBE: careful consideration needs to be given to the possibility of an underlying breast disease and the proper diagnostic steps need to be taken to rule this out. Attributing these abnormalities to hormonal changes and ignoring patient complaints could prove to be devastating.

Mammography:

*A mammogram should always be obtained in post-menopausal women.

**Any persistent palpable nodularity/mass requires tissue diagnosis.

BIRADS Classification:
0   Assessment is incomplete, additional imaging required
1   Negative finding
2   Benign finding
3   Probably benign finding; short follow-up suggested
4   Suspicious abnormality; biopsy should be considered
5   Highly suggested of malignancy; appropriate action should be taken

Ultrasonography:

*Any persisting palpable nodularity/ mass or recurring cyst 3 times, requires tissue diagnosis

Risk Management Recommendations:

RM1:   Obtain and document family and personal medical history
         Document specific findings
         Diagram abnormal findings

RM2:   Document follow-up plan
         Communicate plan and findings with patient
         Tracking system
         Recall system
         Reminder cards
         If MD is referral specialist- write letter of opinion to referring MD outlining evaluation, plan and follow-up
plan

RM3:   Document plan and findings
         Communicate findings and plan with patient
         Write referral letter to specialist: findings, plan, advise, advise and treat or assume care.
         Tracking system
         Via phone/fax if specialist finds abnormal results communicate to referring MD.
         Ordering MD receive results

RM4:   Credentialing
         Informed Consent

         Correlating: Bx results with mammograms and clinical findings.

FIGURE 6.—Key to breast cancer risk prevention algorithm. (Courtesy of Zylstra S, D'Orsi CJ, Ricci BA, et al: Defense of breast cancer malpractice claims. *Breast J* 7:76-90, 2001. Reprinted by permission of Blackwell Science, Inc.)

while the patient is in the office is preferable and may be carried out by fine-needle biopsy, core-needle biopsy, or other means."

W. H. Hindle, MD

Reference

1. Kern KA: The delayed diagnosis of breast cancer: Medicolegal implications and risk prevention for surgeons. *Breast Dis* 12:145-158, 2001.

SUGGESTED READING

Lyon DS: Graduate education in women's health care: Where have all the young men gone? *Curr Women's Health Rep* 2:170-174, 2002.

▶ In the past 2 decades there has been a progressive gender shift in physician training (medical schools and residency) and in clinical practice. This shift is particularly marked in ob-gyn training and practice. For the past decade in the Department of Obstetrics and Gynecology, University of Southern California, LAC+USC Medical Center, Los Angeles, Calif, a typical first year residency "class" would consist of 10 women and 2 men. The resident applicants are selected as objectively as possible based on academics, achievements, and interviews, without regard to gender. During residency, the enthusiasm, compassion and interest in the care and study of the breast are uniformly higher among the women compared to the men. In my experience, these attitudes carry over into clinical practice.

This article[1] summarizes the multifactorial basis of the current gender shift and suggests that a major feature relates to communication and methods of patient satisfaction, both of which can be effectively taught to men as well as women.

Weinberg et al[2] retrospectively reviewed the cases of 2271 women with breast cancer treated at the TriHealth Corporation, Cincinnati, Ohio, and found that male surgeons were 30% more likely to provide women with breast conserving surgery for stages 0, I and IIa,b than female surgeons. Further multifactorial analysis and confirmatory studies from other breast centers would be necessary to document the general validity of this rather surprising result.

William H. Hindle, MD

References

1. Roter DL, Geller G, Bernhadt BA et al: Effects of obstetrician gender on communication and patient satisfaction. *Obstet Gynecol* 93:635-641, 1999.
2. Weinberg E, Woods S, Grannan K, et al: The influence of gender of the surgeon on surgical procedure preference for breast cancer. *Am Surg* 68:398-400, 2002.

Subject Index

A

Abdominal
  hysterectomy, surgical blood loss in, 492

Abortion, 373
  history and breast cancer risk, 526
  induced
    early, mifepristone with vaginal gemeprost or misoprostol for, 379
    IUD insertion after, 366
    methotrexate or mifepristone followed by misoprostol for, 380
    mid-trimester, oral *vs.* vaginal misoprostol for, 381
    misoprostol for, sublingual, 378
    second-trimester, intravaginal misoprostol for, optimization of dosing schedules, 382
  medical *(see* induced *above)*
  missed, medical management of, 375
  spontaneous
    early *(see below)*
    first-trimester, expectant management of, 373
    IUD insertion after, 366
    recurrent *(see below)*
  spontaneous, early
    effects of metformin in polycystic ovary syndrome on, 387
    medical management with mifepristone/misoprostol, 377
    medical management with sublingual misoprostol, 376
    role of ultrasound in expectant management of, 374
  spontaneous, recurrent
    with antiphospholipid antibody, 389
    factor V Leiden and, 384
    pregnancy outcome after, high serum luteinizing hormone and testosterone levels do not predict, 385
    prevention with IV immunoglobulin, 390
    thrombophilia and, 386
    very early, factor V Leiden and G20210A prothrombin mutations as risk factors for, 383

Abscess
  breast, needle aspiration of, 546

Academic
  achievement scores in young adults after very low birth weight, 225

Acupressure
  Korean hand, postoperative nausea and vomiting after gynecologic laparoscopic surgery reduced by, 442

Acyclovir
  regimen, 2-day, for recurrent genital herpes simplex virus type 2 infection, 288

Acyl-CoA
  dehydrogenase deficiency, medium-chain, neonatal screening for, 134

Adenovirus
  infectivity-enhanced, in vivo molecular chemotherapy and noninvasive imaging with (in mice), 463

Adhesion
  molecules expression in placental bed of preeclamptic pregnancies, 19

Adipose
  tissue, fetal, leptin produced by, 5

Adnexa
  torsion, sonographic findings in, 427

Adnexectomy
  bilateral, for endometriosis, recurrence in women on hormone replacement therapy after, 303

Adrenal
  hyperplasia, congenital, prenatal diagnosis of, 156

Adrenomedullin
  circulating, increase in preterm newborns developing intraventricular hemorrhage, 250

Adulthood
  young, outcomes for very low birth weight infants in, 225

African Americans
  stroke in pregnancy and puerperium in, 120

Age
  advancing
    cervical cancer screening and prognosis and, 475
    maternal, and increased risk of cesarean delivery, 183

Agenesis
  müllerian, vaginal creation for, 439

Alcohol
  exposure, prenatal, impact on frontal cortex development in utero, 223

Allograft
  fascia lata in pubovaginal sling surgery for stress incontinence, high failure rate with, 271

venous thromboembolism risk with,
322
Euploidy
preimplantation confirmation by
comparative genomic hybridization,
birth of healthy infant after, 218
Exercise
in pregnant working women, healthy
low-risk, antepartum, intrapartum,
and neonatal significance of, 7
Expectant management
of abortion, spontaneous
early, role of ultrasound in, 374
first-trimester, 373
Extravillous
trophoblast migration, simulation by
IGF-II, mediation by IGF type 2
receptor, 22

F

Factor V Leiden
mutation
low prevalence of large
intraventricular hemorrhage in very
low birth weight infants with, 246
miscarriage and, recurrent, 384
as risk factor for very early recurrent
miscarriage, 383
prevalence, maternal-infant, with severe
preeclampsia, 82
Fallopian tube (*see* Tubal)
Family
history of cancer and oral contraceptive
use and ovarian cancer risk, 352
Fas
expression and Fas ligand expression in
maternal and umbilical cord blood
in preeclampsia, 98
Fascia
lata allograft in pubovaginal sling
surgery for stress incontinence, high
failure rate with, 271
used in colporrhaphy, histologic
examination of, 437
Fat
dietary, and breast cancer risk, 536
Fathers
mortality of, long-term, after
preeclampsia, 86
Fatty acid
oxidation, leptin stimulation by
activation of AMP-activated
protein kinase (in mice), 42
Fecal
incontinence, outcome of
sphincteroplasty combined with
surgery for, 285

Fertility
drugs and risk of ovarian cancer, 336
Fertilization
in vitro (*see* In vitro fertilization)
α-Fetoprotein
maternal, serum, second-trimester
screening for Down syndrome with,
145
Fetus
adipose tissue produces leptin, 5
asphyxia
at delivery, reproductive risk factors
for, 148
intrapartum, prediction and
prevention in preterm pregnancies,
147
brain, metabolic information obtained
by proton magnetic resonance
spectroscopy from, 131
cells circulating in maternal blood,
enrichment, immunomorphological,
and genetic characterization of, 206
complications of pregnancy, 47
death, third-trimester unexplained
intrauterine, association with
inherited thrombophilia, 41
demise, spontaneous (*see* Abortion,
spontaneous)
DNA
cellular and cell-free, kinetics in
maternal circulation during and
after pregnancy, 199
in plasma, maternal, differential DNA
methylation between mother and
fetus as strategy for detecting, 210
Down syndrome, neuronal target genes
of neuron-restrictive silencer factor
in neurospheres derived from, 220
erythrocytes, nucleated
from CVS washings, in first trimester
noninvasive prenatal diagnosis, 209
from maternal blood, diagnosis of
trisomy 21 by use of short tandem
repeat sequences in, 208
gender determination by DNA analysis
in maternal plasma, accuracy of,
203
growth (*see* Growth, fetal)
heart rate
monitoring, electronic, in prediction
and prevention of intrapartum fetal
asphyxia in preterm pregnancies,
147
recordings in maternal type 1
diabetes, computerized analysis of,
150
leptin influences birth weight in twins
with discordant growth, 55

Working
women, healthy low-risk pregnant,
exercise in, antepartum,
intrapartum, and neonatal
significance of, 7

X

X-linked
severe combined immunodeficiency,
sustained correction by ex vivo
gene therapy, 153

Z

Zidovudine
/lamivudine regimens, short-course, in
prevention of mother-to-child
transmission of HIV, 65

resistance mutations in HIV-infected
pregnant women and their
newborns, 64
Zygote
intrafallopian tube transfer *vs.*
blastocyst stage transfer after
repeated implantation failure, 341

Author Index

A

AbdAlla S, 96
Abrams EJ, 71
Adolphson KR, 17
Akhter N, 333
Albayram F, 427
Albert D, 499
Ammann A, 71
Andersen AN, 343
Andersen R, 272
Anderson DF, 8
Apperley JF, 80
Appleton M, 134
Ardekani AM, 454
Ariga H, 199
Armstrong DK, 455
Armstrong K, 499
Arnold DF, 417
Ashok PW, 376, 377
Athanassiou A, 43
Atlas RO, 31
Audibert F, 145
Azam U, 264

B

Backos M, 384, 385
Badrinath P, 45
Bahamondes L, 361
Bahn S, 220
Baird DD, 104
Bajoria R, 55
Baker RS, 15
Banks E, 362
Barkovich AJ, 239
Barnhart KT, 429
Barrett-Connor E, 309
Bartley J, 379
Barton JR, 79
Bauer M, 204
Baxter N, 563
Becher H, 451
Becker-Pergola G, 70
Bedi HS, 239
Beechey-Newman N, 519
Beekman-de Volder HJC, 551
Belloni DR, 409
Benachi A, 206
Benattar C, 145
Benedetti-Panici P, 481
Benyo DF, 106
Beral V, 523
Berenson AB, 310

Berger LA, 284
Bergeron S, 423
Béroud C, 206
Berrington A, 362
Bhaumik M, 428
Bilian X, 368
Binik YM, 423
Bjarnadóttir RI, 359
Blackman D, 421
Blaivas JG, 269
Blessing JA, 471, 472
Bloom SL, 34
Boehler M, 442
Boehringer H, 329
Boer K, 100
Bond CM, 287
Bonidie MJ, 273
Bower C, 213
Brack S, 410
Brady CM, 278
Brady MF, 467
Brain PH, 375
Brateng D, 93, 109
Brehny S, 339
Brewer C, 418
Bristow RE, 455
Brizendine E, 267
Brown A, 379
Brown C, 400
Brown HA, 429
Brown JM, 466
Brown JS, 275, 280
Brown M, 570
Brundage M, 482
Bryant J, 502
Buda A, 462
Burger RA, 457
Burke TW, 479, 487
Busacca M, 393
Busch MP, 199
Byers TE, 112

C

Calhoun BC, 17
Caliskan E, 335
Calvosa C, 272
Cameron AD, 177
Campisi R, 313
Candiani M, 393
Cantù MG, 462
Carbonne B, 383
Carlier F, 153
Carlson A, 156
Carlson KV, 269
Carmina E, 296

Carr DB, 93, 109
Carrell D, 288
Carson LF, 478
Carson SA, 334
Casabonne D, 362
Castellsagué X, 476
Cayol V, 383
Chakraborty C, 22
Challier J-C, 5
Chambers GK, 496
Chan BKS, 322
Chan FY, 77
Chan LY, 406
Chan LYS, 197
Chang-Claude J, 451
Chao J, 452
Chapman KB, 161
Chauveaud A, 433
Chen C-L, 324
Chen K-K, 271
Chen KT, 183
Chen T-M, 499
Cheng Y-M, 403
Cheung AP, 297
Chou C-Y, 403
Christensen RD, 98
Christiansen OB, 390
Christianson RE, 123
Cibelli JB, 161
Cincotta RB, 77
Cirillo PM, 123
Clark AD, 268
Clarke B, 282
Clements NC, 565
Cnattingius S, 232
Cohen AP, 183
Cohn BA, 123
Cohn DE, 491
Coleman RL, 443, 479, 487
Colombo A, 481
Colombo N, 488
Connor JP, 413
Contant T, 412
Cooke GC, 428
Coomarasamy A, 143
Copeland LJ, 491
Cornacchia M, 281
Cornish J, 364
Cowan FM, 242
Craig JC, 389
Creasy GW, 358
Creutzberg CL, 470
Croen LA, 51
Crombie N, 537
Crowther C, 186
Culligan P, 279, 407

BUSINESS REPLY MAIL
FIRST-CLASS MAIL   PERMIT NO 7135   ORLANDO FL

POSTAGE WILL BE PAID BY ADDRESSEE

PERIODICALS ORDER FULFILLMENT DEPT
MOSBY
ELSEVIER SCIENCE
6277 SEA HARBOR DR
ORLANDO FL 32821-9852

VISIT OUR HOME PAGE!
www.mosby.com/periodicals

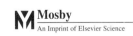

Mosby
An Imprint of Elsevier Science

11830 Westline Industrial Drive
St. Louis, MO   63146   U.S.A.